Myositis: Types, Diagnosis and Treatment

Myositis: Types, Diagnosis and Treatment

Editor: Anthony Griffiths

FOSTER ACADEMICS

www.fosteracademics.com

www.fosteracademics.com

FOSTER ACADEMICS

Cataloging-in-Publication Data

Myositis : types, diagnosis and treatment / edited by Anthony Griffiths.
p. cm.
Includes bibliographical references and index.
ISBN 978-1-64646-629-0
1. Myositis. 2. Myositis--Diagnosis. 3. Myositis--Treatment.
4. Muscles--Diseases. I. Griffiths, Anthony.
RC935.M9 M96 2023
616.743--dc23

Foster Academics,
118-35 Queens Blvd., Suite 400,
Forest Hills, NY 11375, USA

ISBN 978-1-64646-629-0 (Hardback)

Contents

Preface

Every book is initially just a concept; it takes months of research and hard work to give it the final shape in which the readers receive it. In its early stages, this book also went through rigorous reviewing. The notable contributions made by experts from across the globe were first molded into patterned chapters and then arranged in a sensibly sequential manner to bring out the best results.

Any condition that causes inflammation or swelling of the muscles is called myositis. It has various causes, which include inflammatory conditions, injury, infection and immune disorders. Most of the causes of myositis are autoimmune in nature wherein the body attacks its own muscle tissues. Inflammatory conditions such as dermatomyositis, polymyositis, and inclusion body myositis cause severe myositis. Lupus, scleroderma, rheumatoid arthritis are some of the milder forms of myositis. Common cold, flu viruses, and human immunodeficiency virus (HIV) are some viruses that may cause myositis. Its treatment depends on the underlying cause. Myositis caused due to inflammatory conditions requires treatment with drugs such as prednisone, azathioprine and methotrexate that suppress the immune system. This book is compiled in such a manner that it will provide an in-depth knowledge about the types, diagnosis and treatment of myositis. The readers would gain knowledge that would broaden their perspective about this medical condition. The book is appropriate for students seeking detailed information on myositis as well as for experts.

It has been my immense pleasure to be a part of this project and to contribute my years of learning in such a meaningful form. I would like to take this opportunity to thank all the people who have been associated with the completion of this book at any step.

Editor

1

The Value of Effective Lung Ventilation Area Ratio Based on CT Image Analysis is a New Index to Predict the Shorter Outcome of Anti-melanoma Differentiation-Associated Protein 5 Positive Dermatomyositis Associated Interstitial Lung Disease

Changjian Wang[1†], Jinfeng Du[2†], Xilong Mei[3†], Lingchao Guo[1], Fangzhao Li[1], Hong Luo[4] and Fen Li[2*]*

[1] College of Computer, National University of Defense Technology, Changsha, China, [2] Department of Rheumatology and Immunology, The Second Xiangya Hospital of Central South University, Changsha, China, [3] Department of Radiology, The Second Xiangya Hospital of Central South University, Changsha, China, [4] Department of Respiratory and Critical Care Medicine, The Second Xiangya Hospital of Central South University, Changsha, China

***Correspondence:**
Changjian Wang
wangcj@nudt.edu.cn
Fen Li
lifen0731@csu.edu.cn

† These authors have contributed equally to this work and share first authorship*

Background: Anti-melanoma differentiation-associated protein 5 (MDA5) positive dermatomyositis (MDA5$^+$DM) patients have poor outcomes due to rapidly progressive interstitial lung disease (ILD). The accurate assessment of lung involvement is an urgent focus of research.

Methods: A computer-aided lung interstitial image analysis technology has been developed, and a quantitative indicator named effective lung ventilation area ratio (ELVAR) that calculates the proportion of the area outside the lung interstitium in lung tissue has been established. 55 newly diagnosed MDA5$^+$DM patients and 46 healthy individuals, matched for age and gender, were enrolled in this study. MDA5$^+$DM patients were classified into early death group or early survival group according to their survival state within 3 months after diagnosis. Clinical characteristics, laboratory and immunological test results, lung involvement (including ELVAR value) and treatment were compared between early death group and early survival group to determine an index that can predict prognoses of patients with MDA5$^+$DM.

Results: There were significant differences between early death MDA5$^+$DM patients and early survival MDA5$^+$DM patients about 12 indices including age of onset, CRP, ferritin, albumin, and pulmonary involvement including severity of type I respiratory failure at diagnosis, P/F ratio, oxygen supplementation, values of ELVAR, FVC, and DLCO. The results of ROC analysis and correlation analysis showed the value of ELVAR had good diagnostic value and widely correlation with many clinical characteristics. Univariate analysis and Multivariate analysis showed four factors including age of onset, ferritin, value of ELVAR, and oxygen supplementation >4 L/min significantly value for poor prognosis in MDA5$^+$DM patients. A cutoff value of 0.835 about ELVAR had good predictive power for mortality within 3 months in 54.2% of MDA5$^+$DM patients.

Conclusion: The value of ELVAR derived from computed tomography image analysis is a new index that can predict poor outcomes in MDA5$^+$DM patients with rapidly progressive interstitial lung disease.

Keywords: dermatomyositis, anti-melanoma differentiation-associated protein 5 antibody, interstitial lung disease, prognosis, effective lung ventilation area ratio, computer-aided image analysis

INTRODUCTION

Idiopathic inflammatory myopathy (IIM) are heterogenous family of diseases (1). Dermatomyositis (DM) is a subtype of IIM that is characterized by skin rash and myopathy. The incidence of DM in the American population is approximately 1–6 per 100,000 people (2). Although the cause of DM is unknown, recent studies have revealed that anti-melanoma differentiation-associated protein 5 (MDA5) is associated with a subtype of DM (3). MDA5 promotes the production and activation of type I interferon (IFN), which is involved in the pathogenesis of DM (4, 5). Several clinical studies have found that MDA5$^+$DM patients are more likely to develop rapidly progressive interstitial pneumonia (ILD) with life-threatening characteristics (6–9). Even after receiving active drug therapy, MDA5$^+$DM patients may die soon after, and 6-months mortality has been reported to be as high as 59% (10, 11). Therefore, the accurate assessment of prognoses of MDA5$^+$DM patients is an urgent focus of research.

The advantage of high-resolution computed tomography (HRCT) is its ability to detect interstitial pneumonia with mild lesions in the early stage of the disease. The current limitation is the lack of a quantitative method to accurately identify subtle changes in abnormalities. Although several studies on the quantitative analysis of lung interstitial lesions in patients and mice have been conducted (12–16), results have not been convincing. Our study aimed to develop metric tools for clinicians to accurately assess the severity of interstitial pneumonia and establish a methodological plat that combines radiology and computer technology to predict prognoses of patients with MDA5$^+$DM.

MATERIALS AND METHODS

Patient Data Collection

This single-center retrospective study was approved by the ethics committee of the Second Xiangya Hospital of Central South University (approval number: MDA5-IIM2020). All 55 MDA5$^+$DM patients were newly onset and newly diagnosed fulfilling expert consensus from 239th ENMC International Workshop with MDA5 positive characteristic (17). Patients were hospitalized in the ward of Department of Rheumatology and Immunology between January 1st, 2015 and December 31st, 2018. Those who died within 3 months after diagnosis were classified into early death group, and those who had survived more than 3 months after diagnosis were classified into early survival group. Patient survival status was confirmed by medical records or by telephone. The survival status of patients in early survival group was verified 1 year later by telephone. Clinical characteristics, laboratory data, pulmonary involvement, antibody positive, and treatment information were obtained retrospectively from medical records. ILD diagnoses were verified by a radiologist and a respirologist (**Figure 1**). As control group, 46 healthy subjects, matched for age and gender, were included in the study to compare lung HRCT analysis results with the MDA5$^+$DM patients. Our study complied with the Declaration of Helsinki and informed consents were obtained from all subjects (or their legally authorized representative in cases of patient death).

Computer-Aided Analysis of Lung HRCT

ILD include some basic radiology features in HRCT such as reticulations, septal thickening, ground glass opacities, nodules, bronchiectasis and bronchiolectasis, honeycombing, consolidation, etc. All these features showed the differences of density (CT values) in images. Our quantitative analysis method was proposed from difference of CT values in Digital Imaging and Communications in Medicine (DICOM) of HRCT images. Simply, firstly, a special lung segmentation algorithm of interstitial lung disease was developed. Then, high-precision three-dimensional images of lung interstitium were reconstructed to detect interstitial pixels beyond the limit scope of naked eyes. An index named by Effective Lung Ventilation Area Ratio (ELVAR) were calculated indicting pulmonary ventilation function.

Lung Segmentation

The process of lung segmentation was divided into four stages.

1. Lung coarse segmentation stage.

   Original lung HRCT images were collected from lung windows of every 1 mm scan (**Figure 2A**). Due to difference of CT value, the lung tissue can be separated with other human tissues from mediastinum to chest wall. This leaded to the generation of binary lung tissue region images (**Figure 2B**).
2. Lung contour detection stage.

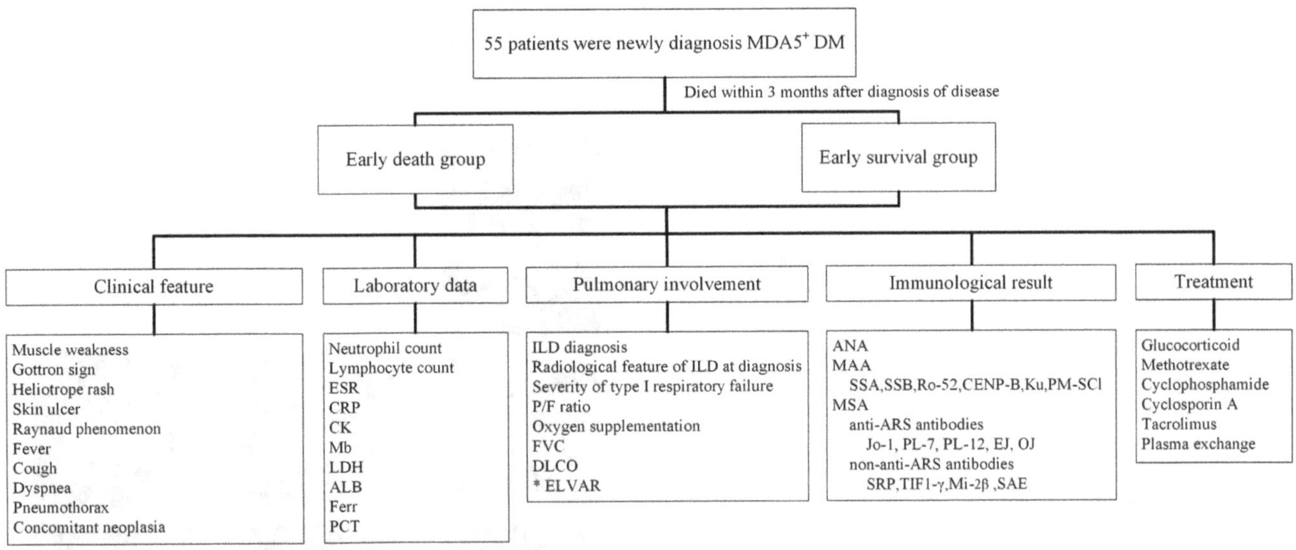

FIGURE 1 | Flow chart of clinical research design for newly diagnosed MDA5+DM patients. ALB, albumin; ANA, antinuclear antibody; ARS, minoacyl-tRNA synthetase; CRP, C reactive protein; CK, creatinine kinase; DLCO, carbon monoxide diffusing capacity; ELVAR, effective lung ventilation area ratio; ESR, erythrocyte sedimentation rate; Ferr, ferritin; FVC, forced vital capacity; ILD, interstitial lung disease; LDH, lactate dehydrogenase; MAA, myositis associated antibody; Mb, Myoglobin; MDA5, melanoma melanoma differentiation associated gene 5; MSA, myositis specific antibody; PCT, procalcitonin; P/F ratio, PaO2/FiO2 ratio; SRP, signal recognition particle; SAE, anti-small ubiquitin-like modifier antibody; TIF1-γ, transcription intermediary factor 1-gamma.

The task of this stage was to draw the outlines of lung based on the coarse segmentation results. Firstly, a Gaussian function was adopted to eliminate noise, hence a transition zone was produced near the lung edge, so the binary lung tissue region images were filtered and smoothed (**Figure 2C**). Subsequently, a Laplace operator was used to produce the inner and outer boundaries on the lung edge. The outer boundary was selected as the candidate lung edge which included all irregular fragments near the boundaries (**Figure 2D**). The lung contour image was finally generated by filling the interior of the candidate lung edge (**Figure 2E**).

3. Lung hole elimination stage.

   Because the lungs are near other organs, such as the heart, spleen, liver, and stomach, an obvious hole can appear in the CT images of the lower part of the lung. The goal of this stage was to detect and eliminate the hole area. Images detecting hole area (**Figure 2D**) were superimposed onto the lung contour images (**Figure 2E**) and were finally shown as **Figure 2F**. Using the region-growing method, the most lateral region of the lung was identified and set as the background, so that only the hole and blood vessels were preserved. Because blood vessels are small, the larger component with more than a specific number of pixels is regarded as the mask hole (**Figure 2G**). The quasi- images of lung with mask hole were obtained by subtracting the mask hole from the lung contour image(**s**).

4. Lung contour shrinkage stage.

   The main objective of this stage was to generate a more accurate lung edge. First the candidate lung edges (**Figure 2E** or **Figure 2H**) were gradually contracted until they were coincided with the zero-crossing boundary, which were regarded as the accurate edges of the lung, therefore the images of lung masks were obtained (**Figure 2I**). An "and" operation on the original image (**Figure 2A**) and its lung mask (**Figure 2I**) would produce accurate lung segmentation result (**Figure 2J**). The total number of lung voxels (L) was obtained by counting the lung pixels from accurate lung segmentation results.

Lung Interstitial Enhancement

Because the lung interstitium was accompanied with blood vessels, and the pixels in the pipeline significantly differed in the direction of curvature, potential lung interstitial pixels not being detected by normally vision could be detected according to their curvature feature. This allowed the identification as many interstitial pixels as possible and the lung interstitial enhancement images were generated (**Figure 2K**). Finally, the total number of interstitium voxels (I) was obtained by counting the pixels of all the lung interstitial enhancement images.

Calculation of Effective Lung Ventilation Area Ratio

Using L, the total number of lung voxels, and I, the total number of interstitial voxels, ELVAR can show pulmonary ventilation function by applying the formula of (L–I)/L (**Figure 2L**), which indirectly correlate with the scope of interstitial lung disease (**Figure 3**), *i.e.*, low value of ELVAR means high scope of lung interstitium and low ventilation function. Using quantitative analysis method of lung segmentation and lung interstitial enhancement, the original lung HRCT images (**Figures 4A1–A4,B1–B4**) could be reconstructed into the lung interstitial enhancement images (**Figures 4C1–C4,D1–D4**) and high-precision three-dimensional images of the lung interstitium (**Figures 4E1–E4**), and the subtle lung interstitial changes

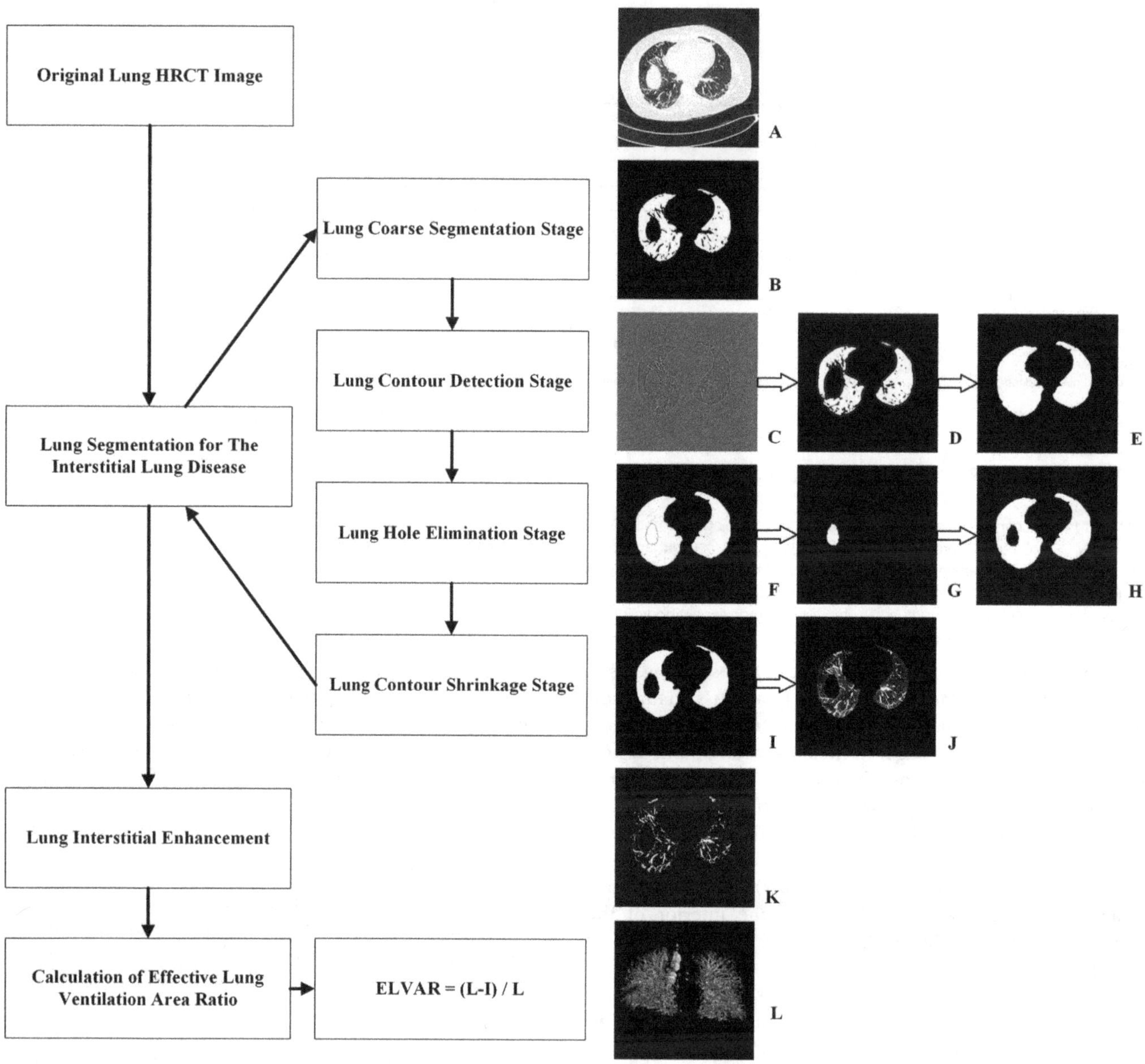

FIGURE 2 | Procedure of computer-aided analysis of lung HRCT. **(A)** Original lung HRCT images were collected; **(B)** Coarse binary lung tissue region images were acquired due to difference of CT value; **(C)** Binary lung tissue region images were filtered and smoothed by Gaussian function; **(D)** Outer boundary of binary lung tissue region images was selected by Laplace operator; **(E)** The interior of lung edge was filled in binary lung tissue region images; **(F)** Images detecting hole area were superimposed onto the lung contour images; **(G)** Images with mask hole were identified; **(H)** Quasi- images of lung with mask hole were obtained by subtracting the mask hole from the lung contour image; **(I)** Images of lung masks with accurate edge were obtained; **(J)** An "and" operation produced accurate lung segmentation images; **(K)** Lung interstitial enhancement images were generated according to curvature feature of lung interstitium; **(L)** ELVAR were calculated by formula of (L–I)/L, L were the total number of lung voxels and I were the total number of interstitial voxels.

can be more easily observed by comparing the images from different patients.

Statistical Analysis

Statistical analysis was performed using the SPSS software version 26.0 (Chicago, IL, USA). Chi-square and Fisher's exact tests were used to compare dichotomous data, and comparisons of continuous variables were performed using Student's *t*-test or Wilcoxon's rank-sum test. Correlation analysis between ELVAR and other variables were applied with Spearman or Kendall. The receiver operator curve (ROC) analysis was performed to evaluate the diagnostic performance of the statistical significance index. Cox proportional hazards regression analysis was used to assess the prognostic factors based on Duration from treatment to death or 1 year. Odds ratios (OR) were presented with 95% confidence intervals (CI). Twelve months of survival curves of different ELVAR values of $MDA5^{+}DM$ patients were drawn

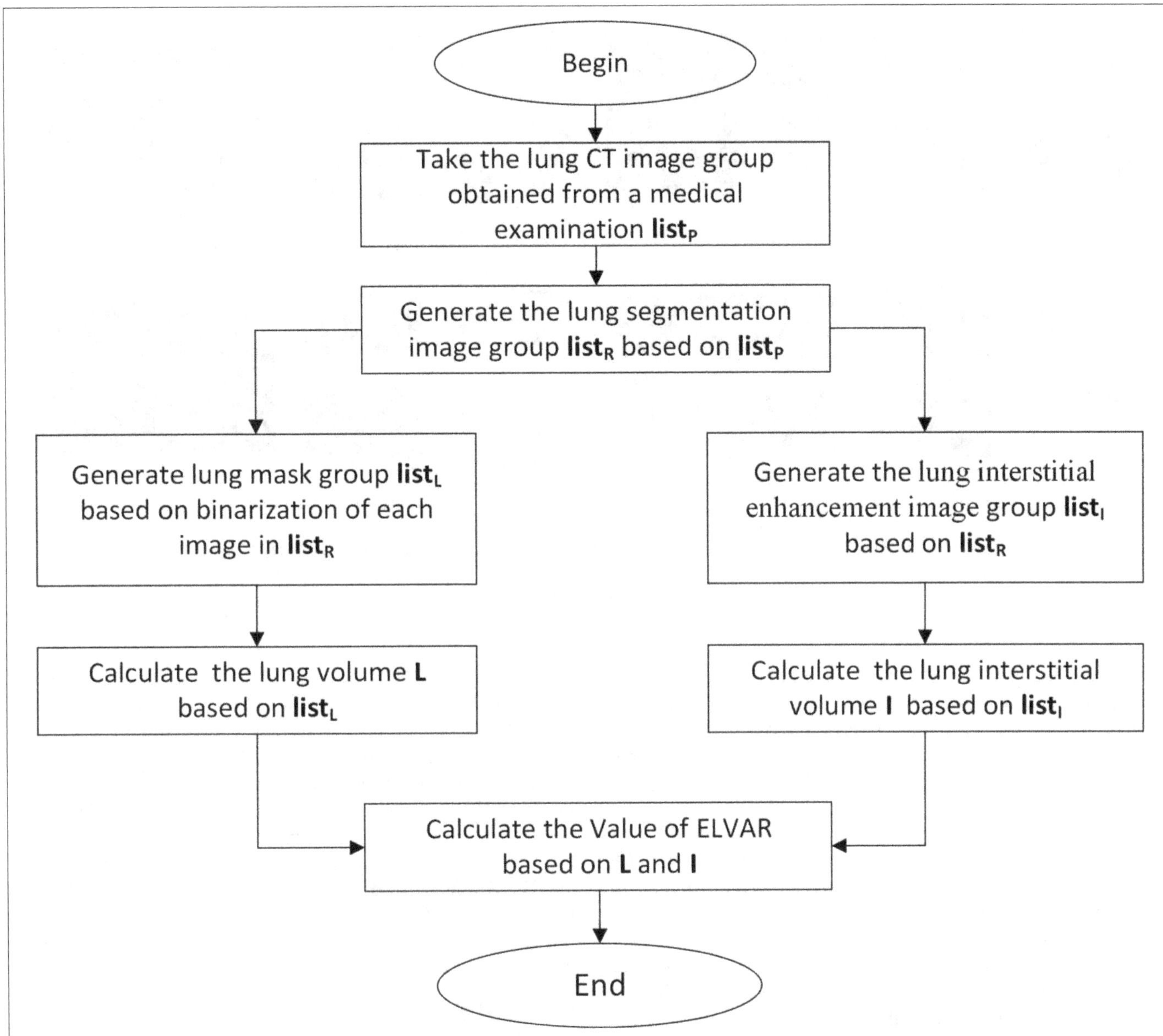

FIGURE 3 | Calculation procedure of Effective Lung Ventilation Area Ratio (ELVAR). List P were original images of lung windows from HRCT **(Figure 2A)**. List R were segmentation results from List P **(Figure 2J)**. List L were data of calculation results of List R in the algorithm program **(Figure 2I)**. List I were data of lung interstitial enhancement of List R in the algorithm program **(Figure 2K)**.

using the Kaplan-Meier method. Two-tailed $p < 0.05$ were considered significant.

RESULTS

Comparisons Between Early Death Group and Early Survival Group

In **Table 1**, the data showed that duration from onset to treatment (months) between early death group and early survival group were 2.0(1.0,3.0) and 2.5(1.5,4.0). Therefore, we had enough evidence to show that our patients were at the early stage of disease. For the 55 $MDA5^{+}DM$ patients, there were no significant difference between two groups in duration from onset to treatment and treatment drugs, which indicted the time of diagnosis and different treatment were not the risk factors leading to different prognosis. There was a significant difference in age of onset between early death group and early survival group (56[47.25,61.75] vs. 50[44,55] years), which suggested that patients with elder age onset had a higher risk of early death. Obviously, the difference among duration from treatment to death or 1 year, mortality within 3 months, mortality within 12 months between above two groups were significant. Serum C reactive protein (CRP) and level of ferritin in early death group (12.29[5.81, 23.65] mg/L

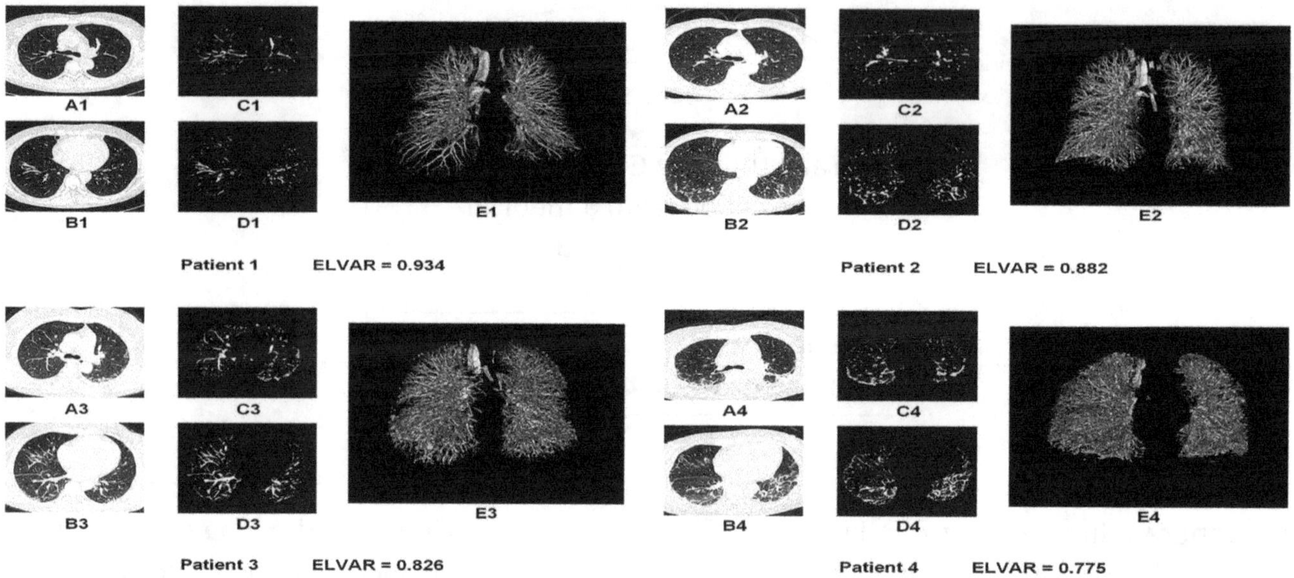

FIGURE 4 | Lung images of four MDA5$^+$DM patients with different value of ELVAR. **(A,B)** Original HRCT images in the different level of lung tissue (A was the section from bifurcation of the trachea and B was the section above the top of diaphragm); **(C,D)** The lung interstitial enhancement images from A and B based on computer aided analysis technique; **(E)** High precision three dimensional images of the lung interstitium from the same person.

and 568.35[481.71, 583.02] ng/ml, respectively) were higher than those in early survival group (4.13[2.21,11.10] mg/L and 452.07[320.44, 561.12] ng/L). However, albumin levels in early death group were lower than those in early survival group (24.40[23.50, 27.35] vs. 30.30[27.60,34.10] g/L), which indicated that MDA5$^+$DM patients in early death group had aggressive systemic involvement. Other characteristics, such as the skin and muscle, laboratory data, myositis-specific autoantibody (MSA), myositis associated autoantibody (MAA) revealed no significant differences between groups (**Table 1**).

For pulmonary involvement, there were no significant differences in cough, pneumothorax, ILD diagnosis, or radiological features of ILD. The values of ELVAR indirectly reflecting the severity of interstitial structure were significantly different between early death group and early survival group (0.7973[0.7458, 0.8338] vs. 0.8685[0.8155, 0.8956], **Figure 5B**). The differences among severity of type I respiratory failure at diagnosis (no, mild and severe), P/F ratio and oxygen supplementation (0 and >4 L/min) between two groups were significantly. The two indices of the lung function test, FVC % predicted (FVC PRED) and DLCO% predicted (DLCO%PRED), were 42 (37, 53) and 35 (28, 46)%, respectively, in early death group, which were lower than those in early survival group (79 [78, 81] and 79 [78, 80]%).

ROC Analysis and Correlation Analysis

The ROC analysis of the eight significantly different indices (i.e., age at onset, CRP, level of ferritin, value of ELVAR, P/F ratio, level of albumin, FVC and DLCO) showed that value of ELVAR, level of albumin and P/F ratio had well diagnostic value for early death within 3 months with higher sensitivity (71.8, 87.2, and 87.2%) and specificity (81.2, 75.0, and 75.0%). FVC and DLCO with lower specificity will be verified with more data in the future because only two patients underwent a lung function test and the remaining 14 patients did not accept the lung function test because of intolerability or early death in the early death group of the study (**Table 2**). As for correlation analysis, level of albumin, value of ELVAR and P/F ratio had different correlation with all indices except for FVC and DLCO, the scope of correlation about value of ELVAR lied in moderate range (**Table 3**). ROC analysis and correlation analysis indicted value of ELVAR had good diagnostic and correlation with clinical characteristics.

Clinical Significance of ELVAR Values

Distribution and Comparison of ELVAR Values Between Healthy Controls and MDA5$^+$DM Patients

Using computer-assisted lung HRCT image analysis, we found that the lungs of MDA5$^+$DM patients differed significantly from those of healthy controls. There were interstitial hyperplasia structures in the outer lung area of patients. In severe cases, it had spread to the middle and upper regions of the lung (**Figure 4**). Results showed that value of ELVAR in healthy controls were higher than those in MDA5$^+$DM patients (0.9351[0.9311, 0.9414] vs. 0.8487[0.8018, 0.8875]; **Figure 5A**).

Difference Between the Lower ELVAR Group and Higher ELVAR Group

The ROC analysis of ELVAR values showed that the best diagnostic cutoff value was 0.835 (**Figure 5C**). Based on this ELVAR cutoff value, 24 MDA5$^+$DM patients were classified into the lower ELVAR group (ELVAR $<$ 0.835) and 31 into the

TABLE 1 | Comparison between early death group and early survival group in MDA5$^+$DM.

Variables	MDA5$^+$DM patients		
	Early death group *N* = 16	**Early survival group *N* = 39**	***P*-value**
Female, n (%)	14(87.5)	28(71.8)	0.217
Age of onset (y)	56(47.25, 61.75)	50(44, 55)	0.033*
Duration from onset to treatment, m	2.0(1.0, 3.0)	2.5(1.5, 4.0)	0.315
Duration from treatment to death or 1 year, m	0.75(0.5, 1.5)	12(12.0, 12.0)	0.000*
Mortality within 3 months, n (%)	16(100)	0 (0)	0.000*
Mortality within 12 months, n (%)	16(100)	1(2.6)	0.000*
Smoking history, n (%)	4(25.0)	4(10.3)	0.163
Clinical feature			
Muscle weakness, n (%)	8(50.0)	25(64.1)	0.337
Gottron sign, n (%)	5(31.3)	9(23.1)	0.531
Heliotrop rash, n (%)	4(25.0)	15(38.5)	0.345
Skin ulcer, n (%)	2(12.5)	12(30.8)	0.162
Raynaud phenomenon, n (%)	0(0.0)	3(7.7)	0.258
Fever, n (%)	7(43.8)	8(20.5)	0.082
Cough, n (%)	2(12.5)	9(23.1)	0.377
Dyspnea, n (%)	12(75.0)	22(56.4)	0.202
Pneumothorax, n (%)	1(6.3)	1(2.6)	0.511
Concomitant neoplasia, n (%)	0(0.0)	1(2.6)	0.522
Laboratory data			
Neutrophil Count, X10^9/L	3.31(2.57, 4.59)	3.29(2.43, 4.86)	0.978
Lymphocyte Count, X10^9/L	0.86(0.45, 1.14)	0.85(0.56, 1.21)	0.670
ESR, mm/hr	43(25, 61)	38.5(28.5, 56.25)	1.000
CRP, mg/L	12.29(5.81, 23.65)	4.13(2.21, 11.10)	0.026*
CK, IU/L	80.10(49.30, 144.23)	84.70(41.50, 191.40)	0.704
LDH, IU/L	382.55(351.30, 535.40)	364.30(266.90, 445.40)	0.069
Myoglobin, ug/L	101(57.65, 111.35)	66.20(38.50, 95.20)	0.132
Albumin, g/L	24.40(23.50, 27.35)	30.30(27.60, 34.10)	0.000*
Ferritin, ng/ml	568.35(481.71, 583.02)	452.07(320.44, 561.12)	0.001*
PCT, ng/ml	0.11(0.053, 0.193)	0.07(0.04, 0.105)	0.089
Pulmonary involvement			
ILD diagnosis, n (%)[&]	16(100)	32(82.1)	0.072
Feature of ILD at diagnosis			
Reticulations, n (%)	3(18.75)	11(28.21)	0.469
Septal thickening, n (%)	8(50.00)	11(28.21)	0.126
Ground glass opacities, n (%)	4(25.00)	9(23.08)	0.880
Nodules, n (%)	5(31.25)	7(17.95)	0.282
Bronchiectasis/Bronchiolectasis, n (%)	1(6.25)	2(5.13)	0.869
Honeycombing, n (%)	1(6.25)	1(2.56)	0.511
Consolidation, n (%)	12(75.00)	22(56.41)	0.202
ELVAR	0.7973(0.7458, 0.8338)	0.8685(0.8155, 0.8956)	0.001*
Severity of type I respiratory failure			
no/mild/moderate/severe, n (%)	4/3/7/2 (25.0/18.8/43.7/12.5)	31/5/3/0 (79.5/12.8/7.7/0.0)	0.000*
no, n (%)	4(25.0)	31(79.5)	0.000*
mild, n (%)	3(18.8)	5(12.8)	0.575
moderate, n (%)	7(43.7)	3(7.7)	0.002*
severe, n (%)	2(12.5)	0(0)	0.026*
P/F ratio, mmHg	226(188, 297.75)	417(312, 476)	0.000*
Oxygen supplementation			
0/1-2/3-4/>4, L/min, n (%)	3/1/6/6 (18.8/6.2/37.5/37.5)	19/8/9/3 (48.7/20.5/23.1/7.7)	0.003*

(Continued)

TABLE 1 | Continued

Variables	MDA5^{+}DM patients		
	Early death group $N = 16$	Early survival group $N = 39$	*P*-value
0L/min, n (%)	3(18.8)	19(48.7)	0.040*
1–2L/min, n (%)	1(6.2)	8(20.5)	0.198
3–4L/min, n (%)	6(37.5)	9(23.1)	0.280
>4L/min, n (%)	6(37.5)	3(7.7)	0.007*
FVC, % PRED	42(37, 53)	79(78, 81)	0.004*
DLCO, % PRED	35(28, 46)	79(78, 80)	0.004*
Antibody positive			
ANA, n (%)	2(12.5)	15(38.5)	0.061
MAA profile	14(87.5)	27(69.2)	0.162
SSA, n (%)	0(0.0)	8(20.5)	0.052
SSB, n (%)	0(0.0)	3(7.7)	0.258
Ro-52, n (%)	14(87.5)	25(64.1)	0.086
CENP-B, n (%)	1(6.3)	1(2.6)	0.511
Ku, n (%)	0(0.0)	1(2.6)	0.522
PM-Scl, n (%)	0(0.0)	2(5.1)	0.361
MSA profile, n (%)	5(31.3)	8(20.5)	0.399
anti-ARS antibodies, n (%)	1(6.3)	4(10.3)	0.642
Jo-1, n (%)	0(0.0)	2(5.1)	0.361
PL-7, n (%)	0(0.0)	1(2.6)	0.522
PL-12, n (%)	0(0.0)	2(5.1)	0.361
EJ, n (%)	0(0.0)	0(0.0)	1.000
OJ, n (%)	1(6.3)	0(0.0)	0.118
Non anti ARS antibodies, n (%)	4(25.0)	6(15.4)	0.405
SRP, n (%)	0(0.0)	2(5.1)	0.361
TIF1-γ, n (%)	1(6.3)	2(5.1)	0.869
Mi-2β, n (%)	3(18.8)	2(5.1)	0.114
SAE, n (%)	0(0.0)	1(2.6)	0.522
Treatment			
Glucocorticoid, <1 /≥1 mg/kg/d, n (%)	6/10(37.5/62.5)	22/17(56.4, 43.6)	0.207
Methotrexate, n (%)	0(0.0)	5(12.8)	0.137
Cyclophosphamide, n (%)	12(75.0)	27(69.2)	0.672
Cyclosporine A, n (%)	1(6.3)	7(17.9)	0.268
Tacrolimus, n (%)	1(6.3)	6(15.4)	0.360
Plasma exchange, n (%)	4(25.0)	3(7.7)	0.083
Single drug or Combination drugs			
1 drug	2(12.5)	6(15.4)	0.785
2 drugs	11(68.8)	20(51.3)	0.240
3 drugs	2(12.5)	11(28.2)	0.217
≥4 drugs	1(6.3)	2(5.1)	0.869

**P* < 0.05.

[&]ILD diagnosis by a radiologist and a respirologist simultaneous.

ANA, antinuclear antibody; CRP, C reactive protein; CK, creatine kinase; DLCO, carbon monoxide diffusing capacity; ELVAR, Efficient Lung Vetilation Area Ratio; ESR, erythrocyte sedimentation rate; FVC, forced vital capacity; ILD, interstitial lung disease; LDH, Lactic dehydrogenase; MDA5, melanoma melanoma differentiation associated gene 5; PCT, procalcitonin; P/F ratio, PaO2/FiO2 ratio; SAE, anti-small ubiquitin-like modifier antibody; SRP, signal recognition particle; TIF1-γ, transcription intermediary factor 1-gamma.

higher ELVAR group (ELVAR ≥ 0.835). The comparison revealed that the rates of mortality within 3 months in the lower and higher ELVAR groups were 54.2 vs. 9.7%, respectively, whereas 12-month mortality rates were 54.2 vs. 12.9%, respectively (**Figure 5D**), which indicated that the ELVAR value was more predictive of early mortality within 3 months. The differences among severity of type I respiratory failure at diagnosis (no), P/F ratio and oxygen supplementation (0 and >4 L/min) between two groups were significantly. For the other indices, dyspnea in lower ELVAR group was more frequent than that in higher ELVAR group (79.2 vs. 48.4%), and lymphocyte count of lower ELVAR group was lower than that of higher

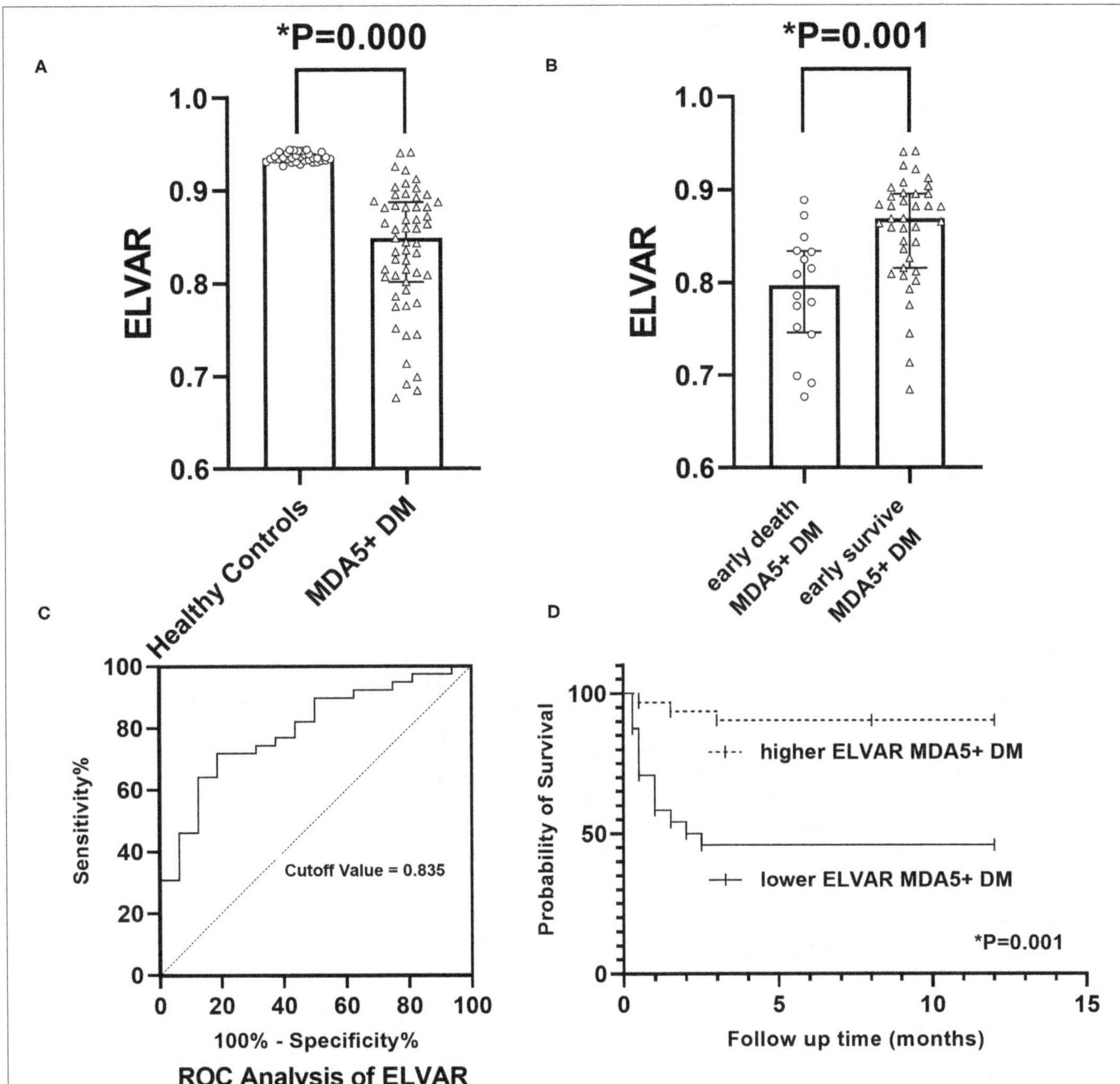

FIGURE 5 | Clinical significance of value of ELVA. **(A)** Comparison of ELVAR values between healthy controls and MDA5$^+$DM patients; **(B)** Comparison of ELVAR values between early death MDA5$^+$DM patients and early survival MDA5$^+$DM patients; **(C)** ROC analysis of ELVAR and best cutoff value was 0.835; **(D)** Comparison of 12-month Kaplan-Meier survival curve between higher ELVAR MDA5$^+$DM patients and lower ELVAR MDA5$^+$DM patients.

ELVAR group (0.65[0.50, 0.87] vs. 0.92[0.63, 1.34] $\times$ 10^9/L; **Table 4**).

ELVAR as a Risk Factor for Poor Prognosis of MDA5$^+$DM Patients

To identify the indicators of poor outcomes in MDA5$^+$DM patients, we performed Cox regression analysis. Results of the univariate analysis revealed that age of onset, CRP, myoglobin, albumin, ferritin, PCT, ELVAR, severity of type I respiratory failure, P/F ratio, oxygen supplementation, FVC and DLCO were significantly associated with poor outcomes. Only four factors including age of onset, ferritin, value of ELVAR and oxygen supplementation >4 L/min showed significantly value for poor prognosis in MDA5$^+$DM patients in the multivariate analysis (**Table 5**). FVC and DLCO were excluded from the multivariate analysis

TABLE 2 | Analysis of ROC by eight significantly different indices between early death group and early survival group.

	Analysis of ROC				
	AUC	Value of cut-off	Sensitivity (%) (C.I.)	Specificity (%) (C.I.)	p value
Age at onset	0.684	54.5	56.3	74.4	0.033*
CRP	0.692	8.51	68.8	74.4	0.026*
Ferritin	0.776	568.34	53.8	96.9	0.004*
ELVAR	0.795	0.835	71.8	81.2	0.001*
P/F ratio	0.822	269.5	87.2	75.0	0.000*
Albumin	0.829	26.65	87.2	75.0	0.000*
FVC#	1.000	64.5	100.0	0.0	0.004*
DLCO#	1.000	61.0	100.0	0.0	0.004*

*$P < 0.05$.

#*Only two patients in early death group accepted lung function test and other 14 patients in early death group didn't accept lung function test for rapidly death or intolerable.*

CRP, C reactive protein; DLCO, carbon monoxide diffusing capacity; ELVAR, Efficient Lung Ventilation Area Ratio; FVC, forced vital capacity; P/F ratio, PaO2/FiO2 ratio.

because of insufficient data due to patient intolerability and early-death patients.

DISCUSSION

It is widely known that the short-term prognosis of MDA5$^+$DM-ILD patients is poor (18). Accurate prediction of MDA5$^+$DM patient outcomes is a key issue in clinical practice. In this study, we established a computer-aided lung interstitial image analysis approach. ELVAR was obtained by calculating the proportion of areas outside the lung interstitium in lung tissue that can indirectly evaluates the severity of lung interstitial lesions. Our results showed that ELVAR values in MDA5$^+$DM patients who died within 3 months after diagnosis were significantly reduced than those who were survival after 3 months. ROC analysis and correlation analysis about value of ELVAR showed that ELVAR values have good predictive power for 3-month mortality and widely correlation with many clinical indices, which indicates that it may be a powerful tool for clinicians to evaluate poor outcomes in MDA5$^+$DM-ILD.

Recently a variety of lung segmentation methods have been advanced (19). According to the different segmentation features used, lung segmentation methods can be divided into threshold-based methods (20), region-based methods (21), and shape-based methods (22). However, these methods had different degrees of partial lung tissue loss. A recent study used deep learning and feature learning to obtain better segmentation results by training with large samples (23). Software package named "CT Pneumonia Analysis" applying in the similar mechanism was used in study by S Ye recently (24). Our design idea was to extent different. We considered deep learning above cannot guarantee the accuracy results for inconsistent diagnosis of complex images and was not feasible for rare diseases such as MDA5$^+$DM. We proposed another lung tissue segmentation method that was suitable for CT images of interstitial lung disease. The lung

TABLE 3 | Correlation analysis between value of ELVAR, level of Albumin, P/F ration and significant different indices from comparison between early death group and early survival group.

Correlation analysis	Value of ELVAR				Level of Albumin				P/F ratio			
	Spearman ρ	P-value	Kendall τ	P-value	Spearmanρ	P- value	Kendallτ	P- value	Spearman ρ	P-value	Kendall τ	P-value
Duration from treatment to death or 1 year	0.488	0.000*			0.502	0.000*			0.511	0.000*		
ELVAR	/	/			0.363	0.006*			0.323	0.016*		
Albumin	0.363	0.006*			/	/			0.433	0.001*		
P/F ratio	0.323	0.016*			0.433	0.001*			/	/		
Ferritin	−0.295	0.029*			−0.391	0.003*			−0.245	0.072		
Age at onset	−0.247	0.069			−0.356	0.008*			−0.211	0.121		
CRP	−0.219	0.108			−0.455	0.000*			−0.322	0.017*		
FVC	−0.010	0.953			−0.046	0.785			0.029	0.865		
DLCO	−0.015	0.928			−0.197	0.236			0.286	0.082		
Mortality within 3 months			0.382	0.001*			0.428	0.000*			0.419	0.000*
Mortality within 12 months			0.363	0.001*			0.429	0.000*			0.399	0.000*
Oxygen supplementation			−0.287	0.006*			−0.219	0.035*			−0.658	0.000*
Severity of type I respiratory failure			−0.287	0.007*			−0.301	0.005*			−0.725	0.000*

*$P < 0.05$.

CRP, C reactive protein; DLCO, carbon monoxide diffusing capacity; ELVAR, Efficient Lung Vetilation Area Ratio; FVC, forced vital capacity; P/F ratio, PaO2/FiO2 ratio.

TABLE 4 | Comparison between lower ELVAR group and higher ELVAR group.

Variables	MDA5⁺DM patients		
	lower ELVAR group *N* = 24	**higher ELVAR group *N* = 31**	***P*-value**
Female, n (%)	20(83.3)	22(71.0)	0.289
Age of onset (y)	53(46.25, 59.25)	52(42, 59)	0.440
Duration from onset to treatment, m	3.0(2.0, 4.0)	2.0(1.0, 3.0)	0.095
Duration from treatment to death or 1 year, m	2.25(0.5, 12.0)	12.0(12.0, 12.0)	0.000*
Mortality within 3 months, n (%)	13(54.2)	3(9.7)	0.000*
Mortality within 12 months, n (%)	13(54.2)	4(12.9)	0.001*
Smoking history, n (%)	3(12.5)	5(16.1)	0.708
Clinical feature			
Muscle weakness, n (%)	12(50.0)	21(67.7)	0.187
Gottron sign, n (%)	7(29.2)	7(22.6)	0.582
Heliotrop rash, n (%)	8(33.3)	11(35.5)	0.869
Skin ulcer, n (%)	6(25.0)	8(25.8)	0.946
Raynaud phenomenon, n (%)	0(0.0)	3(9.7)	0.120
Fever, n (%)	8(33.3)	7(22.6)	0.379
Cough, n (%)	4(16.7)	7(22.6)	0.590
Dyspnea, n (%)	19(79.2)	15(48.4)	0.021*
Pneumothorax, n (%)	1(4.1)	1(3.2)	0.855
Concomitant neoplasia, n (%)	0(0.0)	1(2.6)	0.379
Laboratory data			
Neutrophil Count, $X10^9/L$	3.31(2.67, 4.74)	3.29(2.37, 4.63)	0.754
Lymphocyte Count, $X10^9/L$	0.65(0.50, 0.87)	0.92(0.63, 1.34)	0.022*
ESR, mm/hr	43(31, 62)	32.50(24.50, 56.25)	0.164
CRP, mg/L	9.21(2.60, 18.03)	5.16(2.60, 11.10)	0.222
CK, IU/L	76.20(45.83, 144.23)	87.4(44.6, 201.2)	0.905
LDH, IU/L	378.60(332.80, 525.55)	358.50(268.25, 441.05)	0.157
Myoglobin, ug/L	69.60(49.50, 108.78)	69.4(38.5, 95.2)	0.457
Albumin, g/L	27.40(24.33, 30.83)	29.8(26.7, 34.2)	0.051
Ferritin, ng/ml	519.05(375.45, 570.19)	485.18(357.90, 562.67)	0.131
PCT, ng/ml	0.09(0.053, 0.14)	0.07(0.035, 0.11)	0.214
Pulmonary involvement			
ILD diagnosis, n (%)[&]	22(91.7)	26(83.9)	0.394
Radiological feature of ILD at diagnosis			
Reticulations, n (%)	6(25.0)	8(25.8)	0.946
Septal thickening, n (%)	8(33.3)	11(35.5)	0.869
Ground glass opacities, n (%)	7(29.2)	6(19.4)	0.400
Nodules, n (%)	3(12.5)	9(29.0)	0.145
Bronchiectasis/Bronchiolectasis, n (%)	1(4.2)	2(6.5)	0.714
Honeycombing, n (%)	0(0.0)	2(6.5)	0.209
Consolidation, n (%)	18(75.0)	16(51.6)	0.079
ELVAR	0.7893(0.7442,0.8143)	0.8823(0.8638,0.9025)	0.000*
Severity of type I respiratory failure			
no/mild/moderate/severe, n (%)	11/4/7/2 (45.8/16.7/29.2/8.3)	24/4/3/0 (77.4/12.9/9.7/0)	0.009*
no, n (%)	11(45.8)	24(77.4)	0.017*
mild, n (%)	4(16.7)	4(12.9)	0.697
moderate, n (%)	7(29.2)	3(9.7)	0.066
severe, n (%)	2(8.3)	0(0)	0.105
P/F ratio, mmHg	260(192.5, 419)	417(303, 471)	0.025*

(Continued)

TABLE 4 | Continued

Variables	MDA5+DM patients		
	lower ELVAR group *N* = 24	**higher ELVAR group *N* = 31**	***P*-value**
Oxygen supplementation			
0/1–2/3–4/>4L/min, n (%)	5/5/7/7 (20.8/20.8/29.2/29.2)	17/4/8/2 (54.8/12.9/25.8/6.5)	0.007*
0L/min, n (%)	5(20.8)	17(54.8)	0.011*
1–2L/min, n (%)	5(20.8)	4(12.9)	0.435
3–4L/min, n (%)	7(29.2)	8(25.8)	0.783
>4L/min, n (%)	7(29.2)	2(6.5)	0.025*
FVC, % PRED	79(71,82)	79(78,81)	0.843
DLCO, % PRED	79(77.25,79.75)	79(68.50,80.25)	0.902
Antibody positive			
ANA, n (%)	7(29.2)	10(32.3)	0.807
MAA profile	19(79.2)	22(71.0)	0.493
SSA, n (%)	2(8.3)	6(19.4)	0.255
SSB, n (%)	2(8.3)	1(3.2)	0.412
Ro-52, n (%)	18(75.0)	21(67.7)	0.560
CENP-B, n (%)	1(4.2)	1(3.2)	0.855
Ku, n (%)	0(0.0)	1(3.2)	0.379
PM-Scl, n (%)	2(8.3)	0(0.0)	0.105
MSA profile, n (%)	7(29.2)	6(19.4)	0.400
anti-ARS antibodies, n (%)	2(8.3)	3(9.7)	0.865
Jo-1, n (%)	0(0.0)	2(6.5)	0.209
PL-7, n (%)	0(0.0)	1(3.2)	0.379
PL-12, n (%)	1(4.2)	1(3.2)	0.855
EJ, n (%)	0(0.0)	0(0.0)	1.000
OJ, n (%)	1(4.2)	0(0.0)	0.256
Non-anti-ARS antibodies, n (%)	5(20.8)	5(16.1)	0.657
SRP, n (%)	1(4.2)	1(3.2)	0.855
TIF1-γ, n (%)	1(4.2)	2(6.5)	0.714
Mi-2β, n (%)	2(8.3)	3(9.7)	0.865
SAE, n (%)	1(4.2)	0(0.0)	0.256
Treatment			
Glucocorticoid, <1 /≥1 mg/kg/d, n (%)	12/12(50.0/50.0)	16/15(51.6/48.4)	0.906
Methotrexate, n (%)	2(8.3)	3(9.7)	0.865
Cyclophosphamide, n (%)	19(79.2)	20(64.5)	0.240
Cyclosporine A, n (%)	1(4.2)	7(22.6)	0.057
Tacrolimus, n (%)	2(8.3)	5(16.1)	0.394
Plasma exchange, n (%)	4(16.7)	3(9.7)	0.445
Single drug or Combination drugs			
1 drug	3(12.5)	5(16.1)	0.708
2 drugs	15(62.5)	16(51.6)	0.424
3 drugs	5(20.8)	8(25.8)	0.670
≥ 4 drugs	1(4.2)	2(6.5)	0.714

*$P < 0.05$.

[&] *ILD diagnosis by a radiologist and a respirologist simultaneous.*

ANA, antinuclear antibody; CRP, C reactive protein; CK, creatine kinase; DLCO, carbon monoxide diffusing capacity; ELVAR, Efficient Lung Vetilation Area Ratio; ESR, erythrocyte sedimentation rate; FVC, forced vital capacity; ILD, interstitial lung disease; LDH, Lactic dehydrogenase; MDA5, melanoma melanoma differentiation-associated gene-5; PCT, procalcitonin; P/F ratio, PaO2/FiO2 ratio; SAE, anti-small ubiquitin-like modifier antibody; SRP, signal recognition particle; TIF1-γ, transcription intermediary factor 1-gamma.

edges produced by our method were more accurate than those of above mentioned traditional methods (25). The outstanding feature lying in our computer-aided analysis of lung HRCT were outer boundary of binary lung tissue region images selected by Laplace operator and interstitial enhancement generated according to curvature feature of lung interstitium. Because our imagine analysis had based on high density structure from HRCT, we can apprehension that imagine of normal lung interstitium and abnormal imagine including consolidation, reticulations, septal thickening, ground glass opacities, nodules, bronchiectasis,

TABLE 5 | Univariate analysis and Multivariate analysis of prognostic factors in MDA5^{+}DM patients.

Variable	Univariate analysis		Multivariate analysis	
	HR (95%CI)	*P*- value	HR (95%CI)	*P*- value
Female	0.420(0.095–1.852)	0.252		
Age at onset	2.776(1.031–7.471)	0.043*	9.842(1.434–67.528)	0.020*
Duration from onset to treatment	0.550(0.200–1.515)	0.247		
Mortality within 3 months	0.000(0.000–1.845)	0.069		
Mortality within 12 months	0.001(0.000–1.294)	0.059		
Smoking history	2.309(0.743–7.171)	0.148		
Muscle weakness	0.616(0.231–1.644)	0.334		
Gottron sign	1.311(0.455–3.776)	0.616		
Heliotrop rash	0.598(0.193–1.856)	0.374		
Skin ulcer	0.384(0.087–1.689)	0.205		
Raynaud phenomenon	0.045(0.000–351.921)	0.498		
Fever	2.336(0.869–6.282)	0.093		
Cough	0.527(0.120–2.321)	0.397		
Dyspnea	2.254(0.725–7.002)	0.160		
Pneumothorax	2.142(0.282–16.282)	0.462		
Concomitant neoplasia	0.048(0.000–216181.008)	0.698		
Neutrophil Count	0.272(0.036–2.058)	0.207		
Lymphocyte Count	0.448(0.163–1.237)	0.121		
ESR	0.328(0.093–1.156)	0.083		
CRP	4.665(1.615–13.474)	0.004*	2.172(0.480–9.841)	0.314
CK	5.104(0.674–38.674)	0.115		
LDH	36.822(0.430–3154.017.039)	0.112		
Myoglobin	3.004(1.124–8.031)	0.028*	3.347(0.783–14.306)	0.103
Albumin	0.109(0.035–0.342)	0.000*	0.307(0.053–S1.785)	0.189
Ferritin	7.897(2.862–21.793)	0.000*	11.255(2.084–60.786)	0.005*
PCT	2.793(1.012–7.707)	0.047*	0.954(0.217–4.187)	0.950
ILD diagnosis	25.672(0.061–10818.508)	0.293		
Reticulations	0.630(0.179–2.210)	0.470		
Septal thickening	2.228(0.835–5.940)	0.109		
Ground glass opacities	1.202(0.388–3.730)	0.750		
Nodules	1.542(0.535–4.440)	0.422		
Bronchiectasis/Bronchiolectasis	1.413(0.186–10.712)	0.738		
Honeycombing	2.142(0.282–16.282)	0.462		
Consolidation	2.081(0.671–6.454)	0.205		
ELVAR	0.133(0.038–0.468)	0.002*	0.098(0.017–0.564)	0.009*
Severity of type I respiratory failure				
Mild	7.399(2.370–23.106)	0.001*	0.001(0.000–4.093E+100)	0.995
Moderate	8.453(3.075–23.234)	0.000*	5.369(0.676–42.654)	0.112
Severe	8.516(1.719–42.197)	0.009*	1.062(0.088–12.815)	0.962
P/F ratio	0.095(0.030–0.298)	0.000*	0.000(0.000–4.865E+99)	0.941
Oxygen supplementation				
1–2	3.370(0.958–11.853)	0.058		
3–4	4.802(1.542–14.954)	0.007*	3.476(0.286–42.194)	0.328
>4	3.711(1.337–10.299)	0.012*	0.010(0.001–0.146)	0.001*
FVC	1.000	1.000	NC[&]	
DLCO	1.000	1.000	NC[&]	
ANA	0.296(0.067–1.303)	0.107		
SSA	0.037(0.000–11.180)	0.259		
SSB	0.045(0.000–351.921)	0.498		
RO-52	2.985(0.677–13.150)	0.148		

(Continued)

TABLE 5 | Continued

Variable	Univariate analysis		Multivariate analysis	
	HR (95%CI)	*P*- value	HR (95%CI)	*P*- value
CENP-B	2.142(0.282–16.282)	0.462		
Ku	0.048(0.000–216181.008)	0.698		
PM-Scl	0.047(0.000–2532.428)	0.582		
Jo-1	0.047(0.000–2532.428)	0.582		
PL-7	0.048(0.000–216181.008)	0.698		
PL-12	0.047(0.000–2532.428)	0.582		
OJ	4.085(0.531–31.432)	0.176		
SRP	0.047(0.000–2532.428)	0.582		
TIF1-γ	1.239(0.164–9.388)	0.836		
Mi-2β	2.196(0.625–7.713)	0.220		
SAE	0.048(0.000–216181.008)	0.698		
Glucocorticoid	1.831(0.665–5.043)	0.242		
Methotrexate	0.042(0.000–48.056)	0.378		
Cyclophosphamide	1.176(0.379–3.648)	0.779		
Cyclosporine A	0.363(0.048–2.747)	0.326		
Tacrolimus	0.415(0.055–3.143)	0.395		
Plasma exchange	2.812(0.900–8.787)	0.075		
Single drug or Combination drugs				
1 drug	0.894(0.203–3.935)	0.882		
2 drugs	1.119(0.254–4.923)	0.882		
3 drugs	0.514(0.146–1.804)	0.299		
≥4 drugs	239(0.164–9.388)	0.836		

$^{*}P < 0.05$.

[&] NC, only 2 patients in early death group accepted lung function test and other 14 patients in early death group didn't accept lung function test for rapidly death or intolerable. Hence multivariate analysis didn't include the FVC and DLCO into analysis.

honey combing, cysts could be detected and analysis (26). Because ELVAR was defined with the formula of (L–I)/L (L was the total number of lung voxels and I was the total number of interstitial voxels), which could easily be understood that the level of ELVAR was negative correlation with the scope of abnormal lung interstitium, *i.e.*, high value of ELVAR meant less scope of interstitium and high ventilation, however, the lower value of ELVAR referred to large scope of interstitium and low ventilation which possible indicted poor disease outcome. Finally in our single-center retrospective study, we calculated that value of ELVAR in healthy controls was 0.938 while cut off value of ELVAR by ROC analysis in MDA5$^+$DM-ILD was 0.835. Patients with low ELVAR values (< 0.835) had a 54.2% chance of dying within 3 months, which may be valuable for clinicians to administer more active treatments in these patients.

The prediction value of the pulmonary function test could not be evaluated in this study because 14 patients in early death group did not accept the lung function test for early death or intolerability. In terms of albumin levels, it is widely accepted that patients with hypoalbuminemia do not recover easily; however, there is currently no data to directly verify the relationship between albumin level and prognosis of patients with MDA5$^+$DM. In 2020, a prediction model using CRP and Krebs Von den Lungen-6 (KL-6) combined with the anti-MDA5 antibody was shown to be useful for predicting prognosis of patients with DM-ILD (27). As for ferritin, many studies have shown that serum ferritin levels were not only related to the severity of interstitial pneumonia in patients (28) but also predicted the risk of death (29). Recently, a FLAIR model was developed that combined five clinical indices, which included ferritin, lactate dehydrogenase, MDA5 antibody, HRCT Imagine semi-quantitative score, and rapidly-progressive ILD, to predict amyopathic dermatomyositis survival time (30). This FLAIR model was a multivariable model with rigorously established cutoff values that can be applied by clinicians in a uniform way. The 1-year survival in the discovery and validation cohorts were 34.3% and 15.0% for the high-risk group. This will provide a guidepost for making decisions around how aggressively to immunosuppress (31). Our study showed four factors including age of onset, ferritin, value of ELVAR and oxygen supplementation >4 L/min predicted significantly value for poor prognosis in MDA5$^+$DM patients, which was consistent with FLAIR model to some extent. Above all, these findings highlight the value and importance of quantitative lung involvement of ILD. Our research based on computer-based image analysis technology that attempt to directly quantify lung interstitial lesions, which was simpler and more quantitative than FLAIR's multi-index model, and had a certain degree of innovation.

As an exploratory study that combined computer image analysis and prognosis of MDA5$^+$DM, several limitations may be noticed. First, this was a single-center study, and more data from multi-centers are needed to confirm the efficiency of ELVAR values. Second, the role of ELVAR needs to be verified among different diseases' associated ILD. Third, identification will be needed regarding whether computer-aided analysis of lung HRCT based on Siemens system can be applied to GE or Samsung system.

CONCLUSION

An index named by ELVAR basing on lung segmentation and lung interstitial enhancement was successfully established. The study aimed to assess the role of ELVAR value in predicting early death from interstitial pneumonia secondary to $MDA5^{+}DM$. A retrospective analysis of 46 healthy controls and 55 patients with $MDA5^{+}DM$ from a single center found that the ELVAR value of healthy controls was stable at around 0.938, whereas $MDA5^{+}DM$ patients had lower values. Results showed that early mortality within 3 months of onset in patients with ELVAR values lower than 0.835 was significantly high as 54.2%. This novel index may be valuable for clinicians to efficiently identify severe patients and administer more active treatments.

ETHICS STATEMENT

The studies involving human participants were reviewed and approved by Ethics Committee of Second Xiangya Hospital of Central South University. The patients/participants provided their written informed consent to participate in this study. Written informed consent was obtained from the individual(s) for the publication of any potentially identifiable images or data included in this article.

AUTHOR CONTRIBUTIONS

CW, XM, and FeL designed the research. CW, LG, and FaL developed the computer-aided image analysis technology. XM and HL evaluated the ILD diagnosis of $MDA5^{+}DM$. CW, JD, and FeL were responsible for the statistical analysis. CW and FeL wrote the paper. All authors contributed to the article and approved the submitted version.

REFERENCES

1. András C, Bodoki L, Nagy-Vincze M, Griger Z, Csiki E, Dankó K. Retrospective analysis of cancer-associated myositis patients over the past 3 decades in a hungarian myositis cohort. *Pathol Oncol Res.* (2020) 26:1749–55. doi: 10.1007/s12253-019-00756-4
2. Smoyer-Tomic KE, Amato AA, Fernandes AW. Incidence and prevalence of idiopathic inflammatory myopathies among commercially insured, medicare supplemental insured, and medicaid enrolled populations: an administrative claims analysis. *BMC Musculoskelet Disord.* (2012) 13:103. doi: 10.1186/1471-2474-13-103
3. Dias Junior AG, Sampaio NG, Rehwinkel J. A balancing act: MDA5 in antiviral immunity and autoinflammation. *Trends Microbiol.* (2019) 27:75–85. doi: 10.1016/j.tim.2018.08.007
4. Baechler EC, Bilgic H, Reed AM. Type I interferon pathway in adult and juvenile dermatomyositis. *Arthritis Res Ther.* (2011)13:249. doi: 10.1186/ar3531
5. Ono N, Kai K, Maruyama A, Sakai M, Sadanaga Y, Koarada S, et al. The relationship between type 1 IFN and vasculopathy in anti-MDA5 antibody-positive dermatomyositis patients. *Rheumatology (Oxford).* (2019) 58:786–91. doi: 10.1093/rheumatology/key386
6. Labrador-Horrillo M, Martinez MA, Selva-O'Callaghan A, Trallero-Araguas E, Balada E, Vilardell-Tarres M, et al. Anti-MDA5 antibodies in a large mediterranean population of adults with dermatomyositis. *J Immunol Res.* (2014) 2014:290797. doi: 10.1155/2014/290797
7. Moghadam-Kia S, Oddis CV, Sato S, Kuwana M, Aggarwal R. Anti-melanoma differentiation-associated gene 5 is associated with rapidly progressive lung disease and poor survival in US patients with amyopathic and myopathic dermatomyositis. *Arthritis Care Res (Hoboken).* (2016) 68:689–94. doi: 10.1002/acr.22728
8. Chen F, Wang D, Shu X, Nakashima R, Wang G. Anti-MDA5 antibody is associated with A/SIP and decreased T cells in peripheral blood and predicts poor prognosis of ILD in Chinese patients with dermatomyositis. *Rheumatol Int.* (2012) 32:3909–15s. doi: 10.1007/s00296-011-2323-y
9. Koga T, Fujikawa K, Horai Y, Okada A, Kawashiri SY, Iwamoto N, et al. The diagnostic utility of anti-melanoma differentiation-associated gene 5 antibody testing for predicting the prognosis of Japanese patients with DM. *Rheumatology (Oxford).* (2012) 51:1278–84. doi: 10.1093/rheumatology/ker518
10. Yoshida N, Okamoto M, Kaieda S, Fujimoto K, Ebata T, Tajiri M, et al. Association of anti-aminoacyl-transfer RNA synthetase antibody and anti-melanoma differentiation-associated gene 5 antibody with the therapeutic response of polymyositis/dermatomyositis-associated interstitial lung disease. *Respir Investig.* (2017) 55:24–32. doi: 10.1016/j.resinv.2016.08.007
11. Chen Z, Cao M, Plana MN, Liang J, Cai H, Kuwana M, et al. Utility of anti-melanoma differentiation-associated gene 5 antibody measurement in identifying patients with dermatomyositis and a high risk for developing rapidly progressive interstitial lung disease: a review of the literature and a meta-analysis. *Arthritis Care Res (Hoboken).* (2013) 65:1316–24. doi: 10.1002/acr.21985
12. Kim HG, Tashkin DP, Clements PJ, Li G, Brown MS, Elashoff R, et al. A computer-aided diagnosis system for quantitative scoring of extent of lung fibrosis in scleroderma patients. *Clin Exp Rheumatol.* (2010) 28(5 Suppl 62):S26–35.
13. Goldin JG, Kim GHJ, Tseng CH, Volkmann E, Furst D, Clements P, et al. Longitudinal changes in quantitative interstitial lung disease on computed tomography after immunosuppression in the scleroderma lung study II. *Ann Am Thorac Soc.* (2018) 15:1286–95. doi: 10.1513/AnnalsATS.201802-079OC
14. Bartholmai BJ, Raghunath S, Karwoski RA, Moua T, Rajagopalan S, Maldonado F, et al. Quantitative computed tomography imaging of interstitial lung diseases. *J Thorac Imaging.* (2013) 28:298–307. doi: 10.1097/RTI.0b013e3182a21969
15. Hosein KS, Sergiacomi G, Zompatori M, Mura M. The CALIPER-Revised version of the composite physiologic index is a better predictor

of survival in IPF than the original version. *Lung.* (2020) 198:169–72. doi: 10.1007/s00408-019-00295-4

16. Bell RD, Rudmann C, Wood RW, Schwarz EM, Rahimi H. Longitudinal micro-CT as an outcome measure of interstitial lung disease in TNF-transgenic mice. *PLoS ONE.* (2018) 13:e0190678. doi: 10.1371/journal.pone.0190678
17. Mammen AL, Allenbach Y, Stenzel W, Benveniste O. ENMC 239th workshop study group. 239th ENMC international workshop: classification of dermatomyositis, Amsterdam, the Netherlands, 14–16 december 2018. *Neuromuscul Disord.* (2020) 30:70–92. doi: 10.1016/j.nmd.2019.10.005
18. Wu W, Guo L, Fu Y, Wang K, Zhang D, Xu W, et al. Interstitial lung disease in anti-MDA5 positive dermatomyositis. *Clin Rev Allergy Immunol.* (2021) 60:293–304. doi: 10.1007/s12016-020-08822-5
19. Gerard SE, Herrmann J, Kaczka DW, Musch G, Fernandez-Bustamante A, Reinhardt JM. Multi-resolution convolutional neural networks for fully automated segmentation of acutely injured lungs in multiple species. *Med Image Anal.* (2020) 60:101592. doi: 10.1016/j.media.2019.101592
20. Hu S, Hoffman EA, Reinhardt JM. Automatic lung segmentation for accurate quantitation of volumetric X-ray CT images. IEEE *Trans Med Imaging.* (2001) 20:490–8. doi: 10.1109/42.929615
21. Qi S, van Triest HJ, Yue Y, Xu M, Kang Y. Automatic pulmonary fissure detection and lobe segmentation in CT chest images. *Biomed Eng Online.* (2014) 13:59. doi: 10.1186/1475-925X-13-59
22. Ross JC, Kindlmann GL, Okajima Y, Hatabu H, Díaz AA, Silverman EK, et al. Pulmonary lobe segmentation based on ridge surface sampling and shape model fitting. *Med Phys.* (2013) 40:121903. doi: 10.1118/1.4828782
23. Phellan R, Falcão AX, Udupa JK. Medical image segmentation via atlases and fuzzy object models: improving efficacy through optimum object search and fewer models. *Med Phys.* (2016) 43:401. doi: 10.1118/1.4938577
24. Xu W, Wu W, Zhang D, Chen Z, Tao X, Zhao J, et al. A novel CT scoring method predicts the prognosis of interstitial lung disease associated with anti-MDA5 positive dermatomyositis. *Sci Rep.* (2021) 11:17070. doi: 10.1038/s41598-021-96292-w
25. Guo LC, Wang CJ, Li FZ, He HJ, Li F. Binary surface smoothing for abnormal lung segmentation. *Comput Graph.* (2020) 89:68–76. doi: 10.1016/j.cag.2020.05.011
26. Neji H, Attia M, Affes M, Baccouche I, Ben Miled-M'rad K, Hantous-Zannad S. Interstitial lung diseases: imaging contribution to diagnosis and elementary radiological lesions. *Semin Diagn Pathol.* (2018) 35:297–303. doi: 10.1053/j.semdp.2018.07.001
27. Gono T, Masui K, Nishina N, Kawaguchi Y, Kawakami A, Ikeda K, et al. A multicenter retrospective cohort of Japanese patients with myositis-associated ILD (JAMI) investigators. risk prediction modeling based on a combination of initial serum biomarkers in myositis-associated interstitial lung disease. *Arthritis Rheumatol.* (2020) 73:677–86. doi: 10.1002/art.41566
28. Fujiki Y, Kotani T, Isoda K, Ishida T, Shoda T, Yoshida S, et al. Evaluation of clinical prognostic factors for interstitial pneumonia in anti-MDA5 antibody-positive dermatomyositis patients. *Mod Rheumatol.* (2018) 28:133–140. doi: 10.1080/14397595.2017.1318468
29. Gono T, Kawaguchi Y, Satoh T, Kuwana M, Katsumata Y, Takagi K, et al. Clinical manifestation and prognostic factor in anti-melanoma differentiation-associated gene 5 antibody-associated interstitial lung disease as a complication of dermatomyositis. *Rheumatology (Oxford).* (2010) 49:1713–9. doi: 10.1093/rheumatology/keq149
30. Lian X, Zou J, Guo Q, Chen S, Lu L, Wang R, et al. Mortality risk prediction in amyopathic dermatomyositis associated with interstitial lung disease: the FLAIR model. *Chest.* (2020) 158:1535–45. doi: 10.1016/j.chest.2020.04.057
31. Baker MC, Chung L, Fiorentino DF. A mortality risk score model for clinically amyopathic dermatomyositis-associated interstitial lung disease: will it have the necessary "FLAIR" to improve clinical outcomes? *Chest.* (2020) 158:1307–9. doi: 10.1016/j.chest.2020.06.001

2

ECG Changes Through Immunosuppressive Therapy Indicate Cardiac Abnormality in Anti-MDA5 Antibody-Positive Clinically Amyopathic Dermatomyositis

Takashi Matsuo[1], *Tsuneo Sasai*[1], *Ran Nakashima*[1*], *Yoshihiro Kuwabara*[2], *Eri Toda Kato*[3], *Isao Murakami*[1], *Hideo Onizawa*[4], *Shuji Akizuki*[1], *Kosaku Murakami*[1], *Motomu Hashimoto*[4,5], *Hajime Yoshifuji*[1], *Masao Tanaka*[4], *Akio Morinobu*[1] and *Tsuneyo Mimori*[1,6]

[1] Department of Rheumatology and Clinical Immunology, Kyoto University, Kyoto, Japan, [2] Cancer Control Center, Osaka International Cancer Institute, Osaka, Japan, [3] Department of Cardiovascular Medicine, Kyoto University, Kyoto, Japan, [4] Department of Advanced Medicine for Rheumatic Diseases, Kyoto University, Kyoto, Japan, [5] Department of Clinical Immunology, Graduate School of Medicine, Osaka City University, Osaka, Japan, [6] Takeda General Hospital, Kyoto, Japan

***Correspondence:**
Ran Nakashima
ranran@kuhp.kyoto-u.ac.jp

Anti-melanoma differentiation-associated gene 5 (MDA5) antibody, a dermatomyositis (DM)-specific antibody, is strongly associated with interstitial lung disease (ILD). Patients with idiopathic inflammatory myopathy (IIM) who are anti-MDA5 antibody positive [anti-MDA5 (+)] often experience chest symptoms during the active disease phase. These symptoms are primarily explained by respiratory failure; nevertheless, cardiac involvement can also be symptomatic. Thus, the aim of this study was to investigate cardiac involvement in anti-MDA5 (+) DM. A total of 63 patients with IIM who underwent electrocardiography (ECG) and ultrasound cardiography (UCG) during the active disease phase from 2016 to 2021 [anti-MDA5 (+) group, n = 21; anti-MDA5-negative (-) group, n = 42] were enrolled in the study, and their clinical charts were retrospectively reviewed. The ECG and UCG findings were compared between the anti-MDA5 (+) and anti-MDA5 (-) groups. All anti-MDA5 (+) patients had DM with ILD. The anti-MDA5 (+) group showed more frequent skin ulcerations and lower levels of leukocytes, muscle enzymes, and electrolytes (Na, K, Cl, and Ca) than the anti-MDA5 (-) group. According to the ECG findings obtained during the active disease phase, the T wave amplitudes were significantly lower for the anti-MDA5 (+) group than for the anti-MDA5 (-) group (I, II, and V4–6 lead; $p < 0.01$; aVF and V3, $p < 0.05$). However, the lower amplitudes were restored during the remission phase. Except for the E wave, A wave and Sep e', the UCG results showed no significant differences between the groups. Four patients with anti-MDA5 (+) DM had many leads with lower T wave and cardiac abnormalities (heart failure, diastolic dysfunction, myocarditis) on and after admission. Though anti-MDA5 (+) patients clinically improved after immunosuppressive therapy, some of their ECG findings did not fully recover in remission phase. In conclusion, anti-MDA5 (+) DM appears to show cardiac involvement (electrical activity and function) during the active phase. Further studies are necessary to clarify the actual cardiac condition and mechanism of these findings in patients with anti-MDA5 (+) DM.

Keywords: dermatomyositis, interstitial lung disease, anti-melanoma differentiation-associated gene 5 antibody, electrocardiography, T wave

INTRODUCTION

Idiopathic inflammatory myopathy (IIM) is an autoimmune disease that affects skeletal muscles and various systemic organs, such as the skin, lungs, heart, and joints (1, 2). Currently, myositis-specific autoantibodies (MSAs) and myositis-associated autoantibodies are widely used in clinical practice because they help not only in the diagnosis of IIM, but are also useful for the subcategorization and prediction of the clinical characteristics, disease course, and prognosis of the disease.

The anti-melanoma differentiation-associated gene 5 (MDA5) antibody, which is an MSA, was first reported to be an anti-clinically amyopathic dermatomyositis-140 (anti-CADM-140) antibody specific to CADM in a Japanese cohort in 2005, which showed a strong association with rapidly progressive interstitial lung disease (ILD) (3). The anti-MDA5 antibody can be identified in patients with classic dermatomyositis (DM); however, those with anti-MDA5 antibody (anti-MDA5 [+]) DM/CADM rarely present with critical muscle symptoms, making early detection challenging (4).

Previous studies have shown that 6–75% of the patients with polymyositis (PM)/DM have concomitant cardiac disorders (e.g., heart failure, coronary artery disease, conduction abnormalities, and abnormalities on electrocardiography [ECG] or ultrasound cardiography [UCG]) (5, 6). Nonetheless, there is a paucity of data regarding cardiac involvement in anti-MDA5 (+) DM/CADM (7). Therefore, in this study, we investigated whether cardiac involvement is associated with anti-MDA5 (+) DM/CADM. This is the first report on a specific cardiac abnormality observed in patients with anti-MDA5 (+) DM/CADM.

MATERIALS AND METHODS

Patients and Clinical Data

Patients with PM/DM/CADM who were newly diagnosed and admitted to Kyoto University Hospital for remission induction therapy from March 2016 to September 2021 were enrolled in this study. The patients' medical records were retrospectively reviewed and analyzed. The remission phase was defined as the period during which the steroid dose could be reduced for more than 3 months after treatment without a relapse. All the patients who underwent ECG and UCG were included. PM and DM were diagnosed according to the criteria outlined by Bohan and Peter (1, 2). CADM was diagnosed for the patients who had skin lesions typical of DM, but little or no muscle-related symptoms (8). ILD was diagnosed based on a physical examination, pulmonary function tests, chest radiography, high-resolution chest computed tomography, and the presence of respiratory symptoms. We collected the included patients' laboratory data before treatment (just around the admission date). The patients' serum was screened for MSAs using [35S]methionine-labeled protein/RNA immunoprecipitation and ELISA (MESACUP anti-MDA5, MESACUP anti-TIF1-γ, MESACUP anti-ARS, and MESACUP anti-Mi-2; MBL Co., Ltd., Nagoya, Japan), as previously described (4, 9, 10). We divided the patients into an anti-MDA5 (+) group and an anti-MDA5 (-) group and compared the clinical, laboratory, and physiological data between the two groups.

Ethical Considerations

This study was conducted in accordance with the Declaration of Helsinki and approved by the ethics committee of Kyoto University Graduate School and Faculty of Medicine (approval number: E458). Written informed consent was obtained from all the patients prior to enrollment.

Electrocardiography and Ultrasound Cardiography

ECG and UCG findings were reviewed at the first admission for remission induction. The typical ECG wave forms were analyzed using the QP-170D ECG Viewer software version 9 (Nihon Kohden, Tokyo, Japan). Two cardiologists (Y.K. and E.T.K.) reviewed the ECG and UCG findings. ECG and UCG parameters were then compared between the anti-MDA5 (+) and anti-MDA5 (-) groups.

Statistical Analysis

The differences between the anti-MDA5 (+) and anti-MDA5 (-) groups were analyzed using an unpaired t-test for the continuous variables and a chi-square test for the categorical variables. Data are expressed as the mean ± standard deviation for the continuous variables and as percentages for the categorical variables, unless otherwise noted. All the statistical analyses were performed using the JMP Pro statistical package version 16.0.0 J (SAS Institute Inc., Cary, NC, USA). The differences were considered statistically significant at a two-tailed $p < 0.05$.

RESULTS

Patient Characteristics

Of the 94 enrolled patients with PM/DM/CADM, 63 underwent both ECG and UCG on admission. We divided these patients into an anti-MDA5 (+) group (n = 21) and an anti-MDA5 (-)

group (n = 42), the latter of which comprised fourteen anti-ARS (+), five anti-TIF1-γ (+), seven anti-SRP (+), two anti Mi-2(+), one anti Ku (+), one anti NXP2 (+) and twelve MSA-negative patients. All patients in the anti-MDA5 (+) group had CADM; conversely, all patients in the anti-MDA5 (-) group had PM/DM (**Figure 1**).

We compared the baseline clinical data between the anti-MDA5 (+) and anti-MDA5 (-) groups (**Table 1**). ILD and skin ulcers were observed significantly more frequently in the anti-MDA5 (+) group than in the anti-MDA5 (-) group. White blood cell, lymphocyte, serum creatine phosphokinase, lactate dehydrogenase, aldolase, K, and Ca levels were significantly lower in the anti-MDA5 (+) group than in the anti-MDA5 (-) group ($p < 0.01$). Platelet, AST, ALT, Na, and Cl levels were also significantly lower in the anti-MDA5 (+) group than in the anti-MDA5 (-) group ($p < 0.05$). On or after admission, four patients in the anti-MDA5 (+) group and six patients in the anti-MDA5 (-) group showed obvious cardiac abnormality (e.g., diastolic dysfunction, heart failure, myocarditis).

ECG and UCG Characteristics of Patients With Anti-MDA5 (+) CADM

Next, we analyzed the ECG findings for each group. While the electrolyte levels in all patients were within the normal range on admission, patients with anti-MDA5 (+) CADM tended to show low T waves during the active phase of the disease, but T wave restoration during the remission phase (**Supplementary Figure 1**). At the active phase, the most frequent comment regarding the ECG analysis in the anti-MDA5 (+) group was "non-specific T-wave abnormalities" (57%, 12/21); this is the" low T-wave in multiple leads". The next most frequent comments were "normal range" (19%, 4/21) and "ST-T changes", such as ST depression (19%, 4/21). In the anti-MDA5(-) group, comments included "normal range" (33%, 14/42), "non-specific T-wave abnormalities" (24%, 10/42), and "ST-T changes" (14%, 6/42). We further analyzed the various ECG parameters (including the R and T wave amplitudes, as well as other categories) and compared them between the groups (**Table 2**). There were no significant differences in the heart rate, QT interval, and R wave amplitudes between the anti-MDA5 (+) and anti-MDA5 (-) groups; however, the T wave amplitudes from multiple leads were significantly lower for the anti-MDA5 (+) group than for the anti-MDA5 (-) group (I, II, and V4–6, $p < 0.01$; aVF and V3, $p < 0.05$). The T wave amplitude from the aVR lead, which reflects the reverse direction of the myocardial electrical flow from the other leads, was higher for the anti-MDA5 (+) group than for the anti-MDA5 (-) group ($p < 0.01$). Among the MSA-positive patients (MDA5, ARS, TIF1-γ, SRP), the anti-MDA5 (+) group tended to show a lower T wave amplitude than the patients with ARS, TIF1-γ, and SRP antibody (data not shown).

According to the Minnesota code classification system, a low T wave is defined as a T wave amplitude/R wave amplitude (T/R ratio) <0.1 (11, 12). The T/R ratios for the anti-MDA5 (+) group were lower for some of the leads (V6 $p < 0.01$; II, aVF and V5 $p < 0.05$). The four anti-MDA 5 (+) patients with obvious cardiac abnormality had six or more leads with low T-wave.

Because ILD was found to have been present as a complication in the anti-MDA5 (+) CADM group at a significantly higher frequency (100%) than in the anti-MDA5 (-) group (45.2%), we conducted an additional analysis to examine whether the incidence of ILD affected the ECG findings. First, we compared ECG parameters between the anti-MDA5 (-) patients with and without ILD (n = 22 and 20, respectively). The non ILD group had significantly higher T waves in the III lead, and conversely, significantly lower T waves in the aVL lead. We could not conclude that the presence of ILD was related to the number of lead with low T wave

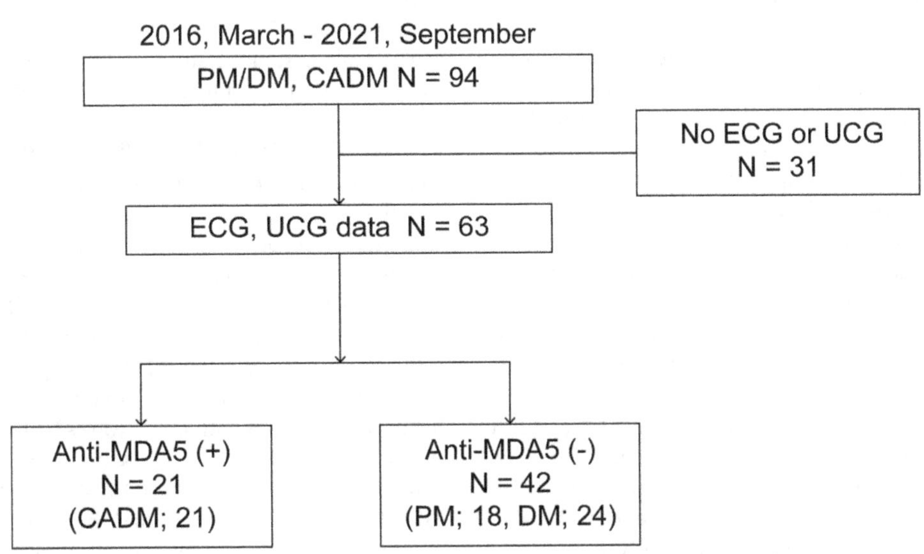

FIGURE 1 | Study flowchart.

TABLE 1 | Patient characteristics.

	MDA5 (+) (N = 21)	MDA5 (-) (N = 42)	p value
Age (years)	55.6 ± 9.6	58.9 ± 16.6	0.4
Female (%)	66.7	73.1	0.59
Disease duration (Months)	6.2 ± 12.4	4.8 ± 3.0	0.49
ILD (%)	100	45.2	<0.01
Heart disease (%)	14.3	12.5	0.8
Malignancy (%)	4.7	16.7	0.18
Skin ulcer (%)	33.3	2.4	<0.01
WBC (/μL)	5959.0 ± 2557.9	8553.1 ± 3625.9	<0.01
Lymphocytes (/μL)	730.0 ± 227.4	1368.6 ± 558.2	<0.01
Neutrophils (/μL)	4677.6 ± 2450.0	6193.1 ± 3394.5	0.08
Platelets (10^4/μL)	23.2 ± 5.8	28.0 ± 8.4	0.03
KL-6 (U/mL)	775.0 ± 292.9	683.5 ± 860.0	0.65
ESR (mm/1 h)	69.7 ± 101.6	40.4 ± 35.9	0.13
CPK (IU/L)	227.7 ± 258.7	3043.3 ± 3724.3	<0.01
LDH (IU/L)	355.8 ± 105.5	617.0 ± 326.1	<0.01
AST (IU/L)	69.7 ± 65.4	123.2 ± 107.3	0.04
ALT (IU/L)	44.1 ± 30.7	83.0 ± 71.9	0.02
CRP (mg/dL)	0.7 ± 0.9	1.2 ± 1.9	0.33
Ferritin (ng/mL)	630.9 ± 664.3	352.7 ± 555.6	0.13
Aldolase (U/L)	7.2 ± 2.1	34.1 ± 29.4	<0.01
Na (mEq/L)	137.2 ± 3.9	139.2 ± 2.3	0.01
K (mEq/L)	3.8 ± 0.3	4.2 ± 0.3	<0.01
Cl (mEq/L)	101.4 ± 4.2	103.5 ± 2.2	0.01
Ca (mg/dl)	8.9 ± 0.3	9.2 ± 0.4	<0.01
TP (g/dL)	6.7 ± 0.4	6.9 ± 0.9	0.38
ALB (g/dL)	3.3 ± 0.5	3.4 ± 0.7	0.46

Statistical significance: $p < 0.05$.
Continuous variables were compared using the unpaired t-test, and are expressed as the mean ± standard deviation. Categorical variables were compared using the chi-square test, and are expressed as percentages (%), unless otherwise noted. Ca refers to corrected total serum calcium (protein-bound calcium, complexed calcium, and ionized calcium). The correction formula is as follows; Corrected Ca value (mg/dl) = serum total Ca value + 4- serum albumin value.
ILD, interstitial lung disease; WBC, white blood cell count; KL-6, Krebs von den Lungen-6; ESR, erythrocyte sedimentation rate; CPK, creatine phosphokinase; LDH, lactate dehydrogenase; AST, aspartate aminotransferase; ALT, alanine aminotransferase; CRP, C-reactive protein; TP, total protein; ALB, albumin.

(**Supplementary Table 1**). Moreover, there were no significant differences in the ECG characteristics between the MDA5 (-) non-ILD group and the acute or subacute ILD (A/S-ILD) groups (n = 22 and 13, respectively; **Supplementary Table 2**). Subsequently, ECG parameters were compared between patients in the anti-MDA5 (+) group (n = 21) and those in the anti-MDA5 (-) group with ILD. The anti-MDA5 (+) group showed a significantly lower T wave than the anti-MDA5 (-) group with ILD (**Supplementary Table 3**). Furthermore, when the anti-MDA5 (-) A/S-ILD group was set as the control group and compared with the anti-MDA5 (+) A/S-ILD group (n=18), the anti-MDA5 (+) A/S-ILD group still showed a significantly lower T wave (**Supplementary Table 4**).

Collectively, the low T wave amplitude recorded on admission was a characteristic feature of the anti-MDA5 (+) group, independent of the presence of ILD.

Next, we analyzed the UCG data (**Table 3**). There appeared to be no difference in the contractile function (left ventricular end-diastolic diameter, left ventricular end-systolic diameter, and left ventricular ejection fraction) between the anti-MDA5 (+) and anti-MDA5 (-) groups. With respect to cardiac diastolic function, the E wave and A wave of the transmitral flow velocity pattern, and movement speed of the mitral valve annulus at the septum (Sep e') were significantly lower ($p <$ 0.05) for the anti-MDA5 (+) group than for the anti-MDA5 (-) group. However, the E/e' ratio was not significantly different between the groups, and no significant differences in the diastolic interventricular septum or left ventricular posterior wall thicknesses were observed; in almost all cases of the anti-MDA5 (+) group, there was normal cardiac function on echo. These results suggest that subclinical damage of the left ventricle exists in patients with anti-MDA5 (+) CADM (13). In this study, two patients (10%) had diastolic dysfunction or diastolic failure in the anti-MDA5 (+) group and three (7%) in the anti-MDA5 (-) group.

Recovery of Low T Waves in Anti-MDA5 (+) CADM After Treatment

For the anti-MDA5 (+) group, we investigated whether ECG changes would be reversible after immunosuppressive therapy. During the active phase of the disease, the number of leads in the 12-lead ECG (not including the aVR lead) that showed a low T wave was higher for the anti-MDA5 (+) group than for the anti-MDA5 (-) group ($p < 0.01$; **Table 4**) upon admission. However, during the remission phase, there was no significant difference in the number of leads with low T waves between the two groups. In summary, the low T wave can be reversible, and this is associated with disease activity in the anti-MDA5 (+) group. Four anti-MDA5 (+) patients who had heart dysfunction improved clinically and still had low T waves even though the number of leads with low T wave decreased. At the remission phase, due to

TABLE 2 | ECG parameters in the active phase.

ECG	HR (bpm)	QT Int (ms)				
MDA5 (+), n = 21	79.5 ± 13.1	369.9 ± 30.4				
MDA5 (-), n = 42	78.9 ± 14.7	374.1 ± 28.0				
p-value	0.43	0.97				
R wave (μV)	**I**	**II**	**III**	**aVR**	**aVL**	**aVF**
MDA5 (+), n = 21	554.8 ± 266.0	757.1 ± 293.1	339.8 ± 313.1	61.4 ± 62.5	284.5 ± 241.7	522.1 ± 299.5
MDA5 (-), n = 42	464.9 ± 234.5	740.- ± 451.8	485.7 ± 444.1	82.6 ± 99.3	274.9 ± 269.9	594.2 ± 444.1
p-value	0.24	0.32	0.09	0.8	0.29	0.17
T wave (μV)						
MDA5 (+), n = 21	85.0 ± 43.0	113.1 ± 84.8	34.3 ± 72.4	-97.4 ± 57.6	27.9 ± 40.8	65.5 ± 78.9
MDA5 (-), n = 42	137.7 ± 63.1	185.8 ± 107.4	40.0 ± 111.8	-159.5 ± 71.0	47.6 ± 72.3	118.6 ± 102.5
p-value	<0.01	<0.01	0.6	<0.01	0.26	0.04
T/R ratio						
MDA5 (+), n = 21	0.21 ± 0.19	0.16 ± 0.16	0.09 ± 0.82	-1.98 ± 1.51	0.04 ± 0.65	0.12 ± 0.19
MDA5 (-), n = 42	0.45 ± 0.54	0.42 ± 0.46	0.32 ± 0.96	-2.70 ± 2.20	0.34 ± 0.92	0.33 ± 0.39
p-value	0.06	0.02	0.35	0.17	0.2	0.03
R wave (μV)	**V1**	**V2**	**V3**	**V4**	**V5**	**V6**
MDA5 (+), n = 21	168.6 ± 102.8	386.4 ± 212.8	596.2 ± 342.2	1206.0 ± 601.0	1627.9 ± 563.9	1286.2 ± 387.8
MDA5 (-), n = 42	221.5 ± 200.1	482.6 ± 375.9	725.0 ± 512.5	1222.7 ± 663.9	1342.4 ± 542.1	1093.7 ± 461.5
p-value	0.08	0.12	0.14	0.64	0.08	0.3
T wave (μV)						
MDA5 (+), n = 21	44.3 ± 116.4	286.7 ± 195.6	315.0 ± 206.7	238.6 ± 192.0	159.8 ± 145.7	114.3 ± 117.1
MDA5 (-), n = 42	27.9 ± 115.3	349.9 ± 222.1	452.1 ± 251.0	405.7 ± 226.6	316.4 ± 180.8	229.5 ± 137.9
p-value	0.6	0.28	0.04	<0.01	<0.01	<0.01
T/R ratio						
MDA5 (+), n = 21	0.30 ± 0.86	0.79 ± 0.64	0.69 ± 0.62	0.28 ± 0.34	0.12 ± 0.13	0.11 ± 0.11
MDA5 (-), n = 42	0.04 ± 1.49	0.96 ± 1.04	0.83 ± 0.69	0.42 ± 0.33	0.30 ± 0.34	0.23 ± 0.15
p-value	0.47	0.25	0.46	0.14	0.02	<0.01

Statistical significance: $p < 0.05$.
The amplitudes of the R and T waves on ECG were calculated for all the leads.
HR, heart rate; QT int, QT interval.

TABLE 3 | UCG parameters in the active phase.

UCG	MDA5 (+) n = 21	MDA5 (-) n = 42	p value
LVEF (%)	67.7 ± 9.5	69.7 ± 6.0	0.31
LVDd (mm)	41.5 ± 4.6	42.4 ± 4.8	0.44
LVDs (mm)	25.9 ± 4.7	25.9 ± 4.1	0.99
IVSTd (mm)	9.3 ± 1.6	9.7 ± 2.7	0.52
PWTd (mm)	9.4 ± 1.7	9.5 ± 1.8	0.94
LADs (mm)	33.8 ± 5.6	32.7 ± 4.2	0.87
E wave (m/sec)	0.58 ± 0.14	0.74 ± 0.23	<0.01
A wave (m/sec)	0.61 ± 0.19	0.74 ± 0.18	0.01
E/A	1.1 ± 0.61	1.1 ± 0.51	0.94
DcT (msec)	218.3 ± 49.4	238.5 ± 73.5	0.27
Sep E/e'	9.5 ± 4.3	9.5 ± 3.7	0.8
Sep e' (cm/sec)	6.7 ± 2.0	8.9 ± 3.9	0.02
Sep a' (cm/sec)	10.3 ± 3.4	10.1 ± 2.1	0.75

Statistical significance: $p < 0.05$.
LVEF, left ventricular ejection fraction; LVDd, left ventricular diameter at end-diastole; LVDs, left ventricular internal dimension in systole; IVSTd, interventricular septal thickness at end-diastole; PWTd, posterior LV wall thickness at end-diastole; LADs, left atrial dimension in systole; E wave, early diastolic filling velocity; A wave, atrial filling velocity; E/A, E wave/A wave ratio; DcT, deceleration time; Sep E/e' ratio, E wave/e' ratio at the septum of the left ventricle; Sep e', peak early diastolic mitral annular velocity at the septum of the left ventricle; Sep a', peak atrial systolic mitral annular velocity at the septum of the left ventricle.

small sample size, there was no significant difference between the groups, but the E wave, A wave, and Sep e' in the anti-MDA5 (+) group were still lower (**Supplementary Table 5**).

Relationship Between the Number of Low T Waves, Clinical Data, and Echocardiography

Next, we performed a sub-analysis to see if the number of T waves was related to clinical and echocardiographic data within the anti-MDA5 (+) group. Regarding ECG findings, we divided patients into three groups, according to the number of leads with low T wave: Group A, 0–2 leads (N = 7); Group B, 3–5 leads (N = 6); and Group C, 6 or more leads (N = 8). Group C showed lower T wave amplitudes at multiple leads (**Supplementary Figure 2**). The results showed no significant difference in the frequency of skin ulcers. Epidemiology at admission showed that the percentage of female patients was 100% (N = 7) in Group A, 83% (N = 5) in Group B, and 25% (N = 2) in Group C. All the four patients who had obvious cardiac abnormality were in Group C and were male. Blood counts showed that the number of WBC and neutrophils, but not lymphocytes and platelets, tended to decrease in Group B

TABLE 4 | Number of leads with a low T wave in the active and remission phases.

		Number of Leads		*p*-value
		0–1	>1	
Active phase	**MDA5 (+)**	2	12	<0.01
	MDA5 (-)	14	7	
Remission phase	**MDA5 (+)**	7	7	n.s.
	MDA5 (-)	9	12	

Statistical significance: $p < 0.05$; n.s., not significant.
"Low T wave" is defined according to the major ECG criteria (Minnesota code) as a T/R ratio <0.1. The T/R ratio at the aVR lead was excluded from the analysis. We counted the number of leads with Low T wave at 11 leads except for aVR (V1-6, I, II, III, aVL, aVF leads) for each patient. '>1' means that there are more than two leads with a low T wave; '0-1' means that there is less than one. The p-value reflects the results of the analysis between the anti-MDA5 (+) and anti-MDA5 (-) groups.

and C (**Supplementary Figure 3**). Blood biochemical tests at admission showed that Group B and C tended to have higher CPK and CRP levels; there seemed to be no difference between the three groups in ferritin and KL-6 levels (**Supplementary Figure 4**). Regarding clinical data and UCG, due to the small sample size, there was no significant difference between the patients that, based on ECG findings, did not completely recover and those that fully recovered (data not shown); the group that did not recover included five men from Group C, including the four patients who had obvious cardiac abnormality.

Collectively, patients with low T wave at multiple leads may develop heart dysfunction or heart failure in anti-MDA5 (+) CADM. The number of leads with low T wave may be associated with some clinical data (e.g., number of WBCs, neutrophils, or levels of CPK and CRP). Even if anti-MDA5 (+) patients achieve remission, some may still have abnormalities on ECG and UCG parameters and cardiac damage.

DISCUSSION

To the best of our knowledge, this is the first report on cardiac involvement in an anti-MDA5 (+) CADM cohort. In this study, we found characteristic subclinical ECG and UCG abnormalities in patients with anti-MDA5 antibodies (a reversible low T wave on ECG and a low E wave, A wave and Sep e' on UCG), suggesting the extent of cardiac damage. Although there were lower levels of electrolytes in the anti-MDA5 (+) group, there were no severe electrolyte abnormalities that could account for the abnormal ECG findings. With respect to the pathophysiology of anti-MDA5 (+) DM/CADM, elevated levels of several cytokines and chemokines, including interleukin (IL)-6, IL-8, IL-10, IP-10, sCD163, YKL-40, and IFN-α, have been reported (14–17). Several inflammatory cytokines, such as TNFα, the IL-1 family, IL-6, IL-8, IL-10, IL-18, and IFNα have also been shown to play a pathological role in various heart diseases (18). IL-8 stimulates the expression of $Na\text{-}K^+$ or Ca^+ channels and affects the flow of Ca^+ or K^+ (19). IL-10, an anti-inflammatory cytokine, correlates with heart inflammation or dysfunction in cardiomyopathy, acute myocarditis, and Takotsubo cardiomyopathy (20–22). Daily IL-18 administration has been reported to induce myocardial dysfunction in BALB/c mice (23), and interferon therapy can lead to reversible cardiomyopathy (24, 25). Thus, a prominent elevated levels of several inflammatory cytokines can cause myocardial impairment in patients with anti-MDA5 (+) DM/CADM.

One hypothesis is that myocardial damage is due to pathological autoantibodies. There have been previous reports of pathological autoantibodies as components of heart damage in mouse models (e.g., anti-myosin antibody, anti-cardiac troponin I antibody) (26). However, it is unclear why anti-MDA5 (+) CADM would have such an abnormal ECG and echocardiography finding. Since the T-wave finding is abnormal, one possibility is that pathological autoantibodies are being produced that causes a defect in ion channels involved in repolarization.

We also speculate that viral infection may be a trigger, with viral-induced myocarditis leading to the development of anti-MDA5 (+) CADM. It has long been suspected that viruses may be involved in the development of PM/DM (e.g., Parvo virus, Coxsackie virus) (27–29). The type1 IFN pathway, which has antiviral effects, is activated in PM/DM (30). There are some reports that seasonality and regionality are related to the development of anti-MDA5 (+) CADM (31, 32). As the phenotype of CADM is different in Asia, Europe, and the United States, the causative virus may be different in each region (33). Thus, environmental factors such as viruses may contribute to the development of the disease. Consistent with this idea, an IFN signature is activated in anti-MDA5 (+) CADM (34).

MDA5 is a viral sensor in the cell, which plays an important role in detecting picornaviruses (e.g., Coxsackie virus) that cause myocarditis and encephalitis (35, 36). During the preparation of this report, COVID-19 became widespread. Recently, there have been increasing reports of an association between COVID-19 infection and autoimmune diseases. COVID-19 infection has been reported to cause the production of autoantibodies and promote the development of autoimmune diseases (37, 38). In COVID-19 infection, MDA5 also acts as a sensor (39), and there has been a report of anti-MDA5 antibody positivity after infection (38). Furthermore, it has been reported that the clinical symptoms, CT images and blood test findings (e.g., hypokalemia, and high levels of ferritin, CPK and CRP) of COVID-19 pneumonia are similar to those of anti-MDA5 (+) CADM (40, 41). COVID-19 infection also results in a high frequency of abnormalities on cardiac MRI and echocardiography, even when the patient is asymptomatic (42, 43). In summary, COVID-19-induced pneumonia and associated autoimmunity provides potential insight into the pathogenesis of anti-MDA5 antibody positive CADM. Since anti-MDA5 (+) CADM was recognized before the spread of COVID-19, we assume that some viruses (recognized by MDA5), which are common in Asia, may be risk factors for the development of anti-MDA5 (+) CADM, including myocardial damage.

We observed that the low T waves recorded in the anti-MDA5 (+) group during the active disease phase were reversible after treatment (**Supplementary Figure 1** and **Table 4**). However, some patients with multiple low T waves developed obvious heart dysfunction and the abnormal T wave did not fully resolve. This suggests that aberrant immune responses associated with anti-MDA5 (+) DM/CADM disease activity affect changes in electrical activity of the heart, leaving some patients with cardiac damage even in remission. We performed a sub-analysis to determine if there was any association between the number of low T waves and clinical data. Although our sample size was small, WBC, neutrophil, CPK and CRP seemed to be associated with the number of leads with low T wave; this may reflect structural damage to the heart. Interestingly, patients with heart dysfunction (e.g., heart failure, myocarditis, and diastolic dysfunction) who had more leads with low T waves were also more likely to be male. The one reported case of anti-MDA5 (+) cardiomyopathy was a 55-year-old man (7). In a model of coxsackie virus myocarditis, males have been reported to be more severely affected (44). In anti-MDA5 (+) DM, muscle, skin, and joint symptoms have been reported to be related to sex (33). One phenotype with high CPK levels and muscle symptoms seemed to be common in male patients (45). Our data suggest that men with anti-MDA5 (+) CADM may be more prone to severe myocardial damage and present low T wave in multiple leads. However, in the patients enrolled, smoking history, hypertension, hyperlipidemia, and diabetes, which are risk factors for heart disease, seemed to be more prevalent in men (data not shown). We would like to collect more cases in the future to clarify the relationship between ECG findings, cardiac function, and clinical data. Investigating the mechanism underlying this electrical abnormality may lead to an understanding of the pathophysiology of anti-MDA5 (+) DM/CADM, which often shows amyopathic or hypomyopathic phenotypes.

In our study, cardiac function was nearly normal for patients with anti-MDA5 antibodies. Some of the UCG parameters (namely, the E wave, A wave and Sep e') showed significant differences between the groups. In the remission phase, the values of E wave, A wave, and Sep e were not significantly different, likely due to the small sample size; however, as in the active phase, they remained lower in the anti-MDA5 (+) group than in the anti-MDA5 (-) group, suggesting that some cardiac damage may remain even after remission. The E wave represents the early diastolic filling velocity, which is one of the transmitral flow velocity patterns. When the left ventricular diastolic function decreases, left ventricular relaxation is delayed, and the E wave also decreases. Sep e' is the peak early diastolic mitral annular velocity at the septum (46). A low Sep e' is an indicator of diastolic disturbance. Previous studies have reported that PM/DM patients are sometimes complicated with left ventricular diastolic dysfunction (LVDD) (12–42%) (6, 47–50). During diastolic dysfunction, the A wave generally tends to be high; therefore, we could not conclude why the A wave was lower in the anti-MDA5 (+) group. The low T-wave and echocardiographic findings suggest that there is an unknown cardiac pathology at this time that does not fit the definition of diastolic dysfunction. In the future, we will try to clarify the cause. Although our findings did not meet the UCG diagnostic criteria for diastolic disturbance (13), our data suggest the possible presence of cardiac involvement in patients with anti-MDA5 antibodies. In our facility, two CADM patients with anti-MDA5 antibodies (10%) and three PM/DM patients (7%) and were diagnosed with LVDD. Although two of the CADM patients with anti-MDA5 antibodies died of respiratory failure, we speculate they may have ultimately had severe heart damage, such as diastolic failure.

We assumed that the ECG results for the anti-MDA5 (+) group were affected by the 100% ILD complication rate in this group; therefore, we conducted a sub-analysis to confirm our hypothesis. Even though ILD was present more frequently in the anti-MDA5 (+) group (**Table 1**), the ECG findings did not show an association with this observation (**Supplementary Tables 1–4**). Few studies have reported abnormal ECG findings in association with PM/DM with LVDD (51). In that sense, the ECG findings for the anti-MDA5-antibody positive patients are unique. ECG records cardiac muscle activity, and the T wave represents the period during which the ventricles transition from systole to diastole. A low T wave may be indicative of an electrical activity alteration and structural change. Further serial functional imaging tests may be useful for identifying the extent of cardiac involvement and understanding the clinical implications of these ECG changes. In the present study, most of the anti-MDA5-antibody positive cases had A/S-ILD, and there were three cases of no A/S-ILD (organizing pneumonia, ILD with chronic course), one of which had multiple leads with low T wave. In our department, we previously certified another six cases of anti-MDA5 (+) non-A/S-ILD, in which a few cases showed the same ECG findings. More cases need to be collected to determine if the ECG findings are also detectable in anti-MDA5 (+) CADM with non-A/S-ILD.

Our study has several limitations. First, this was a retrospective study; therefore, we lacked some clinical data for the included patients. A prospective study is needed to confirm our findings. Second, the clinical implications of a low T wave on ECG, and a low E wave, A wave and Sep e' on UCG, require further assessment. However, our results may provide new insight into whether anti-MDA5 (+) DM/CADM is a multiorgan autoimmune disease. Therefore, further basic investigations are required.

In conclusion, patients with anti-MDA5 antibodies often have specific ECG and UCG findings that indicate subclinical heart involvement. As patients with anti-MDA5 antibodies have a poor prognosis if treatment is delayed, ECG may aid in early detection. Therefore, cardiac function screening and follow-ups for this cohort will be important, even if patients show only slight myocarditis or heart failure.

ETHICS STATEMENT

The studies involving human participants were reviewed and approved by the ethics committee of Kyoto University Graduate School and Faculty of Medicine (approval number: E458). The patients/participants provided their written informed consent to participate in this study.

AUTHOR CONTRIBUTIONS

TaM, YK, and RN designed the study. TaM and TS collected the data. TaM, YK, and EK reviewed the ECG and UCG data. TaM and YK analyzed the data. TaM, YK, EK, and RN interpreted the data. TaM and RN wrote the manuscript. All the authors reviewed and approved the manuscript.

(18K16145 for RN). The funding body had no role in the study design, the collection, analysis, and interpretation of the data, or in the writing of the manuscript.

ACKNOWLEDGMENTS

The authors thank Sachi Ibuki of Kyoto University for preparing the patient samples, as well as Editage (www.editage.com) for English language editing.

REFERENCES

1. Bohan A, Peter JB. Polymyositis and Dermatomyositis. *N Engl J Med* (1975) 292:344–7. doi: 10.1056/NEJM197502132920706
2. Bohan A, Peter JB. Polymyositis and Dermatomyositis. *N Engl J Med* (1975) 292:403–7. doi: 10.1056/NEJM197502202920807
3. Sato S, Hirakata M, Kuwana M, Suwa A, Inada S, Mimori T, et al. Autoantibodies to a 140-Kd Polypeptide, CADM-140, in Japanese Patients With Clinically Amyopathic Dermatomyositis. *Arthritis Rheum* (2005) 52:1571–6. doi: 10.1002/art.21023
4. Nakashima R, Imura Y, Kobayashi S, Yukawa N, Yoshifuji H, Nojima T, et al. The RIG-I-Like Receptor IFIH1/MDA5 Is a Dermatomyositis-Specific Autoantigen Identified by the Anti-CADM-140 Antibody. *Rheumatol (Oxford)* (2010) 49:433–40. doi: 10.1093/rheumatology/kep375
5. Danieli MG, Gelardi C, Guerra F, Cardinaletti P, Pedini V, Gabrielli A. Cardiac Involvement in Polymyositis and Dermatomyositis. *Autoimmun Rev* (2016) 15:462–5. doi: 10.1016/j.autrev.2016.01.015
6. Zhang L, Wang G, Ma L, Zu N. Cardiac Involvement in Adult Polymyositis or Dermatomyositis: A Systematic Review. *Clin Cardiol* (2012) 35:686–91. doi: 10.1002/clc.22026
7. Pau-Charles I, Moreno PJ, Ortiz-Ibáñez K, Lucero MC, Garcia-Herrera A, Espinosa G, et al. Anti-MDA5 Positive Clinically Amyopathic Dermatomyositis Presenting With Severe Cardiomyopathy. *J Eur Acad Dermatol Venereol* (2014) 28:1097–102. doi: 10.1111/jdv.12300
8. Sontheimer RD. Would a New Name Hasten the Acceptance of Amyopathic Dermatomyositis (Dermatomyositis Siné Myositis) as a Distinctive Subset Within the Idiopathic Inflammatory Dermatomyopathies Spectrum of Clinical Illness? *J Am Acad Dermatol* (2002) 46:626–36. doi: 10.1067/mjd.2002.120621
9. Nakashima R, Imura Y, Hosono Y, Seto M, Murakami A, Watanabe K, et al. The Multicenter Study of a New Assay for Simultaneous Detection of Multiple Anti-Aminoacyl-tRNA Synthetases in Myositis and Interstitial Pneumonia. *PloS One* (2014) 9:e85062. doi: 10.1371/journal.pone.0085062
10. Fujimoto M, Murakami A, Kurei S, Okiyama N, Kawakami A, Mishima M, et al. Enzyme-Linked Immunosorbent Assays for Detection of Anti-Transcriptional Intermediary Factor-1 Gamma and Anti-Mi-2 Autoantibodies in Dermatomyositis. *J Dermatol Sci* (2016) 84:272–81. doi: 10.1016/j.jdermsci.2016.09.013
11. Blackburn H, Keys A, Simonson E, Rautaharju P PS. The Electrocardiogram in Population Studies. A Classification System. *Circulation* (1960) 21:1160–75. doi: 10.1161/01.CIR.21.6.1160
12. Rautaharju PM, Surawicz B, Gettes LS, Bailey JJ, Childers R, Deal BJ, et al. AHA/ACCF/HRS Recommendations for the Standardization and Interpretation of the Electrocardiogram: Part IV: The ST Segment, T and U Waves, and the QT Interval: A Scientific Statement From the American Heart Association Electrocardiography and Arrhythmias Committee, Council on Clinical Cardiology; the American College of Cardiology Foundation; and the Heart Rhythm Society: Endorsed by the International Society for Computerized Electrocardiology. *Circulation* (2009) 119:e241–50. doi: 10.1161/CIRCULATIONAHA.108.191096
13. Nagueh SF, Smiseth OA, Appleton CP, Byrd BF, Dokainish H, Edvardsen T, et al. Recommendations for the Evaluation of Left Ventricular Diastolic Function by Echocardiography: An Update From the American Society of Echocardiography and the European Association of Cardiovascular Imaging. *J Am Soc Echocardiogr* (2016) 29:277–314. doi: 10.1016/j.echo.2016.01.011
14. Gono T, Kaneko H, Kawaguchi Y, Hanaoka M, Kataoka S, Kuwana M, et al. Cytokine Profiles in Polymyositis and Dermatomyositis Complicated by Rapidly Progressive or Chronic Interstitial Lung Disease. *Rheumatol (Oxf)* (2014) 53:2196–203. doi: 10.1093/rheumatology/keu258
15. Horai Y, Koga T, Fujikawa K, Takatani A, Nishino A, Nakashima Y, et al. Serum Interferon-α Is a Useful Biomarker in Patients With Anti-Melanoma Differentiation-Associated Gene 5 (MDA5) Antibody-Positive Dermatomyositis. *Mod Rheumatol* (2015) 25:85–9. doi: 10.3109/14397595.2014.900843
16. Jiang L, Wang Y, Peng Q, Shu X, Wang G, Wu X. Serum YKL-40 Level Is Associated With Severity of Interstitial Lung Disease and Poor Prognosis in Dermatomyositis With Anti-MDA5 Antibody. *Clin Rheumatol* (2019) 38:1655–63. doi: 10.1007/s10067-019-04457-w
17. Shirakashi M, Nakashima R, Tsuji H, Tanizawa K, Handa T, Hosono Y, et al. Efficacy of Plasma Exchange in Anti-MDA5-Positive Dermatomyositis With Interstitial Lung Disease Under Combined Immunosuppressive Treatment. *Rheumatology* (2020) 59:3284–92. doi: 10.1093/rheumatology/keaa123
18. Bartekova M, Radosinska J, Jelemensky M, Dhalla NS. Role of Cytokines and Inflammation in Heart Function During Health and Disease. *Heart Fail Rev* (2018) 23:733–58. doi: 10.1007/s10741-018-9716-x
19. Govindaraju V, Michoud MC, Al-Chalabi M, Ferraro P, Powell WS, Martin JG. Interleukin-8: Novel Roles in Human Airway Smooth Muscle Cell Contraction and Migration. *Am J Physiol Cell Physiol* (2006) 291:C957–65. doi: 10.1152/ajpcell.00451.2005
20. Guo Y, Cen Z, Wei B, Wu W, Zhou Q. Increased Circulating Interleukin 10-Secreting B Cells in Patients With Dilated Cardiomyopathy. *Int J Clin Exp Pathol* (2015) 8:8107–14.
21. Izumi T, Nishii M. Diagnostic and Prognostic Biomarkers in Acute Myocarditis. Interleukin-10. *Herz* (2012) 37:627–31. doi: 10.1007/s00059-012-3661-6
22. Santoro F, Tarantino N, Ferraretti A, Ieva R, Musaico F, Guastafierro F, et al. Serum Interleukin 6 and 10 Levels in Takotsubo Cardiomyopathy: Increased

Admission Levels may Predict Adverse Events at Follow-Up. *Atherosclerosis* (2016) 254:28–34. doi: 10.1016/j.atherosclerosis.2016.09.012

23. Woldbaek PR, Sande JB, Strømme TA, Lunde PK, Djurovic S, Lyberg T, et al. Daily Administration of Interleukin-18 Causes Myocardial Dysfunction in Healthy Mice. *Am J Physiol Heart Circ Physiol* (2005) 289:H708–14. doi: 10.1152/ajpheart.01179.2004
24. Condat B, Asselah T, Zanditenas D, Estampes B, Cohen A, O'Toole D, et al. Fatal Cardiomyopathy Associated With Pegylated Interferon/Ribavirin in a Patient With Chronic Hepatitis C. *Eur J Gastroenterol Hepatol* (2006) 18:287–9. doi: 10.1097/00042737-200603000-00010
25. Martin CS, Ionescu LN, Barbu CG, Sirbu AE, Lambrescu IM, Lacau IS, et al. Takotsubo Cardiomyopathy and Transient Thyrotoxicosis During Combination Therapy With Interferon-Alpha and Ribavirin for Chronic Hepatitis C. *BMC Endocr Disord* (2014) 14:10. doi: 10.1186/1472-6823-14-10
26. Caforio ALP, Tona F, Bottaro S, Vinci A, Dequal G, Daliento L, et al. Clinical Implications of Anti-Heart Autoantibodies in Myocarditis and Dilated Cardiomyopathy. *Autoimmunity* (2008) 41:35–45. doi: 10.1080/08916930701619235
27. Prieto S, Grau JM. The Geoepidemiology of Autoimmune Muscle Disease. *Autoimmun Rev* (2010) 9(5):A330-4. doi: 10.1016/J.AUTREV.2009.11.006
28. Svensson J, Holmqvist M, Lundberg IE, Arkema EV. Infections and Respiratory Tract Disease as Risk Factors for Idiopathic Inflammatory Myopathies: A Population-Based Case - Control Study. *Ann Rheum Dis* (2017) 76:1803–8. doi: 10.1136/ANNRHEUMDIS-2017-211174
29. Bax CE, Maddukuri S, Ravishankar A, Pappas-Taffer L, Werth VP. Environmental Triggers of Dermatomyositis: A Narrative Review. *Ann Transl Med* (2021) 9:434–4. doi: 10.21037/ATM-20-3719
30. Higgs BW, Liu Z, White B, Zhu W, White WI, Morehouse C, et al. Patients With Systemic Lupus Erythematosus, Myositis, Rheumatoid Arthritis and Scleroderma Share Activation of a Common Type I Interferon Pathway. *Ann Rheum Dis* (2011) 70:2029–36. doi: 10.1136/ARD.2011.150326
31. Muro Y, Sugiura K, Hoshino K, Akiyama M, Tamakoshi K. Epidemiologic Study of Clinically Amyopathic Dermatomyositis and Anti-Melanoma Differentiation-Associated Gene 5 Antibodies in Central Japan. *Arthritis Res Ther* (2011) 13(6):R214. doi: 10.1186/AR3547
32. Nishina N, Sato S, Masui K, Gono T, Kuwana M. Seasonal and Residential Clustering at Disease Onset of Anti-MDA5-Associated Interstitial Lung Disease. *RMD Open* (2020) 6(2):e001202. doi: 10.1136/RMDOPEN-2020-001202
33. Nombel A, Fabien N, Coutant F. Dermatomyositis With Anti-MDA5 Antibodies: Bioclinical Features, Pathogenesis and Emerging Therapies. *Front Immunol* (2021) 12:773352. doi: 10.3389/FIMMU.2021.773352
34. Pinal-Fernandez I, Casal-Dominguez M, Derfoul A, Pak K, Miller FW, Milisenda JC, et al. Machine Learning Algorithms Reveal Unique Gene Expression Profiles in Muscle Biopsies From Patients With Different Types of Myositis. *Ann Rheum Dis* (2020) 79:1234–42. doi: 10.1136/ANNRHEUMDIS-2019-216599
35. Kato H, Takeuchi O, Sato S, Yoneyama M, Yamamoto M, Matsui K, et al. Differential Roles of MDA5 and RIG-I Helicases in the Recognition of RNA Viruses. *Nature* (2006) 441:101–5. doi: 10.1038/NATURE04734
36. Yoneyama M, Fujita T. RNA Recognition and Signal Transduction by RIG-I-Like Receptors. *Immunol Rev* (2009) 227:54–65. doi: 10.1111/J.1600-065X.2008.00727.X
37. Liu Y, Sawalha AH, Lu Q. COVID-19 and Autoimmune Diseases. *Curr Opin Rheumatol* (2021) 33:155–62. doi: 10.1097/BOR.0000000000000776
38. De Santis M, Isailovic N, Motta F, Ricordi C, Ceribelli A, Lanza E, et al. Environmental Triggers for Connective Tissue Disease: The Case of COVID-19 Associated With Dermatomyositis-Specific Autoantibodies. *Curr Opin Rheumatol* (2021) 33:514–21. doi: 10.1097/BOR.0000000000000844
39. Yin X, Riva L, Pu Y, Martin-Sancho L, Kanamune J, Yamamoto Y, et al. MDA5 Governs the Innate Immune Response to SARS-CoV-2 in Lung Epithelial Cells. *Cell Rep* (2021) 34(2):108628. doi: 10.1016/J.CELREP.2020.108628
40. Moreno-P O, Leon-Ramirez JM, Fuertes-Kenneally L, Perdiguero M, Andres M, Garcia-Navarro M, et al. Hypokalemia as a Sensitive Biomarker of Disease Severity and the Requirement for Invasive Mechanical Ventilation Requirement in COVID-19 Pneumonia: A Case Series of 306 Mediterranean Patients. *Int J Infect Dis* (2020) 100:449–54. doi: 10.1016/J.IJID.2020.09.033
41. Kondo Y, Kaneko Y, Takei H, Tamai H, Kabata H, Suhara T, et al. COVID-19 Shares Clinical Features With Anti-Melanoma Differentiation-Associated Protein 5 Positive Dermatomyositis and Adult Still's Disease. *Clin Exp Rheumatol* (2021) 39:631–8.
42. Puntmann VO, Carerj ML, Wieters I, Fahim M, Arendt C, Hoffmann J, et al. Outcomes of Cardiovascular Magnetic Resonance Imaging in Patients Recently Recovered From Coronavirus Disease 2019 (COVID-19). *JAMA Cardiol* (2020) 5:1265–73. doi: 10.1001/JAMACARDIO.2020.3557
43. Dweck MR, Bularga A, Hahn RT, Bing R, Lee KK, Chapman AR, et al. Global Evaluation of Echocardiography in Patients With COVID-19. *Eur Hear J Cardiovasc Imaging* (2020) 21:949–58. doi: 10.1093/EHJCI/JEAA178
44. Barcena ML, Jeuthe S, Niehues MH, Pozdniakova S, Haritonow N, Kühl AA, et al. Sex-Specific Differences of the Inflammatory State in Experimental Autoimmune Myocarditis. *Front Immunol* (2021) 12:686384. doi: 10.3389/FIMMU.2021.686384
45. Allenbach Y, Uzunhan Y, Toquet S, Leroux G, Gallay L, Marquet A, et al. Different Phenotypes in Dermatomyositis Associated With Anti-MDA5 Antibody: Study of 121 Cases. *Neurology* (2020) 95:70–8. doi: 10.1212/WNL.0000000000009727
46. Paulus WJ, Tschöpe C, Sanderson JE, Rusconi C, Flachskampf FA, Rademakers FE, et al. How to Diagnose Diastolic Heart Failure: A Consensus Statement on the Diagnosis of Heart Failure With Normal Left Ventricular Ejection Fraction by the Heart Failure and Echocardiography Associations of the European Society of Cardiology. *Eur Heart J Eur Heart J* (2007) p:2539–50. doi: 10.1093/eurheartj/ehm037
47. Lu Z, Wei Q, Ning Z, Qian-Zi Z, Xiao-Ming S, Guo-Chun W. Left Ventricular Diastolic Dysfunction - Early Cardiac Impairment in Patients With Polymyositis/Dermatomyositis: A Tissue Doppler Imaging Study. *J Rheumatol* (2013) 40:1572–7. doi: 10.3899/jrheum.130044
48. Gupta R, Wayangankar SA, Targoff IN, Hennebry TA. Clinical Cardiac Involvement in Idiopathic Inflammatory Myopathies: A Systematic Review. *Int J Cardiol Elsevier Ireland Ltd* (2011) 148:261–70. doi: 10.1016/j.ijcard.2010.08.013
49. Wang H, Liu HX, Wang YL, Yu XQ, Chen XX, Cai L. Left Ventricular Diastolic Dysfunction in Patients With Dermatomyositis Without Clinically Evident Cardiovascular Disease. *J Rheumatol* (2014) 41:495–500. doi: 10.3899/jrheum.130346
50. Diederichsen LP, Simonsen JA, Diederichsen AC, Hvidsten S, Hougaard M, Junker P, et al. Cardiac Abnormalities in Adult Patients With Polymyositis or Dermatomyositis as Assessed by Noninvasive Modalities. *Arthritis Care Res* (2016) 68:1012–20. doi: 10.1002/acr.22772
51. Gonzalez-Lopez L, Gamez-Nava JI, Sanchez L, Rosas E, Suarez-Almazor M, Cardona-Muñoz C R-RC. Cardiac Manifestations in Dermato-Polymyositis. *Clin Exp Rheumatol* (1996) 14:373–9.

3

A Commercial Anti-TIF1γ ELISA is Superior to Line and Dot Blot and Should Be Considered as Part of Routine Myositis-Specific Antibody Testing

Ben Mulhearn[1,2*]*, Danyang Li*[1]*, Fionnuala McMorrow*[1]*, Hui Lu*[1]*, Neil J. McHugh*[1] *and Sarah L. Tansley*[1,2]

[1] *Department and Pharmacy and Pharmacology, University of Bath, Bath, United Kingdom,* [2] *Royal National Hospital for Rheumatic Diseases, Royal United Hospitals, Bath, United Kingdom*

Correspondence:
Ben Mulhearn
bm765@bath.ac.uk

Objectives: Anti-TIF1γ is an important autoantibody in the diagnosis of cancer-associated dermatomyositis and the most common autoantibody in juvenile onset dermatomyositis. Its reliable detection is important to instigate further investigations into underlying malignancy in adults. We previously showed that commercial assays using line and dot blots do not reliably detect anti-TIF1γ. We aimed to test a new commercial ELISA and compare with previously obtained protein immunoprecipitation.

Methods: Radio-labelled immunoprecipitation had previously been used to determine the autoantibody status of patients with immune-mediated inflammatory myopathies and several healthy controls. ELISA was undertaken on healthy control and anti-TIF1γ sera and compared to previous immunoprecipitation data.

Results: A total of 110 serum samples were analysed: 42 myositis patients with anti- TIF1γ and 68 autoantibody negative healthy control sera. Anti-TIF1γ was detected by ELISA in 41 out of 42 of the anti-TIF1γ-positive samples by immunoprecipitation, and in none of the healthy controls, giving a sensitivity of 97.6% and specificity of 100%. The false negative rate was 2%.

Conclusion: ELISA is an affordable and time-efficient method which is accurate in detecting anti-TIF1γ.

Keywords: TIF1γ, cancer, autoantibodies, myositis, ELISA - enzyme-linked immunosorbent assay, myositis - diagnosis, dermatomysitis

HIGHLIGHTS

1. Anti-TIF1γ is a key autoantibody in the diagnosis of cancer-associated dermatomyositis and juvenile dermatomyositis
2. ELISA is a quick and easy method in accurately detecting anti-TIF1γ autoantibodies
3. Diagnosis of IIMs should include ANA immunofluorescence, line or dot blot, and anti-TIF1γ ELISA

INTRODUCTION

The ability to detect myositis -specific and -associated antibodies (MSAs and MAAs), which can be found in the sera of 60 – 70% patients with immune-mediated inflammatory myopathies (IIMs) (1), has greatly improved the diagnosis and phenotyping of these rare diseases. Not only do they aid diagnosis, but they also guide further investigation and management (2). For instance, it is well-known that IIMs, and dermatomyositis (DM) in particular, are strongly linked with cancer, with estimates varying between 7 and 32% (3).

Anti-transcription intermediary factor 1γ (TIF1γ) autoantibodies are found in both juvenile dermatomyositis (JDM) and adult IIMs. They are present in 7% of European adults with DM and 20 – 30% of children affected by JDM (2). Strikingly, 38 – 84% of patients adult DM patients ≥ 39 years of age who are TIF1γ-positive in both European and Japanese cohorts develop cancer in the 3 years before and after DM diagnosis (4–6). Anti-TIF1γ detection in patients with a new diagnosis of DM ≥ 39 years of age may therefore prompt a thorough investigation for the detection of cancer and reduce cancer mortality rates, making the accurate detection of anti-TIF1γ a research priority.

Currently the reference standard in the detection of MSAAs is immunoprecipitation (IP) due to its ability to detect well-described and novel autoantibodies. However, this technique is impractical for use in clinical practice owing to its expense and the length of time it takes to reach a result which usually takes a minimum of 2 – 3 weeks. For this reason, several commercially available immunoassays have become available which are low cost, easy to use, and are reported to detect an array of MSAAs. However, these immunoassays are subject to both false positives and false negatives. A number of them have recently been tested by our group and others (7, 8). In particular, anti-TIF1γ was found to be particularly problematic with false negatives found in 40% samples analysed by line blot and 76% by dot blot (7). Espinosa-Ortega et al. (8) also found low concordance between anti-TIF1γ detected by line/dot blot and immunoprecipitation, with a Cohen's kappa of 0.56. This is likely because anti-TIF1γ frequently target a conformational epitope, meaning the tertiary antigen structure is required to remain intact to be recognised by the autoantibody (9). Whereas line and dot blot immunoassays utilise denatured antigen, enzyme-linked immunosorbent assays (ELISAs) maintain the tertiary structure of the protein. Fujimoto et al. (10) recently tested a newly-developed ELISA in a Japanese cohort of patients with a spectrum of IIMs, and found this approach to be highly effective with 100% sensitivity and specificity which was a result comparable to immunoprecipitation.

In this study, we aimed to test the same commercial ELISA kit (Medical & Biological Laboratories Co. Ltd., Nagoya, Aichi, Japan) for the detection of TIF1γ autoantibodies in a European cohort of adult IIM patients and compared results with samples previously analysed using immunoprecipitation.

METHODS

Sample Selection

Myositis serum samples used in this study were chosen as previously described (7) from a biobank of more than 3000 samples collected for research or diagnostic purposes (2, 11). All serum samples had previously been analysed by immunoprecipitation locally and contain at least one MSAA. Twenty-five anti-TIF1γ samples had also been previously analysed by line and dot blot (7). Briefly, sera were stored at -20°C prior to analysis in a facility at the University of Bath. The study had ethical approval through the host Institute (University of Bath EIRA reference number 17-01211). All samples from research cohorts had existing ethics in place.

ELISA

ELISA was performed on 5μL of diluted serum sample as per the manufacturer's instructions (Medical & Biological Laboratories Co. Ltd., Nagoya, Aichi, Japan). All samples were run in duplicate. Briefly, samples were thawed and diluted to a 1:101 concentration and incubated on a microwell plate for 30 minutes. Wells were then incubated with a horseradish peroxidase-conjugated goat anti-human IgG antibody conjugate for 30 minutes followed by a TMB/peroxide substrate for 15 minutes. The reaction was terminated by 0.25 mol/L sulfuric acid. All incubations took place at room temperature with 4 wash cycles between steps. The absorbance of each well was read on a FLUOstar Omega microplate reader (BMG Labtech Ltd., Aylesbury, Buckinghamshire, Great Britain) at 450 nm wavelength. Positive and negative cut off values were calculated according to previous work described by Fujimoto et al. (10) and expressed in arbitrary units (au).

Immunoprecipitation

Radio-immunoprecipitation had been previously undertaken as described by Tansley et al. (7). Briefly, sera were mixed with protein-A-Sepharose beads and a 35(S)methionine radiolabelled K562 cell extract, followed by fractionation by SDS-PAGE and analysis by autoradiography. A characteristic doublet band at 155/140 was read as being positive for TIF1γ (12).

Data Analysis

Statistical analysis was undertaken using Prism 9 version 9.2.0 for macOS (GraphPad Software, LLC., San Diego, CA, USA). Confidence intervals (CI) are expressed at 95%.

RESULTS

A total of 110 serum samples were analysed, of which 42 were known to have anti-TIF1γ and 68 were healthy control sera. Immunoprecipitation data was held for all samples. Diagnoses included DM (n=27), clinically amyopathic DM (n=4), JDM (n=5), polymyositis (n=4), and overlap syndrome (n=2). All HC samples tested were autoantibody negative by immunoprecipitation.

Commercial TIF1γ ELISA Performed as Well as Immunoprecipitation

Forty-one patient samples with anti-TIF1γ tested positive by ELISA as defined by a cut-off point of 32 au. None of the HC samples tested positive using this cut-off point. The remaining anti-TIF1γ positive sample was just under the cut-off for positivity (30.2 au). This gives an area under the ROC curve

(AUC) of 0.988 (CI 0.961 – 1.000, $P < 0.0001$) which is equivalent to sensitivity of 97.6% (CI 87.7% - 99.9%) and a specificity of 100% (CI 94.65% - 100%). In this case, Cohen's Kappa would give a value of 1.

Quantitative results for the ELISA values are shown in **Figure 1**. Briefly, the median ELISA assay result for HC samples was 5.99 au. (median CI 4.74 – 7.87) and for the TIF1γ samples was 128.5 au. (median CI 110.4 – 135.4).

Graph showing the relative ELISA titres for healthy control and TIF1γ samples expressed in arbitrary units for each individual serum sample (circles). Dashed line represents the positive cut-off point as previous described (10). All 68 healthy control (HC) samples were underneath the cut-off and all but one of the 42 TIF1γ samples were above the cut-off. The TIF1γ sample below the cut-off had a weak band in the 140/155 kDa region.

Low Anti-TIF1γ ELISA Titres Are Associated With False Negative Line Blot Results

Given that our group previously tested 25 anti-TIF1γ samples by line blot, we were able to compare ELISA titres in this study with this data to try and understand which samples might test negative by line blot. The results are shown in **Figure 2**. All anti-TIF1γ positive samples by ELISA with low titres (between 30 – 100 au.) tested negative by line blot. However, 3 out of the 9 samples testing negative by line blot had high anti- TIF1γ titres (> 100 au.). The difference in ELISA titres between those testing negative and positive by line blot was statistically significant ($P = 0.0041$, two-tailed Mann-Whitney test), suggesting that lower anti-TIF1γ antibody titres lead to false negative line blot results. Similarly, dot blot samples returned only 7/24 (29%) true

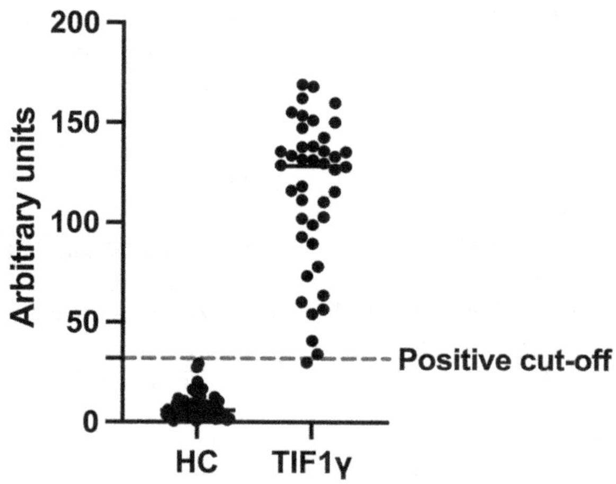

FIGURE 1 | TIF1γ ELISA values for 68 healthy controls and 42 TIF1γ serum samples.

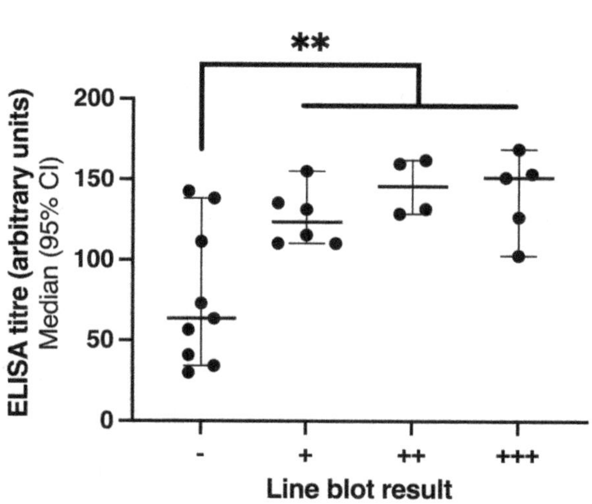

FIGURE 2 | Comparison of anti-TIF1γ ELISA titre and line blot result. **$P \leq 0.01$.

positives out of the anti-TIF1γ samples that tested positive by ELISA and immunoprecipitation.

Graph showing a comparison between anti-TIF1γ ELISA titre and line blot result, as previously tested by our group (7). ELISA titres are expressed in arbitrary units and calculated as per the manufacturer's instructions. Lines and error bars represent median values with 95% confidence intervals. The line blot results are expressed as negative (–), low positive (+), moderately positive (++), and high positive (+++). The median ELISA values for negative, low positive, moderately positive, and high positive results were 63.5 au., 123.5 au., 145.8 au., and 151.2 au., respectively. A two-tailed Mann Whitney test comparing ELISA titres between negative (–) and positive (+, ++, +++) line blots found a statistical difference between the two groups (P = 0.0041).

DISCUSSION

This data has shown that accurate detection of anti-TIF1γ can be achieved by ELISA and confirms the findings made by Fujimoto et al. (10). The accuracy of detection is high and would be acceptable for use in clinical practice. Compared to other cost- and time- effective methods such as line and dot blot which have false negative rate of 40% - 70% (7), this data found that ELISA has a false negative rate of 1/42 (2%). This data has also shown that anti-TIF1γ titre correlates with a positive line blot result. This result is not unexpected given that the line blot is a semi-quantitative method of detecting autoantibodies. Importantly, where ELISA was able to detect samples with low titres of anti-TIF1γ (between 30 – 100 au.), line blot was unable to do so. Line blot also failed to detect some samples with high anti-TIF1g titres (> 100 au.). Taken together, anti-TIF1γ ELISA performs better than line blot in detecting this clinically important autoantibody.

Anti-TIF1γ status by immunoprecipitation was determined by recognition of 155/140kDa bands alongside an anti-TIF1γ standard control. It remains possible that the sample negative by ELISA has an unknown autoantibody with an identical band pattern although this would seem unlikely. Furthermore, the sample produced an ELISA result just below the positive threshold and may simply be a low-titre positive. The ELISA threshold could be adjusted to reduce the likelihood of this occurring, but this is likely to lead to some false positives. The most appropriate cut-off threshold may depend on the clinical context, for example, a low false positive rate may be tolerable in patients with confirmed dermatomyositis to inform the intensity of malignancy screening.

The current study was not designed to investigate the relationship between anti-TIF1γ titres and cancer detection rates. It would, however, be useful to investigate how anti-TIF1γ titre using ELISA correlates with malignancy. Recent work by Fiorentino et al. (13) found anti-TIF1γ titre positively correlated with cancer detection rate in DM, ranging from 8% detection for low titres to 36% detection for high titres. Furthermore, some of our healthy control samples had low anti-TIF1γ titres just below the positive cut-off and it would be of interest to investigate if these healthy subjects had a higher malignancy rate compared to a negative anti-TIF1γ control population.

The detection of anti-TIF1γ in adult DM patients should be considered a red flag for malignancy (4–6). Accurate and timely detection of anti-TIF1γ autoantibodies is therefore vital for these patients to ensure underlying malignancy is diagnosed and treated promptly. We suggest that, when investigating IIMs, anti-TIF1γ ELISA is undertaken alongside, ANA testing and a multiplex immunoblot assay to ensure accurate detection of this important autoantibody.

ETHICS STATEMENT

The studies involving human participants were reviewed and approved by University of Bath EIRA 17-01211. Written informed consent to participate in this study was provided by the participants' legal guardian/next of kin.

AUTHOR CONTRIBUTIONS

Experiments were carried out by BM, HL, FM, and DL. Manuscript was drafted by BM and read by ST and NM. All authors contributed to the article and approved the submitted version.

REFERENCES

1. McHugh NJ, Tansley SL. Autoantibodies in Myositis. *Nat Rev Rheumatol* (2018) 14:290–302. doi: 10.1038/nrrheum.2018.56
2. Betteridge Z, Tansley S, Shaddick G, Chinoy H, Cooper RG, New RP, et al. Frequency, Mutual Exclusivity and Clinical Associations of Myositis Autoantibodies in a Combined European Cohort of Idiopathic Inflammatory Myopathy Patients. *J Autoimmun* (2019) 101:48–55. doi: 10.1016/j.jaut.2019.04.001
3. Aussy A, Boyer O, Cordel N. Dermatomyositis and Immune-Mediated Necrotizing Myopathies: A Window on Autoimmunity and Cancer. *Front Immunol* (2017) 8:992. doi: 10.3389/fimmu.2017.00992
4. Oldroyd A, Sergeant JC, New P, McHugh NJ, Betteridge Z, Lamb JA, et al. The Temporal Relationship Between Cancer and Adult Onset Anti-Transcriptional

Intermediary Factor 1 Antibody-Positive Dermatomyositis. *Rheumatol (United Kingdom)* (2019) 58:650–5. doi: 10.1093/rheumatology/key357

5. Hida A, Yamashita T, Hosono Y, Inoue M, Kaida K, Kadoya M, et al. Anti-TIF1-γ Antibody and Cancer-Associated Myositis: A Clinicohistopathologic Study. *Neurology* (2016) 87:299–308. doi: 10.1212/WNL.0000000000002863
6. Fiorentino DF, Chung LS, Christopher-Stine L, Zaba L, Li S, Mammen AL, et al. Most Patients With Cancer-Associated Dermatomyositis Have Antibodies to Nuclear Matrix Protein NXP-2 or Transcription Intermediary Factor 1γ. *Arthritis Rheum* (2013) 65:2954–62. doi: 10.1002/art.38093
7. Tansley SL, Li D, Betteridge ZE, McHugh NJ. The Reliability of Immunoassays to Detect Autoantibodies in Patients With Myositis is Dependent on Autoantibody Specificity. *Rheumatol (United Kingdom)* (2020) 59:2109–14. doi: 10.1093/rheumatology/keaa021
8. Espinosa-Ortega F, Holmqvist M, Alexanderson H, Storfors H, Mimori T, Lundberg IE, et al. Comparison of Autoantibody Specificities Tested by a Line Blot Assay and Immunoprecipitation-Based Algorithm in Patients With Idiopathic Inflammatory Myopathies. *Ann Rheum Dis* (2019) 78:858–60. doi: 10.1136/ANNRHEUMDIS-2018-214690
9. Targoff IN, Mamyrova G, Trieu EP, Perurena O, Koneru B, O'Hanlon TP, et al. A Novel Autoantibody to a 155-Kd Protein Is Associated With Dermatomyositis. *Arthritis Rheum* (2006) 54:3682–9. doi: 10.1002/art.22164
10. Fujimoto M, Murakami A, Kurei S, Okiyama N, Kawakami A, Mishima M, et al. Enzyme-Linked Immunosorbent Assays for Detection of Anti-Transcriptional Intermediary Factor-1 Gamma and Anti-Mi-2 Autoantibodies in Dermatomyositis. *J Dermatol Sci* (2016) 84:272–81. doi: 10.1016/j.jdermsci.2016.09.013
11. Tansley SL, Simou S, Shaddick G, Betteridge ZE, Almeida B, Gunawardena H, et al. Autoantibodies in Juvenile-Onset Myositis: Their Diagnostic Value and Associated Clinical Phenotype in a Large UK Cohort. *J Autoimmun* (2017) 84:55–64. doi: 10.1016/j.jaut.2017.06.007
12. Fujimoto M, Hamaguchi Y, Kaji K, Matsushita T, Ichimura Y, Kodera M, et al. Myositis-Specific Anti-155/140 Autoantibodies Target Transcription Intermediary Factor 1 Family Proteins. *Arthritis Rheum* (2012) 64:513–22. doi: 10.1002/art.33403
13. Fiorentino DF, Gutierrez-Alamillo L, Hines D, Yang Q, Casciola-Rosen L. Distinct Dermatomyositis Populations are Detected With Different Autoantibody Assay Platforms. *Clin Exp Rheumatol* (2019) 37:1048–51.

4

miR-18a-3p and Its Target Protein HuR May Regulate Myogenic Differentiation in Immune-Mediated Necrotizing Myopathy

Lifang Ye[1,2†], Yu Zuo[1†], Fang Chen[1], Qinglin Peng[1], Xin Lu[1], Guochun Wang[1,2] and Xiaoming Shu[1*]*

[1] *Department of Rheumatology, Key Laboratory of Myositis, China–Japan Friendship Hospital, Beijing, China,* [2] *Peking Union Medical College, Chinese Academy of Medical Sciences, Beijing, China*

***Correspondence:**
Guochun Wang
guochunwang@hotmail.com
Xiaoming Shu
sxm992283@hotmail.com

†These authors have contributed equally to this work

Immune-mediated necrotizing myopathy (IMNM) is characterized by manifestation of myonecrosis and regeneration of muscle fibers; however, the underlying pathogenesis remains unclear. This study aimed to investigate the role and mechanism of miR-18a-3p and its target RNA-binding protein HuR in IMNM. HuR and miR-18a-3p levels were detected in the skeletal muscles of 18 patients with IMNM using quantitative reverse-transcription real-time polymerase chain reaction (qRT-PCR) and western blotting analysis. Human myoblasts were transfected with small interfering RNA targeting HuR and miR-18a-3p mimic or inhibitor. Myogenic differentiation markers, myogenin and myosin heavy chain, were analyzed by qRT-PCR, western blotting analysis, and immunofluorescence staining. The results showed that miR-18a-3p was upregulated (p=0.0002), whereas HuR was downregulated (p=0.002) in the skeletal muscles of patients with IMNM. The expression of miR-18a-3p in patients with IMNM was negatively correlated with those of HuR (r = -0.512, p = 0.029). We also found that disease activity was positively correlated with HuR expression (r = 0.576, p = 0.012) but muscle activity was negatively correlated with miR-18a-3p expression (r = -0.550, p = 0.017). Besides, bioinformatics analysis and dual-luciferase reporter assays suggested that miR-18a-3p could directly target HuR. Cellular experiments showed that overexpression of miR-18a-3p inhibited myogenic differentiation by targeting HuR, whereas inhibition of miR-18a-3p led to opposite results. Therefore, miR-18a-3p and its target protein HuR may be responsible for modulating the myogenic process in IMNM and can thus be therapeutic targets for the same.

Keywords: HuR, miR-18a-3p, RNA binding protein, immune-mediated necrotizing myopathy, myogenic differentiation

---

Abbreviations: IMNM, immune-mediated necrotizing myopathy; UTR, untranslated region; HSMM, human skeletal muscle myoblasts; ELISA, enzyme-linked immunosorbent assay; PGA, physician global assessment; MMT8, manual muscle testing 8; HC, healthy controls; MyoG, myogenin; IIM, idiopathic inflammatory myopathy; RBP, RNA-binding protein; HMGCR, anti-3-hydroxy-3-methylglutaryl-CoA reductase; anti-SRP, anti-signal recognition particle; qRT-PCR, quantitative reverse-transcription real-time polymerase chain reaction.

INTRODUCTION

Immune-mediated necrotizing myopathy (IMNM) is an autoimmune disease that is characterized by severe muscle weakness and myofiber necrosis, but usually low inflammatory cell infiltration and lesser involvement of other organs (1). IMNM consists of three subclasses: anti-signal recognition particle (anti-SRP)-positive, anti-3-hydroxy-3-methylglutaryl-CoA reductase (HMGCR)-positive, and seronegative (2). Myoblast fusion in patients with IMNM is abnormal since the mechanism involved in muscle regeneration is impaired (3); however, the pathogenesis of IMNM is still unclear.

MicroRNAs (miRNA) participate in skeletal muscle differentiation (4). miR-17-92, a highly conserved miRNA cluster, comprises miR-17, miR-20a, miR-18a, miR-19a, miR-19b-1, and miR-92a-1; these miRNAs play an essential role in cell proliferation, differentiation, tumorigenesis, and angiogenesis (5–7). The pathogenic role of miRNAs in many diseases, including autoimmune diseases, has been extensively studied. Previous studies have shown that miRNA expression is abnormal in the peripheral blood mononuclear cells, skeletal muscles, plasma, serum, and lungs of patients with idiopathic inflammatory myopathy (IIM); thus, dysregulated miRNA expression may be involved in disease pathogenesis (8–11). Besides, the expression of inflammatory miRNAs and anti-troponin-targeted miRNAs is increased in mice with severe myositis, indicating that miRNAs are involved in muscle injury, inflammation, and myasthenia (12). Our previous study also revealed that several immune-related miRNAs are correlated with dermatomyositis (13); however, the involvement of miRNAs in IMNM remains unclear.

RNA-binding proteins (RBPs) are known to change the fate or function of bound RNA. Of such RBPs, HuR, a member of the ELAVL1/Hu family, has been reported to modulate the fusion of myoblasts into myotubes during skeletal myogenesis by coordinating the expression of myogenic regulatory factors such as myogenin (MyoG), MyoD, and p21 (14–16). Nevertheless, the role of HuR in IMNM has not been investigated.

In this study, we aimed to explore the role and mechanism of abnormally expressed miR-18a-3p and its target RBP HuR in the myogenesis of patients with IMNM. Our results may help in better understanding the pathogenesis of IMNM and developing effective therapeutic targets.

MATERIALS AND METHODS

Study Population

Patients with IMNM, DM and healthy controls (HCs), who participated in this study, were admitted to the Department of Rheumatology and Physical Examination from 2017 to 2019 in China–Japan Friendship Hospital, Beijing, China. The age and gender of the patients with IMNM were matched with those of the HCs. IMNM was classified according to the pathological criteria described at the 224th European Neuromuscular Center International Workshop (17). This study did not include patients with other autoimmune diseases, tumors, and infections. Skeletal muscle tissue biopsies were obtained from 18 patients with IMNM, 11 patients with DM and 8 HCs. The study was approved by the Ethical Review Committee of the China–Japan Friendship Hospital (2019-25-K19). Before commencing the study, we obtained written informed consent from all patients for the use of their tissues and data.

Clinical Assessment

Detailed results of physical examinations and routine laboratory tests of all patients were recorded at their first visit. Routine laboratory parameters, including the levels of serum C-reactive protein, creatine kinase, alanine aminotransferase, aspartate aminotransferase, and lactate dehydrogenase, and erythrocyte sedimentation rate, were assessed. The damage to the patients with IMNM was evaluated using manual muscle testing 8 (MMT8). A 10 cm visual analog scale (VAS) was used to evaluate the muscle activity component of the myositis disease activity assessment tool (MDAAT-muscle) and physician global assessment (PGA) for disease activity (18).

Serum anti-HMGCR antibodies were detected using an enzyme-linked immunosorbent assay (ELISA) kit (Inova Diagnostics, San Diego, CA, USA). Serum anti-SRP antibodies were detected using a commercially available kit (Euroimmun, Lübeck, Germany).

Myoblast Culture and Differentiation

Human skeletal muscle myoblasts (HSMM) were obtained from Lonza Bioscience (Basel, Switzerland) and cultured using the Clonetics skeletal muscle myoblast cell system (Lonza) in a humidified incubator (Thermo Fisher Scientific, Waltham, MA, USA) at 37°C with 5% CO_2. The cells were seeded in 12-well or 6-well plates and incubated for 18 h before transfection. At 80–90% confluence, the cells were transferred into Dulbecco's modified Eagle medium supplemented with 2% horse serum and 1% penicillin-streptomycin for inducing differentiation.

Cell Transfection

HSMM were seeded in 12-well or 6-well plates; when the cells reached approximately 70% confluence, they were transfected with 100 nM of small interfering RNA targeting HuR (siHuR) or small interfering control RNA (siCtrl), miR-18a-3p mimics or mimics negative control (NC) and miR-18a-3p inhibitor or inhibitor NC (Ribobio, Guangzhou, China) using Lipofectamine 3000 (Invitrogen, Carlsbad, CA, USA) according to the manufacturer's instructions. The culture system was replaced with fresh medium at 12 h post-transfection. The cells were used to stimulate differentiation at 24 h post-transfection.

Dual-Luciferase Reporter Gene Assay

Dual-luciferase reporter gene assay was used to confirm the binding sites of miR-18a-3p and the 3′ untranslated region (UTR) of HuR mRNA. A pmirGLO-HuR-wild type (Hur-WT) or a pmirG-LO-HuR-mutant type (HuR-MUT) and miR-18a-3p mimics or mimics NC were co-transfected into HEK293T cells using Lipofectamine 2000 (Invitrogen). Dual-Glo luciferase assay system (Promega, Madison, WI, USA) was used to measure the luciferase activity in the cell lysates according to the manufacturer's instructions. The ratios of Firefly to Renilla luciferase activities were used as the result of the dual-luciferase reporter gene assay. The experiments were performed in three independent replicates.

Bioinformatics Analysis

The online databases miRwalk (http://mirwalk.umm.uni-heidelberg.de/) and TargetScan (http://www.targetscan.org/vert_72/) were used to search for the targets of miR-18a-3p (19, 20). Venny (https://bioinfogp.cnb.csic.es/tools/venny/index.html) was used to obtain the common targets from above mentioned databases. Heatmap software(ggplot2) was applied to cluster the enrichment terms obtained after Kyoto Encyclopedia of Genes and Genomes-based analysis of the common genes.

RNA Extraction and Quantitative Reverse-Transcription Polymerase Chain Reaction

Trizol (Invitrogen) was used to extract total RNA from the muscle tissues according to the manufacturer's instructions. PrimeScript™ RT reagent Kit (Takara, Otsu, Japan) was used to reverse transcribe RNA into complementary DNA (cDNA). Quantitative reverse-transcription PCR (qRT-PCR) was performed using an ABI 7500 sequence detection system (Applied Biosystems, Foster City, CA) with SYBR Green Master Mix (Qiagen, Hilden, Germany). The thermal conditions were as follows: 95°C for 2 min, followed by 40 cycles at 95°C for 5 s and 60°C for 30 s. *GAPDH* was used as the internal reference of gene expression. Each sample was measured in triplicate. The U6 small RNA was used as the internal reference for estimating the levels of miR-18a-3p and other members in miR-17-92 cluster. All relevant PCR primers used in this study are listed in **Supplementary Table 1**.

Western Blotting Analysis

NE-PER Nuclear and Cytoplasmic Extraction Reagents kit (Thermo Fisher Scientific) was used to extract nuclear-cytoplasmic fraction according to the manufacturer's instructions. NP-40 lysis buffer (Beyotime, Shanghai, China) and phenylmethylsulfonyl fluoride (Solarbio, Beijing, China) were used to obtain total protein. Protein quantification were performed by BCA Protein Assay kit (Thermo Fisher Scientific) as per the manufacturer's instructions. The available protein was denatured with 5× sodium dodecyl sulfate (SDS)-PAGE denatured protein loading buffer (Applygen, Beijing, China) at 98°C for 5 min. Next, SDS-polyacrylamide discontinuous gel electrophoresis was used to separate the denatured protein; then, the protein was transferred to nitrocellulose filter membranes (Millipore, Boston, MA, USA) by wetting transfer method for 90 min. Immunoblotting was conducted using specific antibodies listed in **Supplementary Table 2** and horseradish peroxidase-conjugated secondary antibody. The membranes were visualized using ChemiDoc XRS+ System (Bio-Rad, Hercules, CA, USA), and the grayscale value of the proteins was estimated using Image Lab 6.0.1.

Immunofluorescence Staining

Differentiated HSMM myotubes or primary myotubes were fixed in 95% ethanol. Then, 0.3% Triton X-100 was used for 15 min for cell membrane penetration. The samples were washed three times, for 5 minutes each time, and then blocked with goat serum for 2 h. The samples were then incubated with anti-HuR (1:500; Abcam, Cambridge, MA, USA), anti-MyoG (1:250; Abcam), and anti-myosin heavy chain (MyHC; 1:400; Santa Cruz Biotechnology, Dallas, TX, USA) overnight at 4°C, and then with Alexa 488-conjugated or Alexa 555-conjugated secondary antibody (Abcam) for 30 min at 25°C. Next, 4′,6-diamidino-2-phenylindole (DAPI; Beyotime) was used to stain the cell nuclei, which were observed under a fluorescence microscope (Olympus, Tokyo, Japan). The degree of differentiation was measured by a fusion index, which is defined as the number of nuclei in the myotube and as a percentage of the total nuclei.

Statistical Analysis

Continuous data were expressed as means ± standard deviation for normal distribution or as median and interquartile range for those without normal distribution. Student's *t*-test was used for separating the means of the normal data, whereas Mann–Whitney U test for data that deviated from normal. Spearman's rank-order correlation was used to test correlations of data with non-normal distribution. A p value < 0.05 was considered as statistically significant. SPSS 22.0 (IBM, Armonk, NY, USA) and GraphPad Prism 8.0 (GraphPad Software, San Diego, CA, USA) were used for all statistical analyses.

RESULTS

Clinical Characteristics of Patients With IMNM

The clinical characteristics of the patients with IMNM are presented in **Table 1**. Of the 18 patients with IMNM, 61.1% were female. The average disease onset age was 47.6 years, and the median disease duration was 5 months. 12 patients were positive to the anti-SRP-autoantibody, 2 to the anti-HMGCR-autoantibody, and the remaining four patients were myositis-specific autoantibody negative. The average VAS score was 4.7, and the average MMT8 score was 58.0.

miR-18a-3p Expression in Skeletal Muscles of Patients With IMNM

We found that the expression level of miR-18a-3p was significantly higher in patients with IMNM than in the HCs

TABLE 1 | Clinical features of immune-mediated necrotizing myopathy (IMNM) patients.

Characteristics	Patients (*n* = 18)	HCs (*n* = 8)
Female, no. (%)	11 (61.1%)	5 (62.5%)
Age of onset, mean ± s.d. years	47.6± 15.6	50.8 ± 17.1
Disease duration, median of IQR months	5(2-9.7)	
Clinical features, no. (%)		
Muscle weakness	15 (83.3%)	
Myalgia	6 (33.3%)	
Laboratory data		
MSA, no. (%)		
Anti-SRP- positive	12 (66.6%)	
Anti-HMGCR- positive	2 (11.1%)	
MSA-negative	4 (22.2%)	
CK (IU/L), median (IQR)	3597 (1356-7521)	
ALT (IU/L), median (IQR)	207.5 (61.4-319)	
AST (IU/L), median (IQR)	119.5 (39.7-160.8)	
LDH (IU/L), median (IQR)	674 (426.5-1113)	
ESR (mm/h), median (IQR)	7 (5-20.5)	
CRP (mg/dl), median (IQR)	0.36 (0.25-0.45)	
MMT8, mean ± s.d.	58.0 ± 12.9	
PGA VAS, mean ± s.d.	4.7 ± 1.8	

Average values or numbers of each group are shown. Standard deviation (s.d.), interquartile range (IQR), or percentages are shown. MSA, myositis-specific antibody; IMNM, immune-mediated necrotizing myopathy; SRP, signal recognition particle; HMGCR, 3-hydroxy-3-methyl coenzyme A reductase; CK, creatine kinase; ALT, alanine aminotransferase; AST, aspartate aminotransferase; LDH, lactate dehydrogenase; ESR, erythrocyte sedimentation rate; CRP, C-reactive protein; PGA, physician global assessment; VAS, visual analog scale; MMT8, manual muscle test 8 (0-80).

(p=0.0002) (**Figure 1A**). Since miR-18a-3p is the member of miR-17-92 cluster, and the miR-17-92 cluster participates in skeletal muscle differentiation (7), we further detected the expression of other miRNAs in this cluster in these samples (**Supplementary Figures 1A–E**). The Kyoto Encyclopedia of Genes and Genomes pathway enrichment analysis revealed that the target genes of miR-18a-3p were involved in regulating numerous pathways, ras and mitogen-activated protein kinase (MAPK) signaling pathway are involved in the regulation of myogenic differentiation (21) (**Figure 1B**). Bioinformatics analysis predicted that HuR may be a target gene of miR-18a-3p (**Figure 1C**). Dual-luciferase reporter gene assay showed that overexpression of miR-18a-3p decreased the luciferase activity of the plasmid containing HuR-WT, that is, the luciferase activity of miR-18a-3p binding sequence; however, it did not decrease the activity of HuR-MUT (**Figure 1D**). Furthermore, overexpression of miR-18a-3p strongly suppressed HuR transcription at 24 h post-transfection (**Figure 1E**). Accordingly, western blot analysis showed that the protein levels of HuR were reduced by the transfection of the miR-18a-3p mimics (**Figures 1F, G**). These results demonstrated that miR-18a-3p may directly interact with the predicted target site in HuR.

HuR Expression Levels in Patients With IMNM

Our results showed that the expression level of HuR was significantly reduced in patients with IMNM than in HCs (p=0.002) (**Figure 2A**), but the expression of HuR in DM patients is significantly higher than in HCs (**Supplementary Figure 2**). Western blot analysis revealed a decrease in the protein levels of HuR in patients with IMNM than in the HCs (**Figures 2B, C**). At the same time, miR-18a-3p expressed in patients with IMNM were negatively correlated with those of HuR (r=-0.512, p = 0.029; **Figures 2D**). Furthermore, MyoG was highly expressed in patients with IMNM, and its transcription levels were positively correlated with those of HuR ($r = 0.493, p = 0.037$; **Figures 2E, F**). Besides, the VAS score of patients with IMNM was positively correlated with HuR levels ($r = 0.576, p = 0.012$); however, the muscle activity component of the Myositis Disease Activity Assessment Tool by VAS (MDAAT-muscle) was negatively correlated with miR-18a-3p expression ($r = -0.550, p = 0.017$; **Figures 2G, H**). No association was identified between HuR or miR-18a-3p expression and the MMT8 score.

Involvement of HuR in Myoblast Differentiation

As shown in **Figures 3A, B**, the nuclear abundance of HuR did not change noticeably during differentiation, whereas the cytoplasmatic abundance increased remarkably at the onset of differentiation and remained elevated throughout the process. We observed that the expression levels of MyoG were consistent with those of cytoplasmic HuR; these results were confirmed using immunofluorescence staining of human myoblasts after differentiation (**Figure 3C**). Next, we use siRNA technology to solve the role of HuR in myoblast. Three different siRNAs were designed to target human HuR and transfected in myoblast. The results showed that siHuR effectively down-regulated the mRNA expression in myoblast (**Supplementary Figures 3A**). According to qRT-PCR analysis, transfection of siHuR (100 nM) significantly reduced the cellular level of HuR (>70%) (**Supplementary Figures 3B**). Besides, we observed that transfection of siHuR significantly inhibited the expression levels of HuR and MyoG during differentiation (**Figures 3D, E**). Western blot analysis showed that the protein levels of HuR, MyoG, and MyHC in siHuR-treated myoblasts were significantly decreased when compared with that in the control (**Figures 3F–I**). These results suggested that HuR knockdown could inhibit myoblast differentiation.

HuR Regulation by miR-18a-3p in Myogenic Differentiation

As shown in **Figure 4A**, miR-18a-3p mimics transfection significantly increased miR-18a-3p expression. MyHC immunofluorescence staining on day 5 of differentiation showed that overexpression of miR-18a-3p reduced the fusion rate of myoblasts in comparison to that of the mimics NC (**Figures 4B, C**). Furthermore, miR-18a-3p mimics transfection significantly suppressed the transcription and protein levels of HuR, MyoG, and MyHC (**Figures 4D–F**). The opposite results

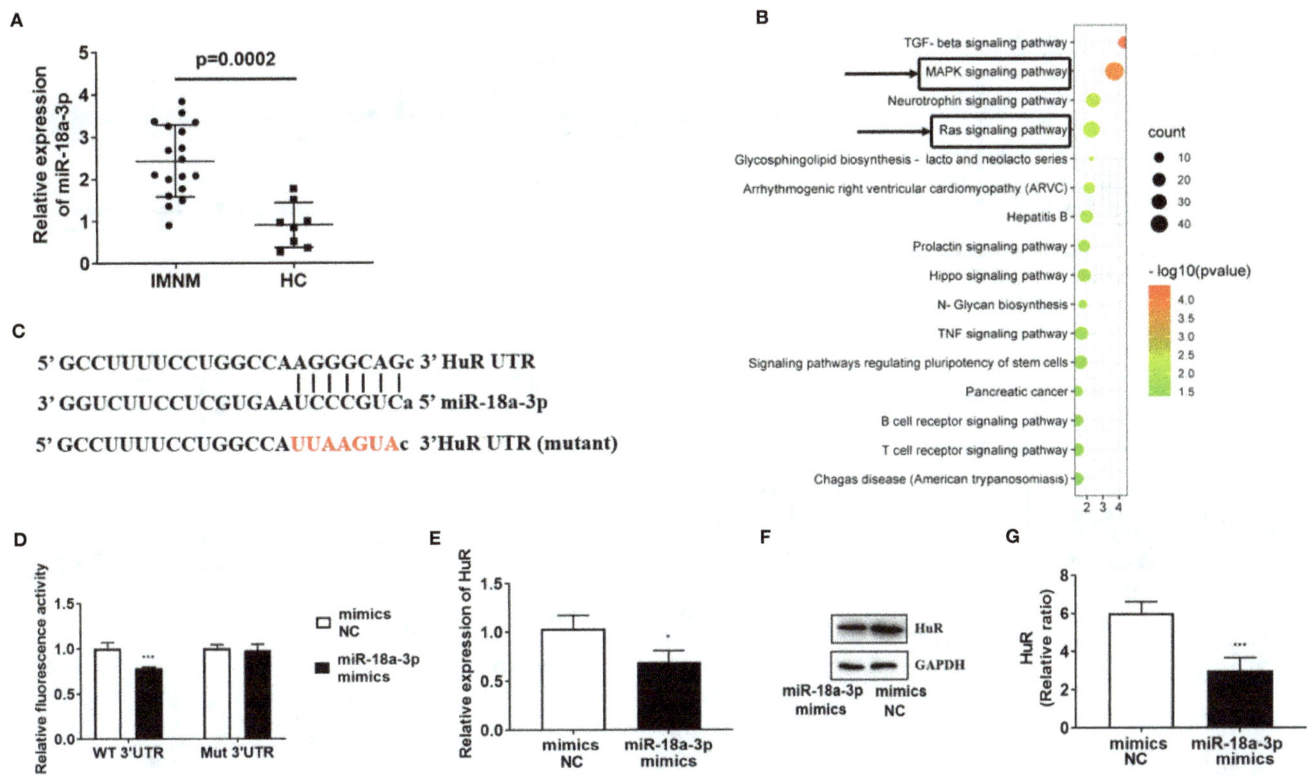

FIGURE 1 | miR-18a-3p is highly expressed in skeletal muscle of patients with immune-mediated necrotizing myopathy (IMNM). **(A)** miR-18a-3p levels in patients with IMNM and healthy controls (HCs) as determined by quantitative reverse-transcription polymerase chain reaction PCR (qRT-PCR). **(B)** Kyoto Encyclopedia of Genes and Genomes (KEGG) pathway analysis of miR-18a-3p target genes. **(C)** Sequence alignment of the 3′ untranslated region (UTR) of HuR mRNA with miR-18a-3p. Nucleotides in deletion mutant (Mut) HuR binding sites are marked in red. **(D)** Effects of miR-18a-3p on the activity of luciferase reporters, bearing wild-type (WT) or Mut on the binding sites of the 3′ UTR of HuR mRNA. **(E)** HuR levels at 24 h post-transfection with miR-18a-3p mimics as determined by qRT-PCR. **(F)** Protein levels of HuR at 24 h post-transfection with miR-18a-3p mimics as determined by western blot analysis. **(G)** Glyceraldehyde 3-phosphate dehydrogenase (GAPDH) was used as an internal control for western blot analysis to normalize the relative protein expression. Relative mRNA expression was estimated using the $2^{-\Delta\Delta Ct}$ method. Data are expressed as means ± standard deviation (SD). *, *** indicate significant differences of $p < 0.05$ and $p < 0.001$, respectively. miR, microRNA; NC, negative control.

were obtained after transfection of the miR-18a-3p inhibitor (**Figures 5A–F**). Our data demonstrated that inhibition of miR-18a-3p might promote myogenic differentiation by targeting HuR.

DISCUSSION

IMNM is a systemic disease characterized by chronic inflammation in muscle tissues, causing weakness and myofiber necrosis (1). In the present study, we explored the role of differentially expressed miRNAs and target genes in regulating the regeneration and differentiation of muscle tissues in patients with IMNM.

miRNA is involved in the regulation of a wide range of developmental and physiological cell processes, including differentiation, proliferation, growth, and apoptosis (22). Previous studies have shown that miRNAs are abnormally expressed in the muscles of patients with IIM and are probably involved in disease pathogenesis. For instance, miR-221, miR-155, miR-146b, miR-214, and miR-222 are upregulated in 10 primary muscle diseases, including IIM (23). Furthermore, miRNAs found in skeletal muscles and myocardium, such as miR-1, miR-133a/b, miR-208, miR-486, miR-206, and miR-499, participate in the myogenic process by modulating the expression of myogenic regulatory factors (24). Of these, the expression of miR-1 and miR-133a/b is decreased in the muscle tissues of patients with IIM and is negatively correlated with that of TNF-α. The latter inhibits the expression of myogenic miRNAs in an NF-κB-dependent manner, suppressing the differentiation of C2C12 myoblasts into myotubes and leading to muscle regeneration (25). In our study, miR-18a-3p was upregulated in patients with IMNM and participated in myogenic differentiation by regulating HuR expression. We also found that miR-18a-3p expression

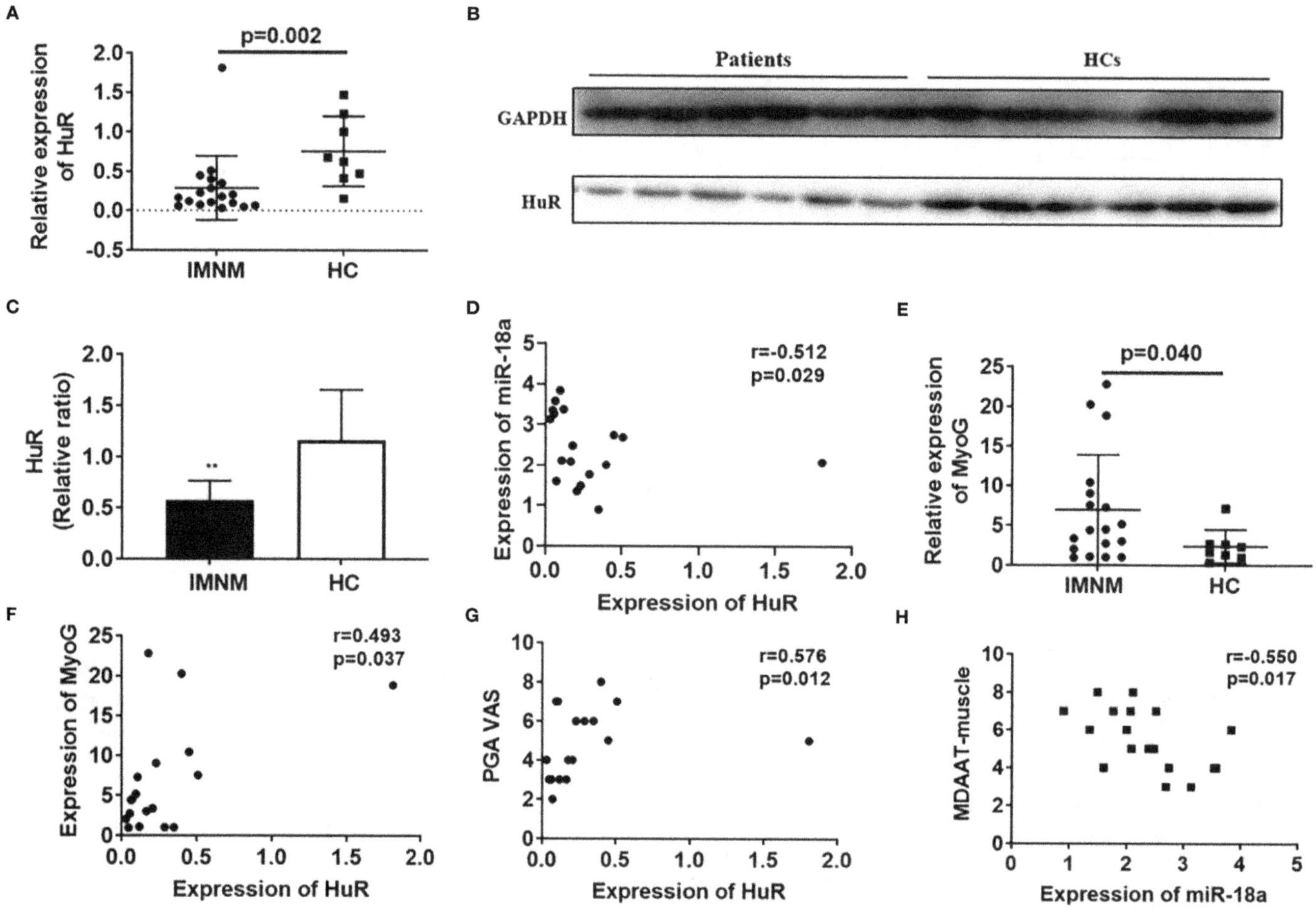

FIGURE 2 | The mRNA and protein levels of HuR are decreased in skeletal muscles of patients with immune-mediated necrotizing myopathy (IMNM). **(A)** mRNA levels of HuR in patients with IMNM and healthy controls (HCs) as determined by qRT-PCR. **(B)** Protein levels of HuR in patients with IMNM and HCs as determined by western blot analysis. **(C)** GAPDH was used as an internal control for western blot analysis to normalize the relative protein expression. **(D)** Correlation of HuR and miR-18a-3p mRNA levels in patients with IMNM. **(E)** mRNA levels of myogenin (MyoG) in skeletal muscles of patients with IMNM and HCs as determined by qRT-PCR. **(F)** Correlation of HuR and MyoG mRNA levels in patients with IMNM. **(G)** Correlation of HuR mRNA levels and Patient Global assessment of disease activity by VAS (0-10). **(H)** Correlation of miR-18a-3p levels and the muscle activity component of the Myositis Disease Activity Assessment Tool by VAS (MDAAT-muscle). Relative mRNA expression was estimated using the $2^{-\Delta\Delta Ct}$ method. Data are expressed as means ± standard deviation (SD). ** indicate significant differences of $p < 0.01$.

was negatively related to the VAS score, revealing the potential role of this miRNA in muscle inflammation and the degenerative pathology of IMNM. A previous study on mice with severe myositis has shown that increased expression of inflammatory miRNAs (miR-146a, miR-142-3p, miR-142-5p, and miR-455-5p) and targeted muscle dystrophins (miR-146a, miR-146b, miR-31, and miR-223) are regulated by NF-κB, and may be related to muscle injury, inflammation, and myasthenia (12). Of note, in our study, we found that the expression of HuR in IMNM was decreased compared to HC, while the expression of HuR in the muscle tissue of DM patients was significantly higher than in the HC. The results of this study further indicate that the muscle damage mechanism of DM may be different from that of IMNM.

The miR-17-92 cluster participates in normal development, skeletal myogenesis, immune disease, cardiovascular disease, and tumorigenesis (26, 27), of which miR-20a, miR-92, and miR-17 regulate the proliferation of myoblasts but inhibit their differentiation by targeting ENH1. Further, miR-17 and miR-20a effectively promote the differentiation of C2C12 cells; whereas miR-18a delays the differentiation of the same cells (7, 28). Here, we use bioinformatics software and luciferase reporter gene detection to show that HuR, a RNA-binding protein, is the direct target of miR-18a-3p. Under the overexpression miR-18a-3p, the expression level of HuR RNA and protein was significantly inhibited, and further inhibit myogenic differentiation. On the contrary, interference of miR-18a-3p promoted the expression of HuR and further promote

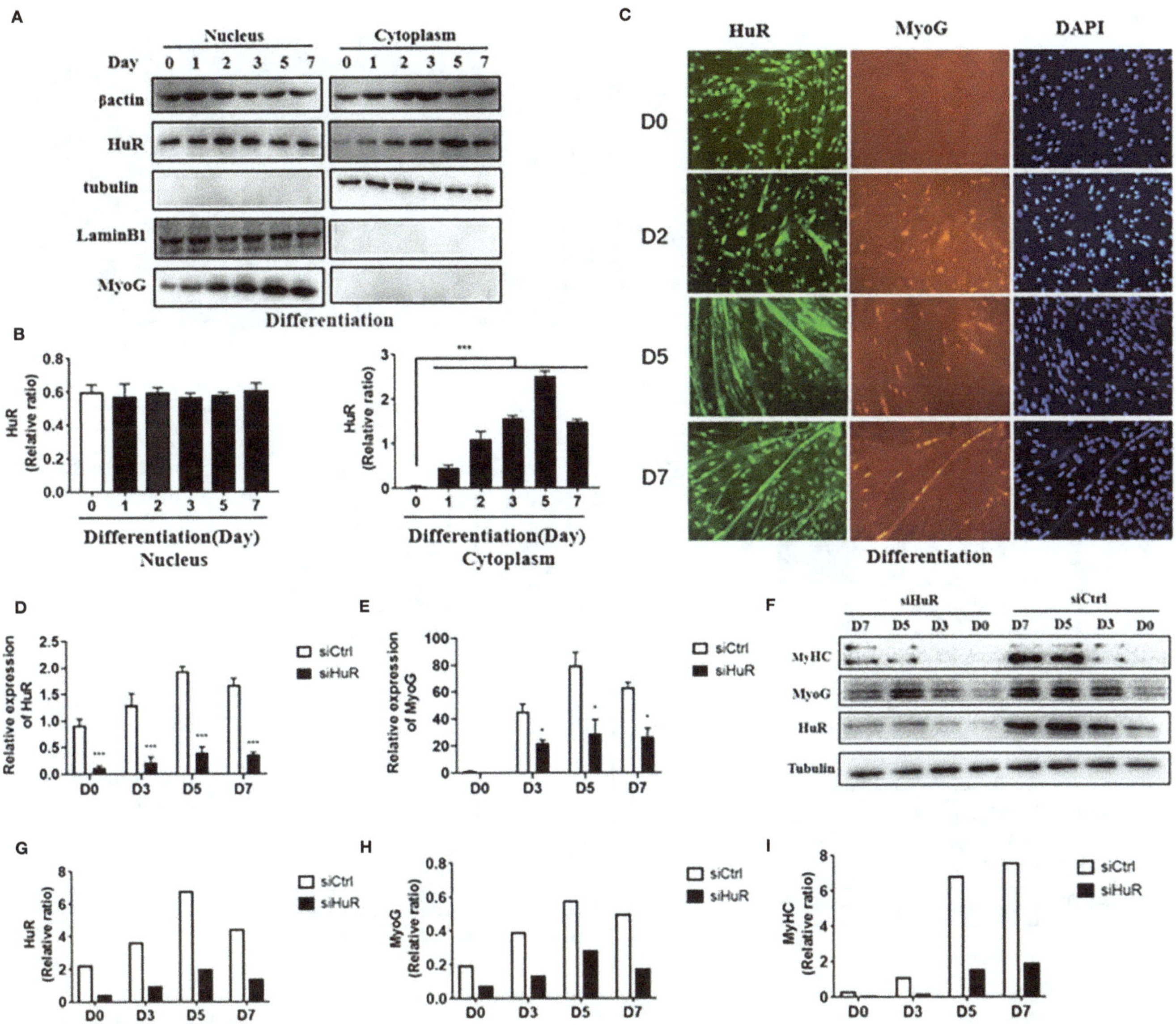

FIGURE 3 | Expression of HuR in human skeletal muscle myoblasts (HSMM) during differentiation. **(A)** Nuclear and cytoplasmic HuR and myogenin (MyoG) protein levels in HSMM during differentiation as determined by western blot analysis. **(B)** HuR levels in the human myoblast nucleus as normalized with lamin-B1 (left) and in the human myoblast cytoplasm as normalized with tubulin (right). **(C)** Immunofluorescence detection of HuR (green) and MyoG (red) in HSMM during differentiation. DAPI (blue) is used as a nuclear stain. Scale bar, 100 μm. **(D)** mRNA levels of HuR post-transfection with small interfering RNA targeting HuR (siHuR) at days 0, 3, 5, and 7 of differentiation as determined by qRT-PCR. **(E)** mRNA levels of MyoG post-transfection with siHuR at days 0, 3, 5, and 7 of differentiation as determined by qRT-PCR. **(F)** Western blot analysis was used to determine HuR, MyoG, and MyHC protein levels post-transfection with siHuR at days 0, 3, 5, and 7 of differentiation. **(G–I)** GAPDH was used as an internal control for western blot analysis to normalize relative protein expression. Relative mRNA expression was estimated using the $2^{-\Delta\Delta Ct}$ method. Data are expressed as means ± standard deviation (SD). *, *** indicate significant differences of $p < 0.05$ and $p < 0.001$, respectively.

myogenic differentiation. In our study, we found that expression of miR-18a-3p in patients with IMNM was negatively correlated with HuR. miR-18a-3p affected myoblast differentiation by downregulating the expression of HuR. In contrast, use of an miR-18a-3p inhibitor led to opposite results.

HuR is an RBP that protects the 3'-UTR of mRNA from decay and degradation by stabilizing the adenylate-uridylate-rich elements. HuR is mainly present in the nucleus, where it combines with the target mRNA, to form a complex that moves to the cytoplasm. When HuR dissociates from the target mRNA, it returns to the nucleus (29). Previous studies have revealed that HuR regulates various myogenic factors, including MyoG, MyoD, and p21, and that its cytoplasmic accumulation is essential in myogenesis (16, 30). In the present

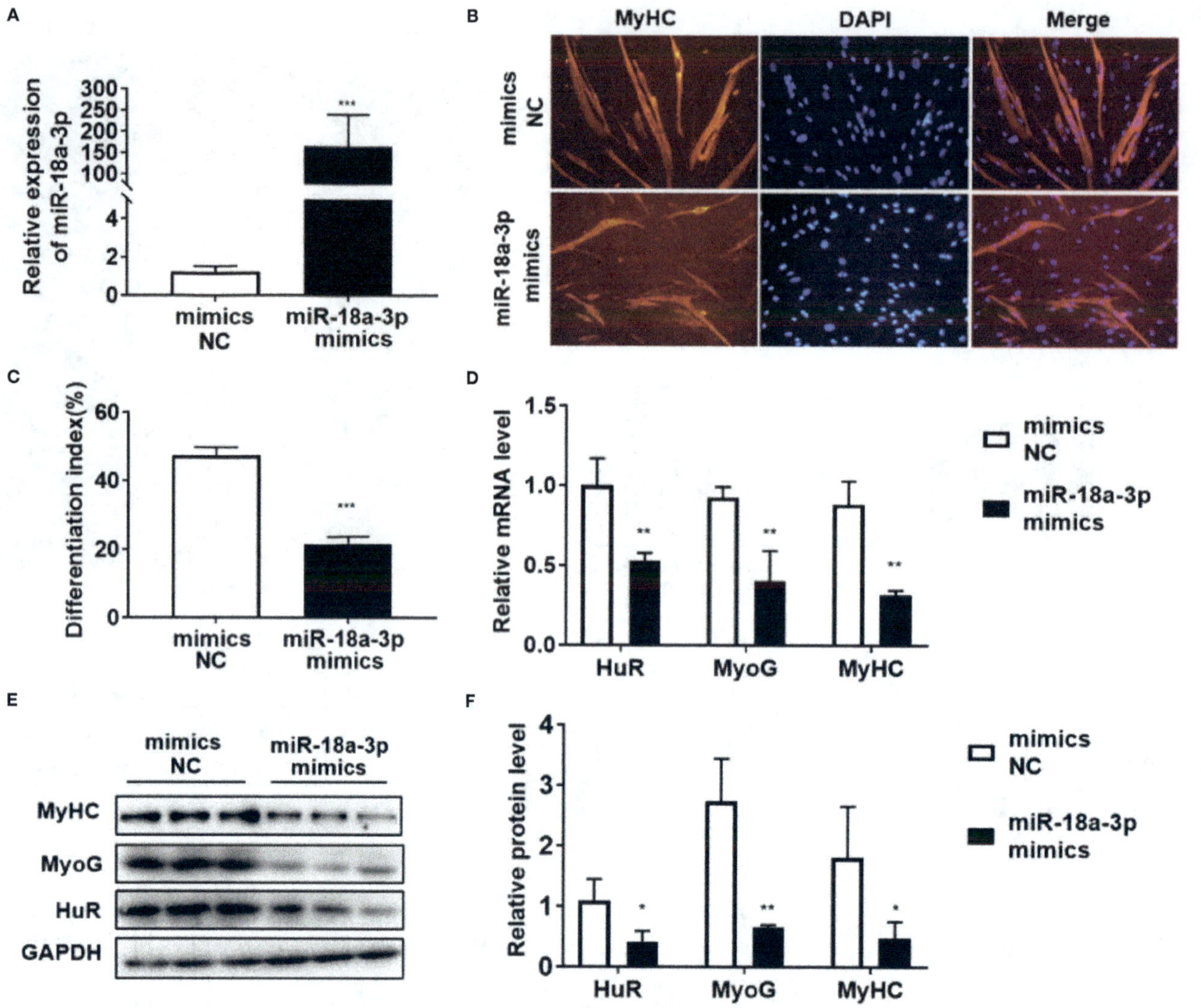

FIGURE 4 | Overexpression of miR-18a-3p inhibits myogenic differentiation. **(A)** miR-18a-3p levels post-transfection with miR-18a-3p mimics at day 5 of differentiation as determined by qRT-PCR. **(B)** Immunofluorescence detection of MyHC (red) in human myoblasts. Scale bar, 100 μm. **(C)** Fusion index (ratio of MyHC positive myotubes with ≥ 2 nuclei to the total number of nuclei). **(D)** mRNA levels of HuR, MyoG, and MyHC post-transfection with miR-18a-3p mimics at day 5 of differentiation as determined by qRT-PCR. **(E, F)** HuR, MyoG, and MyHC protein levels post-transfection with miR-18a-3p mimics at day 5 of differentiation as determined by western blot analysis. Relative mRNA expression was estimated using the $2^{-\Delta\Delta Ct}$ method. Data are expressed as means ± standard deviation (SD). *, **, *** indicate significant differences of $p < 0.05$, $p < 0.01$, and $p < 0.001$, respectively. NC, negative control.

study, we found that the expression of cytoplasmic HuR in myoblasts increased as differentiation progressed and was consistent with that of MyoG. Transfection of siHuR into myoblasts decreased the mRNA and protein levels of MyoG and MyHC in the differentiated myoblasts, thereby inhibiting cell differentiation.

HuR is also involved in the pathogenesis of inflammatory diseases (e.g., rheumatoid arthritis) by binding to the mRNAs of inflammatory cytokines (e.g., TNF-α) (31, 32). We found that the expression of HuR was positively correlated with disease activity in patients with IMNM, suggesting that the participation of this protein in inflammatory response is by stabilizing the mRNAs of inflammatory factors; however, further research is needed to confirm these results.

Overall, our study revealed that miR-18a-3p was significantly upregulated, whereas its target gene HuR was downregulated in the muscle tissues of patients with IMNM compared to DM and HCs. miR-18a-3p were negatively correlated with muscle activity in patients with IMNM, but the expression levels of HuR were positively correlated with disease activity in patients with IMNM. Finally, miR-18a-3p and HuR might regulate myoblast differentiation (**Figure 6**). To the best of our knowledge, this is the first study to report the mechanism of miR-18a-3p inhibiting myogenic differentiation in IMNM.

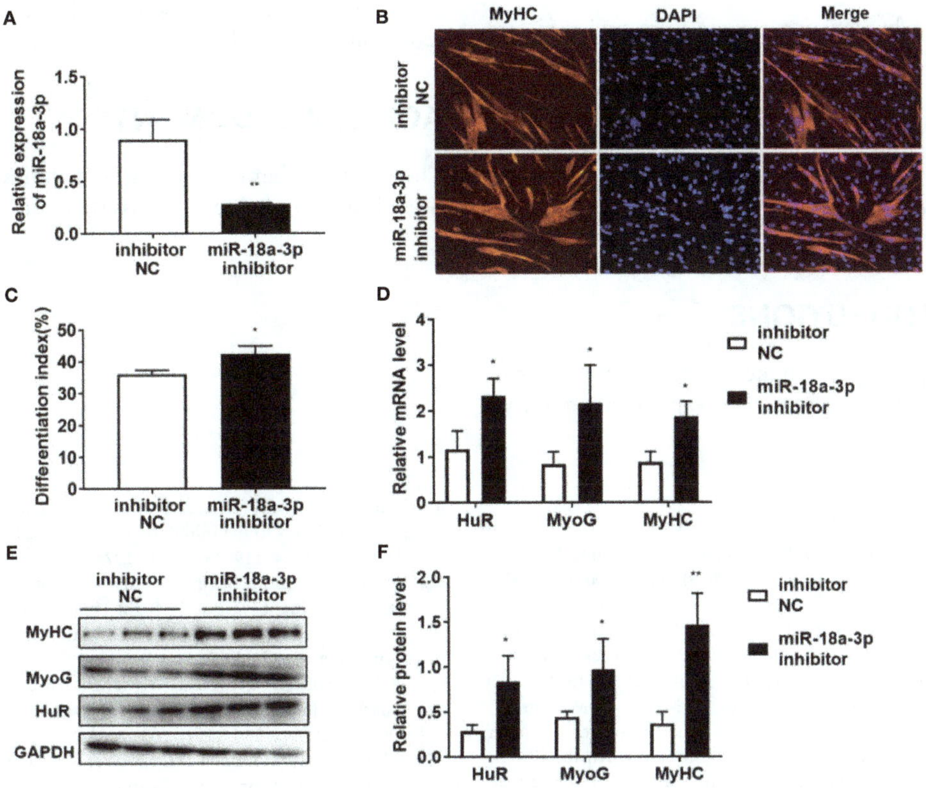

FIGURE 5 | Inhibition of miR-18a-3p promotes myogenic differentiation. **(A)** miR-18a-3p levels post-transfection with miR-18a-3p inhibitor at day 5 of differentiation as determined by qRT-PCR. **(B)** Immunofluorescence detection of MyHC (red) in human myoblasts. Scale bar, 100 μm. **(C)** Fusion index (ratio of MyHC-positive myotubes with ≥ 2 nuclei to the total number of nuclei). **(D)** mRNA levels of HuR, MyoG, and MyHC post-transfection with miR-18a-3p inhibitor at day 5 of differentiation as determined by qRT-PCR. **(E, F)** HuR, MyoG, and MyHC protein levels post-transfection with miR-18a-3p inhibitor at day 5 of differentiation as determined by western blot analysis. Relative mRNA expression was estimated using the $2^{-\Delta\Delta Ct}$ method. Data are expressed as means ± standard deviation (SD). *, ** indicate significant differences of $p < 0.05$ and $p < 0.01$, respectively. NC, negative control.

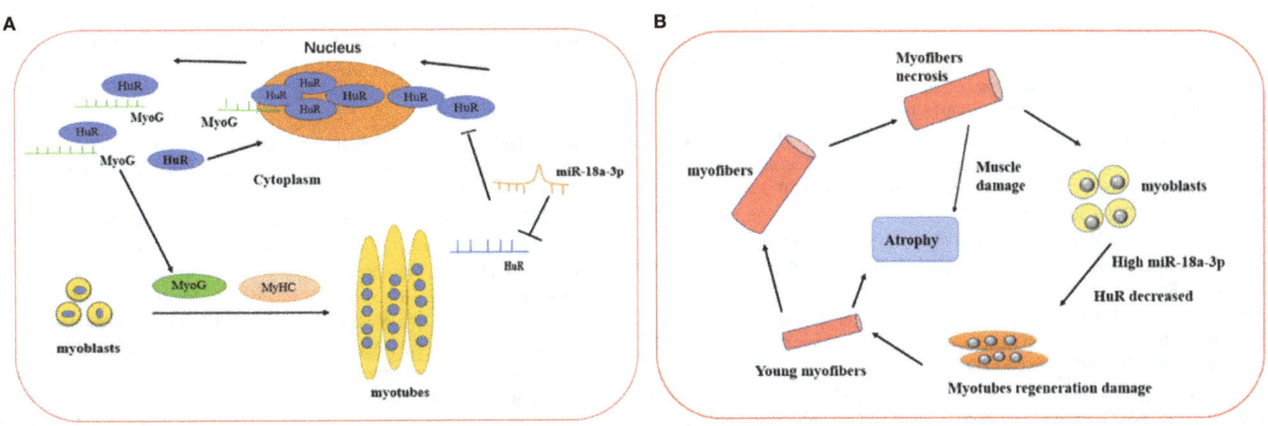

FIGURE 6 | Proposed mechanisms of miR-18a-3p and its target HuR in the IMNM pathogenesis and healthy controls. **(A)** The physical role of miR-18a-3p and HuR in the myogenesis of skeletal muscle. miR-18a-3p is mainly involved in the post-transcriptional regulation of HuR to inhibit HuR expression. HuR is abundantly localized to the cytoplasm in differentiating myoblasts, which promotes the fusion of myoblasts to form myotubes by stabilizing several myogenic regulatory factor mRNAs such as MyoG. After the myogenesis, HuR returns into the nucleus in the differentiated myotubes. **(B)** The proposed mechanisms of miR-18a-3p and HuR in the IMNM pathogenesis. Skeletal muscle was damaged and necrosis, which lead to highly expressed miR-18a-3p and decreased HuR, then myoblast regeneration was impaired by the complex interaction of miR-18a-3p and HuR. Ultimately, the skeletal muscle prompt to atrophy.

ETHICS STATEMENT

The studies involving human participants were reviewed and approved by Ethical Review Committee of the China-Japan Friendship Hospital. The patients/participants provided their written informed consent to participate in this study. Written informed consent was obtained from the individual(s) for the publication of any potentially identifiable images or data included in this article.

AUTHOR CONTRIBUTIONS

LY, YZ, GW, and XS participated in the conception and design of the experiments. LY and YZ performed the experiments and data analysis. LY, YZ, and XS wrote the manuscript. FC, QP, XL, and GW supervised the manuscript. All authors contributed to the article and approved the submitted version.

ACKNOWLEDGMENTS

The authors thank the Central Laboratory of China-Japan Friendship Hospital for their assistance in Western blot imaging.

REFERENCES

1. Pinal-Fernandez I, Casal-Dominguez M, Mammen AL. Immune-Mediated Necrotizing Myopathy. *Curr Rheumatol Rep* (2018) 20(4):21. doi: 10.1007/s11926-018-0732-6
2. Allenbach Y, Benveniste O, Stenzel W, Boyer O. Immune-Mediated Necrotizing Myopathy: Clinical Features and Pathogenesis. *Nat Rev Rheumatol* (2020) 16(12):689–701. doi: 10.1038/s41584-020-00515-9
3. Arouche-Delaperche L, Allenbach Y, Amelin D, Mouly V, Mauhin W, Tchoupou GD, et al. Pathogenic Role of Anti-Signal Recognition Protein and Anti-3-Hydroxy-3-Methylglutaryl-CoA Reductase Antibodies in Necrotizing Myopathies: Myofiber Atrophy and Impairment of Muscle Regeneration in Necrotizing Autoimmune Myopathies. *Ann Neurol* (2017) 81(4):538–48. doi: 10.1002/ana.24902
4. Mok GF, Lozano-Velasco E, Münsterberg A. microRNAs in Skeletal Muscle Development. *Semin Cell Dev Biol* (2017) 72:67–76. doi: 10.1016/j.semcdb.2017.10.032
5. Ventura A, Young AG, Winslow MM, Lintault L, Meissner A, Erkeland SJ, et al. Targeted Deletion Reveals Essential and Overlapping Functions of the miR-17 Through 92 Family of miRNA Clusters. *Cell* (2008) 5):875–86. doi: 10.1016/j.cell.2008.02.019
6. Xiao C, Srinivasan L, Calado DP, Patterson HC, Patterson HC, Zhang B, et al. Lymphoproliferative Disease and Autoimmunity in Mice With Increased miR-17-92 Expression in Lymphocytes. *Nat Immunol* (2008) 9(4):405–14. doi: 10.1038/ni1575
7. Kong D, He M, Yang L, Zhou R, Yan YQ, Liang Y, et al. MiR-17 and miR-19 Cooperatively Promote Skeletal Muscle Cell Differentiation. *Cell Mol Life Sci* (2019) 76(24):5041–54. doi: 10.1007/s00018-019-03165-7
8. Sugiyama Y, Yoshimi R, Takeno M, Kunishita Y, Kishimoto D, Kamiyama R, et al. miR-1 Is a Novel Biomarker for Polymyositis/Dermatomyositis-Associated Interstitial Lung Disease. *Mod Rheumatol* (2020) 30(5):878–83. doi: 10.1080/14397595.2019.1661584
9. Gao S, Luo H, Zhang H, Zuo X, Wang L, Zhu H. Using Multi-Omics Methods to Understand Dermatomyositis/Polymyositis. *Autoimmun Rev* (2017) 16 (10):1044–48. doi: 10.1016/j.autrev.2017.07.021
10. Parkes JE, Day PJ, Chinoy H, Lamb JA. The Role of microRNAs in the Idiopathic Inflammatory Myopathies. *Curr Opin Rheumatol* (2015) 27 (6):608–15. doi: 10.1097/bor.0000000000000225
11. Jiang T, Huang Y, Liu H, Xu Q, Gong Y, Chen Y, et al. Reduced miR-146a Promotes REG3A Expression and Macrophage Migration in Polymyositis and Dermatomyositis. *Front Immunol* (2020) 11:37. doi: 10.3389/fimmu.2020.00037
12. Kinder TB, Heier CR, Tully CB, van der Muelen JH, Hoffman EP, Nagaraju K, et al. Muscle Weakness in Myositis: MicroRNA-Mediated Dystrophin Reduction in a Myositis Mouse Model and Human Muscle Biopsies. *Arthritis Rheumatol* (2020) 72(7):1170–83. doi: 10.1002/art.41215
13. Ye L, Zuo Y, Yang H, Li W. Peng Q, Lu X, et al. Specific Autoantibodies and Clinical Phenotypes Correlate With the Aberrant Expression of Immune-Related MicroRNAs in Dermatomyositis. *J Immunol Res* (2019) 2019:2927061. doi: 10.1155/2019/2927061
14. Van der Giessen K, Di-Marco S, Clair E, Gallouzi IE. RNAi-Mediated HuR Depletion Leads to the Inhibition of Muscle Cell Differentiation. *J Biol Chem* (2003) 278(47):47119–28. doi: 10.1074/jbc.M308889200
15. Von Roretz C, Beauchamp P, Di Marco S, Gallouzi IE. HuR and Myogenesis: Being in the Right Place at the Right Time. *Biochim Biophys Acta* (2011) 1813 (9):1663–67. doi: 10.1016/j.bbamcr.2011.01.036
16. Figueroa A, Cuadrado A, Fan J, Atasoy U, Muscat GE, Muñoz-Canoves P, et al. Role of HuR in Skeletal Myogenesis Through Coordinate Regulation of Muscle Differentiation Genes. *Mol Cell Biol* (2003) 23(14):4991–5004. doi: 10.1128/mcb.23.14.4991-5004.2003
17. Allenbach Y, Mammen AL, Benveniste O, Stenzel W. 224th ENMC International Workshop: Clinico-Sero-Pathological Classification of Immune-Mediated Necrotizing Myopathies. Zandvoort, The Netherlands, 14-16 October 2016. *Neuromuscul Disord* (2018) 28(1):87–99. doi: 10.1016/j.nmd.2017.09.016
18. Rider LG, Feldman BM, Perez MD, Rennebohm RM, Lindsley CB, Zemel LS, et al. Development of Validated Disease Activity and Damage Indices for the Juvenile Idiopathic Inflammatory Myopathies: I. Physician, Parent, and Patient Global Assessments. Juvenile Dermatomyositis Disease Activity Collaborative Study Group. *Arthritis Rheum* (1997) 40(11):1976–83. doi: 10.1002/art.1780401109
19. Kim M, Park Y, Kwon Y, Kim Y, Byun J, Jeong MS, et al. MiR-135-5p-P62 Axis Regulates Autophagic Flux, Tumorigenic Potential, and Cellular Interactions Mediated by Extracellular Vesicles During Allergic Inflammation. *Front Immunol* (2019) 10:738. doi: 10.3389/fimmu.2019.00738
20. Kozomara A, Birgaoanu M, Griffiths-Jones S. Mirbase: From microRNA Sequences to Function. *Nucleic Acids Res* (2019) 47(1):155–62. doi: 10.1093/nar/gky1141
21. Bassel-Duby R, Olson EN. Signaling Pathways in Skeletal Muscle Remodeling. *Annu Rev Biochem* (2006) 75:19–37. doi: 10.1146/annurev.biochem.75.103004.142622
22. Chen W, Liu D, Li QZ, Zhu H. The Function of ncRNAs in Rheumatic Diseases. *Epigenomics* (2019) 11(7):821–33. doi: 10.2217/epi-2018-0135
23. Eisenberg I, Eran A, Nishino I, Moggio M, Lamperti C, Amato A, et al. Distinctive Patterns of microRNA Expression in Primary Muscular Disorders. *Proc Natl Acad Sci USA* (2007) 104(43):17016–21. doi: 10.1073/pnas.0708115104
24. Güller I, Russell AP. MicroRNAs in Skeletal Muscle: Their Role and Regulation in Development, Disease and Function. *J Physiol* (2010) 588 (pt21):4075–87. doi: 10.1113/jphysiol.2010.194175
25. Georgantas RW, Streicher K, Greenberg SA, Greenlees LM, Zhu W, Brohawn PZ, et al. Inhibition of Myogenic microRNAs 1, 133, and 206 by Inflammatory Cytokines Links Inflammation and Muscle Degeneration in Adult Inflammatory Myopathies. *Arthritis Rheumatol* (2014) 66(4):1022–33. doi: 10.1002/art.38292
26. Mogilyansky E, Rigoutsos I. The miR-17/92 Cluster: A Comprehensive Update on Its Genomics, Genetics, Functions and Increasingly Important and Numerous Roles in Health and Disease. *Cell Death Differ* (2013) 20 (12):1603–14. doi: 10.1038/cdd.2013.125

27. Liu QC, Zha XH, Faralli H, Yin H, Louis-Jeune C, Perdiguero E, et al. Comparative Expression Profiling Identifies Differential Roles for Myogenin and P38α MAPK Signaling in Myogenesis. *J Mol Cell Biol* (2012) 4(6):386–97. doi: 10.1093/jmcb/mjs045
28. Qiu H, Liu N, Luo L, Zhong J, Tang Z, Kang K, et al. MicroRNA-17-92 Regulates Myoblast Proliferation and Differentiation by Targeting the ENH1/Id1 Signaling Axis. *Cell Death Differ* (2016) 23(10):1658–69. doi: 10.1038/cdd.2016.56
29. Schultz CW, Preet R, Dhir T, Dixon DA, Brody JR. Understanding and Targeting the Disease-Related RNA Binding Protein Human Antigen R (HuR). *Wiley Interdiscip Rev RNA* (2020) 11(3):e1581. doi: 10.1002/wrna.1581
30. van der Giessen K, Gallouzi IE. Involvement of Transportin 2-Mediated HuR Import in Muscle Cell Differentiation. *Mol Biol Cell* (2007) 18(7):2619–29. doi: 10.1091/mbc.e07-02-0167
31. Suzuki E, Tsutsumi A, Sugihara M, Mamura M, Goto D, Matsumoto I, et al. Expression of TNF-Alpha, Tristetraprolin, T-Cell Intracellular Antigen-1 and Hu Antigen R Genes in Synovium of Patients With Rheumatoid Arthritis. *Int J Mol Med* (2006) 18(2):273–8. doi: 10.3892/ijmm.18.2.273
32. Srikantan S, Gorospe M. HuR Function in Disease. *Front Biosci (Landmark Ed)* (2012) 17:189–205. doi: 10.2741/3921

5

Hsp90 Levels in Idiopathic Inflammatory Myopathies and Their Association With Muscle Involvement and Disease Activity

Hana Štorkánová [1,2†], Sabína Oreská [1,2†], Maja Špiritović [1,3†], Barbora Heřmánková [3†], Kristýna Bubová [1,2†], Olga Kryštůfková [1,2†], Heřman Mann [1,2†], Martin Komarc [4†], Kryštof Slabý [5†], Karel Pavelka [1,2†], Ladislav Šenolt [1,2†], Josef Zámečník [6†], Jiří Vencovský [1,2†] and Michal Tomčík [1,2†]*

[1] Institute of Rheumatology, Prague, Czechia, [2] Department of Rheumatology, 1st Faculty of Medicine, Charles University, Prague, Czechia, [3] Department of Physiotherapy, Faculty of Physical Education and Sport, Charles University, Prague, Czechia, [4] Department of Methodology, Faculty of Physical Education and Sport, Charles University, Prague, Czechia, [5] Department of Rehabilitation and Sports Medicine, 2nd Faculty of Medicine, Charles University and University Hospital Motol, Prague, Czechia, [6] Department of Pathology and Molecular Medicine, 2nd Faculty of Medicine, Charles University and University Hospital Motol, Prague, Czechia

***Correspondence:**
Michal Tomčík
tomcik@revma.cz

Background: Heat shock proteins (Hsp) are chaperones playing essential roles in skeletal muscle physiology, adaptation to exercise or stress, and activation of inflammatory cells. We aimed to assess Hsp90 in patients with idiopathic inflammatory myopathies (IIM) and its association with IIM-related features.

Methods: Hsp90 plasma levels were analyzed in a cross-sectional cohort (277 IIM patients and 157 healthy controls [HC]) and two longitudinal cohorts to assess the effect of standard-of-care pharmacotherapy (n=39 in early disease and n=23 in established disease). Hsp90 and selected cytokines/chemokines were measured by commercially available ELISA and human Cytokine 27-plex Assay.

Results: Hsp90 plasma levels were increased in IIM patients compared to HC (median [IQR]: 20.2 [14.3–40.1] vs 9.8 [7.5–13.8] ng/mL, p<0.0001). Elevated Hsp90 was found in IIM patients with pulmonary, cardiac, esophageal, and skeletal muscle involvement, with higher disease activity or damage, and with elevated muscle enzymes and crucial cytokines/chemokines involved in the pathogenesis of myositis (p<0.05 for all). Plasma Hsp90 decreased upon pharmacological treatment in both patients with early and established disease. Notably, Hsp90 plasma levels were slightly superior to traditional biomarkers, such as C-reactive protein and creatine kinase, in differentiating IIM from HC, and IIM patients with cardiac involvement and interstitial lung disease from those without these manifestations.

Conclusions: Hsp90 is increased systemically in patients with IIM. Plasma Hsp90 could become an attractive soluble biomarker of disease activity and damage and a potential predictor of treatment response in IIM.

Keywords: heat shock protein 90, idiopathic inflammatory myopathies, skeletal muscle involvement, disease activity, disease damage, response to treatment

INTRODUCTION

Idiopathic inflammatory myopathies (IIM) are a heterogeneous group of rare acquired diseases characterized by inflammatory, immune-mediated skeletal muscle involvement associated with mostly painless, symmetric, and predominantly proximal muscle weakness and low muscle endurance. In addition, IIM may also affect the skin and internal organs, mostly the lungs, esophagus, and heart (1). Based on specific clinical and immunological features and histopathology of the skeletal muscle, IIM can be classified into four major subtypes: polymyositis (PM), dermatomyositis (DM), inclusion body myositis (IBM), and immune-mediated necrotizing myopathy (IMNM) (2). Although the exact mechanisms of pathogenesis are still ill-defined, these complex autoimmune disorders are believed to develop as a consequence of abnormal immune activation and non-immune mechanisms, such as autophagy dysregulation, the presence of free radicals, and endoplasmic reticulum (ER) stress (3). ER stress leads to non-immune mediated muscle damage, accumulated unfolded proteins, and imbalanced muscular protein homeostasis (3, 4). Processes caused by ER stress activate heat-shock protein (Hsp) response to protect muscle cells against protein accumulation and inflammation (3, 5).

Heat shock proteins belong to a large family of molecular chaperones, which were discovered upon exposing cells to higher temperatures. Their primary role is to stabilize, activate, and protect proteins against degradation in the proteasome (6). Hsp90 is a highly ubiquitous ATP-dependent molecular chaperone, which is involved in several biological processes, e.g., controlling cell cycle and survival, maintaining homeostasis, stabilizing and activating cellular proteins. It plays an important role in the innate and adaptive immune system through activation and maturation of antigen-presenting cells and induction of pro-inflammatory cytokines [e.g., interleukin (IL)-1β, IL-12, and tumor necrosis factor (TNF)] (6, 7). Hsp90 also participates in autoimmune response, oncogenesis, viral infections, and neurodegenerative diseases (7–10).

To date, only a few studies examined the role of Hsp90 in rheumatic diseases. In rheumatoid arthritis (RA), an association of serum Hsp90 with disease activity and systemic inflammation was found despite the lack of significant differences between patients and healthy controls (11). Similarly, increased Hsp90 expression in peripheral blood mononuclear cells was detected in patients with more active systemic lupus erythematosus (SLE) (12). Our previous study described an increased expression of Hsp90 in the involved skin of scleroderma (SSc) patients and demonstrated its pro-fibrotic properties both *in vitro* and *in vivo* (13). Recently, we demonstrated a potential therapeutic application of Hsp90 inhibitors in SSc and showed increased Hsp90 plasma levels in SSc patients, predominantly in patients with skin and lung involvement (14, 15). In axial spondyloarthritis (ax-SpA), we observed elevated Hsp90 plasma levels, which were associated with inflammation of the sacroiliac joints (16). A potential role of Hsp90 in IIM was investigated by De Paepe et al., who described an increased local expression of Hsp90 in muscle biopsy samples from patients with PM, DM, and IBM, specifically in the regenerating and atrophic muscle fibers, and in macrophages and cytotoxic T-cells actively invading non-necrotic muscle fibers. In spite of the potentially protective effect of Hsp90 expression in regenerating muscle fibers, more evidence suggests the negative and pro-inflammatory role of Hsp90 in IIM (17–19).

Given the lack of organ- and disease-specific biomarkers for IIM, we aimed to examine the systemic levels of Hsp90 in patients with IIM and in healthy individuals, to analyze their association with IIM-related clinical features, and to evaluate their response to pharmacological intervention.

MATERIALS AND METHODS

Patients and Healthy Controls

For the cross-sectional analysis of systemic levels of Hsp90, plasma samples were obtained from 277 Caucasian patients with IIM and 157 healthy Caucasian individuals. In total, two longitudinal cohorts (LC) were included to assess the effect of standard-of-care pharmacological therapy (LC1, LC2). LC1 included consecutively recruited IIM patients from the cross-sectional cohort with a short disease duration (≤ 6 months since the first symptom). Additionally, patients in LC1 had plasma samples and clinical data available at the 6-month and 12-month follow-ups after treatment initiation. LC2 was comprised of consecutively recruited IIM patients with established disease and ongoing treatment. Patients in LC2 had plasma samples and clinical data available at the 6-month follow-up after treatment initiation, and were originally recruited as a control group (i.e., treated with a standard-of-care pharmacotherapy only) in our recently published study on physiotherapy intervention in IIM patients (20). Patients with DM and PM were diagnosed using the Bohan and Peter classification criteria (21), and patients with IMNM fulfilled the definite or probable criteria of the European Neuromuscular Centre (ENMC) (22). Patients with dermatomyositis who developed cancer within three years of the diagnosis were classified as CDM (23). General age-appropriate screening was performed in all IIM patients; it was guided by clinical suspicion and included basic noninvasive examinations, such as chest X-ray, ultrasound of the abdomen, fecal occult blood, and gynecological evaluation or prostate-specific antigen analysis. For patients with DM and positivity of anti-TIF1-γ, anti-NXP2, or anti-SAE, and for patients without other myositis-specific antibodies (MSAs) or myositis-associated antibodies (MAAs), an additional extensive malignancy screening was performed, including serum cancer markers, comprehensive blood tests, whole-body PET-CT or CT scans of the chest, abdomen, and pelvis.

Clinical Evaluation

All patients have been clinically evaluated and treated at the Institute of rheumatology in Prague (IoRP) from 2007 by a board-certified rheumatologist experienced in diagnosing and treating IIM (JV, HM, OK) according to international guidelines (24). Physical functioning and clinical disease activity were assessed by the core set measures of disease activity proposed by the International Myositis Assessment & Clinical Studies Group (IMACS): myositis disease activity assessment tool (MDAAT), which includes the assessment of muscle disease activity (MDA) and physician global assessment of disease activity using the visual analogue scale (VAS), manual muscle testing (MMT) and the health assessment questionnaire (HAQ) (25). In addition to MMT8, we routinely measured muscle strength also in m. triceps brachii and m. iliopsoas. The myositis damage index (MDI) was used to evaluate IIM associated damage (25). All participants gave informed consent prior to participation. Our research was approved by the Ethics Committee of the IoRP. All methods were performed in accordance with the relevant guidelines and regulations.

Laboratory Measurements

Peripheral blood samples were collected into commercially available EDTA-treated tubes, immediately centrifuged, and stored at -80°C until use. Serum levels of C-reactive protein (CRP), creatine phosphokinase (CK), lactate dehydrogenase (LD), alanine aminotransferase (ALT), aspartate aminotransferase (AST), and myoglobin (Mb) were determined using Beckman CoulterAU 680 analyzer (Beckman Coulter, USA). Erythrocyte sedimentation rate (ESR) was measured according to the Fahreus and Westergren method. Antinuclear antibodies (ANA) were detected using indirect immunofluorescence on HEP2 cells (ImmunoConcepts, Sacramento, CA, USA), and the MSAs and MAAs were determined by Myositis Line Immunoassay (IMTEC, Berlin, Germany) (detects anti-Mi-2, anti-PM-Scl, anti-Jo-1, anti-PL-7, anti-PL-12 antibodies) and Myositis Westernblot (Euroimmun, Lübeck, Germany) (detects anti-Mi-2, anti-TIF1-γ, anti-MDA5, anti-NXP2, anti-SAE, anti-Jo-1, anti-SRP, anti-PL-7, anti-PL-12, anti-EJ, anti-OJ antibodies). Plasma Hsp90 was quantified using a commercially available high-sensitive ELISA kit (eBioscience, Vienna, Austria) according to the manufacturer's protocol. The calculated sensitivity is 0.03 ng/mL, and the absorbance value was determined at 450 nm by an ELISA reader (SUNRISE; Tecan, Grödig, Austria). The plasma concentrations of selected cytokines/chemokines were measured by a commercially available Bio-Plex Pro™ human Cytokine 27-plex Assay (BIO-RAD, California, USA) according to the manufacturer's instruction. This kit measures the concentration of 27 cytokines, chemokines or growth factors: interleukin (IL)-1β, IL-1RA, IL-2, IL-4, IL-5, IL-6, IL-7, IL-8, IL-9, IL-10, IL-12 (p70), IL-13, IL-15, IL-17A, eotaxin, fibroblast growth factor (FGF) basic, granulocyte colony-stimulating factor (G-CSF), granulocyte-macrophage colony-stimulating factor (GM-CSF), interferon-γ (IFN-γ), interferon gamma-induced protein (IP)-10, monocyte chemoattractant protein (MCP)-1 (CCL2), macrophage inflammatory proteins (MIP)-1α (CCL3), MIP-1β (CCL4), platelet-derived growth factor (PDGF)-bb, regulated on activation/normal T cell expressed and secreted (RANTES, CCL5), tumor necrosis factor (TNF), and vascular endothelial growth factor (VEGF). The absorbance of the Bio-Plex Pro™ human Cytokine 27-plex Assay (BIO-RAD, California, USA) was established by Luminex BIO-PLEX 200 System (Bio-Rad, California, USA). Samples were measured as duplicates and the mean value was used.

Statistical Analysis

Basic descriptive statistics (mean, median, interquartile range [IQR], skewness, and kurtosis) were computed for all variables, which were subsequently tested for normality using the Kolmogorov–Smirnov and Shapiro-Wilk tests. Differences in interval variables (e.g., Hsp90) were evaluated using the Mann-Whitney U test, while the chi-square test was used to compare frequency counts of categorical variables (e.g., gender). The bivariate relationships between variables under study were assessed using the Spearman correlation coefficient. A correlation coefficient (r) of 0.1 to 0.3 was considered weak, 0.3 to 0.5 was considered moderate, and 0.5 to 1.0 was considered strong. Multivariate regression analysis was used to predict patients' Hsp90 levels by a set of predictors (levels of muscle enzymes, MITAX, and current prednisone equivalent dose). Repeated longitudinal measurements were analyzed by one-way repeated ANOVA followed by *post hoc* comparisons. Diagnostic utility of Hsp90 plasma levels was assessed by the receiver operating characteristic (ROC) curve and area under the curve (AUC) analyses. Data are presented as median (IQR) unless stated otherwise. Statistical significance was set at $p<0.05$. All analyses were conducted using SPSS version 25 (SPSS, Inc., Chicago, IL, USA). Graphs were created using GraphPad Prism 5 (version 5.02; GraphPad Software, La Jolla, CA, USA).

RESULTS

Characteristics of Patients

The cross-sectional study group comprised 104 patients with PM, 104 patients with DM, 42 patients with cancer-associated dermatomyositis (CDM), and 27 patients with IMNM. The clinical and demographic characteristics of this cohort are shown in **Table 1**. The median interval between the diagnosis of cancer and the subsequent diagnosis of DM (n=19) was 24 months, whereas the median interval between the diagnosis of DM and the subsequent confirmation of cancer (n=23) was 3 months. The most prevalent malignancies involved the breast (29%), ovaries (17%), lung (12%), kidney (10%), thymus (10%), and esophagus, urinary bladder, and liver (5% each). Cancer of the cervix, lymph nodes, skin, and large intestines was present in one patient each. The most prevalent antibodies in CDM patients included anti-TIF1-γ (43%), anti-Ro-52 (17%), anti-Mi-2 (12%),

TABLE 1 | Clinical and demographic characteristics of IIM patients and healthy controls: cross-sectional cohort.

Parameters	IIM patients (n=277)	Healthy controls (n=157)	p-value
Sex: Female/Male, n (%)	198 (71)/79 (29)	92 (59)/65 (41)	0.006
Age, years	56.5 (45.9 – 64.4)	46.0 (34.0 – 60.0)	0.001
Clinical features			
Disease duration, years	1.7 (0.6 – 5.9)		
IIM subtype, n (%): PM/DM/	104 (37.5)/104 (37.5)/		
CDM/IMNM	42 (15)/27 (10)		
IIM-associated symptoms, n (%):			
MW/SR/MH/RP/	236 (85)/133 (48)/96 (35)/78 (28)/		
A/ILD/CI/D	76 (27)/126 (45)/50 (18)/120 (43)		
MITAX	0.13 (0.08 – 0.21)		
MYOACT	0.05 (0.02 – 0.12)		
MDI extent	0.08 (0.03 – 0.14)		
MDI severity	0.03 (0.01 – 0.06)		
MDI extended	0.08 (0.00 – 0.13)		
MMT-8	65.0 (55.0 – 74.0)		
HAQ	0.9 (0.3 – 1.5)		
Laboratory features			
Autoantibodies, n (%):			
ANA/Ro-52/Jo-1/TIF1/PM-Scl/	124 (45)/80 (29)/64 (23)/21 (8)/29 (11)/		
Mi-2/Ro-60/HMGCR/SRP/U1RNP/MDA5/	20 (7)/18 (6.5)/14 (5)/10 (4)/9 (3)/6 (2.2)/		
La/PL-7/Ku/SAE/NXP2	4 (1.4)/3 (1.1)/2 (0.7)/2 (0.7)/1 (0.4)		
CRP, mg/L	2.5 (1.3 – 6.3)		
CK, µkat/L	2.6 (0.9 – 12.4)		
LD, µkat/L	4.8 (3.5 – 7.4)		
Current treatment			
Prednisone equivalent dose, mg/day	20.0 (7.5 – 47.5)		
GC/MTX/AZA/	227 (82)/83 (30)/22 (8)/		
CPA/CSA, n (%)	1 (0.3)/5 (2)		

Data are presented as median (inter-quartile range) unless stated otherwise; A, arthritis; ANA, antinuclear antibodies; AZA, azathioprine; CDM, cancer-associated dermatomyositis; CI, cardiac involvement; CK, creatine kinase; CPA, cyclophosphamide; CRP, C-reactive protein; CSA, cyclosporin A; D, dysphagia; DM, dermatomyositis; GC, glucocorticoids; HAQ, Health Assessment Questionnaire; HMGCR, anti-3-hydroxy-3-methylglutaryl-CoA reductase; IIM, idiopathic inflammatory myopathy; ILD, interstitial lung disease; IMNM, immune-mediated necrotizing myopathy; Jo-1, anti-histidyl-tRNA synthetase; Ku, anti-Ku (against the nuclear DNA-dependent protein kinase subunit); La, anti-La (against La(SS-B), a nuclear 47 kD phosphoprotein, associated with small RNA synthesized by RNA polymerase III); LD, lactate dehydrogenase; MDA5, anti-CADM-140 (melanoma differentiation-associated gene 5); MDI, Myositis Damage Index; MH, mechanic's hands; Mi-2, antinuclear helicase 218/240 kDa; MITAX, Myositis Intention to Treat Activity Index; MMT-8, Manual Muscle Testing of eight muscles; MTX, methotrexate; MW, muscle weakness; MYOACT, Myositis Disease Activity Assessment visual analogue scale; NXP2, anti-NXP2 (nuclear matrix protein); PL-7, anti-threonyl-tRNA synthetase; PM, polymyositis; PM-Scl, anti-Pm-Scl (anti-core complex 11-16 proteins); Ro, anti-Ro (52/60kDa, against cytoplasmic RNA and associated peptides); RP, Raynaud's phenomenon; SAE, anti-SUMO1 (small ubiquitin-like modifier 1) activating enzyme; SR, skin rash; SRP, anti-signal recognition particles; TIF1, anti-TIF1 (transcriptional intermediary factor-1); U1RNP, anti-U1-RNP (ribonucleoprotein).

and anti-PM-Scl (5%). Whereas anti-NXP2, anti-Jo-1, and anti-Ro-60 were present only in one patient each; 7 patients (17%) had no detectable MSAs or MAAs.

The first longitudinal cohort (LC1) comprised 39 Caucasian IIM patients from the cross-sectional cohort, including 11 treatment-naïve patients and 28 patients with a short disease duration (median disease duration: 1.2 months), who recently started pharmacological treatment. The clinical and demographic characteristics of this cohort are shown in **Table 2**.

The second longitudinal cohort (LC2) comprised 23 Caucasian IIM patients with established disease (median disease duration: 2.8 years) and ongoing pharmacological treatment. The clinical and demographic characteristics of this cohort are shown in **Supplementary Table 1**.

Plasma Hsp90 in Patients With Idiopathic Inflammatory Myopathies and in Healthy Controls: A Cross-Sectional Analysis

We observed increased plasma levels of Hsp90 in all IIM patients (n=277) compared to healthy individuals (n=157) (median [inter-quartile range]: 20.2 [14.3–40.1] vs 9.8 [7.5–13.8] ng/mL, p<0.0001). Circulating Hsp90 levels were also elevated in all individual subgroups of IIM compared to healthy controls (PM: 19.7 [14.3–42.2], DM: 22.0 [14.1–41.2], CDM: 18.9 [11.7–29.7], IMNM: 19.6 [16.3–45.5] ng/mL, p<0.0001 for all comparisons) (**Figure 1A**). Since healthy controls were significantly younger with a higher proportion of males compared to our IIM cohort (**Table 1**), additional analysis was performed, and all above-mentioned differences remained statistically significant (p<0.001 for all) even after adjusting for age and sex (using a general linear model). Interestingly, no significant differences among all four subsets of IIM were detected (p>0.05 for all comparisons) **(Figure 1A)**.

Hsp90 Plasma Levels in Relation to Disease-Related Features: A Cross-Sectional Analysis

Increased Hsp90 plasma levels were found in male patients and those with IIM-associated interstitial lung disease, cardiac involvement, dysphagia, the positivity of anti-Ro (52kDa) antibodies, and current use of conventional synthetic

TABLE 2 | Baseline clinical characteristics of treatment-naïve and early-disease IIM patients treated with standard-of-care pharmacological therapy: longitudinal cohort 1.

Parameters	Baseline (Month 0) (n=39)	Month 6 (n=39)	Month 12 (n=39)
Sex: Female/Male, n (%)	29 (74)/10 (26)		
Age, years	57.1 (53.2 – 63.3)		
Clinical features			
Disease duration, months	1.2 (0.0 – 2.8)		
IIM subtype, n (%): PM/DM/	13 (33)/18 (46)/		
IMNM	8 (21)		
IIM-associated symptoms, n (%): MW/SR/MH/	39 (100)/24 (62)/14 (36)/		
RP/A/ILD/	10 (26)/10 (26)/26 (67)/		
CI/D	8 (21)/21 (54)		
MITAX	0.2 (0.1 – 0.3)		
MYOACT	0.1 (0.03 – 0.2)		
MDI extent	0.11 (0.03 – 0.13)		
MMT-8	65.0 (55.0 – 71.0)		
HAQ	0.9 (0.4 – 1.4)		
Laboratory features			
Autoantibodies, n (%): ANA/Ro-52/Jo-1/TIF1/	15 (38)/11 (28)/11 (28)/1 (3)/		
PM-Scl/Mi-2/HMGCR/Ro-60/SRP/U1RNP	4 (10)/4 (10)/4 (10)/3(7)//2 (6)/1 (3)		
CRP, mg/L	2.7 (1.3 – 8.1)	2.2 (1.0 – 8.6)	1.6 (0.9 – 15.0)
CK, μkat/L	3.8 (1.3 – 18.3)	1.4 (0.6 – 7.3)	1.4 (0.7 – 3.7)
LD, μkat/L	5.9 (4.0 – 8.5)	4.0 (3.5 – 6.2)	4.1 (3.0 – 4.9)
Current treatment:			
Prednisone equivalent dose, mg/day	20 (0 – 50)	20 (10 – 25)	10 (7.5 – 20)
MTX/AZA, n (%)	9 (23)/3 (8)	14 (36)/5 (13)	12 (31)/9 (23)

Data are presented as median (inter-quartile range) unless stated otherwise; A, arthritis; ANA, antinuclear antibodies; AZA, azathioprine; CDM, cancer-associated dermatomyositis; CI, cardiac involvement; CK, creatine kinase; CRP, C-reactive protein; D, dysphagia; DM, dermatomyositis; HAQ, Health Assessment Questionnaire; HMGCR, anti-3-hydroxy-3-methylglutaryl-CoA reductase; IIM, idiopathic inflammatory myopathy; ILD, interstitial lung disease; IMNM, immune-mediated necrotizing myopathy; Jo-1, anti-histidyl-tRNA synthetase; LD, lactate dehydrogenase; MDI, Myositis Damage Index; MH, mechanic's hands; Mi-2, antinuclear helicase 218/240 kDa; MITAX, Myositis Intention to Treat Activity Index; MMT-8, Manual Muscle Testing of eight muscles; MTX, methotrexate; MW, muscle weakness; MYOACT, Myositis Disease Activity Assessment visual analogue scale; PM, polymyositis; PM-Scl, anti-Pm-Scl (anti-core complex 11-16 proteins); Ro, anti-Ro (52/60kDa, against cytoplasmic RNA and associated peptides); RP, Raynaud's phenomenon; SR, skin rash; SRP, anti-signal recognition particles; TIF1, anti-TIF1 (transcription intermediary factor-1); U1RNP, anti-u1-rnp (ribonucleoprotein).

antirheumatic drugs (csDMARDs) ($p<0.05$ for all comparisons to patients without these features) (**Table 3**). Furthermore, the bivariate analysis demonstrated a significant association of plasma Hsp90 with several clinical and laboratory measures of disease activity and damage. A positive correlation of plasma Hsp90 was found with enzymes reflecting skeletal muscle involvement: lactate dehydrogenase (LD; strong correlation), and aspartate aminotransferase (AST; moderate correlation) (**Figures 1B, C**). In addition, increased plasma Hsp90 was weakly associated with elevated alanine aminotransferase (ALT), decreased muscle strength (decreased MMT-8 total score, specifically in the proximal muscles including m. biceps brachii, m. gluteus maximus, and m. iliopsoas), increased disease activity (MITAX, MYOACT, pulmonary and muscle disease activity, and global disease activity assessed by both the patient and the doctor), increased damage (MDI extent, severity, and extended), and higher current prednisone equivalent dose (**Supplementary Table 2**). Differences in significant disease-related predictors of plasma Hsp90 among individual subtypes of IIM are presented in **Table 4**. To validate the reliability of potential predictors of Hsp90 levels, which were established by the bivariate analysis, three main variables were selected for a multivariate regression analysis model: a composite of muscle enzymes (CK, LD, AST, and ALT), MITAX, and the current prednisone equivalent dose. However, only association with muscle enzymes remained significant ($\beta=0.358$, $p<0.001$) in this multivariate analysis model (**Supplementary Table 2**). Concentrations of extracellular Hsp90 were not significantly affected by other main clinical or laboratory parameters of IIM, such as disease duration (either from the first symptom or from the diagnosis), MSAs, or MAAs (except for anti-Ro-52) (data not shown).

In addition, weak to moderate positive correlations between Hsp90 and several crucial cytokines/chemokines involved in the pathogenesis of IIM were identified by the bivariate analysis, such as IL-1β, IL-6, IL-8, IL-17, interferon (IFN)-γ, C-X-C motif chemokine ligand 10 (CXCL10), monocyte chemoattractant protein 1 (MCP1, CCL2), macrophage inflammatory protein 1-alpha (MIP-1-α, CCL3), MIP-1-β (CCL4), vascular endothelial growth factor (VEGF), and platelet-derived growth factor (PDGF-BB) ($p<0.05$ for all correlations) (**Table 5**).

The Impact of Pharmacotherapy on Plasma Hsp90: A Longitudinal Analysis (LC1 and LC2)

The potential effect of the standard-of-care pharmacotherapy was assessed in two independent cohorts of IIM patients with longitudinally collected blood samples: LC1 comprising treatment naïve patients (n=11) and patients with early disease (n=28) with recently started pharmacological treatment, and LC2 representing patients with established disease (n=23) with ongoing pharmacological treatment.

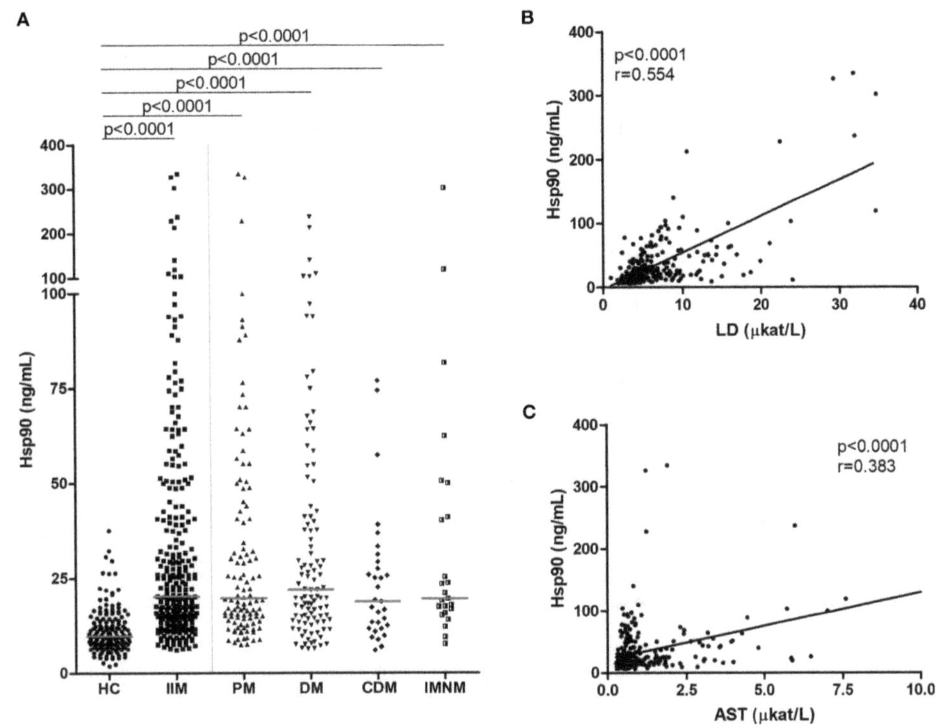

FIGURE 1 | Plasma Hsp90 levels were increased in patients with IIM compared to healthy controls and were associated with serum markers of muscle damage. **(A)** Systemic levels of Hsp90 are significantly elevated in patients with idiopathic inflammatory myopathies (IIM) and individual subtypes of IIM (PM, polymyositis; DM, dermatomyositis; CDM, cancer-associated dermatomyositis and IMNM, immune-mediated necrotizing myopathy) compared to healthy controls (HC). Horizontal bars represent the median. Increased plasma Hsp90 is associated with elevated serum levels of **(B)** lactate dehydrogenase (LD) and **(C)** aspartate aminotransferase (AST).

TABLE 3 | Elevated plasma Hsp90 in subgroups of patients with IIM.

Parameter (number of patients presented with the parameter)	Present median (IQR)	Absent median (IQR)	p-value
Male sex (n=79)	25.3 (15.6 – 50.0)	19.6 (13.4 – 35.6)	0.040
Interstitial lung disease (n=126)	25.4 (15.5 – 50.7)	18.9 (12.8 – 30.3)	0.003
Cardiac involvement (n=50)	27.5 (18.1 – 51.5)	19.3 (13.3 – 39.3)	0.004
Dysphagia (n=120)	25.0 (15.9 – 50.0)	18.2 (13.4 – 34.3)	0.018
Ro-52 (n=80)	29.6 (15.6 – 57.2)	19.2 (13.9 – 31.4)	0.001
csDMARDs (n=111)	22.0 (15.6 – 50.4)	18.9 (12.8 – 32.1)	0.014

csDMARDs, current treatment with conventional synthetic antirheumatic drugs; IIM, idiopathic inflammatory myopathies; IQR, interquartile range; Ro, anti-Ro52 autoantibodies (52 kDa, against cytoplasmic RNA and associated peptides).

In LC1, significantly increased levels of plasma Hsp90 compared to age- and sex-matched healthy controls (n=39) were found in both treatment naïve patients, in patients with early disease, and combined (healthy controls: 8.6 [6.3–11.4], treatment naïve 18.9 [15.2–27.0], early disease 25.1 [14.3–41.1], treatment naïve/early disease 25.1 [15.2–41.1] ng/mL, p<0.0001 for all mentioned comparisons). No significant differences were observed between treatment naïve patients and patients with early disease (p=0.607) (**Figure 2A**). In brief, pharmacological treatment significantly decreased the mean serum levels of LD and CK at month 6 and 12 compared to baseline (LD: by 38% and 48%; CK: by 40% and 69%, respectively, p<0.01 for all comparisons) (**Table 2**). Upon treatment, we found a significant decrease in Hsp90 plasma levels in the whole LC1 at both month 6 and 12 compared to baseline levels (baseline: 25.1 [15.2–41.1], month 6: 7.8 [5.8–11.6], month 12: 7.7 [6.6–11.8] ng/mL, p=0.0001 for both comparisons) (**Figure 2B**). The decrease in plasma Hsp90 levels over 12 months was strongly associated with the decrease in LD over 12 months (r=0.540, p=0.006) (**Figure 2C**). Moreover, baseline Hsp90 was able to predict the change in LD levels at both 6 months (r=0.370, p=0.031) (**Figure 2D**) and 12 months (r=0.458, p=0.021).

In patients with established disease (LC2), we did not observe any significant change in the mean serum levels of LD and CK at month six compared to baseline (LD: -9%, p=0.897; CK: +5%, p=0.154) (**Supplementary Table 1**). However, upon treatment,

TABLE 4 | Significant disease-related predictors of Hsp90 plasma levels in patients with individual subsets of IIM based on bivariate correlations.

	(Spearman's r; p-value)			
Parameter	**PM (n=104)**	**DM (n=104)**	**CDM (n=42)**	**IMNM (n=27)**
C-reactive protein			0.497; 0.007	
Lactate dehydrogenase	0.636; 0.001	0.574; 0.001	0.535; 0.004	0.584; 0.002
Creatine kinase				0.485; 0.014
Aspartate aminotransferase	0.485; 0.001	0.317; 0.001		0.475; 0.019
Alanine aminotransferase	0.234; 0.015		0.395; 0.042	
Manual Muscle Testing 8 (MMT-8) total		-0.210; 0.039		
Myosits intention to treat activity index (MITAX)	0.223; 0.024			0.504; 0.028
Patient disease global activity (PDGA)	0.258; 0.010	0.244; 0.016		
Doctor disease global activity (DGDA)	0.264; 0.008			0.474; 0.040
Pulmonary disease activity		0.232; 0.021		
Muscle disease activity	0.247; 0.012			
Constitutional disease activity	0.250; 0.011			
Myositis damage index (MDI) extent	0.248; 0.025	0.224; 0.049		
Myositis damage index (MDI) extended		0.270; 0.017		
Current prednisone equivalent dose	0.382; 0.001			0.450; 0.036

CDM, cancer-associated dermatomyositis; DM, dermatomyositis; IIM, idiopathic inflammatory myopathies; IMNM, immune-mediated necrotizing myopathy; PM, polymyositis.

TABLE 5 | Cytokines and chemokines involved in the pathogenesis of IIM and their correlation to plasma Hsp90 based on the bivariate analysis in all IIM patients (n=277).

Cytokine/Chemokine	**Spearman's r**	**p-value**
Interleukin 1β	0.188	0.002
Interleukin 6	0.182	0.003
Interleukin 8	0.242	<0.001
Interleukin 17	0.201	0.001
Interferon γ	0.229	<0.001
C-X-C motif chemokine ligand 10 (CXCL10)	0.224	0.001
Monocyte chemoattractant protein 1 (CCL2)	0.161	0.007
Macrophage inflammatory protein 1-α (CCL3)	0.208	<0.001
Macrophage inflammatory protein 1-β (CCL4)	0.229	<0.001
Vascular endothelial growth factor	0.260	<0.001
Platelet-derived growth factor-BB	0.426	<0.001

IIM, idiopathic inflammatory myopathies.

we also detected a significant decrease in plasma Hsp90 levels at month six compared to baseline levels (baseline: 15.7 [9.8–29.5], month 6: 12.9 [9.7–16.6] ng/mL, p=0.042) (**Figure 2E**). In line with the findings in LC1, baseline Hsp90 in LC2 was able to predict the change in LD levels at month six (r=0.447, p=0.037) (**Figure 2F**). In addition, Hsp90 baseline levels also predicted the change in AST and CK levels at month six (r=0.494, p=0.020; r=0.430, p=0.046, respectively).

Performance of Plasma Hsp90 in Comparison to Traditional Soluble Biomarkers

We evaluated the ability of plasma Hsp90 to distinguish IIM patients and its subsets (PM, DM, CDM and IMNM) from HC using the AUC-ROC analysis, and compared it to that of the traditional serum biomarkers such as CRP, CK and LD (**Supplemetary Table 3**). Plasma Hsp90 outperformed serum CRP and CK levels in discriminating between IIM vs. HC (**Supplementary Figure 1A**), as well as between PM vs. HC (**Supplementary Figure 1B**) and DM vs. HC (**Supplementary Figure 1C**), as demonstrated by higher AUC, sensitivity, specificity, and odds ratio (**Supplementary Table 3**). The discriminatory ability between CDM vs. HC (**Supplementary Figure 1D**), and IMNM vs. HC (**Supplementary Figure 1E**) was comparable between Hsp90 and CK (**Supplementary Table 3**). Notably, out of all four biomarkers, plasma Hsp90 attained slightly higher AUC for discriminating between IIM patients with and without interstitial lung disease, and with and without cardiac involvement (**Supplementary Figures 1F-G** and **Supplementary Table 3**).

DISCUSSION

In the present study, we demonstrate elevated systemic levels of Hsp90 in patients with IIM and their association with several disease-related clinical and laboratory features. To date, several different roles of Hsp90 in muscle biology have been proposed. During myogenesis, increased expression of Hsp90 and ubiquitin in regenerating myofibers suggests that both are largely regulated

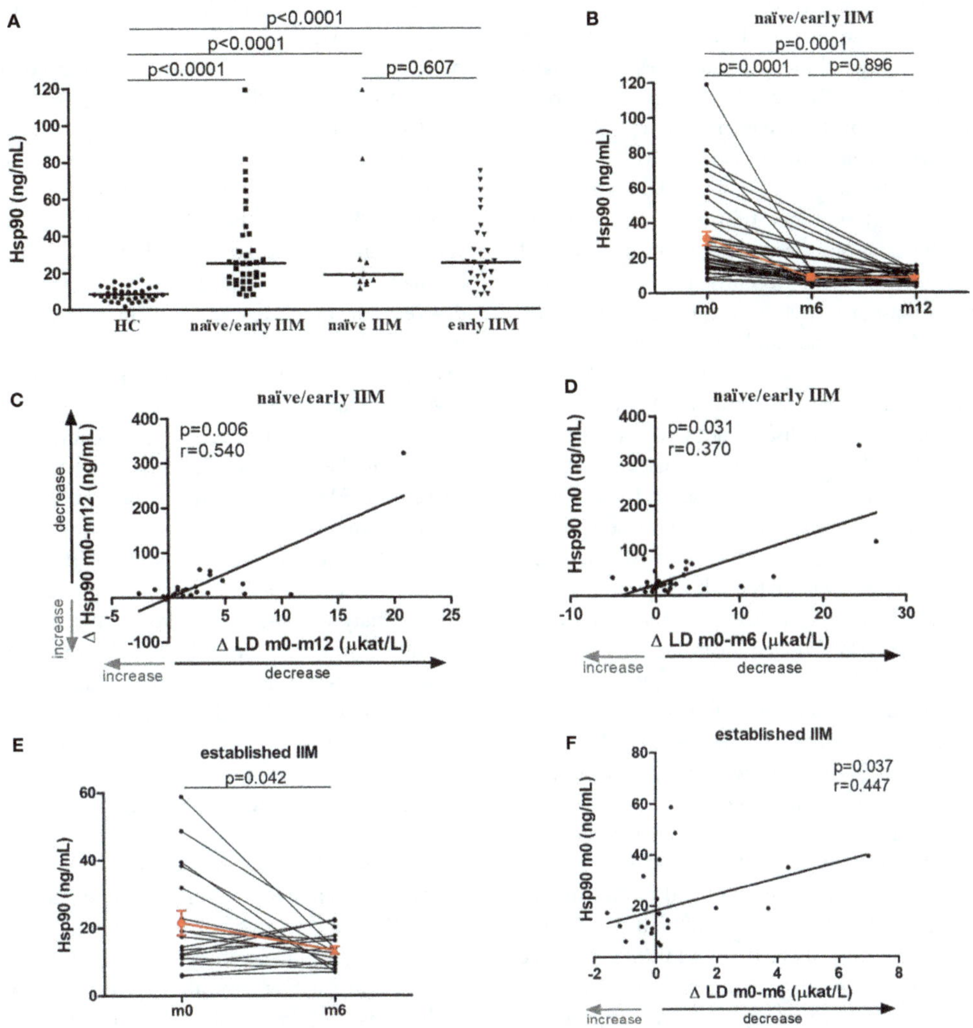

FIGURE 2 | The effect of pharmacotherapy on plasma Hsp90 levels in patients with IIM. **(A)** Plasma Hsp90 levels were increased in both treatment naïve patients with idiopathic inflammatory myopathies (naïve IIM) and patients with short disease duration with recently started pharmacological treatment (early IIM) compared to healthy controls (HC). Horizontal bars represent the median. **(B)** Upon 6 and 12 months of standard-of-care pharmacotherapy, plasma Hsp90 levels significantly decreased in treatment naïve/early IIM patients. **(C)** The 12-month change in Hsp90 was associated with the 12-month change in LD levels. **(D)** Baseline Hsp90 predicted the 6-month change in LD levels. **(E)** In IIM patients with established disease, ongoing standard-of-care pharmacotherapy resulted in a significant decrease in plasma Hsp90 levels over six months. **(F)** Baseline Hsp90 levels were able to predict the 6-month change in the levels of LD. The red line and whiskers represent the mean and standard error of the mean **(B, E)**.

by the activation of developmental mechanisms rather than by any particular disease (26). In damaged muscle fibers, De Paepe et al. propose a general protective role of Hsp90, i.e., counteracting mechanisms involved in the injury of myofibers. Whereas in PM or IBM, they suggest a specific cytotoxic role in the active invasion of myofibers by macrophages and cytotoxic T-cells, which is typically found in these subtypes of IIM (3, 17–19). Furthermore, Hsp90 alpha is secreted by activated endothelial cells and was postulated as a positive regulator of angiogenesis in wound healing (27). We hypothesize that damage to muscle fibers could be associated with an increased formation of a complex of Hsp90 with its client proteins and stabilizing peptides. However, these Hsp90-antigen complexes are recognized by antigen-presenting cells (APCs) such as macrophages or dendritic cells, and are presented by MHC class I or II molecules on APCs to CD8 or CD4 T lymphocytes, which actively invade non-necrotic muscle fibers or infiltrate the perivascular milieu (3, 17, 28). Activation of inflammatory cells leads to a release of pro-inflammatory cytokines and chemokines and an increased production of nitric oxide, which enhances the cytotoxicity of macrophages in myofibers (19, 28, 29).

Hsp are traditionally regarded as intracellular molecules. However, upon necrotic cell death and other stress stimuli, Hsp can be released into the extracellular compartment (29). In line with an increased Hsp90 expression in the involved skeletal muscles demonstrated by de Paepe et al. (17–19), herein, we demonstrate for the first time increased systemic levels of Hsp90 in IIM patients compared to healthy controls. Systemic levels of Hsp90 were comparable among all four IIM subtypes investigated (PM, DM, CDM, IMNM). Since Hsp90 is commonly overexpressed in cancer cells and secreted Hsp90 is believed to promote cancer cell invasion and metastasis (8, 30), it may be surprising that plasma Hsp90 was not actually higher in CDM, possibly due to the different volumes of the involved tissues. Increased plasma Hsp90 does not seem to be specific for IIM. Using the same methodology, our recently published studies demonstrated increased plasma Hsp90 also in patients with axial spondyloarthritis (axSpA) and SSc, and comparable levels in psoriatic arthritis (PsA) when compared to healthy individuals (15, 16). Furthermore, increased plasma Hsp90 in IIM patients was associated with several measures of disease activity (e.g., elevated serum levels of LD, AST and ALT, increased muscle weakness, higher physicians' assessment of global, muscle and pulmonary activity, MITAX, MYOACT) and damage (increased MDI). However, all of these associations (except for that with LD) were weak. Higher plasma Hsp90 was detected in patients with interstitial lung disease (ILD) or anti-Ro-52 antibodies, which are associated with ILD in IIM (31) and cardiac involvement. These findings are in line with a possible role of Hsp90 previously described in SSc-ILD, idiopathic pulmonary fibrosis, heart failure and pathological cardiac remodeling (15, 32–34). Moreover, increased Hsp90 was found in patients with dysphagia and in those currently treated with csDMARDs or with a higher prednisone equivalent dose, which is in line with elevated Hsp90 in patients with higher disease activity. Higher Hsp90 in male IIM patients could be due to a larger muscle mass and higher disease activity in males than in females (MYOACT: 0.08 [0.015-0.135] vs 0.04 [0.02-0.11], respectively, p=0.082). In addition, elevated plasma Hsp90 was weakly associated with increased systemic levels of several key pro-inflammatory and pro-angiogenic cytokines/chemokines implicated in the pathogenesis of IIM, e.g., IL-1β, IL-6, IL-8, IL-17, IFN-γ, CXCL10, CCL2-4, VEGF, and PDGF (1–3, 35–42). However, only the muscle enzymes were confirmed by multivariate analysis as the strongest predictors of plasma Hsp90 in IIM.

Due to the well-known role of Hsp90 in regulating the activity of glucocorticoid receptors (43, 44), the fact that corticosteroids remain the cornerstone therapy in IIM (1, 2), and the positive correlation between plasma Hsp90 and the current prednisone equivalent dose in our cross-sectional cohort, we were interested in analyzing plasma Hsp90 in glucocorticoid naïve IIM patients and assessing the effect of glucocorticoid therapy (with csDMARDs). In treatment naïve IIM patients, plasma Hsp90 was higher than in healthy controls and was comparable to patients with short disease duration, who recently commenced pharmacological treatment (LC1). Interestingly, pharmacological treatment significantly decreased plasma Hsp90 in the pooled treatment naïve/early IIM group (LC1), which was associated with a decline in serum LD levels. A similar decrease in Hsp90 induced by pharmacological therapy was observed in patients with established IIM (LC2). Of particular interest, baseline Hsp90 levels were able to predict the 6-month change in serum LD levels in both LC1 and LC2. Similarly, our recently published study in patients with active SSc-ILD treated with cyclophosphamide demonstrated that baseline Hsp90 predicted the 12-month improvement in diffusing lung capacity for carbon monoxide (DLCO) (15).

Given the lack of organ-specific and disease-specific biomarkers for IIM used in routine clinical practice, we analyzed the diagnostic utility of plasma Hsp90 in IIM and its subsets and compared it to that of traditionally used soluble biomarkers such as CK, LD and CRP (45). Additionally, muscle-derived enzymes such as CK, aldolase, ALT, AST and LD have been used as indirect markers of various conditions causing myolysis, and usually indicate disease activity in patients with IIM (45). Due to their relative muscle specificity, serum CK levels are most frequently used for the diagnosis and monitoring of IIM, while the other markers (such as LD and transaminases) are present in almost all living cells and are far less specific for muscle damage (45). Moreover, elevated serum CRP is rarely seen in IIM, and is mostly observed in IIM-associated arthritis, ILD or cancer (46–48). In contrast, based on our diagnostic utility analysis, plasma Hsp90 outperformed CK and CRP in distinguishing IIM from HC, as well as PM and DM from HC. Of particular interest, plasma Hsp90 attained a slightly higher AUC than CK, LD or CRP in distinguishing IIM patients with ILD and cardiac involvement from those without these manifestations. The latter finding is of some potential, since CRP and ESR are the only routine biochemistry parameters demonstrated to be associated with PM/DM-ILD according to a recent meta-analysis (47). It is also worth mentioning that cardiac troponin isoform I (cTnI) is the only reliable serum marker associated with IIM-related myocardial damage, while other traditional cardiac enzymes need to be interpreted with caution (49, 50).

There are a few limitations to our study. Since IIM is an orphan disease, the number of patients for longitudinal analyses was relatively limited. However, possible selection bias was minimized by consecutive recruitment of patients. Neither aldolase, nor traditional serum markers of myocardial damage were available in our patients for comparative diagnostic utility analysis. Most of the detected associations of plasma Hsp90 with clinical or laboratory parameters of interest were weak and thus need to be interpreted with caution regarding their potential clinical utility. Furthermore, the results of disease activity (MITAX or MYOACT) were unavailable for most of the patients in the longitudinal cohorts at the follow-up examinations, which precluded us from evaluating the associations of the dynamics of plasma Hsp90 with disease activity. Despite these limitations, we believe that our study provides substantial evidence for plasma Hsp90 as a potential biomarker for IIM.

CONCLUSION

In summary, this is the first study demonstrating elevated systemic levels of Hsp90 in patients with IIM and its potential association with several measures of disease activity and tissue damage, including functional impairment of the muscle and organ involvement. Plasma Hsp90 decreased upon pharmacological treatment in IIM patients with both early and established disease, and was able to predict the response to standard-of-care pharmacological therapy. Plasma Hsp90 demonstrated slightly superior ability to discriminate IIM patients from healthy controls, as well as IIM patients with interstitial lung disease or cardiac involvement from those without these manifestations, when compared to traditional soluble biomarkers such as CRP and CK. Thus, plasma Hsp90 could be a potential novel biomarker of disease activity, involvement of the skeletal muscle, lungs and heart, and a promising predictor of treatment response in IIM.

ETHICS STATEMENT

The studies involving human participants were reviewed and approved by Ethics Committee of the Institute of Rheumatology, Na Slupi 450/4, 12800 Prague 2, Czech Republic, with study reference number 5689/2015. The patients/participants provided their written informed consent to participate in this study.

AUTHOR CONTRIBUTIONS

HŠ, MŠ, KS, LŠ, JZ, JV, and MT designed the study. HŠ, SO, MŠ, BH, KB, OK, HM, KS, KP, LŠ, JZ, JV, and MT collected patient data. HŠ, MK, and MT performed the statistical analysis. HŠ and MT prepared the original draft of the manuscript. All authors critically interpreted the results, reviewed the draft version and approved the final manuscript.

ACKNOWLEDGMENTS

The authors would like to thank all patients and healthy controls who participated in the study and Xiao Švec for language editing.

REFERENCES

1. Vencovsky J, Alexanderson H, Lundberg IE. Idiopathic Inflammatory Myopathies. *Rheum Dis Clin North Am* (2019) 45:569–81. doi: 10.1016/j.rdc.2019.07.006
2. Lundberg IE, Miller FW, Tjarnlund A, Bottai M. Diagnosis and Classification of Idiopathic Inflammatory Myopathies. *J Intern Med* (2016) 280:39–51. doi: 10.1111/joim.12524
3. Miller FW, Lamb JA, Schmidt J, Nagaraju K. Risk Factors and Disease Mechanisms in Myositis. *Nat Rev Rheumatol* (2018) 14:255–68. doi: 10.1038/nrrheum.2018.48
4. Rayavarapu S, Coley W, Nagaraju K. Endoplasmic Reticulum Stress in Skeletal Muscle Homeostasis and Disease. *Curr Rheumatol Rep* (2012) 14:238–43. doi: 10.1007/s11926-012-0247-5
5. Ahmed M, Machado PM, Miller A, Spicer C, Herbelin L, He J, et al. Targeting Protein Homeostasis in Sporadic Inclusion Body Myositis. *Sci Transl Med* (2016) 8:331ra41. doi: 10.1126/scitranslmed.aad4583
6. Li J, Buchner J. Structure, Function and Regulation of the Hsp90 Machinery. *BioMed J* (2013) 36:106–17. doi: 10.4103/2319-4170.113230
7. Jackson SE. Hsp90: Structure and Function. *Top Curr Chem* (2013) 328:155–240. doi: 10.1007/128_2012_356
8. Mahalingam D, Swords R, Carew JS, Nawrocki ST, Bhalla K, Giles FJ. Targeting HSP90 for Cancer Therapy. *Br J Cancer* (2009) 100:1523–9. doi: 10.1038/sj.bjc.6605066
9. Geller R, Taguwa S, Frydman J. Broad Action of Hsp90 as a Host Chaperone Required for Viral Replication. *Biochim Biophys Acta* (2012) 1823:698–706. doi: 10.1016/j.bbamcr.2011.11.007
10. Kalia SK, Kalia LV, McLean PJ. Molecular Chaperones as Rational Drug Targets for Parkinson's Disease Therapeutics. *CNS Neurol Disord Drug Targets* (2010) 9:741–53. doi: 10.2174/187152710793237386
11. Procházková L, Hulejová H, Němec P, Šenolt L. Circulating Heat Shock Protein 90 (HSP90) in Patients With Rheumatoid Arthritis and Axial Spondylarthritis. *Ces Revmatol* (2013) 21:164–9.
12. Erkeller-Yuksel FM, Isenberg DA, Dhillon VB, Latchman DS, Lydyard PM. Surface Expression of Heat Shock Protein 90 by Blood Mononuclear Cells From Patients With Systemic Lupus Erythematosus. *J Autoimmun* (1992) 5:803–14. doi: 10.1016/0896-8411(92)90194-u
13. Tomcik M, Zerr P, Pitkowski J, Palumbo-Zerr K, Avouac J, Distler O, et al. Heat Shock Protein 90 (Hsp90) Inhibition Targets Canonical TGF-Beta Signalling to Prevent Fibrosis. *Ann Rheum Dis* (2014) 73:1215–22. doi: 10.1136/annrheumdis-2012-203095
14. Storkanova H, Storkanova L, Navratilova A, Becvar V, Hulejova H, Oreska S, et al. Inhibition of Hsp90 Counteracts the Established Experimental Dermal Fibrosis Induced by Bleomycin. *Biomedicines* (2021) 9:650. doi: 10.3390/biomedicines9060650
15. Storkanova H, Oreska S, Spiritovic M, Hermankova B, Bubova K, Komarc M, et al. Plasma Hsp90 Levels in Patients With Systemic Sclerosis and Relation to Lung and Skin Involvement: A Cross-Sectional and Longitudinal Study. *Sci Rep* (2021) 11:1. doi: 10.1038/s41598-020-79139-8
16. Bubova K, Storkanova H, Oreska S, Spiritovic M, Hermankova B, Mintalova K, et al. Plasma Heat Shock Protein 90 Levels in Patients With Spondyloarthritis and Their Relation to Structural Changes: A Cross-Sectional Study. *biomark Med* (2021) 15:5–13. doi: 10.2217/bmm-2020-0360
17. De Paepe B, Creus KK, Martin JJ, Weis J, De Bleecker JL. A Dual Role for HSP90 and HSP70 in the Inflammatory Myopathies: From Muscle Fiber Protection to Active Invasion by Macrophages. *Ann N Y Acad Sci* (2009) 1173:463–9. doi: 10.1111/j.1749-6632.2009.04812.x
18. Paepe BD, Creus KK, Weis J, Bleecker JL. Heat Shock Protein Families 70 and 90 in Duchenne Muscular Dystrophy and Inflammatory Myopathy: Balancing Muscle Protection and Destruction. *Neuromuscul Disord* (2012) 22:26–33. doi: 10.1016/j.nmd.2011.07.007
19. De Paepe B, De Bleecker JL. The Nonnecrotic Invaded Muscle Fibers of Polymyositis and Sporadic Inclusion Body Myositis: On the Interplay of Chemokines and Stress Proteins. *Neurosci Lett* (2013) 535:18–23. doi: 10.1016/j.neulet.2012.11.064
20. Spiritovic M, Hermankova B, Oreska S, Storkanova H, Ruzickova O, Vernerova L, et al. The Effect of a 24-Week Training Focused on Activities of Daily Living, Muscle Strengthening, and Stability in Idiopathic Inflammatory Myopathies: A Monocentric Controlled Study With Follow-Up. *Arthritis Res Ther* (2021) 23:173. doi: 10.1186/s13075-021-02544-5
21. Bohan A, Peter JB. Polymyositis and Dermatomyositis (First of Two Parts). *N Engl J Med* (1975) 292:344–7. doi: 10.1056/NEJM197502132920706
22. Hoogendijk JE, Amato AA, Lecky BR, Choy EH, Lundberg IE, Rose MR, et al. 119th ENMC International Workshop: Trial Design in Adult Idiopathic Inflammatory Myopathies, With the Exception of Inclusion Body Myositis, 10-12 October 2003, Naarden, The Netherlands. *Neuromuscul Disord* (2004) 14:337–45. doi: 10.1016/j.nmd.2004.02.006

23. Troyanov Y, Targoff IN, Tremblay JL, Goulet JR, Raymond Y, Senecal JL. Novel Classification of Idiopathic Inflammatory Myopathies Based on Overlap Syndrome Features and Autoantibodies: Analysis of 100 French Canadian Patients. *Med (Baltimore)* (2005) 84:231–49. doi: 10.1097/01.md.0000173991.74008.b0
24. Miller FW. New Approaches to the Assessment and Treatment of the Idiopathic Inflammatory Myopathies. *Ann Rheum Dis* (2012) 71:i82–5. doi: 10.1136/annrheumdis-2011-200587
25. Isenberg DA, Allen E, Farewell V, Ehrenstein MR, Hanna MG, Lundberg IE, et al. International Consensus Outcome Measures for Patients With Idiopathic Inflammatory Myopathies. Development and Initial Validation of Myositis Activity and Damage Indices in Patients With Adult Onset Disease. *Rheumatol (Oxford)* (2004) 43:49–54. doi: 10.1093/rheumatology/keg427
26. Bornman L, Polla BS, Gericke GS. Heat-Shock Protein 90 and Ubiquitin: Developmental Regulation During Myogenesis. *Muscle Nerve* (1996) 19:574–80. doi: 10.1002/(SICI)1097-4598(199605)19:5<574::AID-MUS4>3.0.CO;2-8
27. Song X, Luo Y. The Regulatory Mechanism of Hsp90alpha Secretion From Endothelial Cells and its Role in Angiogenesis During Wound Healing. *Biochem Biophys Res Commun* (2010) 398:111–7. doi: 10.1016/j.bbrc.2010.06.046
28. Srivastava P. Roles of Heat-Shock Proteins in Innate and Adaptive Immunity. *Nat Rev Immunol* (2002) 2:185–94. doi: 10.1038/nri749
29. Tsan MF, Gao B. Heat Shock Protein and Innate Immunity. *Cell Mol Immunol* (2004) 1:274–9.
30. Wong DS, Jay DG. Emerging Roles of Extracellular Hsp90 in Cancer. *Adv Cancer Res* (2016) 129:141–63. doi: 10.1016/bs.acr.2016.01.001
31. Ferreira JP, Almeida I, Marinho A, Cerveira C, Vasconcelos C. Anti-Ro52 Antibodies and Interstitial Lung Disease in Connective Tissue Diseases Excluding Scleroderma. *ISRN Rheumatol* (2012) 2012:415272. doi: 10.5402/2012/415272
32. Sontake V, Wang Y, Kasam RK, Sinner D, Reddy GB, Naren AP, et al. Hsp90 Regulation of Fibroblast Activation in Pulmonary Fibrosis. *JCI Insight* (2017) 2:e91454. doi: 10.1172/jci.insight.91454
33. Ranek MJ, Stachowski MJ, Kirk JA, Willis MS. The Role of Heat Shock Proteins and Co-Chaperones in Heart Failure. *Philos Trans R Soc Lond B Biol Sci* (2018) 373:20160530. doi: 10.1098/rstb.2016.0530
34. Garcia R, Merino D, Gomez JM, Nistal JF, Hurle MA, Cortajarena AL, et al. Extracellular Heat Shock Protein 90 Binding to TGFbeta Receptor I Participates in TGFbeta-Mediated Collagen Production in Myocardial Fibroblasts. *Cell Signal* (2016) 28:1563–79. doi: 10.1016/j.cellsig.2016.07.003
35. De Paepe B, Creus KK, De Bleecker JL. Role of Cytokines and Chemokines in Idiopathic Inflammatory Myopathies. *Curr Opin Rheumatol* (2009) 21:610–6. doi: 10.1097/BOR.0b013e3283317b31
36. Moran EM, Mastaglia FL. Cytokines in Immune-Mediated Inflammatory Myopathies: Cellular Sources, Multiple Actions and Therapeutic Implications. *Clin Exp Immunol* (2014) 178:405–15. doi: 10.1111/cei.12445
37. Cerezo LA, Vencovsky J, Senolt L. Cytokines and Inflammatory Mediators as Promising Markers of Polymyositis/Dermatomyositis. *Curr Opin Rheumatol* (2020) 32:534–41. doi: 10.1097/BOR.0000000000000744
38. Martinez CO, McHale MJ, Wells JT, Ochoa O, Michalek JE, McManus LM, et al. Regulation of Skeletal Muscle Regeneration by CCR2-Activating Chemokines is Directly Related to Macrophage Recruitment. *Am J Physiol Regul Integr Comp Physiol* (2010) 299:R832–42. doi: 10.1152/ajpregu.00797.2009
39. Shireman PK, Contreras-Shannon V, Reyes-Reyna SM, Robinson SC, McManus LM. MCP-1 Parallels Inflammatory and Regenerative Responses in Ischemic Muscle. *J Surg Res* (2006) 134:145–57. doi: 10.1016/j.jss.2005.12.003
40. Grundtman C, Tham E, Ulfgren AK, Lundberg IE. Vascular Endothelial Growth Factor Is Highly Expressed in Muscle Tissue of Patients With Polymyositis and Patients With Dermatomyositis. *Arthritis Rheum* (2008) 58:3224–38. doi: 10.1002/art.23884
41. Yoshida K, Ito H, Furuya K, Ukichi T, Noda K, Kurosaka D. Angiogenesis and VEGF-Expressing Cells Are Identified Predominantly in the Fascia Rather Than in the Muscle During the Early Phase of Dermatomyositis. *Arthritis Res Ther* (2017) 19:272. doi: 10.1186/s13075-017-1481-z
42. da Silva TCP, Silva MG, Shinjo SK. Relevance of Serum Angiogenic Cytokines in Adult Patients With Dermatomyositis. *Adv Rheumatol* (2018) 58:17. doi: 10.1186/s42358-018-0018-8
43. Catelli MG, Binart N, Jung-Testas I, Renoir JM, Baulieu EE, Feramisco JR, et al. The Common 90-Kd Protein Component of Non-Transformed '8S' Steroid Receptors is a Heat-Shock Protein. *EMBO J* (1985) 4:3131–5. doi: 10.1002/j.1460-2075.1985.tb04055.x
44. Dalman FC, Scherrer LC, Taylor LP, Akil H, Pratt WB. Localization of the 90-kDa Heat Shock Protein-Binding Site Within the Hormone-Binding Domain of the Glucocorticoid Receptor by Peptide Competition. *J Biol Chem* (1991) 266:3482–90. doi: 10.1016/S0021-9258(19)67821-X
45. Volochayev R, Csako G, Wesley R, Rider LG, Miller FW. Laboratory Test Abnormalities are Common in Polymyositis and Dermatomyositis and Differ Among Clinical and Demographic Groups. *Open Rheumatol J* (2012) 6:54–63. doi: 10.2174/1874312901206010054
46. Xiao Y, Luo H, Zhou B, Dai X, Huang J, Duan L, et al. Comparison of Soluble Urokinase Plasminogen Activator Receptor, Soluble Triggering Receptor Expressed on Myeloid Cells 1, Procalcitonin and C-Reactive Protein in Distinguishing Concurrent Bacterial Infection From Idiopathic Inflammatory Myopathy. *Rheumatol Int* (2017) 37:585–92. doi: 10.1007/s00296-016-3609-x
47. Zhang L, Wu G, Gao D, Liu G, Pan L, Ni L, et al. Factors Associated With Interstitial Lung Disease in Patients With Polymyositis and Dermatomyositis: A Systematic Review and Meta-Analysis. *PloS One* (2016) 11:e0155381. doi: 10.1371/journal.pone.0155381
48. Lu X, Yang H, Shu X, Chen F, Zhang Y, Zhang S, et al. Factors Predicting Malignancy in Patients With Polymyositis and Dermatomyostis: A Systematic Review and Meta-Analysis. *PloS One* (2014) 9:e94128. doi: 10.1371/journal.pone.0094128
49. Aggarwal R, Lebiedz-Odrobina D, Sinha A, Manadan A, Case JP. Serum Cardiac Troponin T, But Not Troponin I, is Elevated in Idiopathic Inflammatory Myopathies. *J Rheumatol* (2009) 36:2711–4. doi: 10.3899/jrheum.090562
50. Kiely PD, Bruckner FE, Nisbet JA, Daghir A. Serum Skeletal Troponin I in Inflammatory Muscle Disease: Relation to Creatine Kinase, CKMB and Cardiac Troponin I. *Ann Rheum Dis* (2000) 59:750–1. doi: 10.1136/ard.59.9.750

GLOSSARY

ALT	alanine aminotransferase
ANA	antinuclear antibodies
ANOVA	analysis of variance
anti-EJ	anti-glycyl-tRNA synthetase
anti-Jo-1	anti-histidyl-tRNA synthetase
anti-MDA5	anti-melanoma differentiation-associated gene 5
anti-Mi-2	antinuclear helicase 218/240 kDa
anti-NXP2	anti-nuclear matrix protein 2
anti-OJ	anti-isoleucyl-tRNA synthetase
anti-PL-12	anti-alanyl-tRNA synthetase
anti-PL-7	anti-threonyl-tRNA synthetase
anti-PM-Scl	anti-core complex 11-16 proteins
anti-SAE	anti-small ubiquitin-like modifier 1
anti-TIF1-γ	anti-transcriptional intermediary factor-1
AST	aspartate aminotransferase
AUC	area under the curve
ax-SpA	axial spondyloarthritis
CDM	cancer-associated dermatomyositis
CK	creatine phosphokinase
CRP	C-reactive protein
csDMARDs	conventional synthetic antirheumatic drugs
DM	dermatomyositis
ENMC	European Neuromuscular Centre
ER	endoplasmic reticulum
ESR	erythrocyte sedimentation rate
FGF	fibroblast growth factor
G-CSF	granulocyte colony-stimulating factor
GM-CSF	granulocyte-macrophage colony-stimulating factor
HAQ	health assessment questionnaire
Hsp	heat-shock protein
IBM	inclusion body myositis
IFN-γ	interferon-γ
IIM	idiopathic inflammatory myopathies
IL	interleukin
IMACS	International Myositis Assessment & Clinical Studies Group
IMNM	immune-mediated necrotizing myopathy
IoRP	Institute of Rheumatology in Prague
IP-10	interferon gamma-induced protein 10
IQR	interquartile range
LC	longitudinal cohort
LD	lactate dehydrogenase
MAAs	myositis-associated autoantibodies
Mb	myoglobin
MCP-1	monocyte chemoattractant protein 1
MDA	muscle disease activity
MDAAT	Myositis Disease Activity Assessment Tool
MDI	myositis damage index
MIP	macrophage inflammatory protein
MITAX	Myositis Intention to Treat Activity Index
MMT	manual muscle testing
MMT-8	manual muscle testing of 8 muscle groups
MSAs	myositis-specific autoantibodies
MYOACT	Myositis Disease Activity Assessment visual analogue scale
PDGF	platelet-derived growth factor
PM	polymyositis
RA	rheumatoid arthritis
RANTES	regulated on activation/normal T cell expressed and secreted
ROC	receiver operating characteristic
SLE	systemic lupus erythematosus
SSc	systemic sclerosis/scleroderma
TNF	tumor necrosis factor
TNF	tumor necrosis factor
VAS	visual analogue scale
VEGF	vascular endothelial growth factor

6

Dermatomyositis With Anti-MDA5 Antibodies: Bioclinical Features, Pathogenesis and Emerging Therapies

*Anaïs Nombel[1], Nicole Fabien[1] and Frédéric Coutant[1,2]**

[1] Immunology Department, Lyon-Sud Hospital, Hospices Civils de Lyon, Pierre-Bénite, France, [2] Immunogenomics and Inflammation Research Team, University of Lyon, Edouard Herriot Hospital, Lyon, France

***Correspondence:**
Frédéric Coutant
frederic.coutant@univ-lyon1.fr*

Anti-MDA5 dermatomyositis is a rare systemic autoimmune disease, historically described in Japanese patients with clinically amyopathic dermatomyositis and life-threatening rapidly progressive interstitial lung disease. Subsequently, the complete clinical spectrum of the disease was enriched by skin, articular and vascular manifestations. Depending on the predominance of these symptoms, three distinct clinical phenotypes with different prognosis are now defined. To date, the only known molecular component shared by the three entities are specific antibodies targeting MDA5, a cytosolic protein essential for antiviral host immune responses. Several biological tools have emerged to detect these antibodies, with drawbacks and limitations for each of them. However, the identification of this highly specific serological marker of the disease raises the question of its role in the pathogenesis. Although current knowledge on the pathogenic mechanisms that take place in the disease are still in their enfancy, several lines of evidence support a central role of interferon-mediated vasculopathy in the development of skin and lung lesions, as well as a possible pathogenic involvement of anti-MDA5 antibodies. Here, we review the clinical and biological evidences in favor of these hypothesis, and we discuss the contribution of emerging therapies that shed some light on the pathogenesis of the disease.

Keywords: myositis, dermatomyositis, idiopathic inflammatory myopathies, MDA5, COVID-19, SARS-CoV-2, autoantibodies, autoantibody

INTRODUCTION

The idiopathic inflammatory myopathies (IIM) are a heterogeneous group of rare connective tissue diseases, characterized by inflammation of several organs and tissues other than the muscles, such as the skin and the lungs. IIM include necrotizing immune-mediated myositis, inclusion body myositis, antisynthetase syndrome and dermatomyositis (DM) (1). These four subgroups are very heterogeneous in their clinical, prognostic and pathological features, which renders the diagnosis and the treatment challenging. However, the discovery and the inclusion of myositis specific autoantibodies (MSA) in the diagnostic algorithm of myositis allowed a better definition of subgroups of patients in terms of clinical phenotypes, prognosis and response to treatment. One of these MSA, the anti-melanoma differentiation-associated gene 5 (MDA5) antibodies (Abs), was originally identified in a specific subset of DM, named clinically amyopathic DM (CADM), associated with an increased risk for rapidly progressive interstitial lung disease (RP-ILD). The clinical presentation of anti-MDA5 DM differs substantially from the other forms of DM, with three distinct clinical phenotypes, according to the predominance of pulmonary, skin-articular or vascular symptoms (2). The pathogenesis of these three forms of anti-MDA5 DM is largely unknown, and to date, the only common molecular characteristic of these entities is the presence in the blood of the patients of Abs targeting the antigen MDA5, a highly specific biomarker of the disease, sometimes difficult to detect with usual techniques. MDA5 is a cytosolic protein, essential for antiviral host immune responses, which functions as a virus RNA sensor and induces, once activated, the production of type I interferons (IFN-I) and pro-inflammatory cytokines by the cell. The pathogenic role of anti-MDA5 Abs is currently unknown, but its involvement in the disease by targeting a critical actor of the immune system could be congruent with the concept of autoimmunity induced by infectious agents.

In this review, we outline the clinical phenotypes of the DM with anti-MDA5 Abs, the distribution and the functions of MDA5, as well as the biological tools available for the detection of anti-MDA5 Abs and their limitations. We focus on recent biological data that provide insight into the pathogenesis of the disease, and we propose a pathophysiological model centered on vascular dysfunction and dysregulated immune system. In this proposed model, we will discuss whether the Abs specific of the disease could be critical players in disease pathogenesis, and not just biomarkers.

CLINICAL SPECTRUM IN ADULTS OF THE DERMATOMYOSITIS WITH ANTI-MDA5 ANTIBODIES

Anti-MDA5 DM is a rare disease representing less than 2% of IIM in Europe (3). Among the subgroup of DM, the prevalence of anti-MDA5 DM ranges from 7 to 60%, with higher prevalence in Asian (11-60%) than in Caucasian (7-16%) (**Table 1**) (1, 4–19). Similar to other autoimmune diseases, anti-MDA5 DM occurs mainly in women, with a female/male ratio that ranges from 0.6 to 7.3 (F/M >1 in 14 out of 16 studies) (**Table 1**) (4–19).

Systemic autoimmune DM are characterized by skin manifestations accompanying or preceding muscle weakness, and, to various extents, lung lesions. The DM associated with anti-MDA5 Abs shares clinical features with DM but also has disease-specific traits. Indeed, the patients with anti-MDA5 DM may have the hallmark cutaneous manifestations of DM, but the disease is also associated with specific skin manifestations. Moreover, the muscle disease is minimal or absent, and pulmonary interstitial lesions may be rapidly progressive which is not the case in other forms of DM.

Muscular Manifestations of Anti-MDA5 Dermatomyositis

Anti-MDA5 DM was first described by Sato et al. in 2005, in a Japanese cohort with CADM and RP-ILD (4). As defined by Sontheimer et al. (20), CADM patients display the hallmark cutaneous manifestations of DM for at least 6 months, without muscle weakness. The hypomyopathic forms of CADM are associated with elevated muscle enzymes and/or abnormalities in EMG or muscle biopsy, whereas amyopathic DM patients have the cutaneous manifestations of DM for at least 6 months, without clinical or biological signs of muscle damage. However, CADM is not sufficient to define anti-MDA5 DM, as not all CADM patients have anti-MDA5 Abs. The proportion of anti-MDA5 Abs positive patients among CADM ranges from 23% to 100%, depending on the cohorts (**Table 1**) (4–7, 9–14, 17, 19). Conversely, the prevalence of CADM among anti-MDA5 Abs positive patients is also very inconsistent (17 to 100%, **Table 1**) (4–19).

When present, muscle damage mainly affects proximal muscles (2, 12). Several histological features of muscle biopsies are shared by different forms of DM, and include perifascicular fiber atrophy, perivascular inflammation, infiltrates of T and B cells, diffuse class I major histocompatibility complex (MHC-I) expression and deposition of complement attack complex (21, 22). In contrast, muscle biopsies of patients with anti-MDA5 DM are often normal or highlight only rare anomalies. Inflammation is absent or scarce and cellular infiltrates, mostly macrophages, cluster focally in the perimysium. MHC-I expression is focal or absent. Complement membrane attack complex deposition is rarely observed. Furthermore, IFN signature in skeletal muscles of patients with anti-MDA5 DM is up-regulated, compared with healthy subjects but lower than patients with anti-MDA5 negative DM (21, 22). These observations are consistent with the mild muscle phenotype frequently associated with anti-MDA5 DM.

Mucocutaneous and Articular Manifestations of Anti-MDA5 Dermatomyositis

The hallmark cutaneous manifestations of the DM spectrum occur with similar prevalence in patients with anti-MDA5 DM. They include periorbital heliotrope (blue–purple) rash with edema, erythematous rash on the face, or the anterior chest (in a V-sign), and back and shoulders (in a shawl sign), violaceous papules or plaques located on the dorsal part of the metacarpophalangeal or interphalangeal joints, called Gottron's papules and cracked palmar fingertips ("mechanic's hands"). It is important to underline here the danger of potential misdiagnosis of patients with anti-MDA5 DM, given the absence of clinical

TABLE 1 | Ethnicity and prevalence of dermatomyositis with anti-MDA5 antibodies.

Country	DM cases* (n)	Anti-MDA5$^+$	Detection technique	CADM among anti-MDA5$^+$	CADM cases (n)	Anti-MDA5$^+$ among CADM	Prevalence of women anti-MDA5$^+$	ILD among anti-MDA5$^+$	RP-ILD among anti-MDA5$^+$	Ref	Publication year
Japan	42	19%	IP/IB/IIF	100%	15	53%	75%	88%	50%	(4)	2005
Japan	30	27%	IP	75%	13	46%	88%	100%	100%	(5)	2009
Japan	65	22%	IP/ELISA	57%	15	53%	79%	100%	71%	(6)	2010
Japan	37	35%	IP/IB	85%	15	73%	69%	92%	54%	(7)	2010
Japan	55	11%	IP	17%	ND	ND	50%	83%	50%	(8)	2011
Japan	376	11%	IP/IB/ELISA	77%	51	65%	79%	93%	65%	(9)	2011
Japan	79	22%	IP/ELISA	82%	21	67%	88%	94%	71%	(10)	2012
China	84	23%	ELISA	26%	8	63%	58%	ND	79%	(11)	2012
China	64	23%	ELISA	80%	32	38%	60%	100%	60%	(12)	2012
China	43	60%	ELISA	35%	9	100%	39%	100%	39%	(13)	2013
China	213	21%	ID	77%	81	42%	71%	82%	64%	(14)	2020
North America	77	13%	IP	50%	ND	ND	88%	67%	20%	(15)	2011
North America	160	7%	IP	46%	ND	ND	73%	73%	ND	(16)	2013
Spain	117	12%	ELISA/IB/IIF	57%	15	53%	64%	64%	57%	(17)	2014
Italy	34	15%	IP-WB/ELISA/IIF	100%	ND	ND	60%	60%	20%	(18)	2014
Brazil	131	16%	ELISA	24%	22	23%	71%	38%	ND	(19)	2018
France	54	9%	IIF/ID	ND	ND	ND	ND	ND	ND	(1)	2018

Selection of cohorts with at least 30 patients (cohorts with JDM patients excluded).
DM, dermatomyositis; CADM, clinically amyopathic dermatomyositis; JDM, juvenile dermatomyositis; ILD, interstitial lung disease; RP-ILD, rapidly progressive interstitial lung disease; IP, immunoprecipitation; IB, immunoblot; IIF, indirect immunofluorescence; ELISA, enzyme-linked immunosorbent assay; WB, western blot; ID, immunodot assay; ND, not done.

evidence of myopathy and also sometimes the similarities of DM-specific manifestations, such as Gottron's papules, with other skin lesions, such as psoriatic lesions (23, 24).

Anti-MDA5 DM is also associated with a more specific cutaneous phenotype, that includes palmar papules and skin ulcerations, reported in both Caucasian (2, 15, 16, 25–28) and Asian populations (9, 10, 12, 29–31). Unlike Gottron's papules, palmar papules are often located on the palmar surface or lateral sides of the fingers, especially over metacarpophalangeal and interphalangeal joints. Many of these lesions have a central ivory coloration, and they are frequently painful. Palmar papules can be associated with hyperkeratosis, and complicated of ulcerations.

Skin ulcerations associated with anti-MDA5 DM usually manifest as deep painful ulcers localized over Gottron's papule, involving the digital pulp and nail folds, or over Gottron's sign on the knees, elbows, or both. The histology of skin ulcerations shows vasculopathy, pauci-inflammatory or characterized by medium vessel wall infiltration with mononuclear cells, and intravascular thrombus (12, 15). Major complications can occur, such as gangrene and osteomyelitis, potentially leading to digital amputation (25, 32, 33).

Less specific auricular skin lesions have also been described in DM with anti-MDA5 Abs, such as antihelix/helix violaceous macules and erythematous auricular papules (34, 35). These particular cutaneous phenotypes, seldom mentioned in the literature, could be clinical markers of poor prognosis, although most previous studies examining auricular skin lesions in the disease have been limited to isolated case reports (36). Other less specific mucocutaneous lesions have been described in DM with anti-MDA5 Abs. They include oral ulcers, panniculitis, alopecia and flagellate erythema (15, 17, 37, 38).

Since 2010, many studies reported the increased prevalence of arthritis (42-82%) and arthralgia in patients with anti-MDA5 DM (2, 9, 15, 16). The arthritis described in the patients closely resembles that found in rheumatoid arthritis, potentially leading to misdiagnosis in the absence of other DM symptoms. They are associated with morning stiffness and are typically symmetric, affecting the small joints of the hands, but also the wrists and the ankles (16, 23, 39). Although rarely described in the literature, the conventional radiography do not show any bone erosion. However, erosions have been exceptionally reported by magnetic resonance imaging (16, 39). When explored, the rheumatoid factor was positive in some cases, but anti-cyclic citrullinated peptide Abs were not detected in any of the patients (27, 39).

Another differential diagnosis of these articular forms of anti-MDA5 DM is the psoriatic arthritis. Indeed arthritis is a common feature associated with psoriasis and some cases of anti-MDA5 DM initially manifest as psoriasiform skin lesions (23, 24, 40). In the literature, one case has been reported of a patient with psoriasiform lesions, associated with severe symmetrical polyarthritis of large and small joints, and a mild proximal weakness in upper and lower extremities. All of these elements initially led to the misdiagnosis of psoriatic arthritis (23). However, thoracic CT scan subsequently showed a bilateral ground-glass pattern, and laboratory tests revealed blood positivity for anti-MDA5 Abs. Thus, the association of arthritis and psoriasiform lesions, associated with weak muscle or pulmonary involvement may lead to a misdiagnosis of psoriatic arthritis, if anti-MDA5 Abs are not explored.

Finally, some patients have a phenotype close to the antisynthetase syndrome (i.e. arthritis, Raynaud's syndrome, mechanic's hands, ILD), further complicating the diagnosis (16, 41).

Lung Manifestations of Anti-MDA5 Dermatomyositis

Anti-MDA5 DM is associated with poor prognosis due to a high prevalence of RP-ILD. ILD is the result of inflammation and fibrosis of the lung parenchyma and specific patterns of ground-glass attenuation are observed on high-resolution computed tomography (42). Significant disparities between association of anti-MDA5 Abs and RP-ILD have been described in the cohorts. For instance, in Japan and in East Asia populations, ILD occurs in 82 to 100% of patients with anti-MDA5 DM, and RP-ILD in 39 to 100% of patients (**Table 1**) (4–14). The incidence of RP-ILD appears less important in Caucasian populations with 38 to 73% of anti-MDA5 DM patients having ILD and 20 to 57% having RP-ILD (**Table 1**) (15–19), some studies reporting a significant association (17, 25) while others do not (15, 16, 19).

It is of importance to note that ILD can be absent at diagnosis and develop many years later, or completely absent in some patients over years of follow-up. Conversely, ILD can sometimes reveals anti-MDA5 DM. For instance, three Japanese patients with ILD and anti-MDA5 Abs, but without cutaneous nor muscular manifestation, had a fatal outcome within two months after onset (43). Similarly, two patients initially hospitalized for fever and dyspnea developed skin symptoms characteristic of DM one month after onset (44).

The mortality rate of patients who develop RP-ILD is reported to be approximately 50%, with most deaths occurring during the very early stages of the illness (6, 7, 9, 10, 13, 43, 45, 46). Some studies suggest that beyond 6 months after onset, disease progression tends to settle down, and relapse seems uncommon (10). However, recurrences have also been described in the form of cutaneous and/or severe respiratory relapse many years after onset and after months of clinical remission and new treatments are needed to contain the exacerbation (47, 48).

Association of Anti-MDA5 Dermatomyositis With Malignancy

Several DM are associated with an increased risk for cancer, such as DM with anti-TIF1γ Abs, and to a lesser extent, DM with anti-NXP2 Abs (3, 49). By contrast, the association of anti-MDA5 DM with cancer has been explored in large cohorts, without any correlation reported (7, 9, 10, 12). However, few cases of cancer have been reported in patients with anti-MDA5 DM (33, 37, 50). Metastatic small cell carcinoma with liver involvement was detected 12 months after anti-MDA5 DM diagnosis in a 60 year-old French woman (50). Another study presented the case of a man diagnosed simultaneously with both anti-MDA5 DM and thyroid cancer (37). Even if no evident causal link is established, these few cases highlight that anti-MDA5 DM and cancer might not be exclusive.

Other Clinical and Biological Features of Anti-MDA5 Dermatomyositis

Among the constitutional symptoms, the fever has been described in up to 74% of anti-MDA5 DM at onset [33-74%] (7–9, 11, 13, 16). Several distinctive features in blood tests are also reported in the disease, such as elevated ferritinemia, with no significant elevation of C-reactive protein. Ferritin levels correlate with the severity of the disease and ILD (6, 7, 51, 52). Liver dysfunction is also recurrently observed in anti-MDA5 DM, as evidenced by elevated levels of alanine transaminase or gamma-glutamyl transferase, without elevated creatine kinase (6, 7, 21, 53). Liver biopsies show steatosis and hepatocyte ballooning (53). Furthermore, liver enzymes might increase as ferritinemia increases and ILD worsens (7). Decreased $CD4^+$ and $CD8^+$ T cell counts and a raised $CD4^+/CD8^+$ ratio are frequently described in peripheral blood of patients with anti-MDA5 DM, even before immunosuppressive treatment (11, 54). When studying the relation between pulmonary lesions and lymphopenia, an increase of $CD4^+$ and $CD8^+$ T cell counts is observed in parallel with pulmonary lesions improvement after treatment. Inversely, $CD4^+$ and $CD8^+$ T cell counts decrease and the $CD4^+/CD8^+$ ratio increases in patients with ILD refractory to treatment (54). Finally, positivity for anti-TRIM21 (Ro52) Abs (55, 56) and older age (14, 29) are indicators of poor prognosis while the female sex and articular form might be factors of good prognosis (57).

Dermatomyositis With Anti-MDA5 Antibodies: Three Distinct Clinical Phenotypes

The heterogeneity of clinical features and outcomes among patients with anti-MDA5 DM prompted to divide the clinical spectrum of anti-MDA5 DM into three distinct clinical subgroups (**Figure 1**) (2). The first one is composed mainly of women with RP-ILD associated with mechanic's hands, with the highest mortality rate (80%). A rheumatologic group (55% of cases) is also made mostly of women with arthralgia or arthritis (83%), less frequent RP-ILD (17%) and a better prognosis. The third clinical phenotype mainly encompasses men with symptoms dominated by skin vasculopathies, including a Raynaud's phenomenon (82%), skin ulcers (77%), digital necrosis (32%) and calcinosis (23%). This last subgroup is frequently associated with proximal muscles weakness (68%), with relatively few RP-ILD (23%) and it is of intermediate prognosis. This classification was already suggested by a

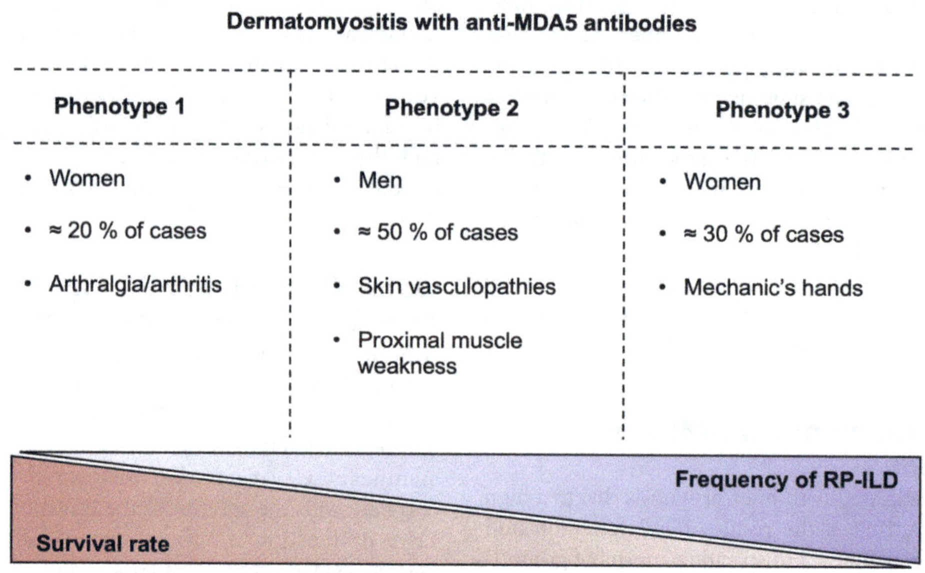

FIGURE 1 | The clinical phenotypes of anti-MDA5 dermatomyositis. Anti-MDA5 dermatomyositis can be divided into three clinical phenotypes with varying degrees of pulmonary damage, which is inversely correlated with the survival. RP-ILD, rapidly progressive interstitial lung disease.

Spanish group in 2014 (17) and could permit an appraisal of the prognosis of patients with anti-MDA5 DM.

JUVENILE DERMATOMYOSITIS ASSOCIATED WITH ANTI-MDA5 ANTIBODIES

Juvenile DM (JDM) is associated with anti-MDA5 Abs in 6 to 12% of cases in European and North American cohorts, and constitutes the third most frequent DM-associated Abs after anti-TIF1γ and anti-NXP2 Abs (56, 58–62). The prevalence of the anti-MDA5 Abs is higher in Japanese cohorts, with 24 to 38% of patients having anti-MDA5 Abs associated JDM (63–65). The anti-MDA5 JDM phenotype is associated with a higher frequency of constitutional symptoms (weight loss, fever and adenopathy) and milder muscle involvement compared to the other forms of JDM (58, 61, 62, 65).

Similarly to the adult form, the specific cutaneous phenotype found in anti-MDA5 DM, i.e. the palmar papules and skin ulcerations, are also observed in anti-MDA5 JDM, as well as arthritis, which is more frequent than in other subtypes of JDM (58, 59, 61, 64). These lesions distinguish anti-MDA5 JDM from the other forms of JDM. The arthritis associated with the juvenile form is similar to the one observed in adults, characterized by symmetrical pain and swelling of the small joints of the hands (58, 66). Anti-MDA5 JDM is also associated with an increased risk of ILD (58, 61, 63–65, 67), which is more frequent compared with other forms of JDM associated with MSA, except for anti-synthetase Abs-associated JDM. RP-ILD appears to be less common (<10%) in Caucasian anti-MDA5 JDM, compared to the adult form (58). Thus, a major difference between the juvenile form and the adult form of the disease in Caucasian patients is observed in terms of outcome, since anti-MDA5 JDM has comparable outcome with the other forms of JDM, but flares are less frequent in this subset of JDM and necessitates less medication (58, 59, 61). The observations on the association between anti-MDA5 Abs JDM and RP-ILD are more contradictory in the Japanese population. Indeed, although some studies report a much higher frequency of RP-ILD in Japanese anti-MDA5 JDM patients associated with a poor prognosis, a recent multicenter study reported only 19% of RP-ILD in a cohort of 31 anti-MDA5 Abs positive patients, with a lower rate of relapse than other MSA positive patients (63, 67, 68).

MDA5 AND ANTI-MDA5 ANTIBODIES

In 2005, Sato et al. reported that Abs found in the sera of patients with CADM react with a cytoplasmic protein of 140 kDa (4). In 2009, the same team described MDA5 as the antigenic target of 140 kDa which is recognized by the Abs found in patients with CADM (69).

MDA5 was initially identified in 2002, as a type I IFN-inducible gene in human melanoma cells, and the first function described for this protein was to induce the death of cancer cells (70). Since this first description, MDA5 is now considered as a key sensor of viral infection, mediating the production by the infected cell of IFN-I and the induction of other genes that collectively establish an antiviral host response. MDA5 is encoded by the gene *IFIH1* (interferon-induced with helicase C domain 1) and is part of the Retinoic acid Inducible Gene-I-like receptor family that detect molecular patterns of viruses that have gained access to the cytosol of the infected cell. More specifically, MDA5 senses preferentially long (> 300 bp) RNA-RNA strand pairs, which are mainly RNA viruses replicative intermediates, although some DNA viruses also produce them during their life cycle (71, 72). MDA5 senses these double-stranded RNA (dsRNA) *via* its RNA helicase domain and a C-terminal domain (CTD), and subsequently transmits a signal *via* its homotypic interacting caspase recruitment domain (CARD). Upon recognition of dsRNA, MDA5 assembles into a filament along the dsRNA axis and adopts a ring-like conformation around dsRNA, allowing MDA5 to bind with a strong affinity to its ligand. MDA5 then interacts with the mitochondrial antiviral signaling protein (MAVS), present on the outer membrane of the mitochondria, peroxisomes and other mitochondria-associated membranes. The interaction between MDA5 and MAVS through their respective CARD leads to the activation of the transcription factors interferon regulatory factor 3 and 7 (IRF3 and IRF7), as well as nuclear factor-kappa B (NF-κB). Phosphorylated IRF3, IRF7 and NF-κB then accumulate in the nuclei where they activate antiviral gene transcription, including IFN-I genes, leading to the production of type I IFN (IFNα and IFNβ) and pro-inflammatory cytokines (73, 74).

By this way, MDA5 is able to detect and limit the replication of several RNA viruses of the picornavirus, flavivirus or coronavirus families, as well as DNA viruses of the herpesvirus family for instance (71, 75). But MDA5 is also able to sense endogenous dsRNA, such as mitochondrial dsRNA generated by bilateral transcription of mitochondrial DNA. This biological mechanism is tightly regulated, by mitochondrial degradasome enzymes such as the polynucleotide phosphorylase (PNPase), avoiding the accumulation of dsRNA and thus deleterious activation of MDA5. As a result, PNPase deficiency can cause a massive accumulation of long mitochondrial dsRNA, escaping into the cytosol and leading ultimately to an uncontrolled activation of MDA5 and an upregulation of interferon-stimulated genes (76). In line with this, patients with hypomorphic mutations in *PNPT1*, the gene that encodes for PNPase, have type I interferonopathies characterized by a constitutive activation of the IFN-I axis (77).

Tissue Distribution and Cellular Location of MDA5

A greater knowledge of the tissue distribution and cellular location of MDA5 is essential to better understand the pathophysiology of anti-MDA5 DM. MDA5 has low tissue specificity in physiological condition (78). A higher expression in the skin and lung tissues of patients with anti-MDA5 DM would be expected compared to expression in muscle tissues. Although studies on MDA5 expression in these target tissues are very rare, MDA5 expression has been shown to be enhanced in skin biopsies of patients with DM, which could offer an element of response to the severe cutaneous symptoms associated with the disease (79).

Defining the cellular location of MDA5 in a pathological context is also critical as pathogenic Abs necessitate to be internalized when the antigenic target is cytosolic, or act by interacting with a protein expressed at the surface of a target cell. At the cellular level, MDA5 was initially described as an intracellular protein found in the cytoplasm of most cells (70). However, Berger et al. studied MDA5 expression and subcellular localization in neutrophils and showed an overexpression of MDA5 both in the cytoplasm and in secretory vesicles as well as a cell surface expression (80). Expression of MDA5 at the surface of other cell types is still being determined. The identification of transient or constitutive expression of MDA5 on the surface of target cells could constitute a critical element in the understanding of the pathogenesis of the disease, in favor of a potential pathogenic role of anti-MDA5 Abs.

Anti-MDA5 Autoantibodies: The Diagnostic Marker

The identification of the anti-MDA5 Abs in CADM was initially performed by immunoprecipitations (IP) of sera from patients incubated with ^{35}S-methionine-labeled K562 cell extracts (4). Since then, radiolabeled IP is considered as the gold standard testing method to detect anti-MDA5 Abs. Although the substitution of radiolabeled antigenic extracts by biotin-labeled recombinant MDA5 constitute a good alternative to bypass the use of radioactive materials (81), IP remains difficult to use in everyday practice, because time-consuming and expensive. Another major issue of IP assay regarding anti-MDA5 Abs identification is the comigration of the MDA5 antigen with other antigens found in DMs, such as the antigens NXP2, TIF1γ and OJ (18, 59, 82). Great expertise is therefore required for correct identification of anti-MDA5 Abs by IP, and alternative interpretation and other assays are therefore required to confirm a serum positivity.

For all the reasons mentioned above, IP is used only in a limited number of medical laboratories, which opted now for qualitative or quantitative alternative assays. Qualitative assays include indirect immunofluorescence (IIF) staining on HEp-2 cells and immunodot assays (so-called line blot or dot blot) (83). IIF staining performed on HEp-2 cells with diluted sera from patients with anti-MDA5 DM can give rise to a characteristic cytoplasmic staining with a finely granular appearance, in rare clustered cells and in one study in all cells (**Figure 2**) (4, 84, 85). This difference could be due to the source of HEp-2 cells differentially expressing MDA5 or to the presence of other Abs. However, the scarcity of positive cells generally observed in the microscope field makes the identification of anti-MDA5 Abs by IIF very touchy, and requires a trained eye. Moreover, this IIF pattern is inconstant. In our personal experience that includes a cohort of 31 anti-MDA5 DM, this particular IIF pattern was observed with 50% of sera. Several nonspecific IIF patterns are otherwise observed and have been described, such as a granular cytoplasmic pattern in all cells (which can mask the typical cytoplasmic pattern), or a nuclear speckled pattern, associated or not with the typical cytoplasmic pattern (**Figure 2**) (4). Finally, anti-MDA5 Abs positive sera can also be negative by IIF (17, 18). IIF results should thus always be interpreted by taking in consideration the clinical context and

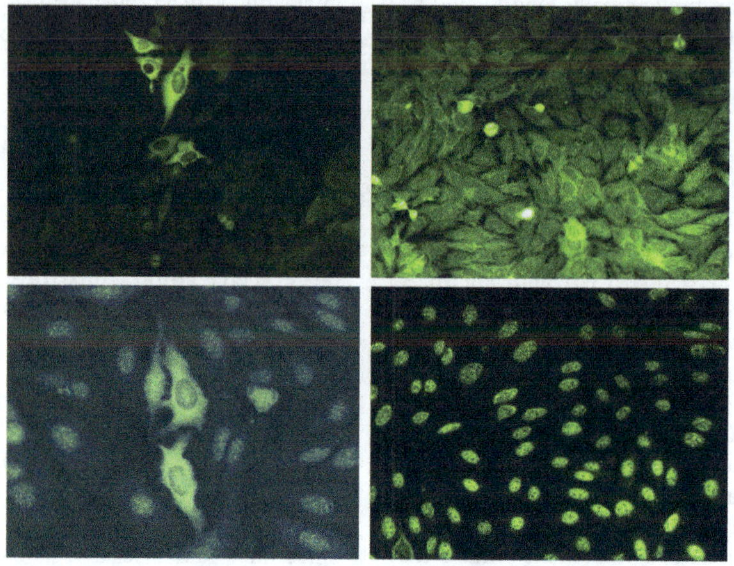

FIGURE 2 | Indirect immunofluorescence patterns of HEp-2 cells stained with anti–MDA5 positive sera. Stainings were performed on HEp-2 cells (Kallestad, Biorad) with sera from patients with anti-MDA5 Abs dermatomyositis. Top left: typical fine granular cytoplasmic staining in rare clustered cells. Top right: granular cytoplasmic pattern in all cells (which can mask the typical cytoplasmic pattern). Bottom left: nuclear speckled pattern, associated with the typical cytoplasmic pattern. Bottom right: isolated nuclear speckled pattern. Note that absence of fluorescence can also be observed with some sera.

other specific assays should be conducted to confirm a positive IIF pattern or to further explore a negative IIF, if there is a strong clinical suspicion of anti-MDA5 DM.

Commercialized immunodot assays (Line blot LIA, Euroimmun, Lübeck, Germany and dot blot D-Tek, BlueDiver, Mons, Belgium) and particle-based multi-analyte technology (PMAT, Inova, Diagnostics, US) can be used for the detection of anti-MDA5 Abs. These specific qualitative assays i.e. Line Blot, Dot blot, have been validated using the IP assay as gold standard, with reported specificity of 96-99% or 98% and sensitivity of 75-93% or 76% respectively. High level of agreement was also found between IP and PMAT (86–88).

Enzyme-linked immunosorbent assays (ELISA) have also been recently developed to detect anti-MDA5 Abs and allow their quantification. An ELISA based on a recombinant MDA5 fusion protein produced in insect cells has shown an analytical sensitivity and specificity of 98% and 100% respectively, compared with IP assays (89). A major benefit of anti-MDA5 Abs ELISA is that it allows a precise quantification of the level of anti-MDA5 Abs in the serum of patients, and a follow-up of its variation during the course of the disease or after the introduction of a therapy.

Anti-MDA5 Autoantibodies: A Tool for Monitoring Disease Activity

The quantification of anti-MDA5 Abs level seems to be a way to predict disease outcome. When comparing surviving and deceased patients, anti-MDA5 Abs levels are significantly lower in surviving patients. Moreover, the outcome of patients with low titers of anti-MDA5 Abs is approximately the same as patients without anti-MDA5 Abs (90). Anti-MDA5 Abs titers also correlate with the severity of the disease, and more particularly with the severity of ILD and cutaneous symptoms. Several Japanese studies reported higher levels of anti-MDA5 Abs in JDM patients with RP-ILD (63, 64, 67). One study reported deep necrotic ulcerations in the patients with the highest anti-MDA5 Abs levels and only superficial cutaneous symptoms in those with the lowest value (12).

Furthermore, the value of the anti-MDA5 Abs could also be useful for the evaluation of the response to treatment. In a Japanese cohort, patients with anti-MDA5 Abs levels greater than 500 units/mL (positivity threshold at 8 units/mL) were resistant to treatment by glucocorticoids/cyclophosphamide or intravenous immunoglobulins, and died (12). Inversely, patients with anti-MDA5 Abs levels lower than 500 units/mL had less severe lung lesions and cutaneous symptoms improved after treatment. Finally, monitoring the Abs levels along the course of the disease could permit to objective a remission or to detect a relapse early. Remission induces the disappearance of anti-MDA5 Abs, whereas it remains elevated in the patients who die or who later relapse (91, 92).

In conclusion, the anti-MDA5 Abs are a critical diagnostic biomarker of the disease and the level of Abs could be an important prognostic and predictive parameter to monitor in patients.

Co-Occurrence of Anti-MDA5 Autoantibodies With Other Autoantibodies

Anti-TRIM21 Abs (also known as anti-Ro52/SSA-52 Abs) are nonspecific Abs encountered in several connective diseases, and also frequently detected in the serum of patients with anti-MDA5 DM, with 27 to 62% of dual-positive patients. These patients seem to develop RP-ILD more frequently and have a less favorable prognosis (15, 16, 55, 56).

A study reported the presence of Abs directed against a nuclear protein, the splicing factor proline/glutamine-rich (SFPQ), in the serum of 27 out of 51 patients (53%) with anti-MDA5 DM (93). SFPQ is a multifunctional nuclear protein of 110 kDa, that participates in diverse molecular functions including transcription regulation, and is also involved in the regulation of host innate immune response to viruses (94, 95). Anti-SFPQ Abs have not been detected in other form of DMs, and were identified at diagnosis in 13 patients, while the others turned positive during the disease course (93). Another study observed an apparition of anti-SFPQ Abs at recurrence (47). The clinical relevance of these Abs is unknown, and they are not researched in current practice.

PATHOGENESIS OF THE DISEASE

Owing to the rarity of anti-MDA5 DM, knowledge on the pathogenic mechanisms of the disease remain limited, but they are believed to occur as a consequence of a particular gene-environmental interaction. Although scarce, several studies have underlined an association of HLA and non-HLA alleles with the disease. Moreover, the identification of seasonal and geographical clustering at disease onset suggests that an infectious agent could be a triggering factor, an attractive hypothesis in view of the antiviral function of the MDA5 antigen. As for the pathogenic mechanisms involved in the disease, since MDA5 is an IFN-I inducible gene, IFN-I could be the starting point for most of the pathophysiological pathways.

Genetic Susceptibility

HLA allele associations have been described in Asian cohorts. The strongest disease association was found with alleles of the type II HLA alleles HLA-DRB1. Analyses of the relationship between type II HLA alleles and anti-MDA5 DM in Chinese cohorts demonstrated a higher frequency of HLA-DRB1*04:01, *12:02 and *12:01 alleles in Chinese patients with anti-MDA5 DM (96, 97). However, different risk factors are observed in particular ethnic groups, including combined frequency of HLA-DRB1*01:01 and *04:05 in Japanese patients (98), with no significant difference for the same alleles in Chinese populations (96). In addition, some alleles such as HLA-DRB1*09:01 have been associated with a worse prognosis in Chinese patients (97). To date, no association between HLA alleles and anti-MDA5 DM has been identified in Caucasian population (99).

Although HLA allele associations differ across ethnic populations, amino acid sequence variations observed in the type II HLA-DRB1 alleles might affect the structure of the antigen-binding groove of the HLA molecule and thereby influence the antigenic repertoire, increasing by this way the disease susceptibility.

One non-HLA locus, an intronic variant of WDFY4, has been recently associated with the anti-MDA5 DM in Japanese patients (100). This variant induces a higher expression of a truncated isoform of the WDFY4 protein. Although the precise biological function of WDFY4 was unknown when this work was published, Kochi et al. demonstrated that the truncated form of WDFY4 markedly enhanced the MDA5-mediated NF-κB activation and cell apoptosis. Interestingly, one year later, Theisen et al. uncovered the function of WDFY4, which is in fact a critical regulator of cross-presentation in the conventional CD1c^{+} dendritic cells (101). This is of particular interest in the context of anti-MDA5 DM since, as it will be discussed later, an inadequate immune response to an infectious agent could be the environmental factor triggering the disease. It is then tempting to speculate that qualitative and/or quantitative alterations of WDFY4 might induce a striking defect in cross-presentation of viral-associated antigens, which may trigger secondarily an aberrant autoimmune response (**Figure 3**).

Other molecular defects, unexplored so far, might also be involved in the pathogenesis of anti-MDA5 DM. For instance, given the role of mitochondrial PNPase in eliminating endogenous dsRNA, local dysregulated expression and/or

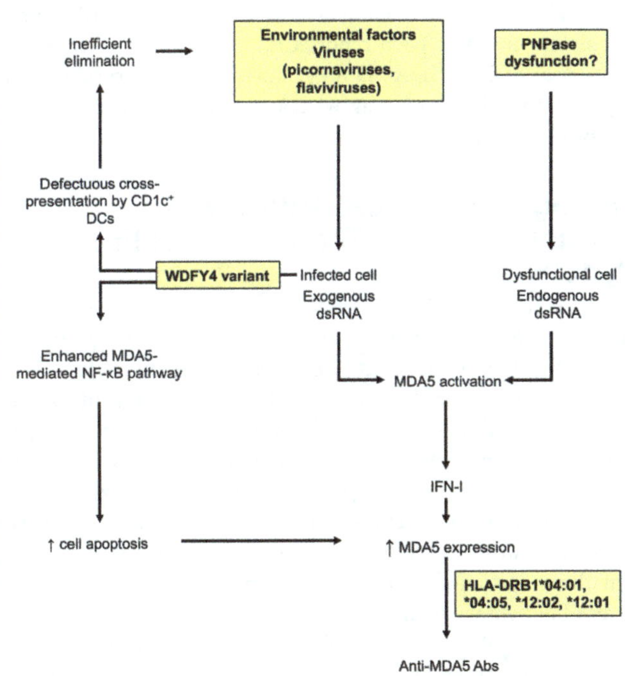

FIGURE 3 | Possible genetic and environmental factors involved in the anti-MDA5 dermatomyositis. Viral double stranded RNA (dsRNA) activates MDA5 in infected cells, leading to type I interferon (IFN-I) production and increased levels of MDA5. Altered WDFY4 impairs antigen cross-presentation by CD1c+ dendritic cells (DCs), favoring an inefficient elimination of infected cells and further activation of MDA5. In parallel, altered WDFY4 also enhances MDA5-mediated nuclear factor-kappa B (NF-κB) pathway leading to the apoptosis of infected cells, and the release of MDA5. Local dysfunctional mitochondrial polynucleotide phosphorylase (PNPase) could lead to intracellular accumulation of endogenous dsRNA, fueling uncontrolled activation and expression of MDA5. Abnormal accumulation of MDA5 may favor a loss of tolerance to MDA5 in an individual with proper genetic background, leading to anti-MDA5 antibodies (Abs).

function of the enzyme could generate an accumulation of endogenous dsRNA, leading to MDA5 activation, IFN-I pathway stimulation and elevated MDA5 expression.

Environmental Factor

The hypothesis of a viral trigger of anti-MDA5 DM is suggested by epidemiological studies that highlighted a seasonal distribution of the disease. Classically, anti-MDA5 DM onset follows a seasonal repartition with an epidemic period in fall and winter, a peak in late winter and spring and a dip in summer, following respiratory virus epidemic period (102, 103). In the hypothesis of a viral infection as a possible initiator of autoimmunity, the scenario could involve an activation of MDA5 in the infected cells, leading to IFN-I production and increased levels of MDA5, followed by an excessive local apoptosis favored by a specific genetic background (intronic variant of WDFY4). The release of the MDA5 antigen into the microenvironment following cell lysis could be the cause of a loss of tolerance towards MDA5, resulting in the production of anti-MDA5 Abs. This mechanism could also be fueled by a defect in the elimination of the virus, due to an inefficient cross-presentation of viral antigens by CD1c$^+$ DCs (**Figure 3**).

It is also interesting to note that a geographical distribution of the disease has also been reported in Japan, with an increased prevalence of anti-MDA5 DM in patients living in rural areas as opposed to urban areas as well as in patients residing near freshwater (103, 104).

Pathogenesis of the Anti-MDA5 Dermatomyositis: The Vasculopathy Hypothesis

Several pieces of evidence point toward a central role of vascular injury in the pathogenesis of anti-MDA5 DM: (i) Patients frequently show typical cutaneous features such as skin ulcers due to severe vasculopathy; (ii) Histopathology of palmar papules, as well as lung tissues highlights vasculopathy (12, 15, 105); (iii) Biomarkers of endothelial dysfunctions have been identified in the sera of patients (106, 107); (iv) Patients exhibited a strong IFN-I signature distributed in the vasculature of the skin (108, 109). It is important to emphasize that these particular features are observed in the skin and the lungs of patients with anti-MDA5 DM but that there is no or few signs of vasculopathy nor of an enhanced IFN-I signature, compared to other DM, in muscle tissue of anti-MDA5 DM patients (21, 22).

Biomarkers of endothelial dysfunctions released in the sera of anti-MDA5 DM patients include endothelin, thrombomodulin, plasminogen activator inhibitor, von Willebrand factor (vWF), soluble vascular cell adhesion molecule-1 and soluble intercellular adhesion molecule-1 (106, 107). Interestingly, serum levels of endothelin and vWF are higher in anti-MDA5 DM patients who have cutaneous ulcers and ILD and IFN-I signature correlates positively with endothelin levels (106). All together, these data suggest that blood vessels exposure to IFN-I in anti-MDA5 DM may lead to endothelial injury, ultimately responsible for the cutaneous and pulmonary lesions associated with this disease.

Vasculopathy and Pulmonary Lesions

Anti-MDA5 DM is associated with an accumulation of activated macrophages (M2) in alveoli (110, 111). Several markers of macrophage activation are elevated in the serum of anti-MDA5 DM patients, such as a soluble form of CD206, which is highly expressed by alveolar macrophages (110, 112). Other soluble markers of activated macrophages, such as a soluble form of CD163, as well as the chitotriosidase and the ferritin, are also found in the sera of patients at significantly higher levels than in other subtypes of DM (110, 111, 113, 114). Neopterin levels, another marker of macrophage activation, are elevated in DM patients with anti-MDA5 Abs in association with RP-ILD and reduced survival. A positive correlation of neopterin levels with ferritin and markers of disease severity, and a negative correlation with pulmonary function have been demonstrated (115). Multiple chemokines can induce the recruitment of M2 macrophages. Among them, the chemokine CX3CL1 (Fractalkine) is of interest in anti-MDA5 DM since its concentration is elevated in sera of patients (116). CX3CL1 secretion can be induced by IFN-I in pulmonary vascular endothelial cells and induces the recruitment of CX3CR1$^+$M2 macrophages in the lungs (117, 118). It is then tempting to speculate that high levels of IFN-I induce endothelial injury leading to the secretion of CX3CL1, responsible for the recruitment of intrapulmonary profibrotic M2 macrophages. Locally, M2 macrophages produce TGF-β to directly promote pulmonary fibrosis, and could be involved in the recruitment of profibrotic CD4$^+$CXCR4$^+$ T cells. In agreement with this, elevated levels of CD4$^+$CXCR4$^+$ T cells are observed in the peripheral blood and the bronchoalveolar lavage fluids of patients with ILD. Locally, the airway epithelial cells and the macrophages are the main sources of the stromal cell derived factor-1 (SDF-1 or CXCL12), the ligand of CXCR4 (119). Once recruited, the CD4$^+$CXCR4$^+$ T cells may promote pulmonary fibroblast proliferation, partly through the release of IL-21, and secondarily by the production of profibrotic agents, namely TGF-β, α-smooth muscle actin and collagen I. IL-21 is known to induce the differentiation of IL-13 producing-CD8$^+$ T cells, which in turn enhance IL-21 production, creating an activation loop (120). IL-13 may fuel pulmonary fibrosis through two mechanisms: direct activation of fibroblast, and stimulation of the synthesis of TGF-β by activated macrophages (121) (**Figure 4**).

Vasculopathy and Cutaneous Lesions

Histology of skin biopsies from patients with anti-MDA5 DM classically show an interface dermatitis, a histopathological pattern characterized by vacuolar changes, apoptotic keratinocytes and infiltration of CD8$^+$ lymphocytes at the dermoepidermal junction (122–124). The interface dermatitis is also a classical feature observed in systemic erythematosus lupus and lichen planus. Another common feature of all these diseases is the enhanced IFN-I signaling into the skin of patients.

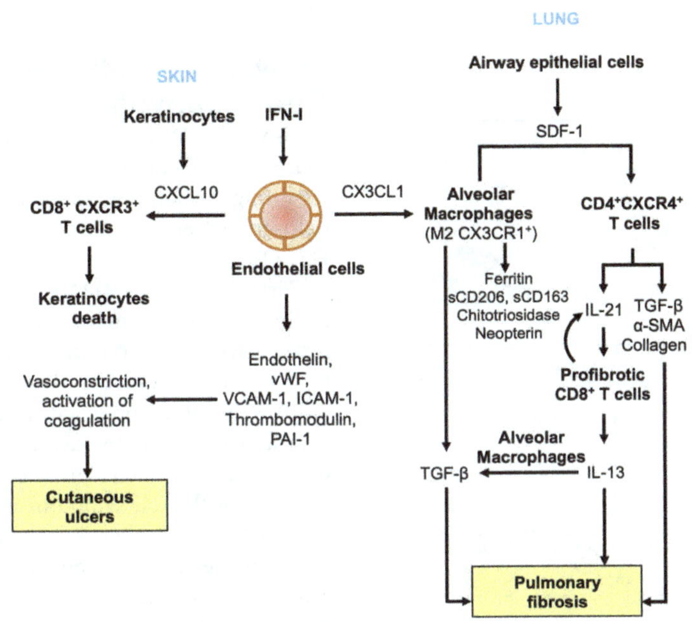

FIGURE 4 | Endothelial dysfunctions and immune alterations in anti-MDA5 dermatomyositis. In the skin, CXCL10, a keratinocyte and endothelial-derived chemokine, induces the recruitment of $CD8^+CXCR3^+$ T cells, potentially autoreactive and leading to keratinocytes death. Endothelin released by injured endothelial cells, is a strong vasoconstrictor which can induce local ischemia responsible for cutaneous ulcers. In the lung, CX3CL1 can be produced by vascular pulmonary endothelial cells following IFN-I exposure. CX3CL1 recruits $CX3CR1^+$ alternative alveolar macrophages (M2). Alveolar M2 macrophages, as well as airway epithelial cells, release stromal cell-derived factor 1 (SDF-1) which induces the accumulation of intrapulmonary $CD4^+CXCR4^+$ T cells. $CD4^+CXCR4^+$ T cells produce profibrotic agents (transformation growth factor-β (TGF-β), α-smooth muscle actin (α-SMA) and collagen I), as well as IL-21, which promotes the differentiation of profibrotic $CD8^+$ T cells. $CD8^+$ T cells secrete IL-13, which stimulates macrophages to produce profibrotic factors.

A common pathophysiological model has therefore been proposed, based on the secretion of keratinocyte-derived CXCL10 following skin exposure to IFN-I (125–128). Consistent with this observation, the expression of CXCL10 as well as the expression of IFN-I induced proteins (ISG15, MxA) are upregulated in the skin of anti-MDA5 Abs positive patients (108, 109, 126, 129). Endothelial cells stimulated by IFN-I could also constitute another source of CXCL10 (130). CXCL10 then induces the recruitment of $CXCR3^+CD8^+$ T cells, potentially autoreactive, responsible for the apoptosis of keratinocytes (125, 126) (**Figure 4**).

In addition, skin biopsies from anti-MDA5 DM patients also show more severe lesions, affecting the deeper layers of skin, down to the dermis. Epidermal necrosis and typical findings of vasculopathy are observed, with vascular fibrin deposition, thickening of the vascular walls and vascular thrombosis of the small and medium vessels (12, 15, 123, 131). Endothelin, released consequently to endothelial injury caused by chronic exposure to IFN-I, acts as a potent vasoconstrictor. It may in part be responsible for the skin ulcers, by inducing a local ischemia, as is the case in other diseases (132). The regression of skin ulcers in patients treated with bosentan, an endothelin-receptor inhibitor, or with a vasodilator drug, such as sildenafil, supports this hypothesis (133–135). In the same way, pro-coagulant factors (e.g. vWF) released by damaged endothelial cell could lead to blood coagulation activation, as evidenced by the vascular fibrin deposits and thromboses observed histologically (**Figure 4**).

Potential Contribution of Anti-MDA5 Antibodies to the Pathogenesis

Whether we consider skin or lung lesions, IFN-I seems to be the starting point for all the pathophysiological pathways described above. Indeed, IFN-I signaling is enhanced in anti-MDA5 DM, in skin and in serum, more than in other DM, suggesting the presence of a specific trigger of the IFN-I pathway in the disease (109, 129, 136). Here we assume that anti-MDA5 Abs could be the cornerstone of the dysregulation of the IFN-I pathway in anti-MDA5 DM. Several observations support this hypothesis: (i) The severity of the disease correlates with the titers of anti-MDA5 Abs (12, 63, 64, 67); (ii) The use of therapies that target the humoral immune response has shown its effectiveness in patients with anti-MDA5 DM (137–141); (iii) MDA5 expression has been shown to be enhanced in skin biopsies of patients (79).

In pathological contexts, MDA5 is overexpressed in altered tissues such as the skin of patients and ectopic expression of MDA5 at the cell surface has been reported (79, 80). In this context, anti-MDA5 Abs could then bind to MDA5-positive cells and induce an inappropriate activation of MDA5, leading to the dysregulation and the chronic activation of the IFN-I pathway in target tissues, worsening the existent lesions. Anti-MDA5 Abs binding to its antigenic target could also induce immune-mediated cytotoxicity by complement fixation or antibody-dependent cytotoxicity, further worsening the lesions (**Figure 5A**). Apart from binding to MDA5 expressed on cell

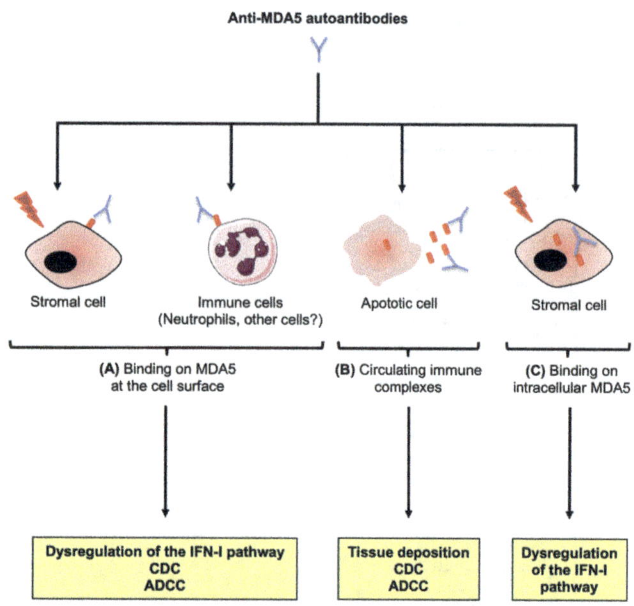

FIGURE 5 | Potential contribution of the anti-MDA5 antibodies to the pathogenesis. Anti-MDA5 antibodies (Abs) may contribute to the pathogenesis in several ways. **(A)** In specific conditions, MDA5 may translocate at the surface of critical stromal cells, or immune cells such as neutrophils. Interaction between the autoAb and the ectopic antigenic target could trigger chronic activation of the type I interferon (IFN-I) signaling pathway, as well as immune mediated cytotoxicity through complement activation (CDC) and/or Ab-dependent cytotoxicity (ADCC). **(B)** Anti-MDA5 Abs could also bind to MDA5 released from apoptotic cells, to form immune complexes that could contribute to immune-mediated damage. **(C)** A cell exposed to a stress (infection, genetic background) overexpresses intracytoplasmic MDA5. Anti-MDA5 Abs might penetrate the cell to bind to MDA5, altering several functional pathways.

surface, anti-MDA5 Abs could also form immune complexes with the MDA5 proteins released from apoptotic skin and/or lung fibroblasts. These immune complexes could then deposit in organs, for example in dermal/lung vessels, inducing more vascular damage (**Figure 5B**). Finally, anti-MDA5 Abs could penetrate cells and interact with cytoplasmic MDA5, similarly to what has been described with other Abs, altering several functional pathways (**Figure 5C**) (142–144).

The isotype and the subclass of anti-MDA5 Abs might also affect their potential pathogenic function. In a Chinese cohort, anti-MDA5 IgA and IgG were the predominant isotypes. Interestingly, anti-MDA5 IgG1 were associated with higher serum ferritin levels, severe interstitial pneumonia, and a higher mortality rate. The combined positivity for anti-MDA5 IgG1 and anti-MDA5 IgG4 was predictive of poor prognosis (145). IgG1 are potent activators of the complement pathway, and as a result, anti-MDA5 IgG1 could be the main subclass involved in the pathogenesis of the disease. The identification of anti-MDA5 IgG4 is more unexpected, as IgG4 are considered non-inflammatory, owing to the unique structure of their hinge region (146). Whether the presence of anti-MDA5 IgG4 in the most severe forms of the disease reflects a modulatory mechanism, although insufficient, remains to be defined.

Similarities Between Anti-MDA5 Dermatomyositis and COVID-19

Anti-MDA5 DM and coronavirus disease 2019 (COVID-19) share several common features, clinical and pathogenic, and exploring the pathophysiological mechanisms of COVID-19 may help to better understand the pathogenesis of anti-MDA5 DM (147).

First, as for anti-MDA5 DM, COVID-19 can be complicated by interstitial pneumonia which can lead to acute respiratory distress syndrome and death. This pulmonary damage is difficult to distinguish from the ILD associated with anti-MDA5 DM (148). Thus, it is important to carefully assess patients with RP-ILD, in particular in the case of a negative RT-PCR test for SARS-CoV-2 (severe acute respiratory syndrome coronavirus 2) as RP-ILD may be the sole symptom at anti-MDA5 CADM onset. Anti-MDA5 DM may then be easily confounded with COVID-19, delaying the diagnosis and treatment. Inversely, patients with positive test for anti-MDA5 Abs, or any other MSA, and who develop acute pneumonia should be tested for SARS-CoV-2 infection, as the infection worsens the patient's condition (149).

Second, anti-MDA5 DM and COVID-19 seem to share several pathogenic mechanisms. Both diseases are characterized by an activation of the IFN-I signaling pathway. However, although in anti-MDA5 DM, dysregulation of the IFN-I axis seems to exacerbate the disease, the role of the IFN-I pathway in COVID-19 appears more complex. MDA5 is a sensor of SARS-CoV-2 in lung cells, and its activation induces an IFN response to eliminate the virus (150–152). The IFN-I pathway plays a major role in the defense against the virus in COVID-19, as illustrated by the impaired IFN-I signaling in severe cases and the presence of anti-IFN-I Abs in the sera of more than 10% of patients with a life-threatening infection (153–156). In this sense, early activation of the IFN-I signaling pathway appears to be an essential weapon against SARS-CoV-2 infection. In contrast, a strong delayed IFN-I response could exacerbate the hyperinflammation associated with the most severe forms of COVID-19 (157, 158).

Another common pathological feature shared by the two diseases is the endothelial injury and the thrombotic manifestations associated with the more severe forms (148, 159, 160). This is highlighted by the presence of markers of endothelial and platelet activation as well as coagulation factors and fibrinolytic enzymes in the serum of patients, such as vWF, thrombomodulin, P-selectin and D-dimer (161). The important systemic inflammatory response and activation of the angiotensin converting enzyme 2 (ACE2), the major cell entry receptor for SARS-CoV-2, expressed on endothelial cells are accountable for these vascular damages (159, 162).

Finally, anti-MDA5 Abs have been identified in the serum of Chinese patients diagnosed with COVID-19 (48.2% of 274 patients), frequently in the most severe cases. Furthermore, the titers of anti-MDA5 Abs appear to correlate with the severity of the disease and were higher in the non-survival cases (163).

These preliminary results should, however, be taken with caution. Indeed, although the titers of anti-MDA5 Abs are statistically higher in the non-survivals infected SARS-CoV-2 patients *versus* the survivals, the orders of magnitude are very low (5.95 ± 5.16 U/mL *vs* 8.22 ± 6.64 U/mL, P = 0.030). In addition, it is well established that common viral infections, as well as SARS-CoV-2 infection, frequently trigger the induction of transient, low-titer, polyspecific autoantibodies (164, 165). In agreement with this, several myositis-specific autoantibodies have been identified as false positives in patients with COVID (166). To what extent these anti-MDA5 Abs are really specific, to what extent they are present in the infection of other RNA viruses or only during the infection by SARS-CoV-2, and what are their implications for the patient in the short and long term are all unanswered questions to be explored.

TREATMENT OF ANTI-MDA5 DERMATOMYOSITIS

Although no recommendations for the management of anti-MDA5 DM exist at this time, a combination immunosuppressive (IS) therapy is wildly used. This intensive IS treatment classically consists of an association of glucocorticoids with a calcineurin inhibitor (cyclosporine A or tacrolimus) or a triple therapy with the addition of intravenous cyclophosphamide or mycophenolate mofetil. However, many cases are refractory to this treatment with a reported overall mortality rate after treatment of 40% (167). Resistance to treatment, beyond worsening clinical signs, can be assessed by monitoring the level of anti-MDA5 Abs, ferritin or IL-18 which tend to stabilize or increase in patients refractory to treatment (51, 91, 168, 169). Other studies evaluating the effectiveness of intensive IS therapy highlighted the importance of beginning the treatment early after the diagnosis to improve the prognosis (91, 170). In addition to being partially efficient, the intense IS bi- or tri-therapy is responsible for several adverse events, mostly infections and renal function alteration. Renal function alteration is mostly due to calcineurin inhibitors and lead to treatment interruption in most cases. Bacterial, viral and fungal infections are reported, the most frequent being the reactivation of cytomegalovirus (29, 46, 171, 172). *Pneumocystis jirovecii* pneumonia is also encountered (29, 173, 174). Whether the infections are the result of IS treatment or of the disease itself is not clear, although DM was associated with a higher risk of developing pneumocystosis in a French retrospective study (175).

Due to the limited effectiveness and frequent adverse events of these treatments, several alternative therapy strategies are currently evaluated to treat refractory cases. The rare studies evaluating alternative therapies, such as the use of vasodilators, inhibitors of the IFN axis, or therapies that target the humoral immune response, illustrate the importance of the dysregulated pathways discussed previously in the pathogenesis of the disease.

Data regarding the improvement of cutaneous lesions after intensive IS treatment are scarce but some case reports of cutaneous lesions refractory to IS drugs have been published (48, 137, 176). As the vascular injury seems to have a central role in the development of skin lesions, drugs such as sildenafil, a vasodilatator, or bosentan, an endothelin-receptor inhibitor, might be added to the IS treatment to treat the skin ulcerations (32, 133–135).

Considering the importance of the IFN-I signaling pathway in anti-MDA5 DM, inhibitors of Janus Kinases (JAK) appear to be a promising treatment for anti-MDA5 DM. Several studies reported the efficacy of tofacitinib and ruxolitinib in patients who experienced a relapse or were refractory to standard treatment (50, 176–179). JAK/STAT signaling pathway is activated by IFNs leading to the transcription of IFN-stimulated genes (ISGs), including MDA5. Tofacitinib and ruxolitinib inhibit this pathway, decreasing MDA5 expression and activation. Furthermore, its effectiveness on refractory forms of ILD reinforces the potential role of IL-21 in the pathophysiology of ILD as JAK-pathway is required for IL-21/IL-21R signaling (119, 180, 181). JAK inhibitors could then be used to treat or prevent severe forms of ILD. Tofacitinib seems well tolerated in most patients but one study reported cytomegalovirus reactivation in 100% of patients, varicella-zoster virus reactivation (60%) and bacterial respiratory infections (80%) (178). Whether these adverse events were caused by the disease or the therapy was not determined. The question remains whether JAK-inhibitors should be administered in patients refractory to classic IS therapy or be initiated at diagnosis to avoid worsening of the disease. A clinical trial including 50 Japanese patients with anti-MDA5 CADM-associated ILD diagnosed for less than 3 months reported a 6-month survival significantly higher (100%) in the group of patients (n=18) who received a glucocorticoid combined with tofacitinb than in the group (n=32) who received conventional immunosuppressive treatment (6-month survival of 78%) (182). JAK inhibitors could therefore have a prominent place in the first-line treatment of anti-MDA5 DM.

A pathogenic role of anti-MDA5 Abs could motivate the use of plasmapheresis, IV immunoglobulins and rituximab. Although evidence is limited to small case series, these therapies seem efficacious (137–141, 183–187), apart from one case report of a patient whose condition worsened after plasma exchange probably due to transfusion-related acute lung injury (188). However, their effectiveness in large cohorts of patients as well as data concerning long-term remission remain to be evaluated.

CONCLUSION

Anti-MDA5 DM is a systemic autoimmune disease that can be divided into 3 clinical subgroups, with different prognosis, linked to the incidence of RP-ILD which is influenced by the ethnic origin of the patients. Recent publications suggest a central role for IFN-I mediated vasculopathy. It might be responsible for both the pulmonary and the cutaneous lesions, through the secretion of endothelial-derived substances inducing the recruitment and the activation of immune cells, *in fine* responsible for the lesions observed in anti-MDA5 DM. Anti-MDA5 Abs might also contribute to the pathogenesis by altering the IFN-I pathway. Of course, further studies need to be conducted to confirm these assumptions. Elucidating the precise role of anti-MDA5 Abs associated to the disease will constitute a crucial step in the understanding of the pathogenesis. An improved knowledge of the pathogenesis of the disease will also undoubtedly pave the way for the development of more effective therapeutic strategies.

AUTHOR CONTRIBUTIONS

AN and FC: writing and figures. FC and NF: concept and proof reading. All authors contributed to the article and approved the submitted version.

REFERENCES

1. Mariampillai K, Granger B, Amelin D, Guiguet M, Hachulla E, Maurier F, et al. Development of a New Classification System for Idiopathic Inflammatory Myopathies Based on Clinical Manifestations and Myositis-Specific Autoantibodies. *JAMA Neurol* (2018) 75:1528–37. doi: 10.1001/jamaneurol.2018.2598
2. Allenbach Y, Uzunhan Y, Toquet S, Leroux G, Gallay L, Marquet A, et al. Different Phenotypes in Dermatomyositis Associated With Anti-MDA5 Antibody: Study of 121 Cases. *Neurology* (2020) 95:e70–8. doi: 10.1212/WNL.0000000000009727
3. Betteridge Z, Tansley S, Shaddick G, Chinoy H, Cooper RG, New RP, et al. Frequency, Mutual Exclusivity and Clinical Associations of Myositis Autoantibodies in a Combined European Cohort of Idiopathic Inflammatory Myopathy Patients. *J Autoimmun* (2019) 101:48–55. doi: 10.1016/j.jaut.2019.04.001
4. Sato S, Hirakata M, Kuwana M, Suwa A, Inada S, Mimori T, et al. Autoantibodies to a 140-Kd Polypeptide, CADM-140, in Japanese Patients With Clinically Amyopathic Dermatomyositis. *Arthritis Rheum* (2005) 52:1571–6. doi: 10.1002/art.21023
5. Fujikawa K, Kawakami A, Kaji K, Fujimoto M, Kawashiri S, Iwamoto N, et al. Association of Distinct Clinical Subsets With Myositis-Specific Autoantibodies Towards Anti-155/140-kDa Polypeptides, Anti-140-kDa Polypeptides, and Anti-Aminoacyl tRNA Synthetases in Japanese Patients With Dermatomyositis: A Single-Centre, Cross-Sectional Study. *Scand J Rheumatol* (2009) 38:263–7. doi: 10.1080/03009740802687455
6. Gono T, Kawaguchi Y, Satoh T, Kuwana M, Katsumata Y, Takagi K, et al. Clinical Manifestation and Prognostic Factor in Anti-Melanoma Differentiation-Associated Gene 5 Antibody-Associated Interstitial Lung Disease as a Complication of Dermatomyositis. *Rheumatology* (2010) 49:1713–9. doi: 10.1093/rheumatology/keq149
7. Nakashima R, Imura Y, Kobayashi S, Yukawa N, Yoshifuji H, Nojima T, et al. The RIG-I-Like Receptor IFIH1/MDA5 Is a Dermatomyositis-Specific Autoantigen Identified by the Anti-CADM-140 Antibody. *Rheumatology* (2010) 49:433–40. doi: 10.1093/rheumatology/kep375
8. Ikeda N, Takahashi K, Yamaguchi Y, Inasaka M, Kuwana M, Ikezawa Z. Analysis of Dermatomyositis-Specific Autoantibodies and Clinical Characteristics in Japanese Patients. *J Dermatol* (2011) 38:973–9. doi: 10.1111/j.1346-8138.2011.01262.x
9. Hamaguchi Y, Kuwana M, Hoshino K, Hasegawa M, Kaji K, Matsushita T, et al. Clinical Correlations With Dermatomyositis-Specific Autoantibodies in Adult Japanese Patients With Dermatomyositis: A Multicenter Cross-Sectional Study. *Arch Dermatol* (2011) 147:391–8. doi: 10.1001/archdermatol.2011.52
10. Koga T, Fujikawa K, Horai Y, Okada A, Kawashiri SY, Iwamoto N, et al. The Diagnostic Utility of Anti-Melanoma Differentiation-Associated Gene 5 Antibody Testing for Predicting the Prognosis of Japanese Patients With DM. *Rheumatology* (2012) 51:1278–84. doi: 10.1093/rheumatology/ker518
11. Chen F, Wang D, Shu X, Nakashima R, Wang G. Anti-MDA5 Antibody Is Associated With A/SIP and Decreased T Cells in Peripheral Blood and Predicts Poor Prognosis of ILD in Chinese Patients With Dermatomyositis. *Rheumatol Int* (2012) 32:3909–15. doi: 10.1007/s00296-011-2323-y
12. Cao H, Pan M, Kang Y, Xia Q, Li X, Zhao X, et al. Clinical Manifestations of Dermatomyositis and Clinically Amyopathic Dermatomyositis Patients With Positive Expression of Anti-Melanoma Differentiation-Associated Gene 5 Antibody. *Arthritis Care Res* (2012) 64:1602–10. doi: 10.1002/acr.21728
13. Chen Z, Cao M, Plana MN, Liang J, Cai H, Kuwana M, et al. Utility of Anti-Melanoma Differentiation-Associated Gene 5 Antibody Measurement in Identifying Patients With Dermatomyositis and a High Risk for Developing Rapidly Progressive Interstitial Lung Disease: A Review of the Literature and a Meta-Analysis. *Arthritis Care Res* (2013) 65:1316–24. doi: 10.1002/acr.21985
14. Li Y, Li Y, Wu J, Miao M, Gao X, Cai W, et al. Predictors of Poor Outcome of Anti-MDA5-Associated Rapidly Progressive Interstitial Lung Disease in a Chinese Cohort With Dermatomyositis. *J Immunol Res* (2020) 2020:1–8. doi: 10.1155/2020/2024869
15. Fiorentino D, Chung L, Zwerner J, Rosen A, Casciola-Rosen L. The Mucocutaneous and Systemic Phenotype of Dermatomyositis Patients With Antibodies to MDA5 (CADM-140). *J Am Acad Dermatol* (2011) 65:25–34. doi: 10.1016/j.jaad.2010.09.016
16. Hall JC, Casciola-Rosen L, Samedy LA, Werner J, Owoyemi K, Danoff SK, et al. Anti-Melanoma Differentiation-Associated Protein 5-Associated Dermatomyositis: Expanding the Clinical Spectrum. *Arthritis Care Res* (2013) 65:1307–15. doi: 10.1002/acr.21992
17. Labrador-Horrillo M, Martinez MA, Selva-O'Callaghan A, Trallero-Araguas E, Balada E, Vilardell-Tarres M, et al. Anti-MDA5 Antibodies in a Large Mediterranean Population of Adults With Dermatomyositis. *J Immunol Res* (2014) 2014:1–8. doi: 10.1155/2014/290797
18. Ceribelli A, Fredi M, Taraborelli M, Cavazzana I, Tincani A, Selmi C, et al. Prevalence and Clinical Significance of Anti-MDA5 Antibodies in European Patients With Polymyositis/Dermatomyositis. *Clin Exp Rheumatol* (2014) 32 (6):891–7.
19. Borges IBP, Silva MG, Shinjo SK. Prevalence and Reactivity of Anti-Melanoma Differentiation-Associated Gene 5 (Anti-MDA-5) Autoantibody in Brazilian Patients With Dermatomyositis. *Bras Dermatol* (2018) 93:517–23. doi: 10.1590/abd1806-4841.20186803
20. Sontheimer RD. MDA5 Autoantibody—Another Indicator of Clinical Diversity in Dermatomyositis. *Ann Transl Med* (2017) 5(7):160. doi: 10.21037/atm.2017.03.94
21. Jiang Y, Liu Y, Zhao Y, Zheng Y, Yu M, Deng J, et al. Mitochondrial Morphology and MAVS-IFN1 Signaling Pathway in Muscles of Anti-MDA5 Dermatomyositis. *Ann Clin Transl Neurol* (2021) 8:677–86. doi: 10.1002/acn3.51311
22. Allenbach Y, Leroux G, Suárez-Calvet X, Preusse C, Gallardo E, Hervier B, et al. Dermatomyositis With or Without Anti-Melanoma Differentiation-Associated Gene 5 Antibodies. *Am J Pathol* (2016) 186:691–700. doi: 10.1016/j.ajpath.2015.11.010
23. Cabezas-Rodríguez I, Morante-Bolado I, Brandy-García A, Queiro-Silva R, Mozo L, Ballina-García FJ. Anti-MDA5 Dermatomyositis Mimicking Psoriatic Arthritis. *Reumatol Clínica* (2018) 14:224–6. doi: 10.1016/j.reuma.2016.10.010
24. Haroon M, Devlin J. Gottrons's Papule in Amyopathic Dermatomyositis Mimicking Psoriasis. *Clin Rheumatol* (2009) 28:1245–6. doi: 10.1007/s10067-009-1244-6

25. Moghadam-Kia S, Oddis CV, Sato S, Kuwana M, Aggarwal R. Antimelanoma Differentiation-Associated Gene 5 Antibody: Expanding the Clinical Spectrum in North American Patients With Dermatomyositis. *J Rheumatol* (2017) 44:319–25. doi: 10.3899/jrheum.160682
26. Hoa S, Troyanov Y, Fritzler M, Targoff I, Chartrand S, Mansour A, et al. Describing and Expanding the Clinical Phenotype of Anti-MDA5-Associated Rapidly Progressive Interstitial Lung Disease: Case Series of Nine Canadian Patients and Literature Review. *Scand J Rheumatol* (2018) 47:210–24. doi: 10.1080/03009742.2017.1334814
27. Gerfaud-Valentin M, Ahmad K, Piegay F, Fabien N, Raphanel B, Cordier J-F, et al. Pneumopathie Infiltrante Diffuse Associée À Une Dermatomyosite Amyopathique Avec Auto-Anticorps Anti-MDA5. *Rev Mal Respir* (2014) 31:849–53. doi: 10.1016/j.rmr.2014.02.010
28. Charrow A, Vleugels RA. Cutaneous Ulcerations in Anti-MDA5 Dermatomyositis. *N Engl J Med* (2019) 381:465. doi: 10.1056/NEJMicm1816147
29. Yamaguchi K, Yamaguchi A, Onuki Y, Itai M, Kashiwagi C, Takehara K, et al. Clinical Features of Dermatomyositis Associated With Anti-MDA5 Antibodies by Age. *Mod Rheumatol* (2020) 31:177–85. doi: 10.1080/14397595.2020.1740400
30. Narang NS, Casciola-Rosen L, Li S, Chung L, Fiorentino DF. Cutaneous Ulceration in Dermatomyositis: Association With Anti-Melanoma Differentiation-Associated Gene 5 Antibodies and Interstitial Lung Disease. *Arthritis Care Res* (2015) 67:667–72. doi: 10.1002/acr.22498
31. So H, Ip RW-K, Wong VT-L, Yip RM-L. Analysis of Anti-Melanoma Differentiation-Associated Gene 5 Antibody in Hong Kong Chinese Patients With Idiopathic Inflammatory Myopathies: Diagnostic Utility and Clinical Correlations. *Int J Rheum Dis* (2018) 21:1076–81. doi: 10.1111/1756-185X.13268
32. Xu A, Lv X, Du F, Dai M. Cutaneous Ulceration and Digital Gangrene in an Anti-MDA5-Positive Overlap Myositis. *Rheumatology* (2021), keab284. doi: 10.1093/rheumatology/keab284
33. Barailler H, Charles S, Goutorbe F, Devaux S. An Unusual Anti–Melanoma Differentiation–Associated Protein 5 Amyopathic Dermatomyositis. *JAAD Case Rep* (2019) 5:383–5. doi: 10.1016/j.jdcr.2019.02.019
34. Okiyama N, Inoue S, Saito A, Nakamura Y, Ishitsuka Y, Fujisawa Y, et al. Antihelix/helix Violaceous Macules in Japanese Patients With Anti-Melanoma Differentiation-Associated Protein 5 (MDA 5) Antibody-Associated Dermatomyositis. *Br J Dermatol* (2019) 180:1226–7. doi: 10.1111/bjd.17431
35. Motegi S, Sekiguchi A, Toki S, Kishi C, Endo Y, Yasuda M, et al. Clinical Features and Poor Prognostic Factors of Anti-Melanoma Differentiation-Associated Gene 5 Antibody-Positive Dermatomyositis With Rapid Progressive Interstitial Lung Disease. *Eur J Dermatol* (2019) 29:511–7. doi: 10.1684/ejd.2019.3634
36. Intapiboon P, Siripaitoon B. Erythematous Auricular Papules in the Fatal Cases of Anti-MDA5 Antibody-Positive Interstitial Lung Disease. *Respir Med Case Rep* (2020) 31:101299. doi: 10.1016/j.rmcr.2020.101299
37. Molina-Ruiz AM, Romero F, Carrasco L, Feltes F, Haro R, Requena L. Amyophatic Dermatomyositis Presenting as a Flagellated Skin Eruption With Positive *MDA5* Antibodies and Thyroid Cancer: A Real Association? *Clin Exp Dermatol* (2015) 40:887–90. doi: 10.1111/ced.12674
38. Watanabe T, Takizawa N, Nagasaka T, Nakamura Y, Ikai H, Yamamoto M, et al. Fatal and Extensive Multiorgan Hemorrhages in Anti-Melanoma Differentiation-Associated Gene 5 Antibody-Positive Dermatomyositis: An Autopsy Case Report. *Med (Baltimore)* (2020) 99:e18600. doi: 10.1097/MD.00000000000186004
39. González-Moreno J, Raya-Cruz M, Losada-Lopez I, Cacheda AP, Oliver C, Colom B. Rapidly Progressive Interstitial Lung Disease Due to Anti-MDA5 Antibodies Without Skin Involvement: A Case Report and Literature Review. *Rheumatol Int* (2018) 38:1293–96. doi: 10.1007/s00296-018-3991-7
40. Rathore U, Haldule S, Gupta L. Psoriasiform Rashes as the First Manifestation of Anti-MDA5 Associated Myositis. *Rheumatology* (2020) 60(7):3483. doi: 10.1093/rheumatology/keaa821
41. Lega J-C, Fabien N, Reynaud Q, Durieu I, Durupt S, Dutertre M, et al. The Clinical Phenotype Associated With Myositis-Specific and Associated Autoantibodies: A Meta-Analysis Revisiting the So-Called Antisynthetase Syndrome. *Autoimmun Rev* (2014) 13:883–91. doi: 10.1016/j.autrev.2014.03.004
42. Tanizawa K, Handa T, Nakashima R, Kubo T, Hosono Y, Watanabe K, et al. HRCT Features of Interstitial Lung Disease in Dermatomyositis With Anti-CADM-140 Antibody. *Respir Med* (2011) 105:1380–7. doi: 10.1016/j.rmed.2011.05.006
43. Sakamoto N, Ishimoto H, Nakashima S, Yura H, Miyamura T, Okuno D, et al. Clinical Features of Anti-MDA5 Antibody-Positive Rapidly Progressive Interstitial Lung Disease Without Signs of Dermatomyositis. *Intern Med* (2019) 58:837–41. doi: 10.2169/internalmedicine.1516-18
44. Ortiz-Santamaria V, Babot A, Ferrer C. Anti-MDA5-Positive Dermatomyositis: An Emerging Entity With a Variable Clinical Presentation. *Scand J Rheumatol* (2017) 46:509–11. doi: 10.1080/03009742.2017.1340512
45. Li Y, Gao X, Li Y, Jia X, Zhang X, Xu Y, et al. Predictors and Mortality of Rapidly Progressive Interstitial Lung Disease in Patients With Idiopathic Inflammatory Myopathy: A Series of 474 Patients. *Front Med* (2020) 7:363. doi: 10.3389/fmed.2020.00363
46. Yamaguchi K, Yamaguchi A, Kashiwagi C, Sawada Y, Taguchi K, Umetsu K, et al. Differential Clinical Features of Patients With Clinically Amyopathic Dermatomyositis Who Have Circulating Anti-MDA5 Autoantibodies With or Without Myositis-Associated Autoantibodies. *Respir Med* (2018) 140:1–5. doi: 10.1016/j.rmed.2018.05.010
47. Endo Y, Koga T, Ishida M, Fujita Y, Tsuji S, Takatani A, et al. Recurrence of Anti-MDA5 Antibody-Positive Clinically Amyopathic Dermatomyositis After Long-Term Remission: A Case Report. *Med (Baltimore)* (2018) 97: e11024. doi: 10.1097/MD.0000000000011024
48. Ishikawa Y, Kasuya T, Fujiwara M, Kita Y. Tofacitinib for Recurrence of Antimelanoma Differentiation-Associated Gene 5 Antibody-Positive Clinically Amyopathic Dermatomyositis After Remission: A Case Report. *Med (Baltimore)* (2020) 99:e21943. doi: 10.1097/MD.0000000000021943
49. Betteridge Z, McHugh N. Myositis-Specific Autoantibodies: An Important Tool to Support Diagnosis of Myositis. *J Intern Med* (2016) 280:8–23. doi: 10.1111/joim.12451
50. Jalles C, Deroux A, Tardieu M, Lugosi M, Viel S, Benveniste O, et al. Dermatomyosite À Anticorps Anti-MDA5 Sévère Associée À Un Cancer Et Contrôlée Par Inhibiteur De JAK. *Rev Méd Interne* (2020) 41:421–4. doi: 10.1016/j.revmed.2020.02.015
51. Gono T, Sato S, Kawaguchi Y, Kuwana M, Hanaoka M, Katsumata Y, et al. Anti-MDA5 Antibody, Ferritin and IL-18 Are Useful for the Evaluation of Response to Treatment in Interstitial Lung Disease With Anti-MDA5 Antibody-Positive Dermatomyositis. *Rheumatology* (2012) 51:1563–70. doi: 10.1093/rheumatology/kes102
52. Fujiki Y, Kotani T, Isoda K, Ishida T, Shoda T, Yoshida S, et al. Evaluation of Clinical Prognostic Factors for Interstitial Pneumonia in Anti-MDA5 Antibody-Positive Dermatomyositis Patients. *Mod Rheumatol* (2018) 28:133–40. doi: 10.1080/14397595.2017.1318468
53. Nagashima T, Kamata Y, Iwamoto M, Okazaki H, Fukushima N, Minota S. Liver Dysfunction in Anti-Melanoma Differentiation-Associated Gene 5 Antibody-Positive Patients With Dermatomyositis. *Rheumatol Int* (2019) 39:901–9. doi: 10.1007/s00296-019-04255-2
54. Huang W, Ren F, Luo L, Zhou J, Huang D, Pan Z, et al. The Characteristics of Lymphocytes in Patients Positive for Anti-MDA5 Antibodies in Interstitial Lung Disease. *Rheumatology* (2020) 59:3886–91. doi: 10.1093/rheumatology/keaa266
55. Huang K, Vinik O, Shojania K, Yeung J, Shupak R, Nimmo M, et al. Clinical Spectrum and Therapeutics in Canadian Patients With Anti-Melanoma Differentiation-Associated Gene 5 (MDA5)-Positive Dermatomyositis: A Case-Based Review. *Rheumatol Int* (2019) 39:1971–81. doi: 10.1007/s00296-019-04398-2
56. Sabbagh S, Pinal-Fernandez I, Kishi T, Targoff IN, Miller FW, Rider LG, et al. Anti-Ro52 Autoantibodies Are Associated With Interstitial Lung Disease and More Severe Disease in Patients With Juvenile Myositis. *Ann Rheum Dis* (2019) 78:988–95. doi: 10.1136/annrheumdis-2018-215004
57. Toquet S, Uzunhan Y, Leroux G, Bonnotte B, Gallay L, Limal N, et al. Facteurs Pronostiques De La Dermatomyosite À Anticorps Anti-MDA5: Sexe Féminin Et Atteinte Articulaire De Bon Pronostic. *Rev Méd Interne* (2018) 39:A114. doi: 10.1016/j.revmed.2018.03.364
58. Tansley SL, Betteridge ZE, Gunawardena H, Jacques TS, Owens CM, Pilkington C, et al. Anti-MDA5 Autoantibodies in Juvenile

Dermatomyositis Identify a Distinct Clinical Phenotype: A Prospective Cohort Study. *Arthritis Res Ther* (2014) 16:R138. doi: 10.1186/ar4600

59. Tansley SL, Simou S, Shaddick G, Betteridge ZE, Almeida B, Gunawardena H, et al. Autoantibodies in Juvenile-Onset Myositis: Their Diagnostic Value and Associated Clinical Phenotype in a Large UK Cohort. *J Autoimmun* (2017) 84:55–64. doi: 10.1016/j.jaut.2017.06.007
60. Mamyrova G, Kishi T, Targoff IN, Ehrlich A, Curiel RV, Rider LG, et al. Features Distinguishing Clinically Amyopathic Juvenile Dermatomyositis From Juvenile Dermatomyositis. *Rheumatology* (2018) 57:1956–63. doi: 10.1093/rheumatology/key190
61. Mamyrova G, Kishi T, Shi M, Targoff IN, Huber AM, Curiel RV, et al. Anti-MDA5 Autoantibodies Associated With Juvenile Dermatomyositis Constitute a Distinct Phenotype in North America. *Rheumatology* (2020) 60(4):1839–49. doi: 10.1093/rheumatology/keaa429
62. Deakin CT, Yasin SA, Simou S, Arnold KA, Tansley SL, Betteridge ZE, et al. Muscle Biopsy Findings in Combination With Myositis-Specific Autoantibodies Aid Prediction of Outcomes in Juvenile Dermatomyositis. *Arthritis Rheumatol* (2016) 68:2806–16. doi: 10.1002/art.39753
63. Kobayashi I, Okura Y, Yamada M, Kawamura N, Kuwana M, Ariga T. Anti-Melanoma Differentiation-Associated Gene 5 Antibody Is a Diagnostic and Predictive Marker for Interstitial Lung Diseases Associated With Juvenile Dermatomyositis. *J Pediatr* (2011) 158:675–7. doi: 10.1016/j.jpeds.2010.11.033
64. Ueki M, Kobayashi I, Takezaki S, Tozawa Y, Okura Y, Yamada M, et al. Myositis-Specific Autoantibodies in Japanese Patients With Juvenile Idiopathic Inflammatory Myopathies. *Mod Rheumatol* (2019) 29:351–6. doi: 10.1080/14397595.2018.1452353
65. Iwata N, Nakaseko H, Kohagura T, Yasuoka R, Abe N, Kawabe S, et al. Clinical Subsets of Juvenile Dermatomyositis Classified by Myositis-Specific Autoantibodies: Experience at a Single Center in Japan. *Mod Rheumatol* (2019) 29:802–7. doi: 10.1080/14397595.2018.1511025
66. Miyamae T, Hara T, Hanaya A, Tani Y, Kishi T, Yamanaka H. Effect of Adalimumab on Refractory Arthritis in Juvenile Idiopathic Inflammatory Myopathy With Anti-MDA5 Autoantibody. *Case Rep Rheumatol* (2018) 2018:1–5. doi: 10.1155/2018/2164312
67. Kobayashi N, Takezaki S, Kobayashi I, Iwata N, Mori M, Nagai K, et al. Clinical and Laboratory Features of Fatal Rapidly Progressive Interstitial Lung Disease Associated With Juvenile Dermatomyositis. *Rheumatology* (2015) 54:784–91. doi: 10.1093/rheumatology/keu385
68. Yamasaki Y, Kobayashi N, Akioka S, Yamazaki K, Takezaki S, Nakaseko H, et al. Clinical Impact of Myositis-Specific Autoantibodies on Long-Term Prognosis of Juvenile Idiopathic Inflammatory Myopathies: Multicentre Study. *Rheumatology* (2021) 60(10):4821–31. doi: 10.1093/rheumatology/keab108
69. Sato S, Hoshino K, Satoh T, Fujita T, Kawakami Y, Fujita T, et al. RNA Helicase Encoded by Melanoma Differentiation-Associated Gene 5 Is a Major Autoantigen in Patients With Clinically Amyopathic Dermatomyositis: Association With Rapidly Progressive Interstitial Lung Disease. *Arthritis Rheum* (2009) 60:2193–200. doi: 10.1002/art.24621
70. Kang DC, Gopalkrishnan RV, Wu Q, Jankowsky E, Pyle AM, Fisher PB. Mda-5: An Interferon-Inducible Putative RNA Helicase With Double-Stranded RNA-Dependent ATPase Activity and Melanoma Growth-Suppressive Properties. *Proc Natl Acad Sci* (2002) 99:637–42. doi: 10.1073/pnas.022637199
71. Kato H, Takeuchi O, Sato S, Yoneyama M, Yamamoto M, Matsui K, et al. Differential Roles of MDA5 and RIG-I Helicases in the Recognition of RNA Viruses. *Nature* (2006) 441:101–5. doi: 10.1038/nature04734
72. Kato H, Takeuchi O, Mikamo-Satoh E, Hirai R, Kawai T, Matsushita K, et al. Length-Dependent Recognition of Double-Stranded Ribonucleic Acids by Retinoic Acid–Inducible Gene-I and Melanoma Differentiation–Associated Gene 5. *J Exp Med* (2008) 205:1601–10. doi: 10.1084/jem.20080091
73. Loo Y-M, Gale M. Immune Signaling by RIG-I-Like Receptors. *Immunity* (2011) 34:680–92. doi: 10.1016/j.immuni.2011.05.003
74. Rehwinkel J, Gack MU. RIG-I-Like Receptors: Their Regulation and Roles in RNA Sensing. *Nat Rev Immunol* (2020) 20:537–51. doi: 10.1038/s41577-020-0288-3
75. Feng Q, Hato SV, Langereis MA, Zoll J, Virgen-Slane R, Peisley A, et al. MDA5 Detects the Double-Stranded RNA Replicative Form in Picornavirus-Infected Cells. *Cell Rep* (2012) 2:1187–96. doi: 10.1016/j.celrep.2012.10.005
76. Linder A, Hornung V. Mitochondrial dsRNA: A New DAMP for MDA5. *Dev Cell* (2018) 46:530–32. doi: 10.1016/j.devcel.2018.08.019
77. Dhir A, Dhir S, Borowski LS, Jimenez L, Teitell M, Rötig A, et al. Mitochondrial Double-Stranded RNA Triggers Antiviral Signalling in Humans. *Nature* (2018) 560:238–42. doi: 10.1038/s41586-018-0363-0
78. The Human Protein Atlas. *Ifih1*. Available at: https://www.proteinatlas.org/ENSG00000115267-IFIH1/tissue (Accessed August 12, 2021).
79. Zahn S, Barchet W, Rehkämper C, Hornung T, Bieber T, Tüting T, et al. Enhanced Skin Expression of Melanoma Differentiation-Associated Gene 5 (MDA5) in Dermatomyositis and Related Autoimmune Diseases. *J Am Acad Dermatol* (2011) 64:988–9. doi: 10.1016/j.jaad.2010.08.004
80. Berger M, Hsieh C-Y, Bakele M, Marcos V, Rieber N, Kormann M, et al. Neutrophils Express Distinct RNA Receptors in a Non-Canonical Way. *J Biol Chem* (2012) 287:19409–17. doi: 10.1074/jbc.M112.353557
81. Hoshino K, Muro Y, Sugiura K, Tomita Y, Nakashima R, Mimori T. Anti-MDA5 and Anti-TIF1-γ Antibodies Have Clinical Significance for Patients With Dermatomyositis. *Rheumatology* (2010) 49:1726–33. doi: 10.1093/rheumatology/keq153
82. Benveniste O, Stenzel W, Allenbach Y. Advances in Serological Diagnostics of Inflammatory Myopathies. *Curr Opin Neurol* (2016) 29:662–73. doi: 10.1097/WCO.0000000000000376
83. Damoiseaux J, Vulsteke J-B, Tseng C-W, Platteel ACM, Piette Y, Shovman O, et al. Autoantibodies in Idiopathic Inflammatory Myopathies: Clinical Associations and Laboratory Evaluation by Mono- and Multispecific Immunoassays. *Autoimmun Rev* (2019) 18:293–305. doi: 10.1016/j.autrev.2018.10.004
84. Fabien N. Anticorps Des Myopathies Autoimmunes: Actualités Des Techniques De Détection Et Intérêt Clinique. *Rev Francoph Lab* (2016) 2016:41–6. doi: 10.1016/S1773-035X(16)30243-X
85. Pacot L, Pouchot J, De Prost N, Senant M, Tartour E, Le Pimpec-Barthes F, et al. Interstitial Lung Disease-Complicated Anti-MDA5 Antibody in Clinically Amyopathic Dermatomyositis Patients: Report of Two Cases With Distinct Clinical Features. *Front Med* (2020) 7:77. doi: 10.3389/fmed.2020.00077
86. Tansley SL, Li D, Betteridge ZE, McHugh NJ. The Reliability of Immunoassays to Detect Autoantibodies in Patients With Myositis is Dependent on Autoantibody Specificity. *Rheumatology* (2020) 59:2109–14. doi: 10.1093/rheumatology/keaa021
87. Cavazzana I, Richards M, Bentow C, Seaman A, Fredi M, Giudizi MG, et al. Evaluation of a Novel Particle-Based Assay for Detection of Autoantibodies in Idiopathic Inflammatory Myopathies. *J Immunol Methods* (2019) 474:112661. doi: 10.1016/j.jim.2019.112661
88. Mahler M, Betteridge Z, Bentow C, Richards M, Seaman A, Chinoy H, et al. Comparison of Three Immunoassays for the Detection of Myositis Specific Antibodies. *Front Immunol* (2019) 10:848. doi: 10.3389/fimmu.2019.00848
89. Sato S, Murakami A, Kuwajima A, Takehara K, Mimori T, Kawakami A, et al. Clinical Utility of an Enzyme-Linked Immunosorbent Assay for Detecting Anti-Melanoma Differentiation-Associated Gene 5 Autoantibodies. *PloS One* (2016) 11:e0154285. doi: 10.1371/journal.pone.0154285
90. Sakamoto S, Okamoto M, Kaieda S, Fujimoto K, Nagata S, Tominaga M, et al. Low Positive Titer of Anti-Melanoma Differentiation-Associated Gene 5 Antibody Is Not Associated With a Poor Long-Term Outcome of Interstitial Lung Disease in Patients With Dermatomyositis. *Respir Investig* (2018) 56:464–72. doi: 10.1016/j.resinv.2018.07.007
91. Muro Y, Sugiura K, Hoshino K, Akiyama M. Disappearance of Anti-MDA-5 Autoantibodies in Clinically Amyopathic DM/interstitial Lung Disease During Disease Remission. *Rheumatology* (2012) 51:800–4. doi: 10.1093/rheumatology/ker408
92. Matsushita T, Mizumaki K, Kano M, Yagi N, Tennichi M, Takeuchi A, et al. Antimelanoma Differentiation-Associated Protein 5 Antibody Level Is a Novel Tool for Monitoring Disease Activity in Rapidly Progressive Interstitial Lung Disease With Dermatomyositis. *Br J Dermatol* (2017) 176:395–402. doi: 10.1111/bjd.14882
93. Hosono Y, Nakashima R, Serada S, Murakami K, Imura Y, Yoshifuji H, et al. Splicing Factor Proline/Glutamine-Rich Is a Novel Autoantigen of Dermatomyositis and Associated With Anti-Melanoma Differentiation-Associated Gene 5 Antibody. *J Autoimmun* (2017) 77:116–22. doi: 10.1016/j.jaut.2016.11.006

94. Greco-Stewart VS, Thibault CS-L, Pelchat M. Binding of the Polypyrimidine Tract-Binding Protein-Associated Splicing Factor (PSF) to the Hepatitis Delta Virus RNA. *Virology* (2006) 356:35–44. doi: 10.1016/j.virol.2006.06.040
95. Landeras-Bueno S, Jorba N, Pérez-Cidoncha M, Ortín J. The Splicing Factor Proline-Glutamine Rich (SFPQ/PSF) Is Involved in Influenza Virus Transcription. *PloS Pathog* (2011) 7:e1002397. doi: 10.1371/journal.ppat.1002397
96. Chen Z, Wang Y, Kuwana M, Xu X, Hu W, Feng X, et al. HLA-DRB1 Alleles as Genetic Risk Factors for the Development of Anti-MDA5 Antibodies in Patients With Dermatomyositis. *J Rheumatol* (2017) 44:1389–93. doi: 10.3899/jrheum.170165
97. Lin J, Zhang Y, Peng Q, Yang H, Shi J, Gu M, et al. Genetic Association of HLA-DRB1 Multiple Polymorphisms With Dermatomyositis in Chinese Population. *HLA* (2017) 90:354–9. doi: 10.1111/tan.13171
98. Gono T, Kawaguchi Y, Kuwana M, Sugiura T, Furuya T, Takagi K, et al. Brief Report: Association of HLA-DRB1*0101/*0405 With Susceptibility to Anti-Melanoma Differentiation-Associated Gene 5 Antibody-Positive Dermatomyositis in the Japanese Population. *Arthritis Rheum* (2012) 64:3736–40. doi: 10.1002/art.34657
99. Rothwell S, Chinoy H, Lamb JA, Miller FW, Rider LG, Wedderburn LR, et al. Focused HLA Analysis in Caucasians With Myositis Identifies Significant Associations With Autoantibody Subgroups. *Ann Rheum Dis* (2019) 78:996–1002. doi: 10.1136/annrheumdis-2019-215046
100. Kochi Y, Kamatani Y, Kondo Y, Suzuki A, Kawakami E, Hiwa R, et al. Splicing Variant of *WDFY4* Augments MDA5 Signalling and the Risk of Clinically Amyopathic Dermatomyositis. *Ann Rheum Dis* (2018) 77:602–11. doi: 10.1136/annrheumdis-2017-212149
101. Theisen DJ, Davidson JT, Briseño CG, Gargaro M, Lauron EJ, Wang Q, et al. WDFY4 Is Required for Cross-Presentation in Response to Viral and Tumor Antigens. *Science* (2018) 362:694–9. doi: 10.1126/science.aat5030
102. Toquet S, Granger B, Uzunhan Y, Mariampillai K, Nunes H, Benveniste O, et al. The Seasonality of Dermatomyositis Associated With Anti-MDA5 Antibody: An Argument for a Respiratory Viral Trigger. *Autoimmun Rev* (2021) 20:102788. doi: 10.1016/j.autrev.2021.102788
103. Nishina N, Sato S, Masui K, Gono T, Kuwana M. Seasonal and Residential Clustering at Disease Onset of Anti-MDA5-Associated Interstitial Lung Disease. *RMD Open* (2020) 6:e001202. doi: 10.1136/rmdopen-2020-001202
104. Muro Y, Sugiura K, Hoshino K, Akiyama M, Tamakoshi K. Epidemiologic Study of Clinically Amyopathic Dermatomyositis and Anti-Melanoma Differentiation-Associated Gene 5 Antibodies in Central Japan. *Arthritis Res Ther* (2011) 13:R214. doi: 10.1186/ar3547
105. Shakshouk H, Deschaine MA, Wetter DA, Drage LA, Ernste FC, Lehman JS. Clinical and Histopathological Features of Adult Patients With Dermatomyositis and MDA5 Autoantibody Seropositivity Status, as Determined by Commercial-Based Testing: A Retrospective, Single-Institution Comparative Cohort Study. *Clin Exp Dermatol* (2021), ced.14870. doi: 10.1111/ced.14870
106. He C, Chen J, Luo X, Yan B. Evaluation of Biomarkers Related to Endothelial Dysfunction: Proof of Vasculopathy in Anti-Melanoma Differentiation-Associated Gene 5 Dermatomyositis. *Clin Exp Rheumatol* (2021) 39:151–7.
107. Funauchi M, Shimadsu H, Tamaki C, Yamagata T, Nozaki Y, Sugiyama M, et al. Role of Endothelial Damage in the Pathogenesis of Interstitial Pneumonitis in Patients With Polymyositis and Dermatomyositis. *J Rheumatol* (2006) 33(5):903–6.
108. Ono N, Kai K, Maruyama A, Sakai M, Sadanaga Y, Koarada S, et al. The Relationship Between Type 1 IFN and Vasculopathy in Anti-MDA5 Antibody-Positive Dermatomyositis Patients. *Rheumatology* (2019) 58:786–91. doi: 10.1093/rheumatology/key386
109. Zhang SH, Zhao Y, Xie QB, Jiang Y, Wu YK, Yan B. Aberrant Activation of the Type I Interferon System may Contribute to the Pathogenesis of Anti-Melanoma Differentiation-Associated Gene 5 Dermatomyositis. *Br J Dermatol* (2019) 180:1090–98. doi: 10.1111/bjd.16917
110. Horiike Y, Suzuki Y, Fujisawa T, Yasui H, Karayama M, Hozumi H, et al. Successful Classification of Macrophage-Mannose Receptor CD206 in Severity of Anti-MDA5 Antibody Positive Dermatomyositis Associated ILD. *Rheumatology* (2019) 58:2143–52. doi: 10.1093/rheumatology/kez185
111. Gono T, Miyake K, Kawaguchi Y, Kaneko H, Shinozaki M, Yamanaka H. Hyperferritinaemia and Macrophage Activation in a Patient With Interstitial Lung Disease With Clinically Amyopathic DM. *Rheumatology* (2012) 51:1336–8. doi: 10.1093/rheumatology/kes012
112. Zhang L, Wang Y, Wu G, Xiong W, Gu W, Wang C-Y. Macrophages: Friend or Foe in Idiopathic Pulmonary Fibrosis? *Respir Res* (2018) 19:170. doi: 10.1186/s12931-018-0864-2
113. Fujisawa T, Hozumi H, Yasui H, Suzuki Y, Karayama M, Furuhashi K, et al. Clinical Significance of Serum Chitotriosidase Level in Anti-MDA5 Antibody–positive Dermatomyositis-Associated Interstitial Lung Disease. *J Rheumatol* (2019) 46:935–42. doi: 10.3899/jrheum.180825
114. Kawasumi H, Katsumata Y, Nishino A, Hirahara S, Kawaguchi Y, Kuwana M, et al. Association of Serum Soluble CD163 With Polymyositis and Dermatomyositis, Especially in Anti-MDA5 Antibody–positive Cases. *J Rheumatol* (2018) 45:947–55. doi: 10.3899/jrheum.170997
115. Peng QL, Zhang YM, Liang L, Liu X, Ye LF, Yang HB, et al. A High Level of Serum Neopterin Is Associated With Rapidly Progressive Interstitial Lung Disease and Reduced Survival in Dermatomyositis. *Clin Exp Immunol* (2020) 199:314–25. doi: 10.1111/cei.13404
116. Takada T, Aoki A, Asakawa K, Sakagami T, Moriyama H, Narita I, et al. Serum Cytokine Profiles of Patients With Interstitial Lung Disease Associated With Anti-CADM-140/MDA5 Antibody Positive Amyopathic Dermatomyositis. *Respir Med* (2015) 109:1174–80. doi: 10.1016/j.rmed.2015.07.004
117. Nakano M, Fujii T, Hashimoto M, Yukawa N, Yoshifuji H, Ohmura K, et al. Type I Interferon Induces CX3CL1 (Fractalkine) and CCL5 (RANTES) Production in Human Pulmonary Vascular Endothelial Cells. *Clin Exp Immunol* (2012) 170:94–100. doi: 10.1111/j.1365-2249.2012.04638.x
118. Ishida Y, Kimura A, Nosaka M, Kuninaka Y, Hemmi H, Sasaki I, et al. Essential Involvement of the CX3CL1-CX3CR1 Axis in Bleomycin-Induced Pulmonary Fibrosis *via* Regulation of Fibrocyte and M2 Macrophage Migration. *Sci Rep* (2017) 7:16833. doi: 10.1038/s41598-017-17007-8
119. Wang K, Zhao J, Chen Z, Li T, Tan X, Zheng Y, et al. CD4+CXCR4+ T Cells as a Novel Prognostic Biomarker in Patients With Idiopathic Inflammatory Myopathy- Associated Interstitial Lung Disease. *Rheumatol (Oxford)* (2019) 58(3):511–21. doi: 10.1093/rheumatology/key341
120. Brodeur TY, Robidoux TE, Weinstein JS, Craft J, Swain SL, Marshak-Rothstein A. IL-21 Promotes Pulmonary Fibrosis Through the Induction of Profibrotic CD8+ T Cells. *J Immunol* (2015) 195:5251–60. doi: 10.4049/jimmunol.1500777
121. Sica A, Mantovani A. Macrophage Plasticity and Polarization: *In Vivo* Veritas. *J Clin Invest* (2012) 122:787–95. doi: 10.1172/JCI59643
122. Kwan C, Milosevic S, Benham H, Scott IA. A Rare Form of Dermatomyositis Associated With Muscle Weakness and Normal Creatine Kinase Level. *BMJ Case Rep* (2020) 13:e232260. doi: 10.1136/bcr-2019-232260
123. Kushnir-Grinbaum D, Cohen-Barak E, Bieber A, Krausz J, Dodiuk-Gad R, Mader R, et al. Toxic Epidermal Necrolysis-Like Dermatomyositis Associated With Antimelanoma Differentiation Antigen 5. *JAAD Case Rep* (2019) 5:91–3. doi: 10.1016/j.jdcr.2018.10.018
124. Joshi R. Interface Dermatitis. *Indian J Dermatol Venereol Leprol* (2013) 79:349. doi: 10.4103/0378-6323.110780
125. Wenzel J, Lucas S, Zahn S, Mikus S, Metze D, Ständer S, et al. CXCR3 <-> Ligand–Mediated Skin Inflammation in Cutaneous Lichenoid Graft-*Versus*-Host Disease. *J Am Acad Dermatol* (2008) 58:437–42. doi: 10.1016/j.jaad.2007.10.647
126. Wenzel J, Schmidt R, Proelss J, Zahn S, Bieber T, Tuting T. Type I Interferon-Associated Skin Recruitment of CXCR3+ Lymphocytes in Dermatomyositis. *Clin Exp Dermatol* (2006) 31:576–82. doi: 10.1111/j.1365-2230.2006.02150.x
127. Wenzel J, Wörenkämper E, Freutel S, Henze S, Haller O, Bieber T, et al. Enhanced Type I Interferon Signalling Promotes Th1-Biased Inflammation in Cutaneous Lupus Erythematosus. *J Pathol* (2005) 205:435–42. doi: 10.1002/path.1721
128. Wenzel J, Zahn S, Bieber T, Tüting T. Type I Interferon-Associated Cytotoxic Inflammation in Cutaneous Lupus Erythematosus. *Arch Dermatol Res* (2009) 301:83–6. doi: 10.1007/s00403-008-0892-8
129. Cassius C, Amode R, Delord M, Battistella M, Poirot J, How-Kit A, et al. MDA5+ Dermatomyositis Is Associated With Stronger Skin Type I Interferon Transcriptomic Signature With Upregulation of IFN-κ

Transcript. *J Invest Dermatol* (2020) 140:1276–9.e7. doi: 10.1016/j.jid.2019.10.020

130. Indraccolo S, Pfeffer U, Minuzzo S, Esposito G, Roni V, Mandruzzato S, et al. Identification of Genes Selectively Regulated by IFNs in Endothelial Cells. *J Immunol* (2007) 178:1122–35. doi: 10.4049/jimmunol.178.2.1122
131. Pau-Charles I, Moreno PJ, Ortiz-Ibáñez K, Lucero MC, Garcia-Herrera A, Espinosa G, et al. Anti-MDA5 Positive Clinically Amyopathic Dermatomyositis Presenting With Severe Cardiomyopathy. *J Eur Acad Dermatol Venereol* (2014) 28:1097–102. doi: 10.1111/jdv.12300
132. Abraham D, Distler O. How Does Endothelial Cell Injury Start? The Role of Endothelin in Systemic Sclerosis. *Arthritis Res Ther* (2007) 9:S2. doi: 10.1186/ar2186
133. Min HK, Kim H-R, Lee S-H, Park S-H, Oh J, Choi K. Refractory Digital Ulcers Treated by Botulinum Toxin and Endothelin Receptor-1 Antagonist in Anti-MDA5-Antibody-Positive Dermatomyositis. *J Clin Neurol* (2020) 16:160. doi: 10.3988/jcn.2020.16.1.160
134. Collantes-Rodríguez C, Jiménez-Gallo D, Ossorio-García L, Villegas-Romero I, Linares-Barrios M. Image Gallery: Cutaneous Ulcers in Anti-MDA 5 Dermatomyositis Successfully Treated With Sildenafil. *Br J Dermatol* (2019) 182:e1. doi: 10.1111/bjd.18376
135. Combalia A, Giavedoni P, Tamez L, Grau-Junyent JM, Mascaró JM. Bosentan for Cutaneous Ulcers in Anti-MDA5 Dermatomyositis. *JAMA Dermatol* (2018) 154:371. doi: 10.1001/jamadermatol.2017.5462
136. Horai Y, Koga T, Fujikawa K, Takatani A, Nishino A, Nakashima Y, et al. Serum Interferon-α Is a Useful Biomarker in Patients With Anti-Melanoma Differentiation-Associated Gene 5 (MDA5) Antibody-Positive Dermatomyositis. *Mod Rheumatol* (2015) 25:85–9. doi: 10.3109/14397595.2014.900843
137. Ogawa Y, Kishida D, Shimojima Y, Hayashi K, Sekijima Y. Effective Administration of Rituximab in Anti-MDA5 Antibody–Positive Dermatomyositis With Rapidly Progressive Interstitial Lung Disease and Refractory Cutaneous Involvement: A Case Report and Literature Review. *Case Rep Rheumatol* (2017) 2017:5386797. doi: 10.1155/2017/5386797
138. So H, Wong VTL, Lao VWN, Pang HT, Yip RML. Rituximab for Refractory Rapidly Progressive Interstitial Lung Disease Related to Anti-MDA5 Antibody-Positive Amyopathic Dermatomyositis. *Clin Rheumatol* (2018) 37:1983–9. doi: 10.1007/s10067-018-4122-2
139. Ge Y, Li S, Tian X, He L, Lu X, Wang G. Anti-Melanoma Differentiation-Associated Gene 5 (MDA5) Antibody-Positive Dermatomyositis Responds to Rituximab Therapy. *Clin Rheumatol* (2021) 40(6):2311–7. doi: 10.1007/s10067-020-05530-5
140. Endo Y, Koga T, Suzuki T, Hara K, Ishida M, Fujita Y, et al. Successful Treatment of Plasma Exchange for Rapidly Progressive Interstitial Lung Disease With Anti-MDA5 Antibody-Positive Dermatomyositis: A Case Report. *Med (Baltimore)* (2018) 97:e0436. doi: 10.1097/MD.0000000000010436
141. Abe Y, Kusaoi M, Tada K, Yamaji K, Tamura N. Successful Treatment of Anti-MDA5 Antibody-Positive Refractory Interstitial Lung Disease With Plasma Exchange Therapy. *Rheumatology* (2020) 59:767–71. doi: 10.1093/rheumatology/kez357
142. Vlahakos D, Foster MH, Ucci AA, Barrett KJ, Datta SK, Madaio MP. Murine Monoclonal Anti-DNA Antibodies Penetrate Cells, Bind to Nuclei, and Induce Glomerular Proliferation and Proteinuria *In Vivo*. *J Am Soc Nephrol* (1992) 2(8):1345–54. doi: 10.1681/ASN.V281345
143. Deng SX, Hanson E, Sanz I. *In Vivo* Cell Penetration and Intracellular Transport of Anti-Sm and Anti-La Autoantibodies. *Int Immunol* (2000) 12:415–23. doi: 10.1093/intimm/12.4.415
144. Douglas J N. Antibodies to an Intracellular Antigen Penetrate Neuronal Cells and Cause Deleterious Effects. *J Clin Cell Immunol* (2013) 04. doi: 10.4172/2155-9899.1000134
145. Chen M, Zhao Q, Diao L, Xue K, Ruan Y, Xue F, et al. Distribution of Anti-Melanoma Differentiation Associated Gene 5 (MDA5) IgG Subclasses in MDA5+ Dermatomyositis. *Rheumatology* (2021) keab268. doi: 10.1093/rheumatology/keab268
146. Della-Torre E, Lanzillotta M, Doglioni C. Immunology of IgG4-Related Disease: Immunology of IgG4-Related Disease. *Clin Exp Immunol* (2015) 181:191–206. doi: 10.1111/cei.12641
147. Giannini M, Ohana M, Nespola B, Zanframundo G, Geny B, Meyer A. Similarities Between COVID-19 and Anti-MDA5 Syndrome: What can We Learn for Better Care? *Eur Respir J* (2020) 56:2001618. doi: 10.1183/13993003.01618-2020
148. Hanley B, Naresh KN, Roufosse C, Nicholson AG, Weir J, Cooke GS, et al. Histopathological Findings and Viral Tropism in UK Patients With Severe Fatal COVID-19: A Post-Mortem Study. *Lancet Microbe* (2020) 1:e245–53. doi: 10.1016/S2666-5247(20)30115-4
149. Quintana-Ortega C, Remesal A, Ruiz de Valbuena M, de la Serna O, Laplaza-González M, Álvarez-Rojas E, et al. Fatal Outcome of Anti-MDA5 Juvenile Dermatomyositis in a Paediatric COVID-19 Patient: A Case Report. *Mod Rheumatol Case Rep* (2021) 5:101–7. doi: 10.1080/24725625.2020.1832755
150. Rebendenne A, Valadão ALC, Tauziet M, Maarifi G, Bonaventure B, McKellar J, et al. SARS-CoV-2 Triggers an MDA-5-Dependent Interferon Response Which Is Unable to Control Replication in Lung Epithelial Cells. *J Virol* (2021) 95(8):e02415–20. doi: 10.1128/JVI.02415-20
151. Yin X, Riva L, Pu Y, Martin-Sancho L, Kanamune J, Yamamoto Y, et al. MDA5 Governs the Innate Immune Response to SARS-CoV-2 in Lung Epithelial Cells. *Cell Rep* (2021) 34:108628. doi: 10.1016/j.celrep.2020.108628
152. Trouillet-Assant S, Viel S, Gaymard A, Pons S, Richard JC, Perret M, et al. Type I IFN Immunoprofiling in COVID-19 Patients. *J Allergy Clin Immunol* (2020) 146(1):206–8.e2. doi: 10.1016/j.jaci.2020.04.029
153. Hadjadj J, Yatim N, Barnabei L, Corneau A, Boussier J, Smith N, et al. Impaired Type I Interferon Activity and Inflammatory Responses in Severe COVID-19 Patients. *Science* (2020) 369:718–24. doi: 10.1126/science.abc6027
154. Zhang Q, Bastard P, Liu Z, Le Pen J, Moncada-Velez M, Chen J, et al. Inborn Errors of Type I IFN Immunity in Patients With Life-Threatening COVID-19. *Science* (2020) 370:eabd4570. doi: 10.1126/science.abd4570
155. Bastard P, Rosen LB, Zhang Q, Michailidis E, Hoffmann H-H, Zhang Y, et al. Autoantibodies Against Type I IFNs in Patients With Life-Threatening COVID-19. *Science* (2020) 370:eabd4585. doi: 10.1126/science.abd4585
156. Goncalves D, Mezidi M, Bastard P, Perret M, Saker K, Fabien N, et al. Antibodies Against Type I Interferon: Detection and Association With Severe Clinical Outcome in COVID-19 Patients. *Clin Transl Immunol* (2021) 10(8):e1327. doi: 10.1002/cti2.1327
157. Lee JS, Shin E-C. The Type I Interferon Response in COVID-19: Implications for Treatment. *Nat Rev Immunol* (2020) 20:585–6. doi: 10.1038/s41577-020-00429-3
158. Lee JS, Park S, Jeong HW, Ahn JY, Choi SJ, Lee H, et al. Immunophenotyping of COVID-19 and Influenza Highlights the Role of Type I Interferons in Development of Severe COVID-19. *Sci Immunol* (2020) 5:eabd1554. doi: 10.1126/sciimmunol.abd1554
159. Nägele MP, Haubner B, Tanner FC, Ruschitzka F, Flammer AJ. Endothelial Dysfunction in COVID-19: Current Findings and Therapeutic Implications. *Atherosclerosis* (2020) 314:58–62. doi: 10.1016/j.atherosclerosis.2020.10.014
160. Siddiqi HK, Libby P, Ridker PM. COVID-19 – A Vascular Disease. *Trends Cardiovasc Med* (2021) 31:1–5. doi: 10.1016/j.tcm.2020.10.005
161. Goshua G, Pine AB, Meizlish ML, Chang C-H, Zhang H, Bahel P, et al. Endotheliopathy in COVID-19-Associated Coagulopathy: Evidence From a Single-Centre, Cross-Sectional Study. *Lancet Haematol* (2020) 7:e575–82. doi: 10.1016/S2352-3026(20)30216-7
162. Evans PC, Rainger GE, Mason JC, Guzik TJ, Osto E, Stamataki Z, et al. Endothelial Dysfunction in COVID-19: A Position Paper of the ESC Working Group for Atherosclerosis and Vascular Biology, and the ESC Council of Basic Cardiovascular Science. *Cardiovasc Res* (2020) 116:2177–84. doi: 10.1093/cvr/cvaa230
163. Liu C, Wang Q, Wang Y, Wang G, Wang L, Chen H, et al. Analysis of the Correlation Between Anti-MDA5 Antibody and the Severity of COVID-19: A Retrospective Study. *medRxiv [Preprint]* (2020) 20164780. doi: 10.1101/2020.07.29.20164780
164. De Santis M, Isailovic N, Motta F, Ricordi C, Ceribelli A, Lanza E, et al. Environmental Triggers for Connective Tissue Disease: The Case of COVID-19 Associated With Dermatomyositis-Specific Autoantibodies. *Curr Opin Rheumatol* (2021) 33:514–21. doi: 10.1097/BOR.0000000000000844
165. Hansen KE, Arnason J, Bridges AJ. Autoantibodies and Common Viral Illnesses. *Semin Arthritis Rheum* (1998) 27:263–71. doi: 10.1016/s0049-0172(98)80047-
166. Gil-Vila A, Perurena-Prieto J, Nolla-Fontana C, Orozco-Galvez O, Miarons-Font M, del Castillo AG, et al. Pos1229 Anti-Mda5 and Antisynthetase

Antibodies Screening in Severe Sars-Cov-2 Pneumonia. Be Aware of False Positive Results. *Ann Rheumatic Dis* (2021) 80:898. doi: 10.1136/annrheumdis-2021-eular.301

167. Romero-Bueno F, Diaz del Campo P, Trallero-Araguás E, Ruiz-Rodríguez JC, Castellvi I, Rodriguez-Nieto MJ, et al. Recommendations for the Treatment of Anti-Melanoma Differentiation-Associated Gene 5-Positive Dermatomyositis-Associated Rapidly Progressive Interstitial Lung Disease. *Semin Arthritis Rheum* (2020) 50:776–90. doi: 10.1016/j.semarthrit.2020.03.007
168. Zohar DN, Seluk L, Yonath H, Shoenfeld Y, Kivity S. Anti-MDA5 Positive Dermatomyositis Associated With Rapidly Progressive Interstitial Lung Disease and Correlation Between Serum Ferritin Level and Treatment Response. *Mediterr J Rheumatol* (2019) 31:75. doi: 10.31138/mjr.31.1.75
169. Osawa T, Morimoto K, Sasaki Y, Matsuda S, Yamana K, Yano R, et al. The Serum Ferritin Level Is Associated With the Treatment Responsivity for Rapidly Progressive Interstitial Lung Disease With Amyopathic Dermatomyositis, Irrespective of the Anti-MDA5 Antibody Level. *Intern Med* (2018) 57:387–91. doi: 10.2169/internalmedicine.8335-16
170. Shu E, Kanoh H, Murakami A, Seishima M. Potential Inhibition of Development of Rapidly Progressive Interstitial Lung Disease by Prompt and Sufficient Immunosuppressive Treatment in Patients With Anti-Melanoma Differentiation-Associated Gene 5 Antibody-Positive Dermatomyositis. *J Dermatol* (2017) 44:e91–2. doi: 10.1111/1346-8138.13659
171. Tsuji H, Nakashima R, Hosono Y, Imura Y, Yagita M, Yoshifuji H, et al. Multicenter Prospective Study of the Efficacy and Safety of Combined Immunosuppressive Therapy With High-Dose Glucocorticoid, Tacrolimus, and Cyclophosphamide in Interstitial Lung Diseases Accompanied by Anti–Melanoma Differentiation–Associated Gene 5–Positive Dermatomyositis. *Arthritis Rheumatol* (2020) 72:488–98. doi: 10.1002/art.41105
172. Matsuda KM, Yoshizaki A, Kuzumi A, Fukasawa T, Ebata S, Yoshizaki-Ogawa A, et al. Combined Immunosuppressive Therapy Provides Favorable Prognosis and Increased Risk of Cytomegalovirus Reactivation in Anti-Melanoma Differentiation-Associated Gene 5 Antibody-Positive Dermatomyositis. *J Dermatol* (2020) 47:483–9. doi: 10.1111/1346-8138.15274
173. Seiller H, Schmutz J-L, Poreaux C, Bursztejn A-C. Dermatomyosite À Anticorps Anti-MDA-5 Compliquée D'une Pneumopathie Interstitielle Et D'une Pneumocystose D'évolution Fatale. *Ann Dermatol Vénéréologie* (2020) 147:862–7. doi: 10.1016/j.annder.2020.08.046
174. Aymonier M, Abed S, Boyé T, Barazzutti H, Fournier B, Morand J-J. Dermatomyosite Associée Aux Anticorps Anti-MDA5 Et Pneumocystose Pulmonaire: Deux Cas D'évolution Fatale. *Ann Dermatol Vénéréologie* (2017) 144:279–83. doi: 10.1016/j.annder.2016.09.677
175. Fillatre P, Decaux O, Jouneau S, Revest M, Gacouin A, Robert-Gangneux F, et al. Incidence of Pneumocystis Jiroveci Pneumonia Among Groups at Risk in HIV-Negative Patients. *Am J Med* (2014) 127:1242. doi: 10.1016/j.amjmed.2014.07.010
176. Wendel S, Venhoff N, Frye BC, May AM, Agarwal P, Rizzi M, et al. Successful Treatment of Extensive Calcifications and Acute Pulmonary Involvement in Dermatomyositis With the Janus-Kinase Inhibitor Tofacitinib – A Report of Two Cases. *J Autoimmun* (2019) 100:131–6. doi: 10.1016/j.jaut.2019.03.003
177. Takatani A, Koga T, Fujita Y, Fukui S, Endo Y, Shimizu T, et al. Efficacy of Tofacitinib for Slowly Progressive Interstitial Lung Disease in a Patient With Anti-MDA5 Antibody-Positive Dermatomyositis. *Clin Immunol* (2020) 215:108451. doi: 10.1016/j.clim.2020.108451
178. Kurasawa K, Arai S, Namiki Y, Tanaka A, Takamura Y, Owada T, et al. Tofacitinib for Refractory Interstitial Lung Diseases in Anti-Melanoma Differentiation-Associated 5 Gene Antibody-Positive Dermatomyositis. *Rheumatology* (2018) 57:2114–9. doi: 10.1093/rheumatology/key188
179. Hosokawa Y, Oiwa H. A Case of Refractory Interstitial Lung Disease in Anti-MDA5–Positive Dermatomyositis That Improved After Switching to Tofacitinib. *J Clin Rheumatol* (2020). doi: 10.1097/RHU.0000000000001645
180. Mehta DS, Wurster AL, Grusby MJ. Biology of IL-21 and the IL-21 Receptor. *Immunol Rev* (2004) 202:84–95. doi: 10.1111/j.0105-2896.2004.00201.x
181. Habib T, Senadheera S, Weinberg K, Kaushansky K. The Common γ Chain (γc) Is a Required Signaling Component of the IL-21 Receptor and Supports IL-21-Induced Cell Proliferation *via* JAK3. *Biochemistry* (2002) 41:8725–31. doi: 10.1021/bi0202023
182. Chen Z, Wang X, Ye S. Tofacitinib in Amyopathic Dermatomyositis–Associated Interstitial Lung Disease. *N Engl J Med* (2019) 381:291–3. doi: 10.1056/NEJMc1900045
183. Scirocco C, Gubbiotti A, Sebastiani A, Sebastiani GD. Rituximab in Antimelanoma Differentiation-Associated Protein-5 Dermatomyositis With Interstitial Lung Disease. *Case Rep Rheumatol* (2020) 2020:8145790. doi: 10.1155/2020/8145790
184. Hisanaga J, Kotani T, Fujiki Y, Yoshida S, Takeuchi T, Makino S. Successful Multi-Target Therapy Including Rituximab and Mycophenolate Mofetil in Anti-Melanoma Differentiation-Associated Gene 5 Antibody-Positive Rapidly Progressive Interstitial Lung Disease With Clinically Amyopathic Dermatomyositis. *Int J Rheum Dis* (2017) 20:2182–5. doi: 10.1111/1756-185X.13136
185. Mao M, Xia S, Guo B, Qian W, Zheng Z, Peng X, et al. Ultra-Low Dose Rituximab as Add-on Therapy in Anti-MDA5-Positive Patients With Polymyositis/Dermatomyositis Associated ILD. *Respir Med* (2020) 172:105983. doi: 10.1016/j.rmed.2020.105983
186. Takahashi R, Yoshida T, Morimoto K, Kondo Y, Kikuchi J, Saito S, et al. Successful Treatment of Anti-MDA5 Antibody-Positive Dermatomyositis-Associated Rapidly Progressive-Interstitial Lung Disease by Plasma Exchange: Two Case Reports. *Clin Med Insights Case Rep* (2021) 14:117954762110363. doi: 10.1177/11795476211036322
187. Silveira MG, Selva-O'Callaghan A, Ramos-Terrades N, Arredondo-Agudelo KV, Labrador-Horrillo M, Bravo-Masgoret C. Anti-MDA5 Dermatomyositis and Progressive Interstitial Pneumonia. *QJM* (2016) 109:49–50. doi: 10.1093/qjmed/hcv068
188. Kagawa H, Tsujino K, Yamamoto Y, Iwai A, Hara R, Matsuki T, et al. Acute Lung Injury After Plasma Exchange in a Patient With Anti-MDA5 Antibody-Positive, Rapidly Progressive, Interstitial Lung Disease: A Case Report. *Respir Med Case Rep* (2020) 29:101016. doi: 10.1016/j.rmcr.2020.101016

7

Case Report: Concurrence of Dermatomyositis and Autoimmune Blistering Diseases: Two Case Reports and a Literature Review

Haixi Wu, Licheng Diao, Ke Xue, Qian Zhao, Xiaoqing Zhao, Qunli Xia, Jie Zheng, Meng Pan and Hua Cao**

Department of Dermatology, Ruijin Hospital, School of Medicine, Shanghai Jiao Tong University, Shanghai, China

***Correspondence:**
Hua Cao
drcaohua@126.com
Meng Pan
pm10633@rjh.com.cn*

Dermatomyositis (DM) is an idiopathic inflammatory myopathy primarily involving skin and muscles. Clinically amyopathic dermatomyositis (CADM), a subset of DM, presents with characteristic cutaneous manifestations without clinical evidence of myositis. Although rare, vesiculobullous eruptions could develop in DM patients. Such "bullous DM" is commonly considered a sign of internal malignancy. However, some cases with similar presentations were diagnosed as autoimmune blistering disease eventually. Herein, we reported two cases of CADM with autoimmune blisters formed. Case 1 presented with vesicles and was diagnosed with CADM initially. However, this patient developed blisters again years later and was diagnosed with "pemphigus foliaceous" (PF) accordingly. Case 2, with a history of nasopharyngeal carcinoma and CADM, developed bullous pemphigoid several days after using a heat patch on her abdomen. The association between disease occurrence and local skin damage might provide more evidence to support the "epitope spreading" hypothesis. Moreover, we reviewed related literature and discussed the differences between the two disease entities in clinical presentations, pathogenesis, therapy, and the risk of complications.

Keywords: dermatomyositis, clinically amyopathic dermatomyositis, bullous dermatomyositis, autoimmune blistering disease, malignancy, interstitial lung disease

INTRODUCTION

Dermatomyositis (DM) is an idiopathic inflammatory myopathy characterized by typical skin lesions and skeletal muscle involvement. Clinically amyopathic dermatomyositis (CADM) is a subset of DM with characteristic cutaneous manifestations and no clinical evidence of myositis (1). These characteristic skin lesions include heliotrope, Gottron's papules, and Gottron's sign. However, vesiculobullous eruptions are rarely observed. If blisters are presented, they are defined as "bullous DM" and are usually considered a sign of internal malignancy (2).

Nevertheless, it was also noted that some mimics can be diagnosed as autoimmune blistering diseases (AIBDs). AIBDs involve a group of dermatoses that autoantibodies bind to antigens in the skin and mucous membranes. AIBDs can be divided into three types, subepidermal split formation (pemphigoid diseases), acantholysis (pemphigus), and dermatitis herpetiformis. Furthermore, the common pemphigoid diseases include bullous pemphigoid (BP), mucous membrane pemphigoid (MMP), and epidermolysis bullosa acquisita (EBA). In contrast, the common pemphigus includes pemphigus vulgaris (PV) and pemphigus foliaceous (PF).

Herein, we reported two cases of CADM with blisters. Case 1 presented with characteristic DM skin lesions and vesicles on the lower back, without muscle weakness or tenderness. The biopsies from erythema and vesicle showed compatible with DM and severe edema of the dermal papilla, respectively. Therefore, the diagnosis of "bullous CADM" was made. Years later, the patient developed blisters and erosions again. This time, the histology, immunohistopathology, and serology tests all suggested the diagnosis of "PF". Case 2, with a medical history of nasopharyngeal carcinoma (NPC) and CADM, this patient developed erythema and dense blisters several days after using a heat patch. "BP" was made with the evidence of histology and serologic findings. These two cases presented with a unique disease progress with different patterns of blister formation and skin damage-triggered AIBD, respectively.

CASE DESCRIPTION

Case 1

In 2017, a 55-year-old Chinese woman presented at the study hospital with 2-month history of skin erythema and 1 week of vesicles. Physical examination showed periorbital erythema, Gottron's papules, Gottron's sign, and erythema on the upper chest and back. Clustered dense vesicles were also observed on her lower back (**Figure 1A**). She had no muscle weakness or muscle tenderness. This patient had a medical history of hypertension and took telmisartan and felodipine for 2 years. Laboratory investigations showed increased levels of lactate dehydrogenase (LDH) [247 IU/L, normal range (NR) 98–192] and aspartate aminotransferase (AST) (50 IU/L, NR 8–40). Myositis-specific antibodies (MSAs) were also positive, including anti-small ubiquitin-like modifier activating enzyme (SAE) and -Jo-1 antibodies (immunoblotting). However, her creatine kinase (CK) was normal (92 IU/L, NR 22–269). No significant abnormality was found on electromyogram (EMG), muscle magnetic resonance imaging (MRI), or muscle biopsy. One skin biopsy from an erythema lesion on the back showed liquefaction of basal cells, edema of the dermal papilla, and mild superficial and middle perivascular lymphocyte infiltration (**Figure 1B**). Another skin biopsy from a vesicle lesion showed severe edema of the dermal papilla and perivascular lymphocyte infiltration (**Figure 1C**). Direct immunofluorescence (DIF) was negative. Screening for interstitial lung disease (ILD) and malignancy was negative. The patient was diagnosed with bullous CADM and treated with methylprednisolone 40 mg/day and hydroxychloroquine 200 mg/day initially. The dose of methylprednisolone was tapered after 2 weeks of treatment due to the significantly reduced skin eruptions and decreased levels of LDH and AST (201 and 16 IU/L, respectively).

Approximately one and a half years later, the patient was hospitalized because of itchy blisters over a month and the dose of prednisone that time was 12.5 mg/day. Physical

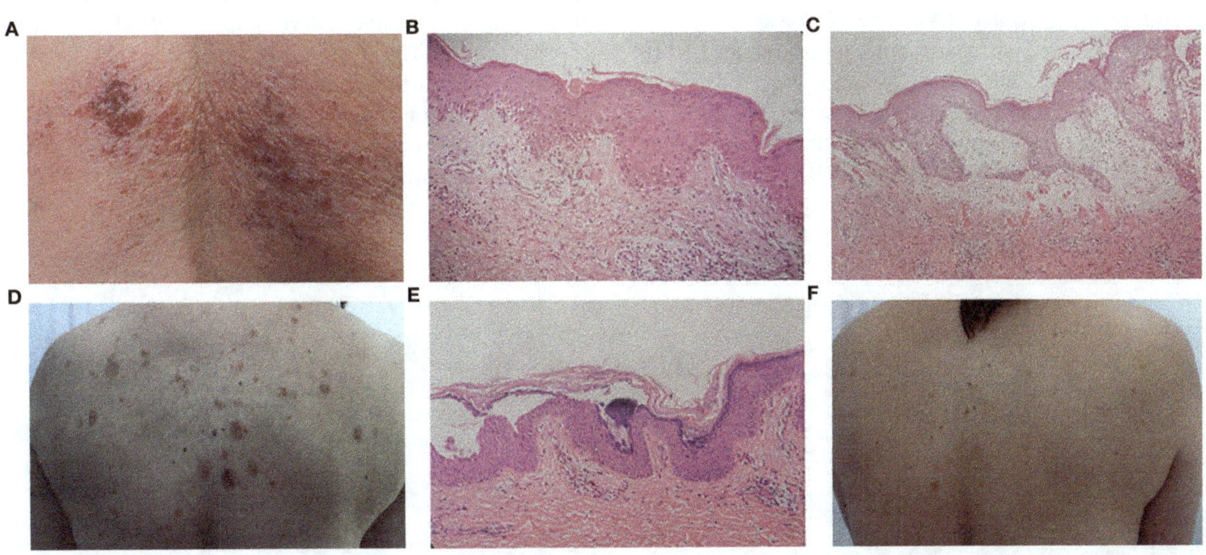

FIGURE 1 | **(A)** Erythema and vesicles formation on the lower back. **(B)** Histology from an erythema on the upper back showed focal parakeratosis of the epidermis, liquefaction of basal cells, edema of dermal papilla, and mild superficial and middle perivascular lymphocyte infiltration. **(C)** Histology from a vesicle on the lower back showed severe edema of dermal papilla and perivascular lymphocyte infiltration. **(D)** Multiple ruptured bullae and erosions on the back. **(E)** Histological examination from a bulla on the abdomen showed acantholysis and intraepidermal bulla formation. **(F)** The patient's condition was stable at the last follow-up.

examination showed some ruptured bullae and erosions on the trunk and extremities (**Figure 1D**). Immunological findings in serum by ELISA showed positive anti-desmoglein (Dsg) 1 antibody (130.5 U/ml, NR ≤20) and negative anti-Dsg3 antibody. Histopathological examination showed acantholysis and intraepidermal bulla formation (**Figure 1E**). DIF revealed intercellular binding of IgG and C3 within the epidermis. Repeat screening for ILD and malignancy was negative. Based on these results, CADM associated with PF was diagnosed. The patient was treated with oral prednisone 12.5 mg/day, methotrexate 7.5 mg/week, and topical halometasone cream. After 2 months, erosions were controlled and the prednisone dose was tapered. At the last follow-up in December 2021, the skin condition was stable with very few skin eruptions (**Figure 1F**).

Case 2

In 2017, a 68-year-old Chinese woman presented a 1-year history of purple erythema on her face. Physical examination showed periorbital and malar purple erythema without muscle weakness or tenderness. She took 2 months of radiotherapy in 2015 due to NPC. Laboratory investigations showed normal levels of muscle enzymes. MSAs showed anti-transcription intermediary factor 1-γ (TIF1-γ) antibody positive (immunoblotting, ELISA), and skin biopsy showed focal liquefaction and degeneration of basal cells, tortuosity of small vessels, and mild perivascular lymphocyte infiltration. Screening for ILD and internal malignancy was negative. The patient was diagnosed with CADM and treated with thalidomide 50 mg/day and hydroxychloroquine 200 mg/day.

This patient developed abdominal bullous eruptions 2 years later after using a heat patch for several days. The eruptions got aggravated and widespread to the whole body within a week. Physical examination showed widespread erythema with bullae and erosions on the trunk, neck, and extremities, including the armpits and groins (**Figure 2A**). The Nikolsky's sign was negative. Immunological findings showed positive anti-BP180 antibody (138.16 U/ml, NR ≤9), while anti-Dsg1, -Dsg3, and -BP230 antibodies were negative. Histology showed a subepidermal bulla and eosinophil infiltration in the bullous fluid and the superficial dermis (**Figure 2B**). Both DIF and indirect immunofluorescence (IIF) were negative. The patient was diagnosed with CADM associated with BP and treated with oral hydroxychloroquine 200 mg/day, minocycline 200 mg/day, and topical halometasone cream. Two months later, the bullous eruptions were controlled (**Figure 2C**). During our latest follow-up in September 2021, this patient presented with no sign of recurrence of BP or malignancy.

DISCUSSION

DM with blister has been reported in different terms in the literature, including DM with vesicle formation, vesiculobullous DM, and bullous DM (3). Apart from this, as reported in this study, there were a total of 14 cases reported so far in the literature that DM patients with blisters turned out to be AIBD eventually (**Table 1**) (4–16).

Fujimoto et al. (14) reported a 39-year-old Japanese woman who presented with PF over 2 years after the onset of CADM. MSAs of that patient showed anti-nuclear matrix protein 2 antibody positive, which is a risk factor of malignancy. Our Case 1 presented a similar disease process with different positive MSAs (i.e., anti- SAE and -Jo-1 antibodies). Additionally, to the best of our knowledge, Case 1 was the first report of vesiculobullous eruptions formed in autoimmune disease at different clinical stages with distinct mechanisms, suggesting that blisters in DM patients could be caused by the aggravation of the primary disease or other autoimmune diseases. Garcia et al. (15) reported a 69-year-old woman who was diagnosed with BP and CADM simultaneously when treated for mucosa-associated lymphoid tissue (MALT) gastric lymphoma. This woman also showed positive anti-melanoma differentiation-associated gene 5 antibody, which is a risk factor of rapid progressive ILD (15). Differently, our Case 2, with a 3-year history of CADM and a 4-year history of NPC, presented with positive anti-TIF1-γ antibody, a biomarker associated with malignancy. Furthermore, Case 2 showed typical progress of BP after using a heat patch, which might imply that the exposure of an antigen caused by local cutaneous damage played an essential role in the pathogenesis.

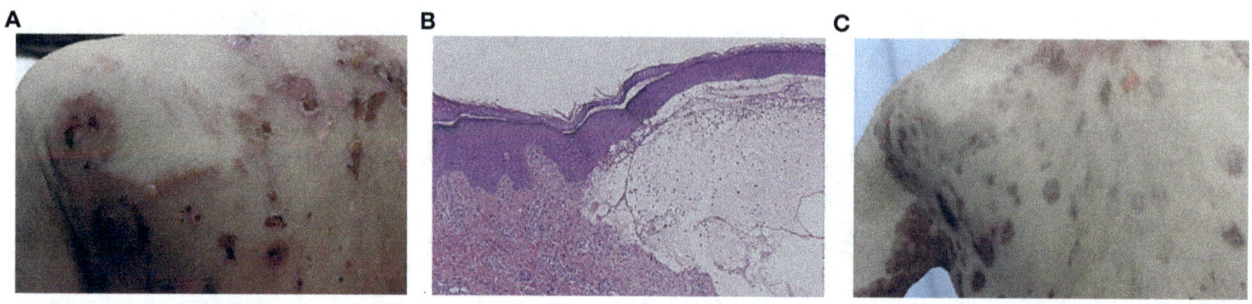

FIGURE 2 | **(A)** Bullae and erosions presented on the back. **(B)** Histology from a bulla on the right forearm showed subepidermal bulla formation and the bullous fluid and the superficial dermis were infiltrated by eosinophils. **(C)** The bullous eruptions were stable 2 months later.

TABLE 1 | A summary of reported cases of DM associated with AIBDs.

	Age	Sex	DM subset	AIBD	Time from onset of DM to AIBD[a]	Possible Trigger	MSAs	ILD	Malignancy
White and Tesar (4)	67	Female	DM	DH	3 years	(-)	/	(-)	(-)
Kalovidouris et al. (5) Case 1[b]	34	Male	DM	DH	-7 years	(-)	Anti-Jo-1 Ab	(-)	(-)
Barrows-Wade and Jordon (6)	56	Female	DM	Linear IgA bullous dermatosis	4 months	(-)	(-)	(-)	(-)
Glover and Leigh (7)	65	Male	DM	BP	Simultaneously	(-)	/	(-)	(-)
Tsukada et al. (8)	70	Male	DM	BP	8 months	(-)	/	(-)	(-)
Narbutt et al. (9)	11	Male	Juvenile DM	PF	2 years	Enalapril	/	(-)	(-)
Yanagi et al. (10)	81	Female	DM	BP	3 months	Surgery	/	(-)	Colon carcinoma
Ahmad and Nabih (11)	53	Female	DM	PF	15 years	Lisinopril	/	(-)	(-)
Black and Marshman (12)	76	Female	DM	PV	3.5 years	(-)	/	(-)	(-)
Thongprasom et al. (13)	36	Female	CADM	PV	-4 years	(-)	/	(-)	(-)
Fujimoto et al. (14)	39	Female	CADM	PF	2 years	(-)	Anti-NXP2 Ab	(-)	(-)
Garcia et al. (15)	69	Female	CADM	BP	Simultaneously	(-)	Anti-MDA5 Ab	(+)	MALT gastric lymphoma
Patsatsi et al. (16) Case 1	51	Female	DM	PV	-8 months	(-)	/	(-)	(-)
Case 2	82	Male	CADM	MMP	-14 years	(-)	/	(+)	(-)
Present Case 1	55	Female	CADM	PF	1.5 years	(-)	Anti-SAE, -Jo-1 Ab	(-)	(-)
Present Case 2	68	Female	CADM	BP	3 years	Heat patch	Anti-TIF1-γ Ab	(-)	NPC

DM, dermatomyositis; AIBDs, autoimmune blistering diseases; MSA, myositis-specific antibody; CADM, clinically amyopathic dermatomyositis; ILD, interstitial lung disease; DH, dermatitis herpetiformis; PV, pemphigus vulgaris; PF, pemphigus foliaceous; BP, bullous pemphigoid; MMP, mucous membrane pemphigoid; NPC, nasopharyngeal carcinoma; MALT, mucosa-associated lymphatic tissue; NXP2, nuclear matrix protein 2; MDA5, melanoma differentiation-associated gene 5; SAE, small ubiquitin-like modifier activating enzyme; TIF1, transcription intermediary factor 1.

[a]Time span from the onset of first symptom assumed to be related to DM to AIBD, the symbol "-" means AIBD occurred before DM.

[b]Case 2 in this literature was polymyositis.

Though both disease entities, bullous DM and AIBD, manifested as blister formation in DM patients, they had respective features to recognize. Moreover, due to the dissimilar pathogenesis, the differences in therapy and risk of complications should be considered. Clinically, blisters in bullous DM patients commonly present an erythema background with negative Nikolsky's sign. Such blisters tend to appear on irritated areas such as the extensors of the arms, knees, upper chest, and back (2). The period of its occurrence is transient and in which there is usually a concurrence of edematous erythema elsewhere. Histopathology of bullous DM commonly presents with papillary dermal edema and mucin deposition with negative DIF. No specific antibodies are detected. However, the vesiculobullous eruptions of AIBDs have unique features of skin manifestation, histopathology, immunopathology, and serum immunology. Pathogenetically, the parallel of bullae and DM was observed (17). It was even postulated that the two clinical forms, edematous and vesiculobullous, could be the same or overlapping manifestations (18). Contrarily, while the AIBD erupted, both of our patients showed no evidence of aggravation of CADM. The association between DM and AIBD remains unknown. AIBD can occur before, simultaneously with, or after the onset of DM. The most acceptable hypothesis for the coexistence of these two autoimmune diseases is epitope spreading. Sequestered antigens being exposed due to tissue damage can lead to a secondary autoimmune disease in some situations (19). Case 2 developed BP after applying a heat patch to her abdomen, which might directly damage the local skin tissue or lead to contact dermatitis. With exposure to autoantigens, this patient may eventually develop BP. Therapeutically, when Case 1 presented vesicles during her first-time hospital visit, we focused on the acute progress of CADM and treated her with methylprednisolone 40 mg/day. However, when she got readmitted to the hospital, we focused on the eruption of AIBD and the therapy was much more prudent. The skin lesions of both cases got relieved after an additional therapy with topical halometasone and immunosuppressant without increasing the corticosteroid.

The primarily fatal complications of DM are malignancy and ILD. The association between bullous DM and malignancy has been validated. It is reported that the risk of developing malignancy in bullous DM can reach as high as 68% (2). As for DM associated with AIBD, among 16 cases (14 cases reported historically and two cases in this study), three of them (18.8%) had a malignant tumor, including colon carcinoma, MALT gastric lymphoma, and NPC. It was notable that all three cases were BP, which accounted for 60% (3/5) among all BP cases. At present, the association between bullous DM and ILD is still uncertain. Among all cases, two of them were diagnosed with ILD (12.5%), and both were diagnosed with CADM. During our last clinical follow-up, Case 1 presented with no sign of malignancy and Case 2 showed no evidence of new malignancy or NPC recurrence. Our follow-up showed no link between blister formation and malignancy in CADM. Nevertheless, a longer follow-up and more cases are warranted for such validations.

ETHICS STATEMENT

Written informed consent was obtained from the individuals for the publication of any potentially identifiable images or data included in this article.

AUTHOR CONTRIBUTIONS

HXW: article writing. LCD: serology tests. KX and QZ: patient management. XQZ: histopathology support. QLX: biopsies. JZ, MP, and HC: article revising. All authors contributed to the article and approved the submitted version.

REFERENCES

1. Sontheimer RD. Dermatomyositis: An Overview of Recent Progress With Emphasis on Dermatologic Aspects. *Dermatol Clin* (2002) 20(3):387–408. doi: 10.1016/s0733-8635(02)00021-9
2. Mitsuya J, Hara H, Hattori A, Matsunaga A, Terui T. Vesicle Formation in Dermatomyositis Associated With Colon Carcinoma. *Clin Exp Dermatol* (2009) 34(7):e221–2. doi: 10.1111/j.1365-2230.2008.03060.x
3. Fujimoto N, Honda S, Wakabayashi M, Hamaguchi Y, Fujimoto M, Tanaka T. Anti-MDA-5 Antibody-Positive Bullous Dermatomyositis With Palmar Papules Complicating Rapidly Progressive Interstitial Lung Disease. *Mod Rheumatol* (2016) 26(4):614–6. doi: 10.3109/14397595.2014.908811
4. White SW, Tesar JT. Dermatomyositis and Dermatitis Herpetiformis. *Arch Dermatol* (1982) 118(8):599–601. doi: 10.1001/archderm.118.8.599
5. Kalovidouris AE, Miller FW, Lawley TJ. Polymyositis/dermatomyositis Associated With Dermatitis Herpetiformis. *Arthritis Rheum* (1989) 32 (9):1179–81. doi: 10.1002/anr.1780320920
6. Barrows-Wade L, Jordon RE, Arnett FC Jr. Linear IgA Bullous Dermatosis Associated With Dermatomyositis. *Arch Dermatol* (1992) 128(3):413–4. doi: 10.1001/archderm.128.3.413
7. Glover M, Leigh I. Dermatomyositis Pemphigoides: A Case With Coexistent Dermatomyositis and Bullous Pemphigoid. *J Am Acad Dermatol* (1992) 27(5 Pt 2):849–52. doi: 10.1016/0190-9622(92)70264-g
8. Tsukada Y, Kawase MK, Murashima A, Kitahora T, Hashimoto T, Komai A. Bullous Pemphigoid Associated With Dermatomyositis Successfully Controlled With Minocycline. *Clin Exp Dermatol* (2003) 28(5):563–4. doi: 10.1046/j.1365-2230.2003.01355.x
9. Narbutt J, Torzecka JD, Sysa-Jedrzejowska A, Pas HH. Pemphigus Foliaceus in an 11-Year-Old Boy With Dermatomyositis: Simple Coincidence or Familial Immunological Background? *Br J Dermatol* (2003) 148(4):838–9. doi: 10.1046/j.1365-2133.2003.05256.x
10. Yanagi T, Kato N, Yamane N, Osawa R. Bullous Pemphigoid Associated With Dermatomyositis and Colon Carcinoma. *Clin Exp Dermatol* (2007) 32 (3):291–4. doi: 10.1111/j.1365-2230.2007.02368.x
11. Ahmad T, Nabih A. Dermatomyositis Followed by Pemphigus Foliaceus: A Case Report and Possible Mechanism. *Rheumatol Rep* (2009) 1(1):e11. doi: 10.4081/rr.2009.e11
12. Black M, Marshman G. Dermatomyositis and Pemphigus Vulgaris: Association or Coincidence? *Australas J Dermatol* (2011) 52(2):e11–4. doi: 10.1111/j.1440-0960.2010.00646.x
13. Thongprasom K, Prasongtanskul S, Fongkhum A, Iamaroon A. Pemphigus, Discoid Lupus Erythematosus, and Dermatomyositis During an 8-Year Follow-Up Period: A Case Report. *J Oral Sci* (2013) 55(3):255–8. doi: 10.2334/josnusd.55.255
14. Fujimoto N, Takayama S, Hamaguchi Y, Fujimoto M, Tanaka T. Pemphigus Foliaceus Associated With Anti-NXP2 Autoantibody-Positive Dermatomyositis. *Acta Derm Venereol* (2014) 94(4):478–9. doi: 10.2340/00015555-1756
15. Garcia B, Dabouz F, Pascal L, Gillard M, Modiano P. [Amyopathic Dermatomyositis (DM) With Anti-MDA5 Antibodies, Associated With Bullous Pemphigoid, Sjogren Syndrome and Gastric MALT Lymphoma]. *Ann Dermatol Venereol* (2017) 144(10):629–33. doi: 10.1016/j.annder.2017.05.009
16. Patsatsi A, Pearson DR, Werth VP. Dermatomyositis in Patients With Autoimmune Blistering Diseases. *Int J Womens Dermatol* (2019) 5(4):256–60. doi: 10.1016/j.ijwd.2019.05.009
17. Nishigori K, Yamamoto T, Yokozeki H. Vesiculo-Bullous Dermatomyositis: Report of Three Cases. *Dermatol Online J* (2009) 15(4):6. doi: 10.5070/D3492472WJ
18. Lozano-Masdemont B, Pulido-Perez A, Parra-Blanco V, Aviles-Izquierdo JA. Edema and Dermatomyositis. Migratory Edema and Edematous and Vesiculobullous Dermatomyositis Overlap. *Reumatol Clin (Engl Ed)* (2018) 14(5):313–4. doi: 10.1016/j.reuma.2017.09.003
19. Chan LS, Vanderlugt CJ, Hashimoto T, Nishikawa T, Zone JJ, Black MM, et al. Epitope Spreading: Lessons From Autoimmune Skin Diseases. *J Invest Dermatol* (1998) 110(2):103–9. doi: 10.1046/j.1523-1747.1998.00107.x

8

Rituximab in the Treatment of Interstitial Lung Diseases Related to Anti-Melanoma Differentiation-Associated Gene 5 Dermatomyositis

Chenjia He[1†], Wenyu Li[2†], Qibing Xie[1] and Geng Yin[1*]*

[1] Department of Rheumatology and Immunology, West China Hospital, Sichuan University, Chengdu, China,
[2] Health Management Center, West China Hospital, Sichuan University, Chengdu, China

***Correspondence:**
Geng Yin
yingeng1975@163.com
Qibing Xie
xieqibing1971@163.com

†These authors have contributed equally to this work*

Objective: The effectiveness of rituximab in anti-melanoma differentiation-associated gene 5 (MDA5) dermatomyositis (DM) with interstitial lung disease (ILD) has been explored only in isolated case reports and small series. This paper aims to review the current evidence regarding rituximab (RTX) use in the treatment of ILD related to anti-MDA5 DM (anti-MDA5 DM-ILD).

Methods: We conducted a review by searching PubMed, Web of Science, Embase, and Cochrane for articles with information on patients with anti-MDA5 DM and RTX treatment, published until August 2021, in English language. The selected studies listed variation in chest high-resolution computed tomography (HRCT) and/or pulmonary function test (PFT) as a primary outcome, in patients with anti-MDA5 DM-related ILD after using RTX.

Results: Of the 145 potentially eligible articles, 17 were selected. The information gathered from a total of 35 patients with anti-MDA5 DM-ILD was reviewed, including 13 men and 22 women. Patient age at onset was 47.60 ± 13.72 years old. A total of 11.43% (4/35) of the patients were found to have chronic ILD (C-ILD) and 88.57% (31/30) exhibited rapidly progressive ILD (RP-ILD). Most patients (29/30) had typical DM rashes. Prior to RTX administration, the majority of patients (27/35) were treated with medium- or high-dose glucocorticoids and at least one additional immunotherapeutic agent. With regard to RTX efficacy for ILD in anti-MDA5 DM, 71.43% (25/35) of the patients responded to treatment. Skin rash also improved in more than half of the patients after RTX treatment. The most common side effects were infections, reported by 37.14% (13/35) of the patients after using RTX.

Conclusion: As a CD20 targeting drug, RTX is a promising therapeutic tool for anti-MDA5 DM-ILD, although the risk of infections should be considered before treatment. Further prospective controlled studies are required to evaluate the optimal RTX treatment regimen.

Systematic Review Registration: https://www.crd.york.ac.uk/prospero/display_record.php?ID=CRD42021289714, identifier CRD42021289714.

Keywords: dermatomyositis, melanoma differentiation-associated gene 5, interstitial lung disease, rituximab, targeting CD20

INTRODUCTION

Dermatomyositis (DM) is an autoimmune inflammatory disease that predominantly affects the muscles of the proximal extremities and the skin. DM is clinically heterogeneous both regarding patient symptoms and the severity of the disease. Myositis-specific autoantibodies (MSAs) are a class of recently discovered biomarkers that are associated to a unique clinical subset of myositis, and are therefore of great value in the classification of the disease, assessment of prognosis, and formulation of treatment plans (1). An important example of MSAs is the anti-melanoma differentiation-associated gene 5 autoantibody (anti-MDA5 autoAb). Patients positive for anti-MDA5 autoantibody (autoAb) typically exhibit cutaneous manifestations and mild or even no myopathy, but frequently are diagnosed with interstitial lung disease (ILD) (2). The prevalence of ILD in patients positive for anti-MDA5 autoAb has been estimated to be 50%–72.7% in reports from Europe and America (3–5) and 82%–100% in studies from Asia (6–10). In addition, the prevalence of patients that develop rapidly progressing ILD (RP-ILD) among the population of patients with anti-MDA5 DM-related ILD (anti-MDA5 DM-ILD) can be as high as 100% (11). More importantly, patients with anti-MDA5 DM usually have a high mortality rate due to relentless RP-ILD and lack of effective treatment. A recent study revealed that the 6-month survival rate of anti-MDA5 DM-ILD patients was only 33% even when treated with immunosuppressants (12).

Currently, there is no universal treatment for anti-MDA5 DM-ILD. Empiric treatment primarily focuses on glucocorticoid administration combined with the commonly used immunosuppressants - cyclophosphamide (CYC), calcineurin inhibitor (CNI) (12). However, there is still a large group of patients with anti-MDA5 DM-ILD who respond poorly to treatment with glucocorticoids and conventional immunosuppressants (13, 14). Hence, there is an urgent need to identify new treatment options for improving the therapeutic effect and prognosis.

CD20 is a transmembrane antigen selectively expressed on pre-B and mature B lymphocytes and is lost when B cells differentiate into plasma cells. In previous years, rituximab (RTX), a chimeric anti-CD20 monoclonal antibody, has been used in the management of B-cell malignancies (15), antineutrophil cytoplasmic antibody (ANCA)-associated renal vasculitis (16), rheumatoid arthritis (RA) (17), and systemic lupus erythematosus (SLE) (18). Although no guidelines on the treatment of myositis-related ILD have been published by the American College of Rheumatology (ACR) or by the European Alliance of Associations for Rheumatology (EULAR), RTX has also been used off-label in patients who did not respond to conventional therapy, based on a postulated pathogenetic role for B cells in anti-MDA5 DM-ILD. It is important to notice that the evaluation of therapeutic efficacy may be challenging in these conditions, since there are only a few case reports and small series in which RTX has been used in anti-MDA5 DM-ILD treatment.

The present paper aims to systematically review the currently available evidence regarding the use of RTX in anti-MDA5 DM-ILD.

METHODS

Literature Search Strategy

This systematic review was registered in PROSPERO (CRD42021289714) and performed according to the Preferred Reporting Items for Systematic Reviews and Meta-Analyses (PRISMA) recommendations (19). Two reviewers conducted a search on PubMed, Web of Science, Embase, and Cochrane databases, in an independent and simultaneous manner, for information on case reports, case series, and case-control studies of patients positive for anti-MDA5 DM and/or RTX treatment, reported until August 2021, in English language. The key retrieval terms included dermatomyositis, anti-MDA5, interstitial lung disease, Rituximab, and CD20 targeting. The detailed search strategy is documented in the supplementary file. The reference list of selected papers was also screened to identify additional studies to be included. **Figure 1** shows the flowchart of the paper selection process.

Inclusion and Exclusion Criteria

Eligible patients in our review fulfilled the following criteria: i) met the Bohan and Peter criteria of DM (21) or Sontheimer's criteria of CADM (22); ii) had positive anti-MDA5 antibody confirmed by immunoblotting assay or ELISA; iii) had confirmed interstitial lung diseases (ILD), defined as ground-glass changes and/or fibrosis noted on high-resolution computed tomography (HRCT) (23). iv) had receive RTX treatment. Subsequently, only cases with complete epidemiological data and therapeutic information were selected. Study designs were either randomized control trials (RCTs), cohort studies, case-control studies, case or case series. Exclusion criteria included suffering from malignancy or other overlapping rheumatic diseases, such as systemic lupus erythematosus (SLE) and systemic sclerosis (SSc).

Data Extraction and Quality Assessment

Data recorded included age, sex, clinical manifestation (pulmonary involvement and/or extrapulmonary manifestations), laboratory data at disease presentation, and administered treatment (e.g., prednisolone, immunosuppressive agents, intravenous immunoglobulin, plasma exchange) previous to RTX administration were also recorded. Additional information collected included the RTX treatment schedule, RTX adverse effects, and clinical response to RTX. Two independent researchers assessed the methodological quality of all studies using the Newcastle-Ottawa Scale (NOS) criteria (24), classified according to the selection of the study groups, the comparability of the groups, and the ascertainment of the outcome. The classification scale ranges from 0 (poor methodological quality) to 9 (optimal methodological quality). Any discrepancies were resolved *via* discussion or consultation with a third researcher.

Response Criteria

Patients were defined as responders if at least one of two criteria were met: i) $\geq$ 10% increase in forced vital capacity (FVC) and/or $\geq$ 15% increase in diffusing capacity of carbon monoxide

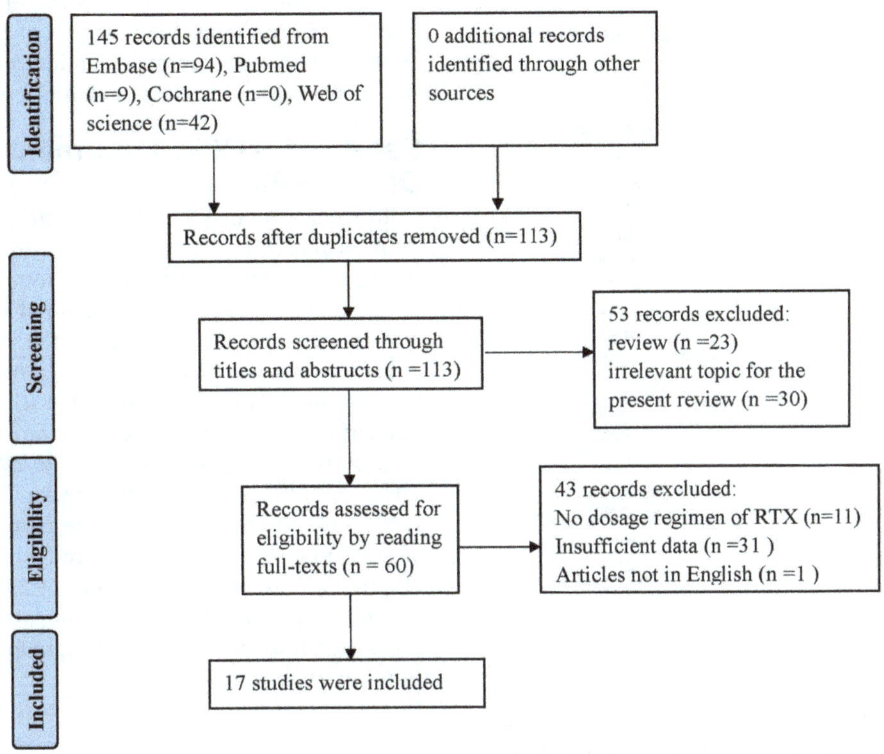

FIGURE 1 | Flow diagram according to Prisma guidelines (20).

(DLCO) (25); ii) improved outcome of lung imaging by either chest X-rays or HRCT (reviewed by a radiologist blinded to the design of the study) (23).

Statistical Analysis

Data are expressed as the mean ± SD. Differences in quantitative parameters between two groups were assessed using the Mann-Whitney U-test. Fisher's exact test was used to compare the trends between groups of qualitative variables. All statistical analyses were performed using Prism 8.3 software (GraphPad Software, La Jolla, CA, USA) and a two-sided p value of 0.05 or less was considered significant.

RESULTS

The bibliographic search conducted to identify cases of anti-MDA5 DM-ILD treated with RTX yielded 145 articles. After screening and eligibility check were conducted, 128 articles were excluded, as detailed in **Figure 1**. Of the 17 articles selected to be included in this review, 16 were case reports and case series, and one was a retrospective case-control study. Clinical data was extracted relating to 35 patients with anti-MDA5 DM-ILD meeting the inclusion criteria (23, 26–41). The demographic characteristics, clinical manifestations, laboratory data, treatment regimen, and outcomes are shown in **Tables 1, 2**.

Clinical Characteristics of Anti-MDA5 DM-ILD Patients Receiving RTX Treatment

The mean age at diagnosis was 47.6 ± 13.72 years. Approximately 62.86% (22/35) of the patients in our study were female and 94.29% (33/35) of patients were Asian. Patients with polymyositis (PM) and/or DM aggravated by ILD can be divided into two main clinical patterns: chronic (C-ILD) and rapidly progressive ILD (RP-ILD) (42), the latter being associated with poorer prognosis. In this study, all enrolled patients had ILD, from which 88.57% (31/35) had RP-ILD, and 11.43% (4/35) had C-ILD. Clinical manifestation data of 30 patients were obtained. Most patients (29/30) had typical DM rashes, such as heliotrope sign (20/30), Gottron's sign (24/30), palmar papules (8/30), V-neck rash (8/30), shawl sign (5/30), mechanic hand (16/30), and ulceration (15/30). Myalgia and muscle weakness were observed in 10 and 9 patients, respectively. There were 20 patients with fever and 14 patients with arthralgia/arthritis. Raynaud's phenomenon was observed in 8 patients (**Table 1**).

Differential Treatment Regimen Across the Anti-MDA5 DM-ILD Patients

Prior to RTX administration, the majority of patients (27/35) in our study were treated with medium or high doses of glucocorticoids and at least one additional immunotherapy treatments, including intravenous cyclophosphamide (18/35,

TABLE 1 | Summary of the general characteristics of 35 patients with anti-MDA5 DM-ILD treated with RTX.

Characteristics	Patients with anti-MDA5 DM-ILD
Demographic	
Age at onset (years), mean ± SD	47.60 ± 13.72
Female, n (%)	22(62.86)
Asian, n (%)	33(94.29)
ILD, n (%)	35 (100)
C-ILD, n (%)	4(11.43)
RP-ILD, n (%)	31(88.57)
Cutaneous involvement	29/30
Heliotrope rash	20/30
Gottron's papules or sign	24/30
Palmar papules	8/30
V-neck rash	8/30
Shawl sign	5/30
Mechanic hand	16/30
Ulceration	15/30
Myalgia	10/30
Muscle weakness	9/30
Fever	20/30
Arthralgia/arthritis	14/30
Raynaud's phenomenon	8/30

RTX, rituximab; DM, dermatomyositis; MDA5, melanoma differentiation-associated gene 5; ILD, interstitial lung disease; RP-ILD, rapidly progressive interstitial lung disease; C-ILD, chronic interstitial lung disease.

51.43%), calcineurin inhibitor (18/35, 51.43%), intravenous immunoglobulin (8/35, 22.86%), mycophenolate mofetil (8/35, 22.86%), polymyxin B hemoperfusion treatment (2/35, 5.71%), plasmapheresis (1/35, 2.86%), methotrexate (1/35, 2.86%), azathioprine (1/35, 2.86%), hydroxychloroquine (1/35, 2.86%), and thalidomide (1/35, 2.86%). In this study, 19 patients were treated with two or more immunotherapy treatments. Remarkably, three patients received five treatment modalities. Approximately 42.86% (15/35) of patients were treated with the lymphoma schedule or lymphoma-like schedule (350–375 mg/m^2 every 1 or 2 weeks) and 17.14% (6/35) of patients received the rheumatology schedule (500–1000 mg every 2 weeks). Other schedules included 500–550 mg RTX every week in 5 (14.29%) patients. In addition to the above conventional regimens, 9 anti-MDA5 DM-ILD patients were treated with a novel low-dose RTX regimen (100 mg per week)(**Table 2**).

Efficacy of RTX for Anti-MDA5 DM-ILD Patients

Considering the efficiency of RTX treatment for ILD in anti-MDA5 DM patients, 71.43% (25/35) of patients presented a response to treatment (assessed by chest HRCT and/or PFT). In the C-ILD subgroup, 75% (3/4) of the patients presented a response to RTX, while 70.97% (22/34) of patients in the RP-ILD subgroup presented a response to RTX. Among the low-dose and conventional-dose RTX subgroups, the response rate to treatment was 77.78% (7/9) and 69.23% (18/31), respectively (**Table 3**). Ferritin data were collected from 24 patients in this study. The levels of ferritin were significantly higher in the RTX treatment responsive subgroup than in the non-responsive subgroup (P=0.0196)(supplementary Fig 1). Seventeen patients had decreased ferritin levels after RTX treatment. A decrease of anti-MDA5 autoAb titers observed in patients 17, 25 and 27 after RTX treatment, while data from other patients were not available. Considering the outcome of cutaneous involvement, 19 patients showed improvement, including reduced degree and size of skin rash or healing of skin ulcers.

Safety of RTX in Treatment of Anti-MDA5 DM-ILD Patients

With regard to safety of RTX in anti-MDA5 DM-ILD patients, infusion reactions were not reported in any of the cases under study, and the most common side effects were infections. A total of 16 infection were reported by 13 patients, after RTX. Noteworthy, 56.25% (9/16) of the infection events were pulmonary infections, and more than half of them were caused by cytomegalovirus (CMV) (**Table 4**). The infection rate of patients in the low-dose and conventional-dose RTX subgroups was 55.56% (5/9) and 30.77% (8/26), respectively. The survival rates among patients with C-ILD and RP-ILD were 100% (4/4) and 64.52% (20/31), respectively. The survival rates of patients in the low-dose and conventional-dose RTX subgroups were 66.67% (6/9) and 69.23% (18/26), respectively (**Table 3**). The survival rates of patients in the RTX treatment responsive and non-responsive subgroups were 92% (23/25) and 10% (1/10), respectively (**Table 5**).

DISCUSSION

The hallmarks of anti-MDA5 DM are the presence of autoantibodies targeting MDA5 and unique cutaneous features, as well as an elevated risk of ILD. The underlying pathogenesis is not yet fully understood. T and B lymphocytes (23, 43–47), neutrophils (48, 49), macrophages (50, 51), type I interferon (IFN-I) (52, 53) and "Cytokines storm" [which is similarity with SARS-CoV-2 infection (54)] were thought to be involved in the development of the disease (**Figure 2**). MDA5 protein, as a pattern recognition receptor (PRR), can recognizes viral double-stranded RNA (dsRNA) then activates IFN-I pathway (55) and induces the production of proinflammatory cytokines by the cell. Indeed, the aberrant activation of the type I interferon system has been demonstrated in anti-MDA5 DM in previous studies (52, 53). While MDA5 protein is also an IFN-inducible protein (56), so activation of the IFN-I system can further promote the production of MDA5 protein. Abnormal accumulation of MDA5 protein may lead to a loss of tolerance to MDA5, resulting in the production of anti-MDA5 autoAb. As for how anti-MDA5 autoAbs play their potentially pathogenic role is less well understood and is only briefly described here in light of a recent review on the subject (47). In pathological contexts, MDA5 is strong expressed in skin tissue of DM patients (57) and detectable in cytoplasmic, cell surface, and secretory vesicles in neutrophils (58). Hence, some scholars have speculated that anti-MDA5 Abs can bind to MDA5 on cell surface and induce an inappropriate activation of MDA5, resulting in chronic activation of the IFN-I pathway. Apart from binding to MDA5 expressed on cell surface, they suggested anti-MDA5 Abs could also form immune complexes with the MDA5 proteins released from apoptotic cell and interact

TABLE 2 | Clinical course of 35 patients with anti-MDA5 DM-ILD using RTX.

Patient no./ Age at Entry, Years/Sex	Previous Therapy	RTX Treatment Schedule	Co-Intervention with RTX	Ferritin Levels at Admission/After RTX (ng/ml)	Outcome of Skin Rash	Outcome of Lung (Chest CT or PFT)	RTX Response/ Outcome of Survival	Ref.
1/36/F	PSL, IVCY, CNI, MMF	375 mg/m^2 i.v. at Day 0,Day 14	PSL 1mg/kg/d, MMF, CNI	77/10.8	Not improved	Chest CT improved, DLCO rose to 72.8% from 55% after RTX	Success/ alive	1 (23)
2/59/M	PSL	375 mg/m^2 i.v. at Day 0,Day 14	PSL 1mg/kg/d, IVIG, CNI	1119.3/110.7	improved	Chest CT improved, DLCO rose to 61.3% from 33.8% after RTX	Success/ alive	
3/24/M	PSL, CNI, MTX, IVCY	375 mg/m^2 i.v. at Day 0,Day 14	PSL 1mg/kg/d, CNI	749.8/366.5	improved	Chest CT improved after RTX	Success/ alive	
4/41/F	PSL, IVCY, IVIG	375 mg/m^2 i.v. at Day 0,Day 14	PSL 2mg/kg/d, IVCY	276.1/N.A.	Not improved	Chest CT deteriorated	Failure/died	
5/37/F	PSL, IVCY, MMF,IVIG	375 mg/m^2 i.v. at Day 0,Day 14	PSL 2mg/kg/d, IVIG	1811/118	Not improved	Chest CT improved after RTX	Success/ alive	
6/51/M	mPSL, AZA,IVCY	375 mg/m^2 i.v. at Day 0,Day 14	PSL 2mg/kg/d, IVIG	1433.5/1169	improved	Chest CT deteriorated	Failure/died	
7/56/F	mPSL, IVCY, CNI	375 mg/m^2 i.v. at Day 0, Day 14	PSL 1mg/kg/d, CNI	490.2/53.3	improved	Chest CT improved, DLCO rose to 71% from 36.6% after RTX	Success/ alive	1 (23)
8/53/F	PSL, IVCY	100mg/w i.v. (for 4 ws)	PSL 1mg/kg/d, CNI	187.1/11.5	improved	Improvement in chest CT, PFT was initially not completed because of dyspnea. After RTX, DLCO rose to 70.1%	Success/ alive	
9/28/M	mPSL, IVIG	100mg/w i.v. (for 4 ws)	PSL 1mg/kg/d, CNI	4676/24.4	improved	Improvement in chest CT, PFT was initially not completed because of dyspnea. After RTX, DLCO rose to 95.8%	Success/ alive	
10/36/F	mPSL, CNI, IVIG	100mg/w i.v. (for 4 ws)	PSL 1mg/kg/d, CNI	1141.2/36.3	improved	Chest CT improved after RTX	Success/ alive	
11/39/M	PSL, MMF, THD, IVCY	100mg/w i.v. (for 2 ws)	PSL 1mg/kg/d	1042.8/789	improved	Chest CT deteriorated	Failure/died	
12/49/F	PSL, MMF, CNI, IVCY, IVIG	In Ref.2, three in four patients use RTX 1g i.v. at Day 0, Day 14; one in four patients use RTX 500mg/w i.v. (for 4 ws)	PSL	N.A./23	improved	Chest CT improved, FVCrose to 67% from 39% after RTX	Success/ alive	2 (26)
13/50/M	PSL, MMF, IVCY, CNI		PSL, CNI	N.A./260	improved	Chest CT improved, FVCrose to 105% from 76% after RTX	Success/ alive	
14/38/M	PSL, MMF, CNI, IVIG		PSL	2844/902	improved	Chest CT unchanged, FVC rose to 121% from 94% after RTX	Success/ alive	
15/48/M	PSL, CNI		PSL	N.A./170	improved	Chest CT improved, DLCO rose to 72% from 54% after RTX	Success/ alive	
16/71/F	mPSL 1g×3d, followed by PSL 1mg/kg/d, CNI, IVCY, IVIg, PMX	350mg/m^2/w i.v. (for 4 ws)	PSL, CNI	3149.8/253.1	improved	Chest CT improved after RTX	Success/ alive	3 (27)
17/48/M	mPSL 1g×3d, followed by PSL 1mg/kg/d, CNI, IVCY	350mg/m^2/w i.v. (for 4 ws)	PSL, CNI	781/186	improved	Chest CT improved after RTX	Success/ alive	4 (28)
18/71/F	mPSL 1g×3d,followed by PSL 1mg/kg/d,CNI, IVCY	350mg/m^2/w i.v. (for 2 ws)	PSL, CNI	507/1740	Not improved	Chest CT deteriorated	Failure/died	5 (29)
19/69/F	mPSL 1g×3d, followed by PSL 1mg/kg/d, CNI	350mg/m^2/w i.v. (for 2 ws)	PSL, CNI, IVCY	219/1930	Not improved	Chest CT deteriorated	Failure/died	
20/57/M	PSL 1mg/kg/d, CNI, IVCY, PMX, MMF	550mg/w i.v. (for 4 ws)	PSL, CNI, MMF, IVIG	1178/continued to decrease	N.A.	Chest CT improved after RTX	Success/ alive	6 (30)
21/49/F	PSL, HCQ	1g i.v. at Day0,Day 14	PSL, IVIG, CTX, CNI, EMCO	N.A./N.A.	N.A.	Chest CT deteriorated, Initial PFT results showed FVC and DLCO were 87.5% and 59% respectively	Failure/died	7 (31)
22/55/F	mPSL 500mg/week	375mg/m^2/w (for 4 ws)	PSL 1mg/kg/d, CNI	1630/N.A.	improved	Chest CT improved, FVC rose to 88% from 60% after RTX	Success/ alive	8 (32)
23/64/F	mPSL 500mg×3d, followed by mPSL 40-80mg/d, CNI, IVCY, IVIG	375mg/m^2 (use twice)	mPSL 500mg×3d, followed by mPSL 40-80mg/d, CNI, IVIG	300/	N.A.	Chest CT deteriorated, Initial PFT results showed FVC and DLCO were 83.2% and 68.6% respectively	Failure/died	9 (33)
24/70/F	mPSL pulse therapy, followed by PSL, CNI, IVCY	375mg/m^2/w (for 4 ws)	PSL, CNI	N.A./N.A.	improved	Chest CT improved after RTX	Success/ alive	10 (34)
25/29/F	mPSL 1g×3d, followed by PSL 45mg/d, CNI, IVCY, PE	375mg/m^2/w (for 4 ws)	PSL 40mg/d, CNI	77/decrease	improved	Chest CT unchanged	Failure/alive	11 (35)
26/50/F	PSL 25mg/d, MMF	1g i.v. at Day0,Day 14	PSL 12.5mg/d	N.A./N.A.	improved	Chest CT improved, DLCO rose to 56% from 42% after RTX	Success/ alive	12 (36)
27/62/M	mPSL pulse therapy, followed by PSL 60mg/ d, IVCY, CNI	500 mg i.v. at Day 3,Day 10, Day 17	mPSL pulse therapy, IVCY, CNI, TOF(5mg bid),PE(days 1,7, 8, 9)	6711.3/normal	N.A.	Chest CT improved after RTX	Success/ alive	13 (37)
28/37/F	mPSL pulse therapy, followed by PSL 50mg/ d	500 mg/w i.v.	mPSL pulse therapy, IVCY, CNI, TOF, PE	412.2/N.A.	N.A.	Chest CT improved after RTX	Success/ alive	14 (38)
29/42/F	mPSL 1g×3d, mechanical ventilation	500 mg/w i.v. (only once)	None	169.4/N.A.	N.A.	Chest CT deteriorated	Failure/died	15 (39)

(Continued)

TABLE 2 | Continued

Patient no./ Age at Entry, Years/Sex	Previous Therapy	RTX Treatment Schedule	Co-Intervention with RTX	Ferritin Levels at Admission/After RTX (ng/ml)	Outcome of Skin Rash	Outcome of Lung (Chest CT or PFT)	RTX Response/ Outcome of Survival	Ref.
30/16/F	mPSL 1g×3d, followed by PSL1mg/kg/d, CNI	1g i.v. at Day 1, Day 15	IVCY, IVIG	2006/normal	improved	Chest CT improved, DLCO rose to 80% from 59% after RTX	Success/ alive	16 (40)
31/44/M	GC	100 mg i.v. (only once)	GC, CNI, Other treatments are not mentioned	N.A./N.A.	N.A.	Chest CT improved after RTX	Success/ alive	17 (41)
32/36/F	GC	100 mg i.v. (only once)	GC, CNI, Other treatments are not mentioned	N.A./N.A.	N.A.	Chest CT improved after RTX	Success/ alive	17 (41)
33/55/F	GC	100 mg i.v. (only once)	GC, CNI, Other treatments are not mentioned	N.A./N.A.	N.A.	Chest CT improved after RTX	Success/ died	
34/59/M	GC	100 mg i.v. (only once)	GC, CNI, Other treatments are not mentioned	N.A./N.A.	N.A.	Chest CT improved after RTX	Success/ died	
35/37/F	GC	100 mg i.v. (only once)	GC, CNI, Other treatments are not mentioned	N.A./N.A.	N.A.	Chest CT deteriorated	Failure/died	

RTX, rituximab; PSL, prednisolone; mPSL, methylprednisolone; IVCY, intravenous cyclophosphamide; IVIG, intravenous immunoglobulin; CNI, calcineurin inhibitors; MMF, mycophenolate mofetil; MTX, methotrexate; AZA, azathioprine; TOF, tofacitinib; THD, thalidomide; PMX, polymyxin B hemoperfusion treatment; HCQ, hydroxychloroquine; PE, plasma exchange; w/ws, week/weeks; m, month; i.v., intravenous; N.A., not available; PFT, pulmonary function testing; FVC, forced vital capacity; DLCO, diffusing capacity of carbon monoxide; MAS, macrophage activation syndrome; HBV, Hepatitis B Virus; TB, tuberculosis; RFP, rifampin; success/failure, interstitial lung disease respond/did not respond to RTX treatment.

TABLE 3 | Effiacy and safety data of the 35 patients with anti-MDA5 DM-ILD treated with RTX.

	Pattern of ILD		RTX Treatment Schedule	
	C-ILD	**RP-ILD**	**Low-Dose RTX**	**Conventional-Dose RTX**
Total	4	31	9	26
Mean age, years (mean ± SD)	34.75 ± 11.30	49.26 ± 13.25	43 ± 10.46	49.19 ± 14.51
Female, n (%)	3 (75)	19 (61.29)	5 (55.56)	17 (65.39)
Response to RTX Treatment, n (%)	3 (75)	22 (70.97)	7 (77.78)	18 (69.23)
Infection, n(%)	N.A.	N.A.	5 (55.56)	8 (30.77)
Survival, n (%)	4 (100)	20 (64.52)	6 (66.67)	18 (69.23)

RTX, rituximab; DM, dermatomyositis; MDA5, melanoma differentiation-associated gene 5; ILD, interstitial lung disease; RP-ILD, rapidly progressive interstitial lung disease; C-ILD, chronic interstitial lung disease; N.A., not available.

with cytoplasmic MDA5, which may similar to other Abs described previously (59, 60). In the lungs, the chemokine CX3CL1 can be produced by vascular endothelial cells when exposed to IFN-I and induce recruitment of CX3CR1^{+} M2 macrophages (61, 62). Local production of transformation growth factor-β (TGF-β) by M2 macrophages directly promotes pulmonary fibrosis. Moreover, there is a CD4^{+}CXCR4^{+} T cell subset in anti-MDA5 DM-ILD, which can produce profibrotic agents (TGF-β, α-smooth muscle actin (α-SMA), collagen I, and IL-21) (46). In addition, the process of activated neutrophils releasing neutrophil extracellular traps (NETs) could expose autoantigens that have the potential to break immune tolerance and lead to production of autoantibodies (63). In recent years, accumulating evidence suggested that B lymphocytes may play a critical role in the pathogenesis of anti-MDA5 DM-ILD. First, plasma cells that secrete antibodies derive from B lymphocytes, while multiple studies have already demonstrated that anti-MDA5 autoantibodies are closely related to disease activity and ILD in patients with anti-MDA5 DM (64, 65); Secondly, B cell activating factor (BAFF) is a member of the tumor necrosis factor (TNF) superfamily, playing a key role in the

TABLE 4 | Summary of infections in the patients comprised in the present study.

Infection Type	Number of Iinfection Events	Remarks
Upper respiratory infection	2	Occurred in patients 31, 32.
Pulmonary infection	9	Occurred in patients 4, 6, 11, 13, 14, 27, 32, 33, 34; Five of them were CMV infection.
Urinary tract infection	2	Occurred in patient 27, the other one is unknown.
Appendicitis	1	N.A.
Skin infection	1	Occurred in patient 12.
Herpes infection	1	N.A.

CMV, cytomegalovirus; N.A., not available.

TABLE 5 | Clinical data between RTX treatment responsive and non-responsive subgroups in 35 patients with anti-MDA5 DM-ILD.

	RTX Treatment Responsive	RTX Treatment Non-Responsive
Total	25	10
Mean age, years (mean ± SD)	46.96 ± 13.68	49.20 ± 14.41
Female, n (%)	14 (56%)	8 (80%)
C-ILD, n (%)	3 (12%)	1 (10%)
RP-ILD, n (%)	22 (88%)	9 (90%)
Survival, n (%)	23 (92%)	1 (10%)

RTX, rituximab; DM, dermatomyositis; MDA5, melanoma differentiation-associated gene 5; ILD, interstitial lung disease; RP-ILD, rapidly progressive interstitial lung disease; C-ILD, chronic interstitial lung disease.

survival and balance of peripheral B cells and plasma cells. It not only promotes the maturation of B cells, but also regulates immunoglobulin class-switching (66, 67). Data from Kobayashi et al. showed that juvenile dermatomyositis (JDM) patients with a high titer of anti-MDA5 autoantibodies had higher levels of BAFF than those with low titers (68). Another study noted that higher levels of BAFF were detected in patients positive for anti-MDA5 autoantibodies, when compared to negative patients, and that the levels of BAFF correlated positively with the titers of anti-MDA5 autoantibodies. The same study also indicates that the BAFF level of anti-MDA5 DM patients aggravated by ILD was significantly higher than anti-MDA5 DM patients not suffering from ILD, and the level of BAFF was parallel with KL-6, an indicator of the severity of ILD, suggesting that patients with anti-MDA5 DM complicated with severe ILD tend to have higher levels of serum BAFF (52); Thirdly, a recent study by Shuang Ye et al. revealed that the peripheral percentage of $CD4^+CXCR4^+T$ cells is relevant to the severity of ILD in idiopathic inflammatory myopathy (IIM), especially to anti-MDA5 DM-ILD. Furthermore, they confirmed that the circulating $CD4^+CXCR4^+T$ cell subset expresses high levels of IL-21 (46), which can induce the differentiation of B cells into plasmablasts by binding to the IL-21 receptor on the surface of B cells (69).

Based on the possible causative role of B cells, targeting CD20 in the treatment of anti-MDA5 DM-ILD seems to be of great importance. Hence, RTX is empirically used as a therapeutic agent for patients with anti-MDA5 DM-ILD. All currently published studies on the efficacy of RTX in the treatment of anti-MDA5 DM-ILD are case reports, case series, or case-control studies. The present work offers a systematic review of the effects of RTX in 35 anti-MDA5 DM-ILD patients. The clinical response after using RTX for ILD could be defined by the improvement of chest HRCT and/or PFT. After RTX treatment, 71.43% (25/35) of patients responded positively, according to chest HRCT and/or PFT. According to the data here analyzed, anti-MDA5 DM patients with RP-ILD (22/31, 70.97%) had a lower rate of response to RTX than C-ILD (3/4, 75.0%) patients. We also observed that patients in the low-dose RTX subgroup (7/9, 77.78%) had a higher response rate than patients in the conventional-dose RTX subgroup (18/26, 69.23%). In addition, patients with anti-MDA5 DM usually exhibit typical cutaneous manifestations. Previous studies that assessed the efficacy of RTX for cutaneous lesions in anti-MDA5 DM patients have demonstrated different therapeutic effects (70, 71). In our study, skin rash improved in more than half of the patients that used RTX, whereas the rate of response to RTX treatment on cutaneous lesions in anti-MDA5 DM patients cannot be accurately calculated due to the unavailability of information on some cases. Further large-sample studies are required to evaluate the efficacy of RTX on the cutaneous lesions of patients with anti-MDA5 DM. Similarly, we observed that ferritin levels decreased in more than half of the patients, after RTX treatment. A study by Gono et al. showed that ferritin level is a poor prognostic factor in RP-ILD patients with anti-MDA5 DM, and also indicated that ferritin concentrations are useful for the evaluation of the response to treatment in patients with anti-MDA5 DM-ILD (72). This indicates that the condition of most patients in our study improved after RTX. Considering the results described above and the fact that all patients in our study received glucocorticoids and/or immunosuppressants prior to RTX treatment and had poor response to these drugs, RTX may be an effective treatment for anti-MDA5 DM-ILD resistant to glucocorticoids and multiple immunotherapies.

From a safety perspective, 37.14% (13/35) of patients developed infection after RTX therapy, and four patients died of pulmonary infection in our study. Although there seems to be an increased risk of clinical infections after RTX treatment, the rate of infection is poorly correlated with the types of immune diseases and is closely correlated with low hypogammaglobulinemia, neutropenia, $CD4^+$ T cell dysfunction, etc. (73). Recently, a registry-based study estimated at 30% the efficacy and safety for RTX treatment in anti-synthetase syndrome, which was similar to the rate of infections after RTX administration in anti-MDA5 DM-ILD in the present review. In addition, 55.56% (5/9) of the patients in the low-dose subgroup were infected, which proved to be higher than the percentage of infections in the conventional-dose subgroup (30.77%) (8/26). This is most likely due to the fact that 6 patients who received low-dose RTX in Reference 17 were not included (due to lack of chest HRCT and/or PFT data), which led to biases in the results. Given that the response rate to RTX treatment of patients to in the low-dose subgroup (77.78%) was also higher than that of patients from the conventional-dose subgroup, and that this low-dose RTX regimen has been successfully used in several other immune diseases (74–76), we speculate that low-dose RTX (100 mg per week) may lead to a better therapeutic response than the conventional dose regimen. However, due to the limited number of patients in our study, whether low-dose RTX is recommended for anti-MDA5 DM-ILD remains to be verified in larger sample trials.

To our knowledge, the data on anti-MDA5 DM-ILD patients treated with RTX reviewed in this study were larger than those in previous studies, and we describe the detailed regimen used for

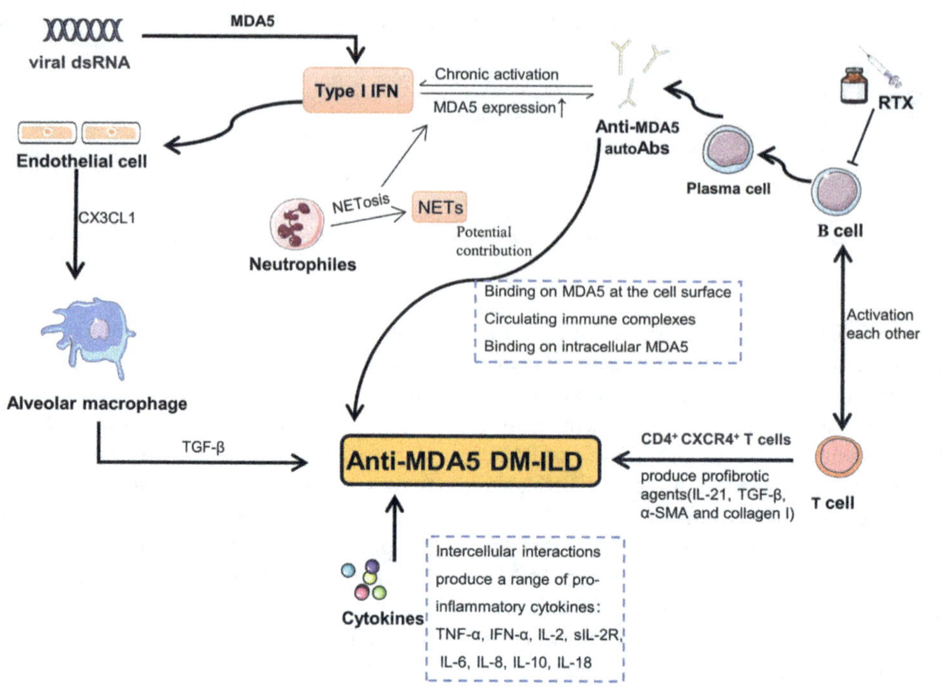

FIGURE 2 | Schematic representation of the hypothesized pathogenesis in anti-MDA5 DM-ILD. MDA5 protein can recognizes viral dsRNA then activates IFN-I pathway. Activation of the IFN-I system promote the production of MDA5 and cause MDA5 overexpression. Abnormal accumulation of MDA5 protein may lead to a loss of immune tolerance, resulting in the production of anti-MDA5 autoAb. Anti-MDA5 autoAbs may potential contribute to the pathogenesis through binding to MDA5 on cell surface, forming immune complexes, and interacting with cytoplasmic MDA5. In the lungs, CX3CL1 can be produced by endothelial cells when exposed to IFN-I and induce recruitment of alveolar M2 macrophages. Local production of TGF-β by M2 macrophages directly promotes pulmonary fibrosis. $CD4^{+}CXCR4^{+}$ T cell subset in anti-MDA5 DM-ILD can produce profibrotic agents (TGF-β, α-SMA, collagen I, and IL-21). The process of activated neutrophils releasing NETs could expose MDA5 autoantigens. MDA5, melanoma differentiation-associated gene 5; DM, dermatomyositis; ILD, interstitial lung disease; autoAb, autoantibody; RTX, rituximab; dsRNA, double-stranded ribose nucleic acid; NETs, neutrophil extracellular traps; NETosis, neutrophil extracellular traps externalization process; IFN-I, type I interferon; TGF-β, transformation growth factor-β; α-SMA, α-smooth muscle actin.

RTX administration. In addition, we evaluated the changes in ILD through HRCT and/or PFT, providing more evidence for the efficacy and safety of RTX in the treatment of anti-MDA5 DM-related ILD. However, there are some limitations to this study. First, the statistical analysis of the results was limited by the small sample size, which is not easy to circumvent due to the rarity of the disease. Second, the appropriate timing of RTX administration was not demonstrated in the present study. Third, the information of anti-MDA5 autoAb titers before and after RTX treatment were not available in most cases. Finally, multiple immunosuppressants were administered prior to RTX therapy in most patients, which may prevent the attribution of improvement to RTX treatment alone.

In summary, this systematic review allows us to conclude that as a CD20 targeting drug, RTX has a good response in the treatment of ILD related to anti-MDA5 DM. Combined with the current evidence that B cells may be involved in the pathogenesis of this disease, we suggest that RTX could be a promising treatment for anti-MDA5 DM-ILD. Also, patients with anti-MDA5 DM-ILD often have a condition with worse prognosis and were treated with multiple immunosuppressants previously or simultaneously to RTX administration, the risk of infection, especially opportunistic infections, should be considered during the use of RTX, and a low dose of RTX (100 mg every week) may also be applied; In addition, belimumab, a human monoclonal antibody targeting BAFF, may also be considered as a candidate therapy for anti-MDA5 DM-ILD, since some cases in our study showed poor response to RTX treatment. Finally, further prospective controlled clinical studies are required to evaluate the status and optimal regimen of RTX in anti-MDA5 DM-ILD.

AUTHOR CONTRIBUTIONS

QX, GY, and CH conceived the study. CH designed the study forms. GY and QX guided this study. CH and WL searched the literature and screened the studies for inclusion, extracted data, and assessed methodological quality. CH, WL, GY, and QX organized and analyzed data. All authors drafted and revised the manuscript. All authors contributed to the article and approved the submitted version.

REFERENCES

1. McHugh NJ, Tansley SL. Autoantibodies in Myositis. *Nat Rev Rheumatol* (2018) 14(5):290–302. doi: 10.1038/nrrheum.2018.56
2. Kurtzman DJB, Vleugels RA. Anti-Melanoma Differentiation-Associated Gene 5 (MDA5) Dermatomyositis: A Concise Review With an Emphasis on Distinctive Clinical Features. *J Am Acad Dermatol* (2018) 78(4):776–85. doi: 10.1016/j.jaad.2017.12.010
3. Hall JC, Casciola-Rosen L, Samedy LA, Werner J, Owoyemi K, Danoff SK, et al. Anti-Melanoma Differentiation-Associated Protein 5-Associated Dermatomyositis: Expanding the Clinical Spectrum. *Arthritis Care Res (Hoboken)* (2013) 65(8):1307–15. doi: 10.1002/acr.21992
4. Moghadam-Kia S, Oddis CV, Sato S, Kuwana M, Aggarwal R. Anti-Melanoma Differentiation-Associated Gene 5 Is Associated With Rapidly Progressive Lung Disease and Poor Survival in US Patients With Amyopathic and Myopathic Dermatomyositis. *Arthritis Care Res (Hoboken)* (2016) 68 (5):689–94. doi: 10.1002/acr.22728
5. Ceribelli A, Fredi M, Taraborelli M, Cavazzana I, Tincani A, Selmi C, et al. Prevalence and Clinical Significance of Anti-MDA5 Antibodies in European Patients With Polymyositis/Dermatomyositis. *Clin Exp Rheumatol* (2014) 32 (6):891–7.
6. Cao H, Pan M, Kang Y, Xia Q, Li X, Zhao X, et al. Clinical Manifestations of Dermatomyositis and Clinically Amyopathic Dermatomyositis Patients With Positive Expression of Anti-Melanoma Differentiation-Associated Gene 5 Antibody. *Arthritis Care Res (Hoboken)* (2012) 64(10):1602–10. doi: 10.1002/acr.21728
7. Nakashima R, Imura Y, Kobayashi S, Yukawa N, Yoshifuji H, Nojima T, et al. The RIG-I-Like Receptor IFIH1/MDA5 is a Dermatomyositis-Specific Autoantigen Identified by the Anti-CADM-140 Antibody. *Rheumatol (Oxford)* (2010) 49(3):433–40. doi: 10.1093/rheumatology/kep375
8. Hamaguchi Y, Kuwana M, Hoshino K, Hasegawa M, Kaji K, Matsushita T, et al. Clinical Correlations With Dermatomyositis-Specific Autoantibodies in Adult Japanese Patients With Dermatomyositis: A Multicenter Cross-Sectional Study. *Arch Dermatol* (2011) 147(4):391–8. doi: 10.1001/archdermatol.2011.52
9. Motegi SI, Sekiguchi A, Toki S, Kishi C, Endo Y, Yasuda M, et al. Clinical Features and Poor Prognostic Factors of Anti-Melanoma Differentiation-Associated Gene 5 Antibody-Positive Dermatomyositis With Rapid Progressive Interstitial Lung Disease. *Eur J Dermatol* (2019) 29(5):511–7. doi: 10.1684/ejd.2019.3634
10. Li Y, Li Y, Wu J, Miao M, Gao X, Cai W, et al. Predictors of Poor Outcome of Anti-MDA5-Associated Rapidly Progressive Interstitial Lung Disease in a Chinese Cohort With Dermatomyositis. *J Immunol Res* (2020) 2020:2024869. doi: 10.1155/2020/2024869
11. Fujikawa K, Kawakami A, Kaji K, Fujimoto M, Kawashiri S, Iwamoto N, et al. Association of Distinct Clinical Subsets With Myositis-Specific Autoantibodies Towards Anti-155/140-kDa Polypeptides, Anti-140-kDa Polypeptides, and Anti-Aminoacyl tRNA Synthetases in Japanese Patients With Dermatomyositis: A Single-Centre, Cross-Sectional Study. *Scand J Rheumatol* (2009) 38(4):263–7. doi: 10.1080/03009740802687455
12. Tsuji H, Nakashima R, Hosono Y, Imura Y, Yagita M, Yoshifuji H, et al. Multicenter Prospective Study of the Efficacy and Safety of Combined Immunosuppressive Therapy With High-Dose Glucocorticoid, Tacrolimus, and Cyclophosphamide in Interstitial Lung Diseases Accompanied by Anti-Melanoma Differentiation-Associated Gene 5-Positive Dermatomyositis. *Arthritis Rheumatol* (2020) 72(3):488–98. doi: 10.1002/art.41105
13. Chen F, Li S, Wang T, Shi J, Wang G. Clinical Heterogeneity of Interstitial Lung Disease in Polymyositis and Dermatomyositis Patients With or Without Specific Autoantibodies. *Am J Med Sci* (2018) 355(1):48–53. doi: 10.1016/j.amjms.2017.07.013
14. Yoshida N, Okamoto M, Kaieda S, Fujimoto K, Ebata T, Tajiri M, et al. Association of Anti-Aminoacyl-Transfer RNA Synthetase Antibody and Anti-Melanoma Differentiation-Associated Gene 5 Antibody With the Therapeutic Response of Polymyositis/Dermatomyositis-Associated Interstitial Lung Disease. *Respir Investig* (2017) 55(1):24–32. doi: 10.1016/j.resinv.2016.08.007
15. Kimani S, Painschab MS, Kaimila B, Kasonkanji E, Zuze T, Tomoka T, et al. Safety and Efficacy of Rituximab in Patients With Diffuse Large B-Cell Lymphoma in Malawi: A Prospective, Single-Arm, Non-Randomised Phase 1/2 Clinical Trial. *Lancet Glob Health* (2021) 9(7):e1008–e16. doi: 10.1016/S2214-109X(21)00181-9
16. Jones RB, Tervaert JW, Hauser T, Luqmani R, Morgan MD, Peh CA, et al. Rituximab Versus Cyclophosphamide in ANCA-Associated Renal Vasculitis. *N Engl J Med* (2010) 363(3):211–20. doi: 10.1056/NEJMoa0909169
17. Edwards JC, Szczepanski L, Szechinski J, Filipowicz-Sosnowska A, Emery P, Close DR, et al. Efficacy of B-Cell-Targeted Therapy With Rituximab in Patients With Rheumatoid Arthritis. *N Engl J Med* (2004) 350(25):2572–81. doi: 10.1056/NEJMoa032534
18. Cervera R, Mosca M, Rios-Garces R, Espinosa G, Trujillo H, Bada T, et al. Treatment for Refractory Lupus Nephritis: Rituximab vs Triple Target Therapy. *Autoimmun Rev* (2019) 18(12):102406. doi: 10.1016/j.autrev.2019.102406
19. Moher D, Liberati A, Tetzlaff J, Altman DG, Group P. Preferred Reporting Items for Systematic Reviews and Meta-Analyses: The PRISMA Statement. *PloS Med* (2009) 6(7):e1000097. doi: 10.1371/journal.pmed.1000097
20. Page MJ, McKenzie JE, Bossuyt PM, Boutron I, Hoffmann TC, Mulrow CD, et al. The PRISMA 2020 Statement: An Updated Guideline for Reporting Systematic Reviews. *BMJ* (2021) 372:n71. doi: 10.1136/bmj.n71
21. Bohan A, Peter JB. Polymyositis and Dermatomyositis (First of Two Parts). *N Engl J Med* (1975) 292(7):344–7. doi: 10.1056/NEJM197502132920706
22. Sontheimer RD. Would a New Name Hasten the Acceptance of Amyopathic Dermatomyositis (Dermatomyositis Sine Myositis) as a Distinctive Subset Within the Idiopathic Inflammatory Dermatomyopathies Spectrum of Clinical Illness? *J Am Acad Dermatol* (2002) 46(4):626–36. doi: 10.1067/mjd.2002.120621
23. Ge Y, Li S, Tian X, He L, Lu X, Wang G. Anti-Melanoma Differentiation-Associated Gene 5 (MDA5) Antibody-Positive Dermatomyositis Responds to Rituximab Therapy. *Clin Rheumatol* (2021) 40(6):2311–7. doi: 10.1007/s10067-020-05530-5
24. Stang A. Critical Evaluation of the Newcastle-Ottawa Scale for the Assessment of the Quality of Nonrandomized Studies in Meta-Analyses. *Eur J Epidemiol* (2010) 25(9):603–5. doi: 10.1007/s10654-010-9491-z
25. American Thoracic Society. Idiopathic Pulmonary Fibrosis: Diagnosis and Treatment. International Consensus Statement. American Thoracic Society (ATS), and the European Respiratory Society (ERS). *Am J Respir Crit Care Med* (2000) 161(2 Pt 1):646–64. doi: 10.1164/ajrccm.161.2.ats3-00
26. So H, Wong VTL, Lao VWN, Pang HT, Yip RML. Rituximab for Refractory Rapidly Progressive Interstitial Lung Disease Related to Anti-MDA5 Antibody-Positive Amyopathic Dermatomyositis. *Clin Rheumatol* (2018) 37 (7):1983–9. doi: 10.1007/s10067-018-4122-2
27. Koichi Y, Aya Y, Megumi U, Shunichi K, Masafumi S, Hiroaki M, et al. A Case of Anti-MDA5-Positive Rapidly Progressive Interstitial Lung Disease in a Patient With Clinically Amyopathic Dermatomyositis Ameliorated by Rituximab, in Addition to Standard Immunosuppressive Treatment. *Modern Rheumatol* (2017) 27(3):536–40. doi: 10.3109/14397595.2015.1014140
28. Ogawa Y, Kishida D, Shimojima Y, Hayashi K, Sekijima Y. Effective Administration of Rituximab in Anti-MDA5 Antibody-Positive Dermatomyositis With Rapidly Progressive Interstitial Lung Disease and Refractory Cutaneous Involvement: A Case Report and Literature Review. *Case Rep Rheumatol* (2017) 2017:5386797–. doi: 10.1155/2017/5386797
29. Tokunaga K, Hagino N. Dermatomyositis With Rapidly Progressive Interstitial Lung Disease Treated With Rituximab: A Report of 3 Cases in Japan. *Internal Med* (2017) 56(11):1399–403. doi: 10.2169/internalmedicine.56.7956
30. Hisanaga J, Kotani T, Fujiki Y, Yoshida S, Takeuchi T, Makino S. Successful Multi-Target Therapy Including Rituximab and Mycophenolate Mofetil in Anti-Melanoma Differentiation-Associated Gene 5 Antibody-Positive Rapidly Progressive Interstitial Lung Disease With Clinically Amyopathic Dermatomyositis. *Int J Rheumatic Dis* (2017) 20(12):2182–5. doi: 10.1111/1756-185x.13136
31. Alqatari S, Riddell P, Harney S, Henry M, Murphy G. MDA-5 Associated Rapidly Progressive Interstitial Lung Disease With Recurrent Pneumothoraces: A Case Report. *BMC Pulm Med* (2018) 18(1):59. doi: 10.1186/s12890-018-0622-8

32. Hoa S, Troyanov Y, Fritzler MJ, Targoff IN, Chartrand S, Mansour AM, et al. Describing and Expanding the Clinical Phenotype of Anti-MDA5-Associated Rapidly Progressive Interstitial Lung Disease: Case Series of Nine Canadian Patients and Literature Review. *Scand J Rheumatol* (2018) 47(3):210–24. doi: 10.1080/03009742.2017.1334814
33. Tamai K, Tachikawa R, Otsuka K, Ueda H, Hosono Y, Tomii K. Early Pulmonary Involvement of Anti-CADM-140 Autoantibody-Positive Rapidly Progressive Interstitial Lung Disease Preceding Typical Cutaneous Symptoms. *Intern Med* (2014) 53(21):2515–9. doi: 10.2169/internalmedicine.53.2769
34. Nishizawa T, Kida G, Tsukahara Y, Emoto K, Tsumiyama E, Kriiwa S, et al. A Case of Rapidly Progressive Interstitial Pneumonia in Association With Amyopathic Dermatomyositis With Elevated Titers of Anti-MDA-5 Antibody, Successfully Treated With Rituximab in Addition to Standard Immunosuppressive Therapy. *Am J Respir Crit Care Med* (2018) 197: A6475.
35. Kishida D, Sakaguchi N, Ueno K-I, Ushiyama S, Ichikawa T, Yoshinaga T, et al. Macrophage Activation Syndrome in Adult Dermatomyositis: A Case-Based Review. *Rheumatol Int* (2020) 40(7):1151–62. doi: 10.1007/s00296-020-04590-9
36. Scirocco C, Gubbiotti A, Sebastiani A, Sebastiani GD. Rituximab in Antimelanoma Differentiation-Associated Protein-5 Dermatomyositis With Interstitial Lung Disease. *Case Rep Rheumatol* (2020) 2020:8145790–. doi: 10.1155/2020/8145790
37. Machiyama T, Shirai T, Fujita Y, Sato H, Fujii H, Ishii T, et al. Successful Concomitant Therapy With Tofacitinib for Anti- Melanoma Differentiation Associated Gene 5 Antibody-Positive Rapidly Progressive Interstitial Lung Disease With Poor Prognostic Factors: A Case Report and Literature Review. *Med: Case Rep Study Protoc* (2021) 2(1):e0026. doi: 10.1097/md9.0000000000000026
38. Akiyama C, Shirai T, Sato H, Fujii H, Ishii T, Harigae H. Association of Various Myositis-Specific Autoantibodies With Dermatomyositis and Polymyositis Triggered by Pregnancy. *Rheumatol Int* (2021). doi: 10.1007/s00296-021-04851-1
39. Mehta AA, Paul T, Cb M, Haridas N. Anti-MDA5 Antibody-Positive Dermatomyositis With Rapidly Progressive Interstitial Lung Disease: Report of Two Cases. *BMJ Case Rep* (2021) 14(4):e240046. doi: 10.1136/bcr-2020-240046
40. Yeung T-W, Cheong K-N, Lau Y-L, Tse K-CN. Adolescent-Onset Anti-MDA5 Antibody-Positive Juvenile Dermatomyositis With Rapidly Progressive Interstitial Lung Disease and Spontaneous Pneumomediastinum: A Case Report and Literature Review. *Pediatr Rheumatol* (2021) 19(1):103. doi: 10.1186/s12969-021-00595-1
41. Mao M-M, Xia S, Guo B-P, Qian W-P, Zheng Z-X, Peng X-M, et al. Ultra-Low Dose Rituximab as Add-on Therapy in Anti-MDA5-Positive Patients With Polymyositis/Dermatomyositis Associated ILD. *Respir Med* (2020) 172:105983. doi: 10.1016/j.rmed.2020.105983
42. Ye S, Chen XX, Lu XY, Wu MF, Deng Y, Huang WQ, et al. Adult Clinically Amyopathic Dermatomyositis With Rapid Progressive Interstitial Lung Disease: A Retrospective Cohort Study. *Clin Rheumatol* (2007) 26(10):1647–54. doi: 10.1007/s10067-007-0562-9
43. Mukae H, Ishimoto H, Sakamoto N, Hara S, Kakugawa T, Nakayama S, et al. Clinical Differences Between Interstitial Lung Disease Associated With Clinically Amyopathic Dermatomyositis and Classic Dermatomyositis. *Chest* (2009) 136(5):1341–7. doi: 10.1378/chest.08-2740
44. Zou J, Li T, Huang X, Chen S, Guo Q, Bao C. Basiliximab may Improve the Survival Rate of Rapidly Progressive Interstitial Pneumonia in Patients With Clinically Amyopathic Dermatomyositis With Anti-MDA5 Antibody. *Ann Rheum Dis* (2014) 73(8):1591–3. doi: 10.1136/annrheumdis-2014-205278
45. Matsushita T, Kobayashi T, Kano M, Hamaguchi Y, Takehara K. Elevated Serum B-Cell Activating Factor Levels in Patients With Dermatomyositis: Association With Interstitial Lung Disease. *J Dermatol* (2019) 46(12):1190–6. doi: 10.1111/1346-8138.15117
46. Wang K, Zhao J, Chen Z, Li T, Tan X, Zheng Y, et al. CD4+CXCR4+ T Cells as a Novel Prognostic Biomarker in Patients With Idiopathic Inflammatory Myopathy-Associated Interstitial Lung Disease. *Rheumatol (Oxford)* (2019) 58 (3):511–21. doi: 10.1093/rheumatology/key341
47. Nombel A, Fabien N, Coutant F. Dermatomyositis With Anti-MDA5 Antibodies: Bioclinical Features, Pathogenesis and Emerging Therapies. *Front Immunol* (2021) 12:773352. doi: 10.3389/fimmu.2021.773352
48. Zhang S, Shen H, Shu X, Peng Q, Wang G. Abnormally Increased Low-Density Granulocytes in Peripheral Blood Mononuclear Cells are Associated With Interstitial Lung Disease in Dermatomyositis. *Mod Rheumatol* (2017) 27 (1):122–9. doi: 10.1080/14397595.2016.1179861
49. Peng Y, Zhang S, Zhao Y, Liu Y, Yan B. Neutrophil Extracellular Traps may Contribute to Interstitial Lung Disease Associated With Anti-MDA5 Autoantibody Positive Dermatomyositis. *Clin Rheumatol* (2018) 37(1):107–15. doi: 10.1007/s10067-017-3799-y
50. Gono T, Miyake K, Kawaguchi Y, Kaneko H, Shinozaki M, Yamanaka H. Hyperferritinaemia and Macrophage Activation in a Patient With Interstitial Lung Disease With Clinically Amyopathic DM. *Rheumatol (Oxford)* (2012) 51 (7):1336–8. doi: 10.1093/rheumatology/kes012
51. Horiike Y, Suzuki Y, Fujisawa T, Yasui H, Karayama M, Hozumi H, et al. Successful Classification of Macrophage-Mannose Receptor CD206 in Severity of Anti-MDA5 Antibody Positive Dermatomyositis Associated ILD. *Rheumatol (Oxford)* (2019) 58(12):2143–52. doi: 10.1093/rheumatology/kez185
52. Zhang SH, Zhao Y, Xie QB, Jiang Y, Wu YK, Yan B. Aberrant Activation of the Type I Interferon System may Contribute to the Pathogenesis of Anti-Melanoma Differentiation-Associated Gene 5 Dermatomyositis. *Br J Dermatol* (2019) 180(5):1090–8. doi: 10.1111/bjd.16917
53. Horai Y, Koga T, Fujikawa K, Takatani A, Nishino A, Nakashima Y, et al. Serum Interferon-Alpha is a Useful Biomarker in Patients With Anti-Melanoma Differentiation-Associated Gene 5 (MDA5) Antibody-Positive Dermatomyositis. *Mod Rheumatol* (2015) 25(1):85–9. doi: 10.3109/14397595.2014.900843
54. Giannini M, Ohana M, Nespola B, Zanframundo G, Geny B, Meyer A. Similarities Between COVID-19 and Anti-MDA5 Syndrome: What can We Learn for Better Care? *Eur Respir J* (2020) 56(3):2001618. doi: 10.1183/13993003.01618-2020
55. Rehwinkel J, Gack MU. RIG-I-Like Receptors: Their Regulation and Roles in RNA Sensing. *Nat Rev Immunol* (2020) 20(9):537–51. doi: 10.1038/s41577-020-0288-3
56. Kang DC, Gopalkrishnan RV, Wu Q, Jankowsky E, Pyle AM, Fisher PB. Mda-5: An Interferon-Inducible Putative RNA Helicase With Double-Stranded RNA-Dependent ATPase Activity and Melanoma Growth-Suppressive Properties. *Proc Natl Acad Sci USA* (2002) 99(2):637–42. doi: 10.1073/pnas.022637199
57. Zahn S, Barchet W, Rehkamper C, Hornung T, Bieber T, Tuting T, et al. Enhanced Skin Expression of Melanoma Differentiation-Associated Gene 5 (MDA5) in Dermatomyositis and Related Autoimmune Diseases. *J Am Acad Dermatol* (2011) 64(5):988–9. doi: 10.1016/j.jaad.2010.08.004
58. Berger M, Hsieh CY, Bakele M, Marcos V, Rieber N, Kormann M, et al. Neutrophils Express Distinct RNA Receptors in a Non-Canonical Way. *J Biol Chem* (2012) 287(23):19409–17. doi: 10.1074/jbc.M112.353557
59. Vlahakos D, Foster MH, Ucci AA, Barrett KJ, Datta SK, Madaio MP. Murine Monoclonal Anti-DNA Antibodies Penetrate Cells, Bind to Nuclei, and Induce Glomerular Proliferation and Proteinuria. *vivo J Am Soc Nephrol* (1992) 2(8):1345–54. doi: 10.1681/ASN.V281345
60. Deng SX, Hanson E, Sanz I. *In Vivo* Cell Penetration and Intracellular Transport of Anti-Sm and Anti-La Autoantibodies. *Int Immunol* (2000) 12 (4):415–23. doi: 10.1093/intimm/12.4.415
61. Ishida Y, Kimura A, Nosaka M, Kuninaka Y, Hemmi H, Sasaki I, et al. Essential Involvement of the CX3CL1-CX3CR1 Axis in Bleomycin-Induced Pulmonary Fibrosis *via* Regulation of Fibrocyte and M2 Macrophage Migration. *Sci Rep* (2017) 7(1):16833. doi: 10.1038/s41598-017-17007-8
62. Nakano M, Fujii T, Hashimoto M, Yukawa N, Yoshifuji H, Ohmura K, et al. Type I Interferon Induces CX3CL1 (Fractalkine) and CCL5 (RANTES) Production in Human Pulmonary Vascular Endothelial Cells. *Clin Exp Immunol* (2012) 170(1):94–100. doi: 10.1111/j.1365-2249.2012.04638.x
63. Thieblemont N, Wright HL, Edwards SW, Witko-Sarsat V. Human Neutrophils in Auto-Immunity. *Semin Immunol* (2016) 28(2):159–73. doi: 10.1016/j.smim.2016.03.004
64. Matsushita T, Mizumaki K, Kano M, Yagi N, Tennichi M, Takeuchi A, et al. Antimelanoma Differentiation-Associated Protein 5 Antibody Level is a Novel Tool for Monitoring Disease Activity in Rapidly Progressive Interstitial Lung Disease With Dermatomyositis. *Br J Dermatol* (2017) 176 (2):395–402. doi: 10.1111/bjd.14882

65. Chen Z, Cao M, Plana MN, Liang J, Cai H, Kuwana M, et al. Utility of Anti-Melanoma Differentiation-Associated Gene 5 Antibody Measurement in Identifying Patients With Dermatomyositis and a High Risk for Developing Rapidly Progressive Interstitial Lung Disease: A Review of the Literature and a Meta-Analysis. *Arthritis Care Res (Hoboken)* (2013) 65(8):1316–24. doi: 10.1002/acr.21985
66. Groom JR, Fletcher CA, Walters SN, Grey ST, Watt SV, Sweet MJ, et al. BAFF and MyD88 Signals Promote a Lupuslike Disease Independent of T Cells. *J Exp Med* (2007) 204(8):1959–71. doi: 10.1084/jem.20062567
67. Stohl W. Biologic Differences Between Various Inhibitors of the BLyS/BAFF Pathway: Should We Expect Differences Between Belimumab and Other Inhibitors in Development? *Curr Rheumatol Rep* (2012) 14(4):303–9. doi: 10.1007/s11926-012-0254-6
68. Kobayashi N, Kobayashi I, Mori M, Sato S, Iwata N, Shigemura T, et al. Increased Serum B Cell Activating Factor and a Proliferation-Inducing Ligand Are Associated With Interstitial Lung Disease in Patients With Juvenile Dermatomyositis. *J Rheumatol* (2015) 42(12):2412–8. doi: 10.3899/jrheum.140977
69. Spolski R, Leonard WJ. Interleukin-21: A Double-Edged Sword With Therapeutic Potential. *Nat Rev Drug Discov* (2014) 13(5):379–95. doi: 10.1038/nrd4296
70. Girard C, Vincent T, Bessis D. [Dermatomyositis and Acute Interstitial Lung Disease Associated With MDA-5 Antibodies: An Atypical Case]. *Ann Dermatol Venereol* (2013) 140(10):628–34. doi: 10.1016/j.annder.2013.04.083
71. Clottu A, Laffitte E, Prins C, Chizzolini C. Response of Mucocutaneous Lesions to Rituximab in a Case of Melanoma Differentiation Antigen 5-Related Dermatomyositis. *Dermatology* (2012) 225(4):376–80. doi: 10.1159/000346573
72. Gono T, Sato S, Kawaguchi Y, Kuwana M, Hanaoka M, Katsumata Y, et al. Anti-MDA5 Antibody, Ferritin and IL-18 are Useful for the Evaluation of Response to Treatment in Interstitial Lung Disease With Anti-MDA5 Antibody-Positive Dermatomyositis. *Rheumatol (Oxford)* (2012) 51 (9):1563–70. doi: 10.1093/rheumatology/kes102
73. Christou EAA, Giardino G, Worth A, Ladomenou F. Risk Factors Predisposing to the Development of Hypogammaglobulinemia and Infections Post-Rituximab. *Int Rev Immunol* (2017) 36(6):352–9. doi: 10.1080/08830185.2017.1346092
74. Li Y, Shi Y, He Z, Chen Q, Liu Z, Yu L, et al. The Efficacy and Safety of Low-Dose Rituximab in Immune Thrombocytopenia: A Systematic Review and Meta-Analysis. *Platelets* (2019) 30(6):690–7. doi: 10.1080/09537104.2019.1624706
75. Yang CS, Yang L, Li T, Zhang DQ, Jin WN, Li MS, et al. Responsiveness to Reduced Dosage of Rituximab in Chinese Patients With Neuromyelitis Optica. *Neurology* (2013) 81(8):710–3. doi: 10.1212/WNL.0b013e3182a1aac7
76. Wang BJ, Wang CJ, Zeng ZL, Yang Y, Guo SG. Lower Dosages of Rituximab Used Successfully in the Treatment of Anti-NMDA Receptor Encephalitis Without Tumour. *J Neurol Sci* (2017) 377:127–32. doi: 10.1016/j.jns.2017.04.007

9

Simultaneously Developed Amyopathic Dermatomyositis and Autoimmune Sclerosing Cholangitis – A Coincidence or a Shared Immunopathogenesis?

Tomislav Ledenko[1†], *Iva Sorić Hosman*[1*†], *Marijana Ćorić*[2,3] *and Alenka Gagro*[3,4]

[1] Department of Pediatrics, Zadar General Hospital, Zadar, Croatia, [2] Department of Pathology and Cytology, University Hospital Centre Zagreb, Zagreb, Croatia, [3] School of Medicine, University of Zagreb, Zagreb, Croatia, [4] Division of Pulmonology, Allergology, Immunology and Rheumatology, Department of Pediatrics, Children's Hospital Zagreb, Zagreb, Croatia

***Correspondence:**
Iva Sorić Hosman
isoric.zd@gmail.com

[†]These authors have contributed equally to this work and share first authorship

Inflammatory rheumatic diseases (IRD) and autoimmune liver diseases (AILD) share many similarities regarding epidemiology, genetics, immunology and therapeutic regimens, so it is not surprising that approximately 20% of patients with AILD are diagnosed with an IRD as well. Clinical features and biochemical hallmarks of IRD and AILD often intertwine and cross diagnostic criteria. Therefore, the real distinction of underlying disorders in a patient with these comorbidities may be challenging. The present report is the first report of simultaneously developed juvenile dermatomyositis (JDM) and autoimmune sclerosing cholangitis (ASC) with both entities fulfilling the latest guidelines for a definite diagnosis. Both of these diagnoses are difficult to definitely establish since ASC has a similar serologic profile as autoimmune hepatitis and liver histological analysis is frequently non-specific, whereas clinically amyopathic JDM diagnosis depends mostly on classical dermatological symptoms, while the rest of the diagnostic criteria, including the necessity for skin or muscle biopsy and the presence of myositis specific antibodies, are still not uniformed. In spite of these challenges, our patient clearly met European League Against Rheumatism/American College of Rheumatology classification criteria for CAJDM and The European Society for Pediatric Gastroenterology, Hepatology and Nutrition diagnostic criteria for ASC. Since elevated serum transaminases, the presence of serum antinuclear antibodies and hypergammaglobulinemia could be explained as a part of both JDM and ASC, the underlying pathophysiology remains debatable. Intriguingly, JDM and ASC share genetic predisposition including human leukocyte antigen allele DRB1*0301 and tumor necrosis factor α 308A allele. Furthermore, both humoral and cellular components of the adaptive immune system contribute to the pathogenesis of JDM and ASC. Moreover, recent findings indicate that the loss of the CD28 expression on T-cells plays a significant role in their pathogenesis along with the Th17 immune pathway. Despite these common features that suggest shared autoimmunity, AILD and autoimmune myositis are traditionally studied and managed independently. The lack of therapies that target the underlying cause results in a high rate of adverse events due to unspecific immunosuppressive therapy. Shared autoimmunity is an ideal area to develop new, targeted immunotherapy that would hopefully be beneficial for more than one disease.

Keywords: juvenile dermatomyositis, amyopathic dermatomyositis, autoimmune liver disease, autoimmune sclerosing cholangitis, shared autoimmunity, myositis specific antibodies

INTRODUCTION

Juvenile dermatomyositis (JDM) is an autoimmune inflammatory disease affecting skeletal muscle tissue and skin, with an incidence of 3.2 per million children per year (1, 2). Clinically amyopathic JDM (CAJDM), or more recently called skin-predominant JDM, is DM subphenotype which includes hallmark cutaneous manifestations of DM without muscle weakness lasting for at least 6 months, affecting only around 10% of all JDM patients (3, 4). Autoimmune sclerosing cholangitis (ASC) is autoimmune liver disease (AILD) affecting intrahepatic and extrahepatic bile ducts, with an incidence of 1 per million children per year (5). The diagnosis is based on elevated liver enzymes, serological profile similar to autoimmune hepatitis (AIH) and bile duct lesions visualized on cholangiography (6). Therefore, a concomitant development of both of these autoimmune diseases in the same patient is exceptional.

Among patients with autoimmune myositis (AIM), elevated serum liver enzymes are a common phenomenon. Patients with DM frequently have simultaneously elevated creatine kinase (CK), aspartate aminotransferase (AST) and alanine aminotransferase (ALT) at the presentation, usually of skeletal muscle origin. Serum transaminases usually normalize proportionally to CK serum level (7). Consequently, concomitantly elevated CK, AST and ALT may be attributed to myositis leaving a concurrent liver disease unrecognized, while elevated transaminases without a determination of serum CK level may be misdiagnosed as a liver disease.

Along with elevated liver enzymes, patients with AIM as well as those with AILD often have positive antinuclear antibodies (ANA) and hypergammaglobulinemia. Therefore, in a case of increased transaminases without elevation of serum CK in patients with myositis, additional liver disease should be excluded. Here we report an extraordinary case of JDM and ASC co-occurrence and discuss shared clinical, biochemical, immunological and genetic features of these two distinct clinical entities.

CASE REPORT

A 16-years old, previously healthy boy presented at our Department of Pediatrics with a 12-months history of skin rash. There was no history of photosensitivity, oral ulcers, alopecia, Raynaud's phenomenon, joint pain, morning stiffness, fever, myalgia or weight loss. Physical examination revealed characteristic cutaneous features of DM including Gottron's papules (multiple erythematous papules over the dorsal aspect of metacarpophalangeal and interphalangeal joints, **Figure 1**), Gottron's sign (violaceus macules over extensor surfaces of elbows and medial malleoli), heliotrope rash (violaceous erythema of the eyelids or periorbital skin) and the malar rash, including the nose bridge (**Figure 2**). The rest of the physical

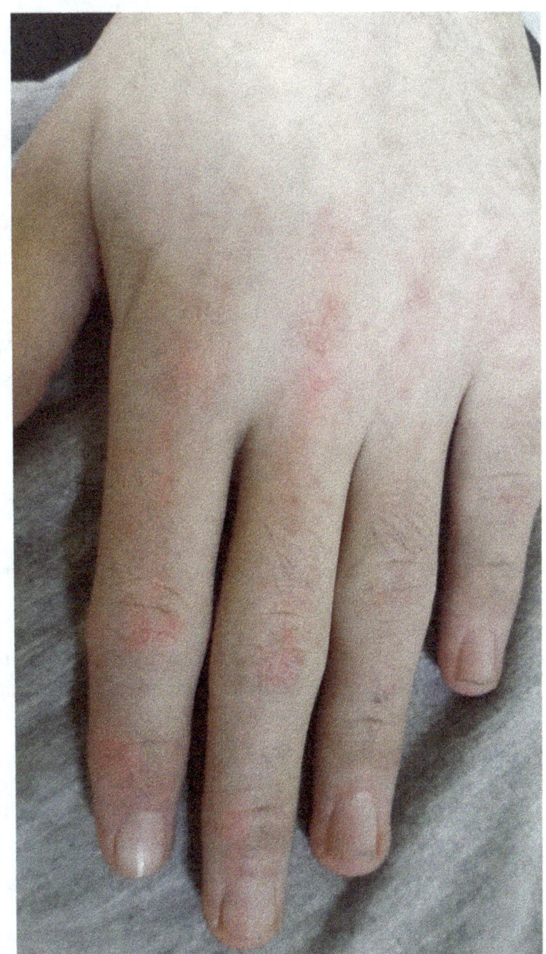

FIGURE 1 | Characteristic cutaneous features of DM called Gottron's papules (multiple erythematous papules over the dorsal aspect of metacarpophalangeal and interphalangeal joints).

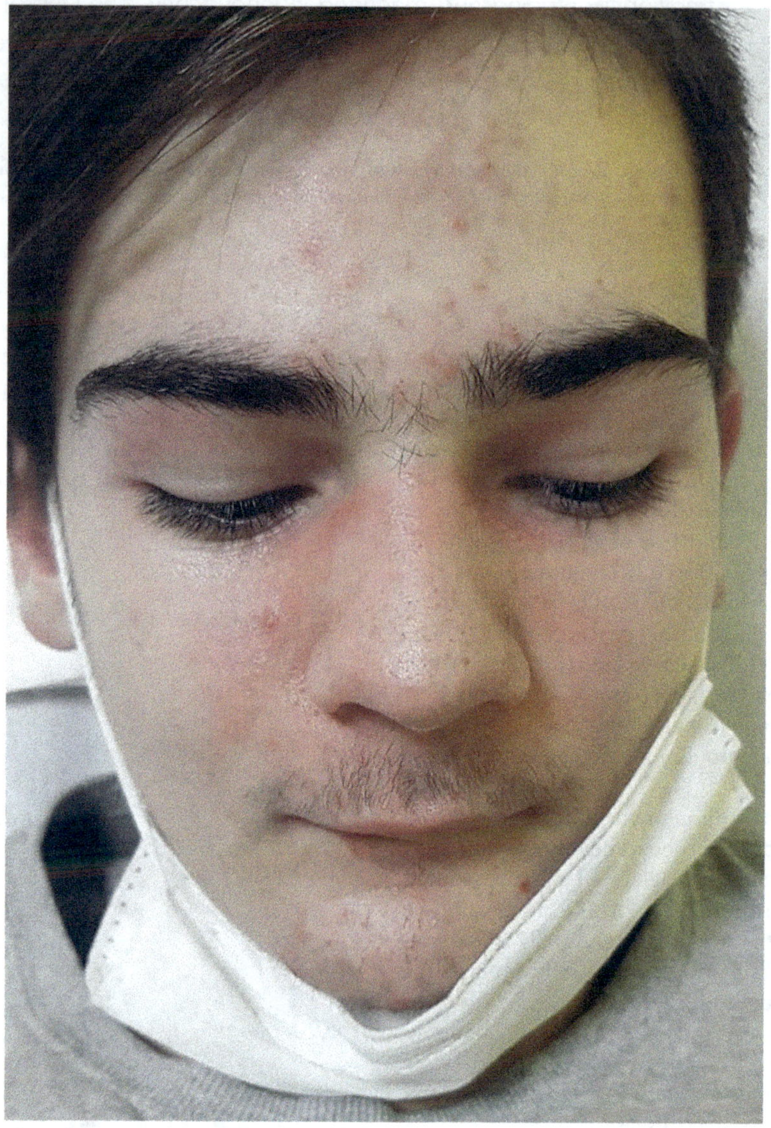

FIGURE 2 | Characteristic cutaneous features of DM called heliotrope rash (violaceous erythema of the eyelids or periorbital skin) and the malar rash.

examination was unremarkable. There was no clinically detectable muscle weakness. Chest radiograph, echocardiogram and renal ultrasound were normal.

Laboratory investigations were: C-reactive protein 4.2 mg/l (normal <3 mg/l), erythrocyte sedimentation rate 11 mm/h (normal <12 mm/h), AST 69 U/l (normal 10–42 U/l), ALT 107 U/l (normal 10–37 U/l), γ-glutamyltransferase 178 U/l (normal 10-43 U/l). Serum CK levels and lactate dehydrogenase were within normal range (233 U/l and 287 U/l, respectively). Fecal calprotectin was 316 mcg/g and fecal occult blood test was negative. Immunoglobulin (Ig) G levels were increased up to 22.1 g/l (normal 7-16 g/l) as well as total serum protein and albumin to globulin ratio. The rest of the laboratory findings where within the reference range, including blood count, coagulogram, urea, creatinine, alkaline phosphatase, bilirubin, complement (C3, C4), anti-tissue transglutaminase antibodies, rheumatoid factor, anti- cyclic citrullinated peptide antibodies, alpha1-antitrypsin, copper, ceruloplasmin and urine analysis (including proteinuria and copperuria). Hepatitis A, B, C, EBV, CMV, Toxoplasma and HSV1 serology as well as quantiferone test were negative.

Immunological blood tests revealed positive ANA, while antibodies against double-strained DNA and extractable nuclear antigens were negative. Furthermore, cytoplasmic (c-) and atypical perinuclear (a p-) anti-neutrophil cytoplasmic antibodies (ANCA) were positive, whereas p-ANCA were firstly negative, but on a second examination were positive. Anti-cardiolipin (ACA), anti-beta2 glycoprotein I (B2GPI) and anti- glycoprotein 210 (gp210) antibodies were also positive. Anti-liver/kidney microsomal type 1(LKM-1), anti-liver cytosol type 1 (LC-1), anti-smooth muscle antibodies (SMA), anti-soluble liver antigen (SLA) and anti-mitochondral (AMA) antibodies were all negative. Amongst myositis specific antibodies (MSA) only anti-transcriptional intermediary factor 1 gamma (anti-TIF1γ) antibodies were positive.

Although serum CK levels were within normal range, electromyography showed occasional polyphasy and decreased action potential amplitudes on both peroneal nerves. Furthermore, our patient was positive for myositis specific anti-TIF1γ antibodies, which are, according to the most recent guidelines, an additional criterion for diagnosing skin-predominant DM (8, 9). Based on the European League Against Rheumatism/American College of Rheumatology (EULAR/ACR) classification criteria for idiopathic inflammatory myopathies and more recently proposed classification criteria by the Delphi project group our patient was diagnosed with CAJDM (**Tables 1, 2**) (2, 8).

Since there was no correlation between serum transaminases and CK levels, other source of transaminases, rather than skeletal muscles, was suspected. Abdominal ultrasound revealed dilated common bile duct and magnetic resonance cholangiopancreatography (MRCP) confirmed distended common and intrahepatic bile ducts (**Figure 3**). Finally, histological analysis of the liver biopsy specimen showed a dense mononuclear cell infiltration with peripheral piecemeal necrosis in 1 out of the total 10 portal places encompassed within the specimen (**Figure 4**). Although the histological finding was non-specific, it was compatible with the diagnosis of ASC. Based on the European Society for Pediatric Gastroenterology Hepatology and Nutrition (ESPGHAN) scoring system ASC diagnosis was finally established (**Table 3**) (6).

After being diagnosed with both CAJDM and ASC, our patient was managed in an interdisciplinary manner. Since high-dose steroid is the preferred initial treatment for both JDM and ASC, the patient commenced prednisone at a dose of 60 mg/day. The dose was gradually decreased in parallel to the decline of serum transaminases. Azathioprine (100 mg/day) was added as a steroid-sparing agent (6, 9). According to the ESPGHAN protocol, ursodeoxycholic acid (UDCA, 750 mg/day) was also administered (6). Because of the deterioration of skin symptoms despite a good patient's compliance, 6 months after the therapy initiation, hydroxychloroquine (200 mg/day), which is recommended for skin predominant JDM by the Children's Arthritis and Rheumatology Research Alliance (CARRA), was added to the therapy regimen (10). Eventually, the treatment resulted in clinical and laboratory improvement. Since the patient's follow-up to this date is only a year long, further interdisciplinary monitoring is planned.

TABLE 1 | Clinical practice guidance table for the diagnosis of juvenile dermatomyositis (9) and results in our patient.

EXAMINATION	FINDING	FINDINGS IN OUR PATIENT
1) Dermatological symptom	a) Heliotrope rash: reddish purple edematous erythema in the eyelids, unilateral or bilateral b) Gottron's signs: Erythematous or violaceous macules on extensor surface of the finger joints with hyperkeratosis and dermatrophy c) Erythema of extensor surfaces of the joints of the elbow, knee etc.*[1]. d) Findings of skin biopsy consistent with dermatomyositis*[2]	a) + b) + c) + d) ND
2) Muscular symptom	Muscle weakness of proximal muscles in upper or lower extremities*[3]	–
3) Imaging	Findings indicating myositis with MRI: High intensity on T2 weighted/fat suppression MRI and normal intensity on T1 weighted MRI	ND
4) Biochemical examination	Elevated serum level of muscle enzymes (creatine kinase or aldolase)	–
5) Immunological examination	Positive result for myositis-specific autoantibodies*[4]	+
6) Pathological examination	Pathological findings indicating myositis with muscle biopsy (degeneration of muscle fibers and cellular infiltration)	ND
7) Exclusions	Myositis caused by infections, eosinophilic myositis, autoinflammatory diseases with rash similar to DM such as Nakajo-Nishimura syndrome, drug-induced myopathy, myopathy due to endocrine abnormality or congenital anomaly, muscle symptoms due to electrolyte abnormality, muscular dystrophy and other congenital muscular diseases, muscle weakness due to central or peripheral neuropathy, psoriasis, eczema, and other related diseases with other causes such as allergy.	–
DIAGNOSIS	**Classical JDM**: The presence of 1 or more items of (1) dermatological symptoms (a) to (c) (2), muscular symptom and 2 or more items of (3) to (6) during the follow-up without any of items of (7).	-
	JHDM: The presence of 1 or more items of classical dermatological symptoms (a) to (c), and 1 or more items of findings indicating myositis (3) to (6) without clinical muscle weakness without any of items of (7).	+
	JADM: The presence of 1 or more items of classical dermatological symptoms (a) to (c) without any evidences of myositis (2) to (6) without any of items of (7).	-
	JPM: The presence of 3 or more items of (2) to (6) without dermatological symptoms (1) without any of items of (7).	-

*[1]*Ulcerative lesions or secondary infection may modify the appearance of rash.*

*[2]*Hyperkeratosis, vacuolation of basal keratinocytes, deposition of melanin, perivascular lymphocyte infiltration, increased dermal edema, mucin deposition and thickening or atrophy of skin are observed, but it is difficult to differentiate JDM from SLE by pathological findings alone. Thus, single symptom is not adopted as a dermatological finding.*

*[3]*Muscle weakness ranges from mild ones (e.g., stumbling, new onset of difficulties in exercise) to advanced ones (e.g., difficulties in standing up from sitting position or rolling over in the bed).*

*[4]*Although only anti-Jo-1 antibodies could be measured at the time of revision of these guidelines, anti-ARS, anti-MDA5, anti-Mi-2, and anti-TIFI-γ antibodies are currently listed on the national health insurance price list.*

[+], *Positive finding; -, Negative finding; ND, not done; JDM, juvenile dermatomyositis; JHDM, juvenile hypomyopathic dermatomyositis; JADM, juvenile amyopathic dermatomyositis; JPM, juvenile polymyositis.*

TABLE 2 | EULAR/ACR classification criteria table for adult and juvenile idiopathic inflammatory myopathies and their major subgroups (2) and score in our patient.

Variable	Finding	Without muscle biopsy	With muscle biopsy	Score in our patient
Age of onset	Age of onset of first symptom assumed to be related to the disease ≥ 18 years and < 40 years	1.3	1.5	0
	Age of onset of first symptom assumed to be related to the disease ≥ 40 years	2.1	2.2	0
Muscle weakness	Objective symmetric weakness, usually progressive, of the proximal upper extremities	0.7	0.7	0
	Objective symmetric weakness, usually progressive, of the proximal lower extremities	0.8	0.5	0
	Neck flexors are relatively weaker than neck extensors	1.9	1.6	0
	In the legs proximal muscles are relatively weaker than distal muscles	0.9	1.2	0
Skin manifestations	Heliotrope rash: Purple, lilac-colored or erythematous patches over the eyelids or in a periorbital distribution, often associated with periorbital edema	3.1	3.2	3.1
	Gottron's papules: Erythematous to violaceous papules over the extensor surfaces of joints, which are sometimes scaly. May occur over the finger joints, elbows, knees, malleoli and toes	2.1	2.7	2.1
	Gottron's sign: Erythematous to violaceous macules over the extensor surfaces of joints, which are not palpable	3.3	3.7	3.3
Other clinical manifestations	Dysphagia or esophageal dysmotility	0.7	0.6	0
Laboratory measurements	Anti-Jo-1 (anti-histidyl-tRNA synthetase) autoantibody present	3.9	3.8	0
	Elevated serum levels of creatine kinase (CK) or lactate dehydrogenase (LDH) or aspartate aminotransferase (AST) or alanine aminotransferase (ALT)	1.3	1.4	1.3
Muscle biopsy features-presence of:	Endomysial infiltration of mononuclear cells surrounding, but not invading, myofibres		1.7	0
	Perimysial and/or perivascular infiltration of mononuclear cells		1.2	0
	Perifascicular atrophy		1.9	0
	Rimmed vacuoles		3.1	0
TOTAL SCORE	Probability of IIM without muscle biopsy=1/[1+exponential(5.33–score)] or probability of IIM including muscle biopsy=1/[1+exponential(6.49–score)] or by using a web calculator at www.imm.ki.se/biostatistics/calculators/iim			**9.8 → 99% probability of IIM diagnosis (JDM subgroup)**

IIM, idiopathic inflammatory myositis; JDM, juvenile dermatomyositis.

With an aggressive early treatment, 30–50% of patients have the potential to reach remission within 2–3 years of disease onset with a mortality rate of less than 4%, whereas 40-60% of patients have a persistently active disease leading to complications like calcinosis, persistent muscle weakness, skin or muscle atrophy and lipodystrophy (11). Based on Single Hub and Access point for pediatric Rheumatology in Europe (SHARE) recommendations, biologics that include intravenous immunoglobulin (IVIG) in immunomodulatory dosage as well as B cell depletion therapy (rituximab) may be a useful adjunct for resistant or refractory disease. IVIG are given to patients with prominent skin features and it usually takes 2-3 months of therapy for the clinical improvement. The effect of rituximab can take up to 26 weeks to be seen. Anti-TNF agents may also be considered in a refractory disease; infliximab or adalimumab are favored over etanercept. The SHARE group recommends withdrawing treatment if a patient has been off steroids and in remission on a disease-modifying antirheumatic drug a minimum of 1 year (11).

DISCUSSION

Classification and Diagnosis

Skin-predominant DM or CADM can be challenging to diagnose since, until recently, it has not been recognized by the most of classification guidelines in the field. As a consequence, more than a half of these patients have had an alternate diagnosis prior to eventually being diagnosed with DM, with a median diagnostic delay of 15 months. The most common alternate diagnosis was systemic lupus erythematosus (SLE) (12). This is not surprising considering skin lesions occur very early in the disease course in both SLE and DM and show a similar distribution. In order to resolve the existing classification dilemma for patients with CADM, the latest EULAR/ACR classification criteria for inflammatory myopathies include three DM associated skin manifestations: Gottron's sign, Gottron's papules and heliotrope rash (2). In spite of this enormous improvement, approximately 26% of patients with CADM still do not meet criteria for a definite classification (13). For this reason, additional efforts have been made to develop skin-focused classification criteria. With the identification of MSA, new phenotypes have been characterized depending on the type of cutaneous lesions, autoantibody profile, systemic involvement and outcome (14). The presence of MSA has been proposed as an additional criterion when classifying patients with CADM (8, 9).

Our patient was diagnosed with CAJDM based on hallmark cutaneous manifestations of DM (Gottron's papules, Gottron's sign, heliotrope rash) lasting for more than 6 months with no clinical signs of myositis. Since he had electromyographic signs of muscle involvement and positive MSA, skin biopsy was not performed, even though EULAR/ACR classification guidelines recommend skin biopsy in patients without muscle involvement. However, the EULAR/ACR criteria do not include MSA except for anti-Jo-1 autoantibody, whereas the latest guidelines include positive anti-TIF1γ autoantibodies as an additional criterion (8, 9). CAJDM includes two subphenotypes named amyopathic JDM and hypomyopathic JDM, with the latter group having evidence of subclinical myositis upon laboratory, electrophysiological and/or radiologic evaluation (15). Accordingly, our patient appertains to the hypomyopathic group. Analysis of hypomyopathic DM

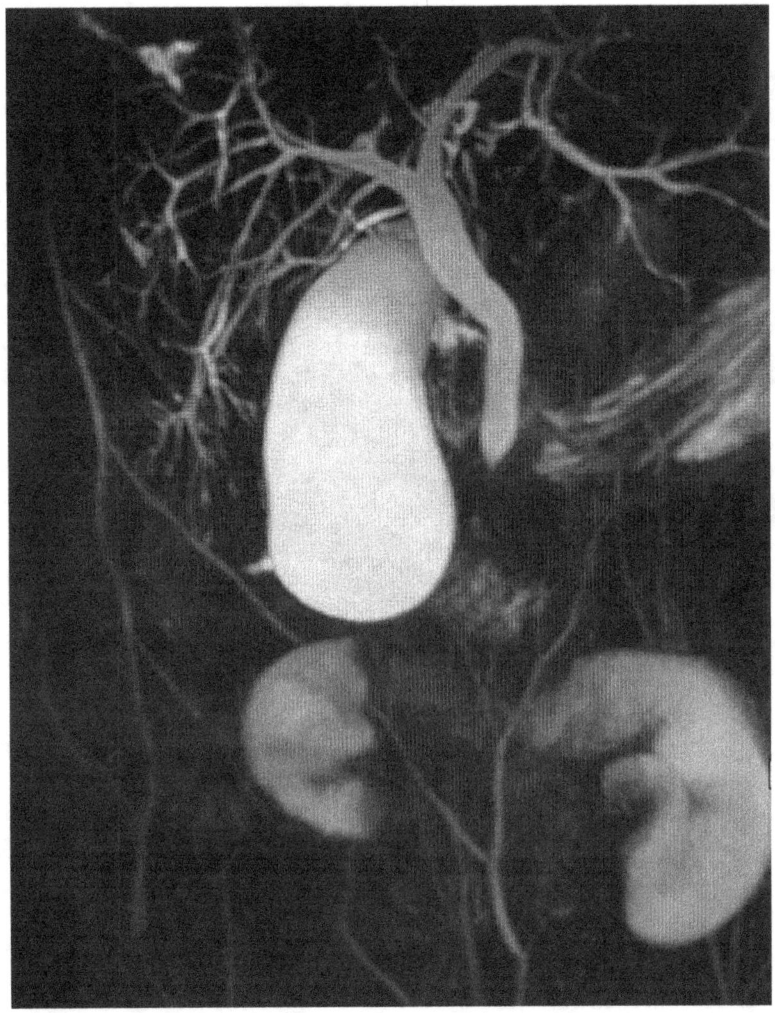

FIGURE 3 | Distended common bile duct and intrahepatic bile ducts **on** magnetic resonance cholangiopancreatography (MRCP).

patients in the literature shows that none of the reported adult or juvenile hypomyopathic DM patients, despite of laboratory (abnormal CK), electrophysiological (abnormal EMG) and/or radiologic (MRI) evidence of myositis, developed clinically significant myositis during a mean follow-up exceeding 5 years (15–18). Therefore, the presence of subclinical myositis is not predictive of a future clinically significant myositis.

Elevated transaminases are frequently found in patients with AIM. This elevation generally follows the trend of serum CK level suggesting the skeletal muscle, rather than the liver, as the source of transaminases. Approximately 80% of all patients with AIM have elevated serum transaminases at the time of presentation and their serum level normalization following the normalization of CK levels, confirming the strong correlation between CK level and transaminases (7, 19). Therefore, evaluation for additional liver disease is not routinely required. However, if elevated liver enzymes do not follow serum CK level, further evaluation is required. A wide range of hepatic disorders in patients with AIM have been reported, including fatty liver, hepatic congestion, non-specific reactive hepatitis and AILD (20). Mostly reported concomitant rheumatic diseases in patients with AILD are SLE, rheumatoid arthritis, Sjogren's syndrome and systemic sclerosis, while concurrent AIM is extremely rarely observed. Only a few cases of AIH type 1 patients with polymyositis have been reported to this date (21–27) and only one case each AIH type 1 (28) and AIH-primary biliary cirrhosis overlap syndrome (29) associated with DM. However, all of the reported patients were adults and had at least one additional autoimmune disease. To our knowledge, the present case is the first report of concomitant DM and ASC (or even AILD in general) development in pediatric population.

ASC affects about a half of children presenting with AILD. These patients usually have the same serological profile and liver histology as AIH but with an abnormal cholangiography finding already at presentation (30, 31). Since approximately 25% of the children with ASC have no histological features suggesting bile duct involvement, cholangiography is crucial for diagnosis. However, International Autoimmune Hepatitis Group

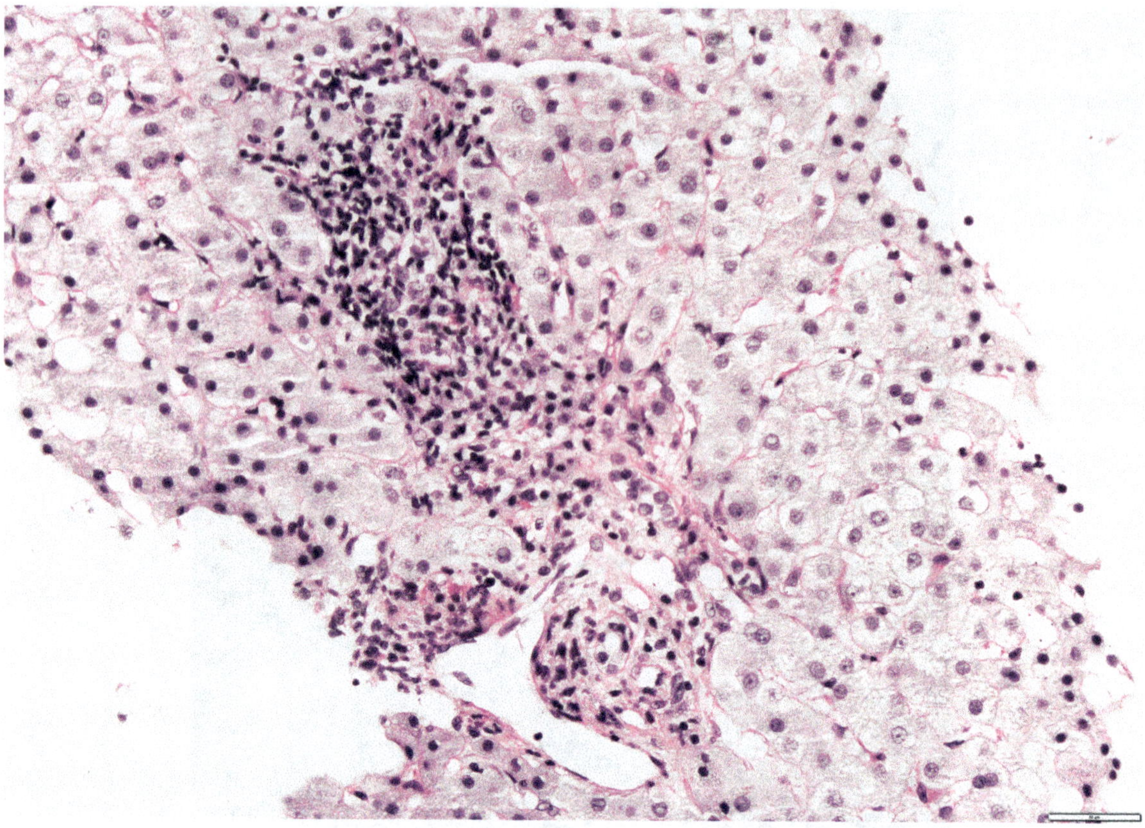

FIGURE 4 | Liver biopsy shows mononuclear infiltration of portal tract with focal interface hepatitis (PAS-D stain, magnification 200x).

TABLE 3 | ESPGHAN table of scoring criteria for the diagnosis of juvenile autoimmune liver disease (6) and results in our patient.

VARIABLE	CUT-OFF	POINTS		OUR PATIENT
		AIH	ASC	
ANA	≥ 1:20#	1	1	+
and/or SMA*	≥ 1:80	2	2	–
Anti-LKM-1* or	≥ 1:10#	1	1	–
	≥ 1:80	2	1	–
Anti-LC-1	Positive#	2	1	–
Anti-SLA	Positive#	2	2	–
pANNA	Positive	1	2	+
IgG	> ULN	1	1	–
	> 1.20 ULN	2	2	+
Liver histology	Compatible with AIH	1	1	+
	Typical of AIH	2	2	–
Absence of viral hepatitis (A,B,E,EBV), NASH, Wilson disease & drug exposure	Yes	2	2	+
Presence of extrahepatic autoimmunity	Yes	1	1	+
Family history of autoimmune disease	Yes	1	1	–
Cholangiography	Normal	2	-2	–
	Abnormal	-2	2	+
TOTAL POINTS		≥ 7: probable AIH; ≥ 8: definite AIH	≥ 7: probable ASC; ≥ 8: definite ASC	6 for AIH 11 for ASC

AIH, autoimmune hepatitis; ASC, autoimmune sclerosing cholangitis; ANA, anti-nuclear antibody; SMA, anti-smooth muscle antibody; anti-LKM-1, anti-liver kidney microsomal antibody type 1; anti-LC-1, anti-liver cytosol type 1; anti-SLA, anti-soluble liver antigen; IgG, immunoglobulin G; EBV, Epstein Barr virus; NASH, non-alcoholic steatohepatitis; ULN, upper limit of normal.

**Antibodies measured by indirect immunofluorescence on a composite rodent substrate (kidney, liver, stomach).*

#Addition of points achieved for ANA, SMA, anti-LKM-1, anti-LC-1 and anti-SLA autoantibodies cannot exceed a maximum of 2 points.

(IAIHG) scoring systems do not include cholangiography at the disease onset (32). A prospective study showed that almost a half of the children whit serological and histological features of AIH have bile duct damage demonstrable by cholangiography (30). Therefore, although cholangiography in adults is recommended in a case of cholestasis, it is mandatory in children with AIH or ASC regardless of cholestatic enzyme levels and abnormal cholangiography findings have been proposed as an additional criterion when diagnosing ASC (6). Although in our patient the liver histology was not typical of AIH, it was compatible with AIH and MRCP was abnormal. Additional fulfilled ESPGHAN criteria for ASC diagnosis in our patient were positive ANA, apANCA, high titer IgG, presence of extrahepatic autoimmunity and the absence of viral hepatitis, non-alcoholic steatohepatitis, Wilson's disease and drug exposure (6).

Autoantibodies

ANA positivity is common in a number of autoimmune liver and rheumatic diseases, as well as in up to 15% of healthy individuals (33). MSA, on the other hand, are highly specific antibodies for AIM and are not identifiable in other rheumatic diseases (34). Our patient was positive with anti-TIF1γ, the most common MSA identifiable in 20 -35% of JDM patients (34, 35). Patients with CADM more frequently have anti-TIF1γ autoantibodies than DM patients (75 vs. 37%) (36). This autoantibody is associated with more severe cutaneous lesions, rash in photo-exposed pattern, a chronic disease course, focal or generalized lipodystrophy and milder muscle involvement (35, 37–40). Raynaud's phenomenon and arthritis, as well as interstitial lung disease, are less frequent in anti-TIF1γ positive patients, but adults seem to have a much higher risk (>5x) for an associated internal malignancy (paraneoplastic DM), whereas anti-TIF1γ positive juvenile patients have a decreased association with internal malignancy (11, 41).

Antiphospholipid antibodies, including anti-cardiolipin (ACA) and anti-beta 2 glycoprotein I (anti-B2GPI) antibodies, exhibit a broad range of target specificities and affinities and can be positive in a wide range of autoimmune diseases. Though they have not been associated with DM, anti-B2GPI antibodies are frequently positive in patients with AILD and are associated with a large bile-duct involvement, increased mortality and increased cholangiocarcinoma risk in these patients (42). Interestingly, our patient was also positive with anti-gp210 antibodies, autoantibodies against the nuclear pore complex protein, which are highly specific of primary biliary cholangis (PBC), but have not been associated with other liver (autoimmune or non-autoimmune) or non-liver autoimmune diseases (43). In patients with PBC, positive anti-gp210 antibodies are an independent predictor of poor prognosis, a more rapid disease progression and a lower 5-year transplant-free survival compared to anti-gp210 negative patients. Furthermore, the degree of anti-gp210 expression is positively correlated with the intensity of inflammation around small bile ducts. The persistence of anti-gp210 after UDCA treatment is a risk factor for the progression to end-stage hepatic failure, whereas the disappearance of anti-gp210 after therapy indicates a more favorable clinical course in PBC (43). However, a possibility of a prognostic role of positive anti-gp210 antibodies in patients with ASC remains to be investigated.

Perinuclear ANCA (pANCA), though commonly associated with ASC, were initially negative in our patient, but on a second examination were positive, possibly due to the fact that the presence of ANA may interfere with pANCA detection, since neutrophil nuclei are stained by ANA, masking the perinuclear staining by pANCA (44). Atypical pANCA (or perinuclear anti-neutrophil nuclear antibodies, pANNA) have been associated with both ASC and AIH with a higher prevalence in patients with ASC (30, 45) and are included in both IAIHG and ESPGHAN criteria for AILD diagnosis. Even though the clinical significance of ANCA in these disorders remains unclear, detection of pANCA in a pediatric patient with hepatitis of unknown etiology points toward the diagnosis of AIH or ASC with the cholangiography finding crucial for the distinction between these two clinical entities.

Autoimmune Mechanisms and Genetic Predisposition

In both ASC and JDM, along with humoral immunity, features of cellular immunity also play a prominent role in the disease development. Autoantibodies may be the actual pathogenic agents or they may occur secondary as a consequence of tissue damage by autoreactive T cells.

Defective regulatory T cells ($CD4^+CD25^+$ T cells) play a major role in the loss of tolerance that leads to autoimmune disease since these cells control the process of autoantigen recognition by preventing proliferation of autoreactive T cells. In children with AILD, regulatory T cells are defective in number and function compared with healthy controls and even when compared between patients at disease onset and those in remission (46). Regulatory T cells in children with AILD produce interferon (IFN) -γ and interleukin (IL)-17 and thereby sustain inflammation and hepatic damage. This is reflected in peripheral blood and liver by increased number of Th17 cells, IFN-γ and IL-17 (47). Intriguingly, an increased expression of these cells and cytokines was also found in serum, muscle and skin tissue of patients with DM (48, 49). In addition to that, one study found even higher gene expression of Th17 related cytokines in JDM than DM patients, indicating that Th17 pathway plays a more prominent role in the pathogenesis of JDM than DM (50).

Furthermore, these two distinct clinical entities share genetic predisposition. Both ASC and JDM are associated with higher frequency of HLA-DRB1*0301 allele (51–53). In HLA-DRB1*0301-positive individuals, TNF-α and IFN-γ secretion is increased (54). Furthermore, both JDM and ASC patients have a higher frequency of the TNFα-308A allele than healthy controls and this genotype is associated with a higher serum and local (muscle fibres and liver, respectively) expression of TNFα (55, 56). TNF-α induces CD28 loss in T cells (57). The loss of CD28 expression on $CD8^+$ T-cells, or so-called aging of T-cells, appears to play an important role in the pathogenesis of both JDM and ASC. $CD8^+CD28^-$ T cells are apoptosis-resistant and are easily triggered to produce proinflammatory cytokines, mostly IFN-γ and TNF-α (57). In JDM patients, a high frequency of these cells is present in circulation and muscle tissue (58), whereas in AILD patients these cells accumulate in liver and localize around bile ducts (57). CD28⁻ T cells can increase adhesion molecule expression on biliary epithelial cells and, consequently, contribute to the activation of cytolitic mechanisms leading to cholangiocyte apoptosis (57).

On top of all that, disease onset in both ASC and JDM has been associated with infective agents as a trigger. Most of the JDM patients (>60%) report symptoms of a respiratory or gastrointestinal infection around 3 months before the disease onset (59), while in ASC pathogenesis a possible role of bacteria has been proposed, since atypical pANCA cross-react with the bacterial cell division protein (60). In addition to that, a molecular mimicry has been described with protein products of the Escherichia coli mutY gene and Salmonella typhimurium mutB gene and the gp210 epitope, suggesting that anti-gp210 antibodies may arise by molecular mimicry of bacterial antigenic determinants (61). However, since defective regulatory T cells, increased IL-17 production, HLA-DRB1*0301 allele, TNFα-308A allele and an infective trigger are a common findings in a wide range of autoimmune disease, these shared autoimmune mechanisms and genetic predisposition do not necessary mean a shared autoimmunity.

Considering the important role TNF-α clearly has in the pathogenesis of both ASC and JDM, TNF-α inhibitors might be effective in both of these diseases as well as in a case of their co-existence. Indeed, effectiveness of infliximab has been reported in both refractory AILD and JDM (62–64). However, a number of reports on anti-TNF-α-induced AIH and AIM has been published (65–68), highlighting the dual effects that anti-TNF-α agents might have. This paradox of anti-TNF-α therapy has been mainly attributed to the disruption of the regulatory role of TNF-α signaling in immune pathways (68). In addition to that, the high risk for serious infections is a well-recognized side effect of anti-TNF-α therapy (63, 68), making TNF-α antagonists a therapeutic option only for refractory cases of AIH. A better understanding of the TNF-α role in the pathogenesis of these diseases is a prerequisite to introducing TNF-α-blockers to therapy. Furthermore, considering both of these diseases show defective regulatory T cells, introducing sirolimus (a therapeutic agent that selectively expands regulatory T cells) could be beneficial for more than one disease (69). Further research is required to elucidate benefits of biologic therapy for ASC and JDM.

CONCLUSION

ASC and CAJDM are rare diseases that are challenging to diagnose and treat separately, but even more of a diagnostic and therapeutic challenge when coexisting. Since scoring systems for classification include interfering features like liver enzyme abnormalities, hypergammaglobulinemia and abnormal titer of serum ANA, the question of concomitant development of these two clinical entities in the same patient remains debatable. In addition to the mentioned interfering data, histological examination of a liver biopsy specimen in ASC and skin biopsy specimen in JDM often may not be helpful for a correct diagnosis due to a lack of specificity.

The present report is, to the best of our knowledge, the first report of simultaneously developed JDM and ASC with both entities fulfilling the latest guidelines for a definite diagnosis. Intriguingly, although extremely rarely associated, these two distinct clinical entities share multiple immunopathogenic features as well as genetic susceptibility factors. The present report emphasizes the need for further research in order to better understand underlying pathogenesis and resolve the remaining dilemmas in the field of shared autoimmunity. Furthermore, in inflammatory rheumatic diseases affecting the skin, including JDM, a more detailed characterization of skin lesions, serological markers and their correlation with disease outcomes and therapeutic responses is an imperative for a more individualized approach.

The coexistence of autoimmune liver and rheumatic diseases represents an ideal area for investigating and developing new therapeutic agents and personalized treatments. Research goals for the future should include further elucidation of shared autoimmune pathways across the spectrum of autoimmune diseases what will eventually lead to the identification of novel therapeutic targets. Targeted immunotherapy aimed at shared components of immunopathogenesis in frequently associated autoimmune diseases would be highly beneficial for more than one disease and would, consequently, minimize potential adverse effects of treating each comorbidity separately.

ETHICS STATEMENT

Written informed consent was obtained from the individual(s), and minor(s)' legal guardian/next of kin, for the publication of any potentially identifiable images or data included in this article.

AUTHOR CONTRIBUTIONS

TL conceived the study and defined the concept. TL and AG cared for the patient and extracted the data from the hospital. MĆ performed the histological analysis. TL and IS wrote the initial draft of the manuscript. AG and MĆ reviewed the manuscript and contributed to the final draft. All authors contributed to the article and approved the submitted version.

REFERENCES

1. Meyer A, Meyer N, Schaeffer M, Gottenberg JE, Geny B, Sibilia J. Incidence and Prevalence of Inflammatory Myopathies: A Systematic Review. *Rheumatology* (2015) 54:50–63. doi: 10.1093/rheumatology/keu289
2. Lundberg IE, Tjärnlund A, Bottai M, Werth VP, Pilkington C, Visser M, et al. European League Against Rheumatism/American College of Rheumatology Classification Criteria for Adult and Juvenile Idiopathic Inflammatory Myopathies and Their Major Subgroups [Published Correction Appears in Ann Rheum Dis. 2018 Sep;77(9):E64]. *Ann Rheum Dis* (2017) 76(12):1955–64. doi: 10.1136/annrheumdis-2017-211468
3. Bendewald MJ, Wetter DA, Li X, Davis MDP. Incidence of Dermatomyositis and Clinically Amyopathic Dermatomyositis: A Population-Based Study in Olmsted County, Minnesota. *Arch Dermatol* (2010) 146:26–30. doi: 10.1001/archdermatol.2009.328
4. Oberle EJ, Bayer ML, Chiu YE, Co DO. How Often are Pediatric Patients With Clinically Amyopathic Dermatomyositis Truly Amyopathic? *Pediatr Dermatol* (2017) 34:50–7. doi: 10.1111/pde.13013
5. Deneau M, Jensen MK, Holmen J, Williams MS, Book LS, Guthery SL. Primary Sclerosing Cholangitis, Autoimmune Hepatitis, and Overlap in Utah Children: Epidemiology and Natural History. *Hepatology* (2013) 58(4):1392–400. doi: 10.1002/hep.26454
6. Mieli-Vergani G, Vergani D, Baumann U, Czubkowski P, Debray D, Dezsofi A, et al. Diagnosis and Management of Pediatric Autoimmune Liver Disease: ESPGHAN Hepatology Committee Position Statement. *J Pediatr Gastroenterol Nutr* (2018) 66(2):345–60. doi: 10.1097/MPG.0000000000001801
7. Mathur T, Manadan AM, Thiagarajan S, Hota B, Block JA. Serum Transaminases are Frequently Elevated at Time of Diagnosis of Idiopathic Inflammatory Myopathy and Normalize With Creatine Kinase. *J Clin Rheumatol* (2014) 20(3):130–2. doi: 10.1097/RHU.0000000000000038
8. Concha JSS, Pena S, Gaffney RG, Patel B, Tarazi M, Kushner CJ, et al. Skin Myositis Delphi Group. Developing Classification Criteria for Skin-Predominant Dermatomyositis: The Delphi Process. *Br J Dermatol* (2020) 182(2):410–7. doi: 10.1111/bjd.18096
9. Kobayashi I, Akioka S, Kobayashi N, Iwata N, Takezaki S, Nakaseko H, et al. Clinical Practice Guidance for Juvenile Dermatomyositis (JDM) 2018-Update. *Mod Rheumatol* (2020) 30(3):411–23. doi: 10.1080/14397595.2020.1718866
10. Kim S, Kahn P, Robinson AB, Lang B, Shulman A, Oberle EJ, et al. Childhood Arthritis and Rheumatology Research Alliance Consensus Clinical Treatment Plans for Juvenile Dermatomyositis With Skin Predominant Disease. *Pediatr Rheumatol Online J* (2017) 15(1):1. doi: 10.1186/s12969-016-0134-0
11. Bellutti Enders F, Bader-Meunier B, Baildam E, Constantin T, Dolezalova P, Feldman BM, et al. Consensus-Based Recommendations for the Management of Juvenile Dermatomyositis. *Ann Rheum Dis* (2017) 76(2):329–40. doi: 10.1136/annrheumdis-2016-209247
12. Da Silva DM, Patel B, Werth VP. Dermatomyositis: A Diagnostic Dilemma. *J Am Acad Dermatol* (2018) 79(2):371–3. doi: 10.1016/j.jaad.2017.12.074
13. Patel B, Khan N, Werth VP. Applicability of EULAR/ACR Classification Criteria for Dermatomyositis to Amyopathic Disease. *J Am Acad Dermatol* (2018) 79(1):77–83.e1. doi: 10.1016/j.jaad.2017.12.055
14. Calvao J, Azeiteiro A, Gonçalo M. The Importance of New Specific Autoantibodies in Dermatomyositis. *Rev Soc Port Dermatol Venereol* (2019) 77(1):15e24. doi: 10.29021/spdv.77.1.1021
15. Gerami P, Walling HW, Lewis J, Doughty L, Sontheimer RD. A Systematic Review of Juvenile-Onset Clinically Amyopathic Dermatomyositis. *Br J Dermatol* (2007) 157(4):637–44. doi: 10.1111/j.1365-2133.2007.08055.x
16. Eisenstein DM, Paller AS, Pachman LM. Juvenile Dermatomyositis Presenting With Rash Alone. *Pediatrics* (1997) 100:391–2. doi: 10.1542/peds.100.3.391
17. El-Azhary R, Pakzad SY. Amyopathic Dermatomyositis: Retrospective Review of 37 Cases. *J Am Acad Dermatol* (2002) 46:560–5. doi: 10.1067/mjd.2002.120620
18. Gerami P, Schope JM, McDonald L, Walling HW, Sontheimer RD. A Systematic Review of Adult Onset Clinically-Amyopathic Dermatomyositis (Syn. Dermatomyositis Sine Myositis): A Missing Link Within the Spectrum of the Idiopathic Inflammatory Myopathies. *J Am Acad Dermatol* (2006) 54:597–613. doi: 10.1016/j.jaad.2005.10.041
19. Edge K, Chinoy H, Cooper RG. Serum Alanine Aminotransferase Elevations Correlate With Serum Creatine Phosphokinase Levels in Myositis. *Rheumatol (Oxford)* (2006) 45(4):487–8. doi: 10.1093/rheumatology/kel009
20. Matsumoto T, Kobayashi S, Shimizu H, Nakajima M, Watanabe S, Kitami N, et al. The Liver in Collagen Diseases: Pathologic Study of 160 Cases With Particular Reference to Hepatic Arteritis, Primary Biliary Cirrhosis, Autoimmune Hepatitis and Nodular Regenerative Hyperplasia of the Liver. *Liver* (2000) 20(5):366–73. doi: 10.1034/j.1600-0676.2000.020005366.x
21. Kurihara Y, Shishido T, Oku K, Takamatsu M, Ishiguro H, Suzuki A, et al. Polymyositis Associated With Autoimmunehepatitis, Primary Biliary Cirrhosis, and Autoimmune Thrombocytopenic Purpura. *Mod Rheumatol* (2011) 21:325–9. doi: 10.3109/s10165-010-0397-0
22. Ko KF, Ho T, Chan KW. Autoimmune Chronic Active Hepatitis and Polymyositis in a Patient With Myasthenia Gravis and Thymoma. *J Neurol Neurosurg Psychiatry* (1995) 59:558–59. doi: 10.1136/jnnp.59.5.558
23. Stefanidis I, Giannopoulou M, Liakopoulos V, Dovas S, Karasavvidou F, Zachou K. A Case of Membranous Nephropathy Associated With Sjögren Syndrome, Polymyositis and Autoimmune Hepatitis. *Clin Nephrol* (2008) 70:245–50. doi: 10.5414/CNP70245
24. Lis-Swiety A, Brzezinska-Wcislo L, Pierzchala E, Wcislo-Dziadecka D. Systemic Sclerosis-Polymyositis Overlap Syndrome Accompanied by Autoimmune Hepatitis and Sarcoidosis of Mediastinal Lymphnodes. *J Eur Acad Dermatol Venereol* (2006) 20:107–8. doi: 10.1111/j.1468-3083.2005.01321.x
25. Marie I, Levesque H, Courtois H, Francois A, Riachi G. Polymyositis, Cranial Neuropathy, Autoimmune Hepatitis, and Hepatitis C. *Ann Rheum Dis* (2000) 59(10):839–40. doi: 10.1136/ard.59.10.839a
26. Hounoki H, Shinoda K, Ogawa R, Taki H, Tsuneyama K, Tobe K. Simultaneously Developed Polymyositis and Autoimmune Hepatitis. *BMJ Case Rep* (2011) 2011:1–3. doi: 10.1136/bcr.09.2011.4763
27. Salman-Monte TC, Carrión-Barberà I, García CP, Beltrán JG, Monfort J. Inflammatory Myopathy and Autoimmune Hepatitis in a Patient With a Flare of Systemic Lupus Erythematosus: An Exceptional Association. *Eur J Rheumatol* (2018) 5(3):197–200. doi: 10.5152/eurjrheum.2018.17135
28. De Souza FH, Barros TB, de Moraes MT, Missumi LS, Lima FR, Levy-Neto M, et al. Hepatite Autoimune E Dermatomiosite: Uma Rara Associação [Autoimmune Hepatitis and Dermatomyositis: A Rare Association]. *Acta Reumatol Port* (2012) 37(3):264–7.
29. Pamfil C, Candrea E, Berki E, Popov HI, Radu PI, Rednic S. Primary Biliary Cirrhosis-Autoimmune Hepatitis Overlap Syndrome Associated With Dermatomyositis, Autoimmune Thyroiditis and Antiphospholipid Syndrome. *J Gastrointest Liver Dis* (2015) 24(1):101–4. doi: 10.15403/jgld.2014.1121.cpa
30. Gregorio GV, Portmann B, Karani J, Harrison P, Donaldson PT, Vergani D, et al. Autoimmune Hepatitis/Sclerosing Cholangitis Overlap Syndrome in Childhood: A 16-Year Prospective Study. *Hepatology* (2001) 33(3):544–53. doi: 10.1053/jhep.2001.22131
31. Mieli-Vergani G, Vergani D. Sclerosing Cholangitis in Children and Adolescents. *Clin Liver Dis* (2016) 20:99–111. doi: 10.1016/j.cld.2015.08.008
32. Alvarez F, Berg PA, Bianchi FB, Bianchi L, Burroughs AK, Cancado EL, et al. International Autoimmune Hepatitis Group Report: Review of Criteria for Diagnosis of Autoimmune Hepatitis. *J Hepatol* (1999) 31(5):929–38. doi: 10.1016/s0168-8278(99)80297-9
33. Selmi C, Ceribelli A, Generali E, Scirè CA, Alborghetti F, Colloredo G, et al. Serum Antinuclear and Extractable Nuclear Antigen Antibody Prevalence and Associated Morbidity and Mortality in the General Population Over 15 Years. *Autoimmun Rev* (2016) 15(2):162–6. doi: 10.1016/j.autrev.2015.10.007
34. Rider LG, Nistala K. The Juvenile Idiopathic Inflammatory Myopathies: Pathogenesis, Clinical and Autoantibody Phenotypes, and Outcomes. *J Intern Med* (2016) 280:24–38. doi: 10.1111/joim.12444
35. Tansley SL, Simou S, Shaddick G, Betteridge ZE, Almeida B, Gunawardena H, et al. Autoantibodies in Juvenile-Onset Myositis: Their Diagnostic Value and Associated Clinical Phenotype in a Large UK Cohort. *J Autoimmun* (2017) 84:55–64. doi: 10.1016/j.jaut.2017.06.007
36. Mamyrova G, Kishi T, Targoff IN, Ehrlich A, Curiel RV, Rider LG. Childhood Myositis Heterogeneity Collaborative Study Group. Features Distinguishing Clinically Amyopathic Juvenile Dermatomyositis From Juvenile Dermatomyositis. *Rheumatol (Oxford)* (2018) 57(11):1956–63. doi: 10.1093/rheumatology/key190
37. Bingham A, Mamyrova G, Rother KI, Oral E, Cochran E, Premkumar A, et al. Predictors of Acquired Lipodystrophy in Juvenile-Onset Dermatomyositis

and a Gradient of Severity. *Med (Baltimore)* (2008) 87:70–86. doi: 10.1097/MD.0b013e31816bc604

38. Rider LG, Shah M, Mamyrova G, Huber AM, Rice MM, Targoff IN, et al. The Myositis Autoantibody Phenotypes of the Juvenile Idiopathic Inflammatory Myopathies. *Med (Baltimore)* (2013) 92:223–43. doi: 10.1097/MD.0b013e31829d08f9
39. Gunawardena H, Wedderburn LR, North J, Betteridge Z, Dunphy J, Chinoy H, et al. Clinical Associations of Autoantibodies to a P155/140 kDa Doublet Protein in Juvenile Dermatomyositis. *Rheumatol (Oxford)* (2008) 47:324–8. doi: 10.1093/rheumatology/kem359
40. Deakin CT, Yasin SA, Simou S, Arnold KA, Tansley SL, Betteridge ZE, et al. UK Juvenile Dermatomyositis Research Group Muscle Biopsy Findings in Combination With Myositis-Specific Autoantibodies Aid Prediction of Outcomes in Juvenile Dermatomyositis. *Arthritis Rheum* (2016) 68 (11):2806–16. doi: 10.1002/art.39753
41. Best M, Molinar N, Chasset F, Vincent T, Cordel N, Bessis D. Use of Anti-Transcriptional Intermediary Factor-1 Gamma Autoantibody in Identifying Adult Dermatomyositis Patients With Cancer: A Systematic Review and Meta-Analysis. *Acta Derm Venereol* (2019) 99(3):256–62. doi: 10.2340/00015555-3091
42. Jendrek ST, Gotthardt D, Nitzsche T, Widmann L, Korf T, Michaels MA, et al. Anti-GP2 IgA Autoantibodies are Associated With Poor Survival and Cholangiocarcinoma in Primary Sclerosing Cholangitis. *Gut* (2017) 66:137–44. doi: 10.1136/gutjnl-2016-311739
43. Cristoferi L, Gerussi A, Invernizzi P. Anti-Gp210 and Other Anti-Nuclear Pore Complex Autoantibodies in Primary Biliary Cholangitis: What We Know and What We Should Know. *Liver Int* (2021) 41(3):432–5. doi: 10.1111/liv.14791
44. Deniziaut G, Ballot E, Johanet C. Antineutrophil Cytoplasmic Auto-Antibodies (ANCA) in Autoimmune Hepatitis and Primary Sclerosing Cholangitis, Clin. *Res Hepatol Gastroenterol* (2013) 37:105–7. doi: 10.1016/j.clinre.2012.07.008
45. Mulder AH, Horst G, Haagsma EB, Limburg PC, Kleibeuker JH, Kallenberg CG. Prevalence and Characterization of Neutrophil Cytoplasmic Antibodies in Autoimmune Liver Diseases. *Hepatology* (1993) 17:411–7. doi: 10.1002/hep.1840170310
46. Liberal R, Grant CR, Longhi MS, Mieli-Vergani G, Vergani D. Regulatory T Cells: Mechanisms of Suppression and Impairment in Autoimmune Liver Disease. *IUBMB Life* (2015) 67(2):88–97. doi: 10.1002/iub.1349
47. Liberal R, Grant CR, Yuksel M, Graham J, Kalbasi A, Ma Y, et al. Regulatory T-Cell Conditioning Endows Activated Effector T Cells With Suppressor Function in Autoimmune Hepatitis/Autoimmune Sclerosing Cholangitis. *Hepatology* (2017) 66(5):1570–84. doi: 10.1002/hep.29307
48. Bilgic H, Ytterberg SR, Amin S, McNallan KT, Wilson JC, Koeuth T, et al. Interleukin-6 and Type I Interferon-Regulated Genes and Chemokines Mark Disease Activity in Dermatomyositis. *Arthritis Rheum* (2009) 60(11):3436–46. doi: 10.1002/art.24936
49. Wong D, Kea B, Pesich R, Higgs BW, Zhu W, Brown P, et al. Interferon and Biologic Signatures in Dermatomyositis Skin: Specificity and Heterogenecity Across Diseases. *PloS One* (2012) 7(1):e29161. doi: 10.1371/journal.pone.0029161
50. López De Padilla CM, Crowson CS, Hein MS, Pendegraft RS, Strausbauch MA, Niewold TB, et al. Gene Expression Profiling in Blood and Affected Muscle Tissues Reveals Differential Activation Pathways in Patients With New-Onset Juvenile and Adult Dermatomyositis. *J Rheumatol* (2017) 44 (1):117–24. doi: 10.3899/jrheum.160293
51. Junge N, Tiedau M, Verboom M, Hallensleben M, Blasczyk R, Schlue J, et al. Human Leucocyte Antigens and Pediatric Autoimmune Liver Disease: Diagnosis and Prognosis. *Eur J Pediatr* (2016) 175(4):527–37. doi: 10.1007/s00431-015-2662-x
52. Wang P, Su H, Underhill J, Blackmore LJ, Longhi MS, Grammatikopoulos T, et al. Autoantibody and Human Leukocyte Antigen Profiles in Children With Autoimmune Liver Disease and Their First-Degree Relatives. *J Pediatr Gastroenterol Nutr* (2014) 58(4):457–62. doi: 10.1097/MPG.0000000000000245
53. O'Hanlon TP, Rider LG, Mamyrova G, Targoff IN, Arnett FC, Reveille JD, et al. HLA Polymorphisms in African Americans With Idiopathic Inflammatory Myopathy: Allelic Profiles Distinguish Patients With Different Clinical Phenotypes and Myositis Autoantibodies. *Arthritis Rheum* (2006) 54(11):3670–81. doi: 10.1002/art.22205
54. Lio D, Candore G, Romano GC, D'Anna C, Gervasi F, Di Lorenzo G, et al. Modification of Cytokine Patterns in Subjects Bearing the HLA-B8,DR3 Phenotype: Implications for Autoimmunity. *Cytokines Cell Mol Ther* (1997) 3(4):217–24.
55. Fedczyna TO, Lutz J, Pachman LM. Expression of TNFalpha by Muscle Fibers in Biopsies From Children With Untreated Juvenile Dermatomyositis: Association With the TNFalpha-308A Allele. *Clin Immunol* (2001) 100 (2):236–9. doi: 10.1006/clim.2001.5063
56. Chaouali M, Azaiez MB, Tezeghdenti A, Lagha A, Yacoubi-Oueslati B, Ghazouani E, et al. Association of TNF-α-308 Polymorphism With Susceptibility to Autoimmune Hepatitis in Tunisians. *Biochem Genet* (2018) 56(6):650–62. doi: 10.1007/s10528-018-9867-4
57. Liaskou E, Jeffery LE, Trivedi PJ, Reynolds GM, Suresh S, Bruns T, et al. Loss of CD28 Expression by Liver-Infiltrating T Cells Contributes to Pathogenesis of Primary Sclerosing Cholangitis. *Gastroenterology* (2014) 147(1):221–232.e7. doi: 10.1053/j.gastro.2014.04.003
58. Murata K, Dalakas MC. Expression of the Costimulatory Molecule BB-1, the Ligands CTLA-4 and CD28, and Their mRNA in Inflammatory Myopathies. *Am J Pathol* (1999) 155(2):453–60. doi: 10.1016/s0002-9440(10)65141-3
59. Pachman LM, Lipton R, Ramsey-Goldman R, Shamiyeh E, Abbott K, Mendez EP, et al. History of Infection Before the Onset of Juvenile Dermatomyositis: Results From the National Institute of Arthritis and Musculoskeletaland Skin Diseases Research Registry. *Arthritis Rheum* (2005) 53(2):166–72. doi: 10.1002/art.21068
60. Terjung B, Spengler U. Atypical P-ANCA in PSC and AIH: A Hint Toward a "Leaky Gut"? *Clin Rev Allergy Immunol* (2009) 36:40–51. doi: 10.1007/s12016-008-8088-8
61. Nickowitz RE, Worman HJ. Autoantibodies From Patients With Primary Biliary Cirrhosis Recognize a Restricted Region Within the Cytoplasmic Tail of Nuclear Pore Membrane Glycoprotein Gp210. *J Exp Med* (1993) 178 (6):2237–42. doi: 10.1084/jem.178.6.2237
62. Riley P, McCann LJ, Maillard SM, Woo P, Murray KJ, Pilkington CA. Effectiveness of Infliximab in the Treatment of Refractory Juvenile Dermatomyositis With Calcinosis. *Rheumatol (Oxford)* (2008) 47(6):877–80. doi: 10.1093/rheumatology/ken074
63. Weiler-Normann C, Schramm C, Quaas A, Wiegard C, Glaubke C, Pannicke N, et al. Infliximab as a Rescue Treatment in Difficult-to-Treat Autoimmune Hepatitis. *J Hepatol* (2013) 58(3):529–34. doi: 10.1016/j.jhep.2012.11.010
64. Rajanayagam J, Lewindon PJ. Infliximab as Rescue Therapy in Paediatric Autoimmune Hepatitis. *J Hepatol* (2013) 59(4):908–9. doi: 10.1016/j.jhep.2013.05.046
65. Rodrigues S, Lopes S, Magro F, Cardoso H, Horta e Vale AM, Marques M, et al. Autoimmune Hepatitis and Anti-Tumor Necrosis Factor Alpha Therapy: A Single Center Report of 8 Cases. *World J Gastroenterol* (2015) 21(24):7584–8. doi: 10.3748/wjg.v21.i24.7584
66. Mostamand S, Schroeder S, Schenkein J, Miloh T. Infliximab-Associated Immunomediated Hepatitis in Children With Inflammatory Bowel Disease. *J Pediatr Gastroenterol Nutr* (2016) 63(1):94–7. doi: 10.1097/MPG.0000000000001137
67. Kim NN, Lio PA, Morgan GA, Jarvis JN, Pachman LM. Double Trouble: Therapeutic Challenges in Patients With Both Juvenile Dermatomyositis and Psoriasis. *Arch Dermatol* (2011) 147(7):831–5. doi: 10.1001/archdermatol.2011.49
68. Saitis A, Gatselis N, Zachou K, Dalekos GN. Use of Tnfα Antagonists in Refractory AIH: Revealing the Unforeseen. *J Hepatol* (2013) 59(1):197–8. doi: 10.1016/j.jhep.2013.02.029
69. Kurowski J, Melin-Aldana H, Bass L, Alonso EM, Ekong UD. Sirolimus as Rescue Therapy in Pediatric Autoimmune Hepatitis. *J Pediatr Gastroenterol Nutr* (2014) 58(1):e4–6. doi: 10.1097/MPG.0b013e318291feaa

10

Incidence and Distinct Features of Immune Checkpoint Inhibitor-Related Myositis From Idiopathic Inflammatory Myositis: A Single-Center Experience With Systematic Literature Review and Meta-Analysis

Naoki Hamada[1†], Ayaka Maeda[1†], Kaoru Takase-Minegishi[1‡], Yohei Kirino[1*‡], Yumiko Sugiyama[1], Ho Namkoong[2], Nobuyuki Horita[3], Ryusuke Yoshimi[1], Hideaki Nakajima[1] and YCU irAE Working Group*

[1] Department of Stem Cell and Immune Regulation, Yokohama City University Graduate School of Medicine, Yokohama, Japan, [2] Department of Infectious Diseases, Keio University School of Medicine, Tokyo, Japan, [3] Chemothrapy Center, Yokohama City University Hospital, Yokohama, Japan

***Correspondence:**
Kaoru Takase-Minegishi
kaoru_t@yokohama-cu.ac.jp
Yohei Kirino
kirino@yokohama-cu.ac.jp

†These authors have contributed equally to this work and share first authorship

‡These authors have contributed equally to this work and share last authorship

Immune checkpoint inhibitor (ICI)-related myositis is a rare, potentially fatal condition that warrants further studies. Its incidence, clinical features, and prognosis remain poorly understood. To address these gaps, we conducted a systematic review and meta-analysis to evaluate the risk of myositis associated with ICI for solid tumors by analyzing phase III randomized controlled trials of anti-programmed death-1/ligand-1 (PD-1/PD-L1) and anti-cytotoxic T-lymphocyte antigen-4 (CTLA-4). To complement this analysis with clinical data, we evaluated published ICI case reports along with cases from our institutional registry. This registry comprised 422 patients treated with ICIs alone or in combination from September 2014 to June 2021. The analysis revealed an incidence of ICI-related myositis in 6,838 patients in 18 randomized controlled trials of 0.38% (odds ratio 1.96; 95% confidence interval 1.02–3.75) for patients receiving ICIs compared with controls. Detailed analysis of 88 cases from the literature search and our registry showed that myositis induced by PD-1 inhibitors was more frequent than that induced by anti-CTLA-4 agents, revealing a clinically diverse trend including myasthenia gravis and myocarditis. Importantly, having ptosis at the time of onset was significantly associated with the development of concomitant myocarditis (odds ratio 3.81; 95% CI 1.48–9.83), which is associated with poor prognosis. Regarding treatment, most patients received glucocorticoids, and some received immunosuppressants. Our study revealed the incidence of ICI-mediated myositis and the clinical features of myocarditis, highlighting the need for recognition and early intervention.

Keywords: immune checkpoint inhibitor (ICI), irAE, autoimmune, myocarditis, myositis

INTRODUCTION

Immune checkpoint inhibitors (ICIs) have revolutionized cancer treatment by exerting anti-tumor effects on various types and stages of cancer that cannot be achieved with existing drugs, and numerous clinical trials are underway to expand indications (1). However, treatment response to ICIs is variable in terms of both efficacy and adverse effects (2, 3). Autoimmune reactions to various organs—immune-related adverse events (irAEs)—are observed in patients treated with ICIs (4, 5). The phenotypes of irAEs vary and it is currently impossible to predict how often they will occur, and in which organs. ICI-related myositis is rare but has been reported to be potentially fatal (6).

A review by Kadota et al. (7) reported that myositis occurred in patients receiving anti-programmed death-1 (PD-1) alone, anti-cytotoxic T-lymphocyte antigen-4 (CTLA-4) alone, and with combination therapy. Mean time from ICI initiation to the onset of ICI-related myositis was 4 weeks. Causes of death were myocarditis, respiratory paralysis, and cancer progression. In patients without myocarditis or respiratory muscle paralysis, creatine kinase (CK) levels normalized after ICI discontinuation and administration of immunosuppressive drugs, and the prognosis of myositis was good. The review suggested that the clinical features of ICI-related myositis can be divided into two subsets: new onset of myositis as an irAE, and onset of idiopathic inflammatory myositis (IIM). However, because of its rarity, the incidence, clinical features, and prognosis of ICI-related myositis are still poorly understood.

A systematic review on myocarditis has been published (8), but, to our knowledge, no meta-analysis on this topic has been conducted. Since the 2019 publication of the Kadota et al. review (7) many additional cases have been reported, thus there is the opportunity to clarify some of the questions about this condition. With this aim, we conducted a systematic review on ICI-related myositis. To clarify the detailed clinical features of ICI-related myositis, we searched the literature for case reports together with data from the Yokohama City University ICI registry. Here, we report the incidence, clinical features, and potential predictors of fatal myocarditis in these patients.

MATERIALS AND METHODS

Systematic Review and Meta-Analysis of Randomized Controlled Trials

The systematic review was conducted following the Preferred Reporting Items for Systematic Reviews and Meta-Analyses guidelines (9, 10) and was registered in the University Hospital Medical Information Network Center Clinical Trial Registry (Japan) as UMIN000044960 (11). Institutional Review Board approval and patient informed consent were waived for the systematic review and meta-analysis due to nature of the study.

In the electronic search, we systematically searched PubMed, EMBASE, the Cochrane Central Register of Controlled Trials, and Web of Science Core Collection (up to August 16 2021) for randomized controlled trials (RCTs) reporting the risk of myositis associated with ICIs for the treatment of patients with solid tumors. Search formulae are presented in Supplementary Text 1. Two investigators (AM, KT-M) independently screened candidate articles by checking the title and abstract after uploading the citation list into Endnote X9 software (Thomson Reuters, Philadelphia, PA, USA). Inclusion criteria were as follows: (1) phase III RCT study design; (2) the experimental group was treated with at least one type of ICI with or without other systemic chemotherapy and the control group with non-ICIs; (3) three-arm studies where an ICI was included in at least one arm; (4) patients clinically diagnosed with any solid tumor; and (5) the study included the incidence of myositis. Exclusion criteria were as follows: (1) systematic review or meta-analyses; (2) retrospective analyses; (3) single prospective cohort studies with no control group; (4) ICI two-drug combination therapy; (5) republished research literature; (6) studies with no or insufficient safety results at the time of the literature search; and (7) studies published in languages other than English. Only full-text papers were used for analysis. Disagreements in assessing cases or data were resolved *via* discussion between the two investigators.

Odds ratios (ORs) of any-grade myositis between the ICI treatment arm and non-ICI arm were calculated using a random-effect model meta-analysis. Heterogeneity was assessed using I^2 statistics and P-values. Heterogeneity was indicated by I^2 wherein 0% indicated no heterogeneity and 100% indicated the strongest heterogeneity. Statistical analyses were performed using Review Manager 5.3 (Cochrane Community, London, UK). The Cochrane Risk of Bias Tool was used to evaluate the risk of bias for each RCT (12). The quality of the RCTs was independently assessed by two reviewers (AM, KT-M).

Patients and Design of the Yokohama City University Institutional Database

Consecutive cancer patients (excluding those in clinical trials) who received ICIs (nivolumab, pembrolizumab, ipilimumab, atezolizumab, or durvalumab) for approved cancer types at the collaborative research department of Yokohama City University Hospital between December 2014 and May 2021 were included. The study was approved by the ethics committee of Yokohama City University (A200500004). In this study, we included patients treated with ICI monotherapy or combination therapy. Demographic, clinical, and treatment data were obtained from clinical charts. The study followed the Ethical Guidelines for Epidemiology Research, published by the Japanese Ministry of Health, Labour and Welfare, and had an opt-out strategy.

Literature Review of Case Reports

We searched the literature for cases of ICI-related myositis using PubMed on September 7, 2021. 'ICI-related myositis' was defined according to the previously reported literature review (7). Cases clinically diagnosed as myositis were included in the analysis, but cases with focal myositis, such as orbital myositis, were excluded. We searched PubMed using the following terms: (pembrolizumab OR nivolumab OR ipilimumab) AND (myositis

OR myopathy OR myopathies OR dermatomyositis OR polymyositis). Additional related articles were identified through a manual search of the bibliographies of the included studies to ensure that all relevant studies and recent reviews were included.

Data from case reports were divided into two groups: myositis alone, and concomitant myocarditis. Clinical characteristics, the type of ICI, autoantibody status, management, and outcome were evaluated and compared between two groups.

Clinical data were analyzed using both univariate and multivariate analysis. Comparisons of frequencies were made by Fisher's exact test, or by chi-square test if there were three or more categories for each variable. Continuous variables were compared using Mann-Whitney U test. Logistic regression models were used to identify multivariate predictors of myocarditis, after adjusting for the effects of age and gender. Values of $p<0.05$ were considered significant. Statistical analyses were performed using software IBM/SPSS Statistics version 22 (Armonk, NY).

RESULTS

Incidence and Risk of ICI-Related Myositis in the Systematic Review and Meta-Analysis

Of 5,471 candidate articles, 120 were potentially eligible after abstract and title screening. From these 120, 19 studies were excluded, and 101 articles were reviewed in detail. Studies of 93 RCTs were insufficient to assess the incidence of myositis. Finally, 18 RCTs (13–30) were included in this meta-analysis (**Figure 1**). Characteristics of the included studies are

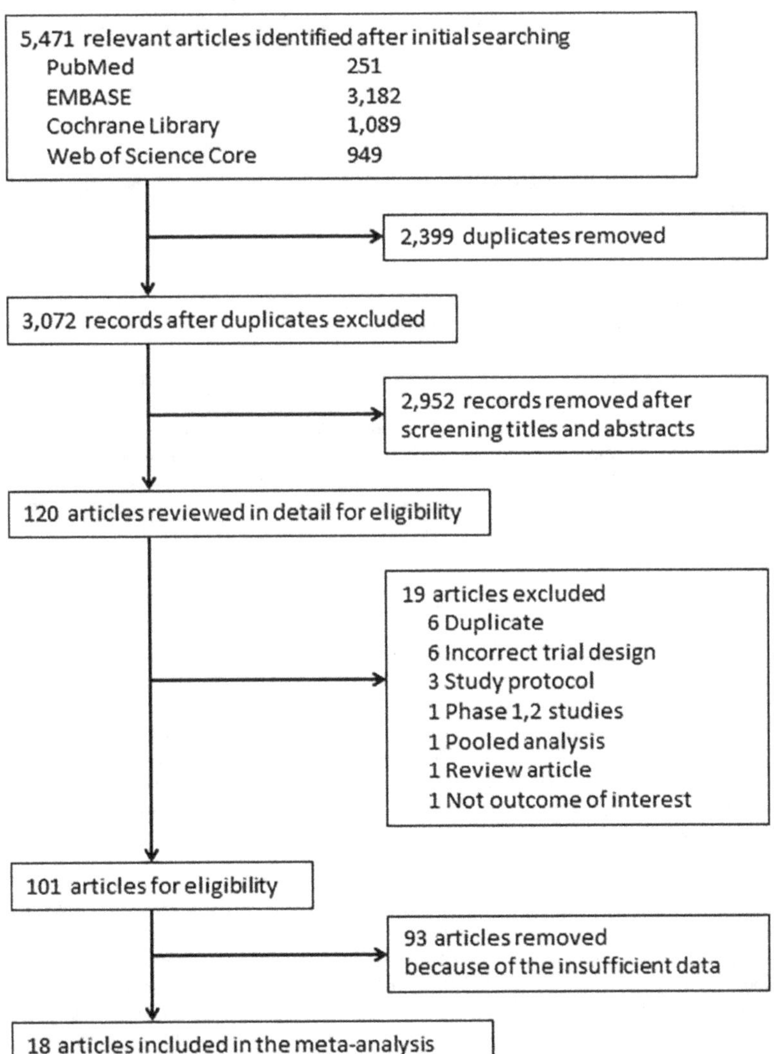

FIGURE 1 | PRISMA flow diagram for the meta-analysis. Study selection process according to the Preferred Reporting Items for Systematic Reviews and Meta-Analyses (PRISMA) guidelines.

summarized in **Table 1**. Visual inspection of the funnel plot was assessed (**Supplementary Figure 1**). The overall risk of bias for most studies evaluated was also low (**Supplementary Figure 2**). There was no clear risk of publication bias in the included studies.

A total of 33 events of any-grade myositis were observed in 12,866 participants (ICI treatment arm, n = 6,838; non-ICI treatment arm, n = 6,028) from 18 RCTs. Twenty-six events were observed in the ICI arm and seven events were observed in the non-ICI arm. Among the 26 ICI-related myositis, 11 events were caused by anti-PD-1, 13 by anti-programmed death ligand 1 (PD-L1), and two by anti-CTLA-4, suggesting that any ICI can elicit this condition. We calculated OR and 95% CI to compare PD-1/PD-L1 and CTLA-4 blockade therapies. There was no significant difference in frequencies of myositis between two groups (OR 1.07; 95% CI: 0.27-9.41). The overall incidence of ICI-related myositis was 0.38% (26 of 6,838), and did not seem to be affected by the cancer type or ICI regimen. We found that myositis was significantly increased with ICI treatment compared with non-ICI treatment (OR, 1.96; 95% confidence interval [CI] 1.02–3.75; $p = 0.04$; $I^2 = 0\%$) (**Figure 2**). These data suggest that ICI-related myositis may be an important component of irAEs in patients receiving ICI therapy.

Summary of Single Center Analysis

Meta-analysis provides epidemiological data such as the incidence of ICI-related myositis, but it is difficult to analyze detailed clinical characteristics. To understand the prognosis of ICI-related myositis, we first examined our institutional database. A total of 422 patients were identified. Among these, 365 cases were treated with a PD-1 or PD-L1 inhibitor alone, nine were treated with a CTLA-4 inhibitor alone, and 47 cases were treated with a PD-1 inhibitor and CTLA-4 inhibitor combination. There were three cases of ICI-related myositis (incidence 0.71%). Baseline characteristics are shown in **Supplementary Table 1**. All three patients were Asian Japanese and one was female, with mean age 71 ± 6.6 years. Mean treatment duration prior to ICI-related myositis was 13.7 weeks (range 3–34). These patients had muscle weakness with elevated CK with a clinical diagnosis of ICI-related myositis.

TABLE 1 | Overview of the included studies in the meta-analysis.

First author	Year	Cancer types	Cancer status	Study setting	ICI arm	Non-ICI arm	Number of patients			
							ICI		Non-ICI	
							All	Myositis	All	Myositis
André (12)	2020	MSI-High Colorectal	Advanced	First-line	Pembrolizumab	Chemotherapy	153	1	143	0
Eggermont (13)	2018	Melanoma	Resected stage III	Adjuvant	Pembrolizumab	Placebo	509	1	502	0
Ferris (14)	2016	HNSCC	Recurrent	After platinum-based chemotherapy	Nivolumab	MTX, Docetaxel, or Cetuximab	236	0	111	1
Galsky (15)	2020	Urothelial	Metastatic	First-line	Atezolizumab + platinum-based chemotherapy	Placebo + platinum-based chemotherapy	453	3	390	1
Gutzmer (16)	2020	Melanoma	Advanced	First-line	Atezolizumab	Placebo	230	1	281	0
Kojima (17)	2020	Esophageal	Advanced	Second-line	Pembrolizumab	Chemotherapy	314	1	296	0
Kuruvilla (18)	2021	HL	Relapsed or refractory	Second or later line	Pembrolizumab	Brentuximab	148	1	152	0
Miles (19)	2021	TNBC	Metastatic	First-line	Atezolizumab + PTX	Placebo + PTX	431	1	218	0
Mittendorf (20)	2020	TNBC	Stage II-III	First-line	Atezolizumab	Placebo	164	1	167	0
Moore (21)	2021	Ovarian	Ssage III-IV	Neoadjuvant	Atezolizumab + CBDCA + PTX + Bevacizumab	Placebo + CBDCA + PTX + Bevacizumab	642	4	644	5
Powles (22)	2018	Urothelial	Advanced or metastatic	After platinum-based chemotherapy	Atezolizumab	Vinflunine, PTX, or Docetaxel	459	1	443	0
Powles (23)	2020	Urothelial	Advanced or metastatic	First-line	Avelumab + BSC	BSC alone	344	1	345	0
Reck (24)	2016	SCLC	Extensive-stage	First-line	Ipilimumab + CDDP/CBDCA + VP-16	Placebo + CDDP/ CBDCA + VP-16	562	2	561	0
Rini (25)	2019	RCC	Advanced	First-line	Pembrolizumab + Axitinib	Sunitinib	429	2	425	0
Rini (26)	2019	RCC	Metastatic	First-line	Atezolizumab + Bevacizumab	Sunitinib	451	1	446	0
Rudin (27)	2020	SCLC	Stage IV	First-line	Pembrolizumab + EP	Placebo + EP	223	1	223	0
Schmid (28)	2020	TNBC	Stage II-III	First-line	Pembrolizumab + chemotherapy	Placebo + Chemotherapy	781	3	389	0
Winer (29)	2021	TNBC	Metastatic	Second or later line	Pembrolizumab	Chemotherapy	309	1	292	0

MSI-H, microsatellite-instability–high; NSCLC, non-small cell lung cancer; HNSCC, head-and-neck squamous cell cancer; TNBC, triple-negative breast cancer; SCLC, small cell lung cancer; RCC, renal cell carcinoma; ICI, immune checkpoint inhibitor; PTX, paclitaxel; CBDCA, carboplatin; BSC, best supportive care; CDDP, cisplatin; VP-16, etoposide; EP, etoposide and platinum; MTX, methotrexate.

Study or Subgroup	ICI Events	ICI Total	Control Events	Control Total	Weight	Odds Ratio M-H, Random, 95% CI
André, T. 2020	1	153	0	143	4.1%	2.82 [0.11, 69.86]
Eggermont, A. M. M. 2018	1	509	0	502	4.1%	2.96 [0.12, 72.95]
Ferris, R. L. 2016	0	236	1	111	4.1%	0.16 [0.01, 3.85]
Galsky, M.D. 2020	3	453	1	390	8.2%	2.59 [0.27, 25.03]
Gutzmer, R. 2020	1	230	0	281	4.1%	3.68 [0.15, 90.76]
Kojima, T. 2020	1	314	0	296	4.1%	2.84 [0.12, 69.92]
Kuruvilla, J. 2021	1	148	0	152	4.1%	3.10 [0.13, 76.75]
Miles, D. 2021	1	431	0	218	4.1%	1.52 [0.06, 37.53]
Mittendorf, E. A. 2020	1	164	0	167	4.1%	3.07 [0.12, 75.99]
Moore, K. N. 2021	4	642	5	644	24.3%	0.80 [0.21, 3.00]
Powles, T. 2018	1	459	0	443	4.1%	2.90 [0.12, 71.42]
Powles, T. 2020	1	344	0	345	4.1%	3.02 [0.12, 74.33]
Reck, M. 2016	2	562	0	561	4.6%	5.01 [0.24, 104.57]
Rini, B. I. 2019-1	2	429	0	425	4.6%	4.98 [0.24, 103.97]
Rini, B. I. 2019-2	1	451	0	446	4.1%	2.97 [0.12, 73.18]
Rudin, C. M. 2020	1	223	0	223	4.1%	3.01 [0.12, 74.37]
Schmid, P. 2020	3	781	0	389	4.8%	3.50 [0.18, 67.97]
Winer, E. P. 2021	1	309	0	292	4.1%	2.84 [0.12, 70.10]
Total (95% CI)		**6838**		**6028**	**100.0%**	**1.96 [1.02, 3.75]**
Total events	26		7			

Heterogeneity: Tau² = 0.00; Chi² = 5.90, df = 17 (P = 0.99); I² = 0%
Test for overall effect: Z = 2.03 (P = 0.04)

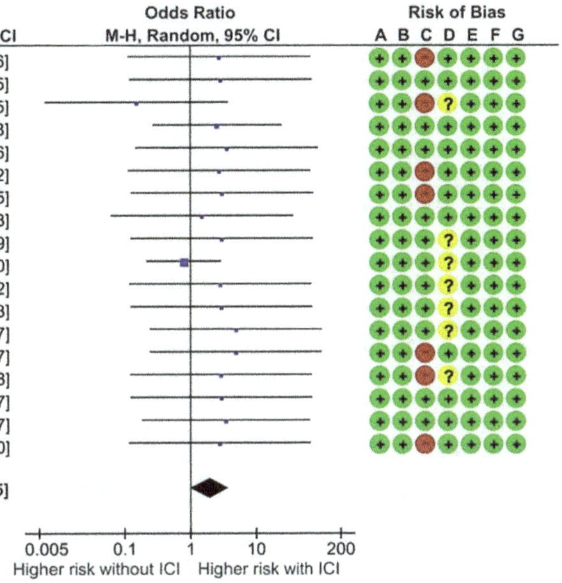

Risk of bias legend
(A) Random sequence generation (selection bias)
(B) Allocation concealment (selection bias)
(C) Blinding of participants and personnel (performance bias)
(D) Blinding of outcome assessment (detection bias)
(E) Incomplete outcome data (attrition bias)
(F) Selective reporting (reporting bias)
(G) Other bias

FIGURE 2 | Forest plot with risk of bias summary for incidence of immune checkpoint inhibitor-related myositis.

All were treated with glucocorticoids and other drugs were initiated. However, two patients died (one with pneumonia and one with tumor progression). Patient details are shown in **Supplementary Text 2**.

Clinical Features and Prognosis of ICI-Related Myositis

To clarify the clinical features of ICI-related myositis in a larger patient population, we evaluated the clinical features of published case reports of ICI-related myositis. Of 75 candidate articles, 63 were identified as eligible (31–93). A further 14 relevant articles (7, 94–106) were added through hand searching. Among the 77 articles, 30 were from Japan, 23 were from USA, five were from France and four were from Canada and Australia (**Supplementary Table 1**). A total of 85 myositis cases associated with at least one ICI were identified. We combined these with the three cases from our institutional database so 88 cases were analyzed in total (precise clinical information of these three patients is noted in the Supplementary Text 2). The most frequent cancer types were lung cancer and melanoma (28 and 27 cases, respectively), followed by urothelial carcinoma. Treatment regimens were as follows: pembrolizumab (anti-PD-1; 37 cases), nivolumab (anti-PD-1; 29 cases), ipilimumab (anti-CTLA-4; four cases), and nivolumab plus ipilimumab (14 cases). Estimated onset time of myositis after ICI administration was 5.6 ± 6.1 weeks and the appearance of autoantibodies varied.

All cases except one were treated with glucocorticoids. Thirty-three patients died, of which 19 deaths were associated with myositis. Because myocarditis is known to be a frequent and fatal complication of ICI-related myositis (107), we compared clinical features of patients with and without myocarditis. Thirty-six of the 88 cases (40.9%) were complicated by myocarditis, confirming the high incidence of myocarditis in ICI-related myositis (**Table 2**).

There were some significant differences in clinical characteristics in the group that developed myocarditis. First, we analyzed overall ICI use and found that the occurrence of myocarditis was significantly affected by the type of ICI regimen (p=0.015), but was underpowered to detect an association with a specific regimen. Second, in terms of clinical features at the time of myositis onset, ptosis and respiratory muscle paralysis (type II respiratory failure) were significantly more frequent in the myocarditis group (p=0.007; OR 3.81; 95% CI 1.48–9.83 and p=0.001; OR 5.43; 95% CI 2.07–14.26, respectively). The ORs were calculated from multivariate logistic regression analysis, which also revealed that ptosis and respiratory muscle paralysis were independently associated with the development of myocarditis (p=0.031; OR 2.97; 95% CI 1.10–8.02 and p=0.003; OR 4.54; 95% CI: 1.68–12.23, respectively,

TABLE 2 | Clinical features and prognosis of immune checkpoint inhibitor-related myositis.

		Total (n = 88)	Myocarditis (+) (n = 36)	Myocarditis (-) (n = 52)	*P* value	OR	95% CI
Age	Mean, years	68.0	71.9	65.3	0.089		
	Median, years	71	73.5	70.5			
Gender	Male, n	62	27	35	0.484	1.46	0.56-3.77
	Female, n	26	9	17			
Onset date	Mean, weeks	5.6	4.4	6.5	0.462		
	Median, weeks	3.8	3.7	3.9			
Cancer type, (n)		Melanoma (27)	Melanoma (12)	Melanoma (15)	0.075		
		NSCLC (28)	NSCLC (7)	NSCLC (21)			
		UTC (12)	UTC (8)	UTC (4)			
		HNC (3)	HNC (0)	HNC (3)			
		RCC (4)	RCC (2)	RCC (2)			
		HL (2)	HL (0)	HL (2)			
		Others (12)	Others (7)	Others (5)			
ICI, (n)		Nivolumab (29)	Nivolumab (8)	Nivolumab (21)	0.015		
		Pembrolizumab (37)	Pembrolizumab (16)	Pembrolizumab (21)			
		Nivolumab + Ipilimumab (14)	Nivolumab + Ipilimumab (8)	Nivolumab + Ipilimumab (6)			
		Ipilimumab (4)	Ipilimumab (0)	Ipilimumab (4)			
		Others (4)	Others (4)	Others (4)			
Clinical presentation							
	Ptosis, n (%)	45/84 (54)	24/33 (73)	21/51 (41)	0.007	3.81	1.48-9.83
	Ophthalmoplegia, n (%)	28/72 (39)	13/24 (54)	15/48 (31)	0.076	2.60	0.95-7.13
	Dysphasia, n (%)	33/80 (41)	15/31 (48)	18/49 (37)	0.355	1.61	0.65-4.02
	Respiratory muscle paralysis, n (%)	34/82 (41)	21/32 (66)	13/50 (26)	0.001	5.43	2.07-14.26
	Limb weakness, n (%)	79/84 (94)	28/33 (85)	51/51 (100)	0.008	0.05	0.00-0.94
	Rhabdomyolysis, n (%)	8/88 (9)	5/36 (14)	3/52 (6)	0.264	2.63	0.59-11.81
	Myasthenia gravis, n (%)	34/88 (39)	19/36 (53)	15/52 (29)	0.028	2.76	1.13-6.70
	Interstitial lung disease, n (%)	2/88 (2)	0/36 (0)	2/52 (4)	0.511	0.28	0.01-5.94
	Cutaneous manifestations*1, n (%)	16/88 (18)	0/36 (0)	16/52 (31)	<0.001	0.03	0.00-0.52
Other irAEs, (n)			Thyroiditis (2)	Hypothyroidism (2)			
			Diarrhea (1)	Thyroiditis (2)			
				Rheumatoid arthritis (1)			
				Colitis (1)			
				Cerebral meningitis (1)			
Autoantibody							
	Anti-AChR, n (%)	17/37 (46)	8/21 (38)	9/16 (56)	0.331	0.48	0.13-1.80
	Anti-striated muscle, n (%)	14/15 (93)	11/12 (92)	3/3 (100)	1.000	1.10	0.04-33.38
	Anti-TIF1γ, n (%)	6/6	0/0	6/6			
Treatment							
	PSL, n (%)	87/88 (99)	36/36 (100)	51/52 (98)	1.000	2.13	0.08-53.67
	IVIG, n (%)	43/88 (49)	19/36 (53)	24/52 (46)	0.665	1.30	0.56-3.06
	Apheresis, n (%)	25/88 (28)	17/36 (47)	8/52 (15)	0.002	4.92	1.81-13.35
	Bio (Infliximab or Rituximab), n (%)	7/88 (8)	6/36 (17)	1/52 (2)	0.017	10.20	1.17-88.84
	Immunosuppressants, (n)		MTX (2), Tac (1), MMF (3)	MTX (3), Tac (3), AZA (1), HCQ (1)			
	Pyridostigmine*2, n (%)	12/89 (13)	5/37 (14)	7/52 (13)			
Outcome							
	Recovery of myositis, n (%)	55/81 (68)	12/29 (41)	43/52 (83)	<0.001	0.15	0.05-0.41
Prognosis							
	All deaths, n (%)	33/85 (39)	18/34 (53)	15/51 (29)	0.041	2.70	1.09-6.66
	Directly caused by myositis, n (%)	19/33 (58)	15/18 (83)	4/15 (27)	0.002	13.75	2.54-74.30
	Infection related to myositis, n (%)	4/33 (12)	1/18 (6)	3/15 (20)	0.308	0.24	0.02-2.54
	Progression of a cancer, n (%)	13/33 (39)	3/18 (17)	10/15 (67)	0.005	0.10	0.02-0.52
	Other reasons, n (%)	1/33 (3)	1/18 (6)	0/15 (0)			

*NSCLC, non-small cell lung cancer; UTC, urothelial carcinoma; HNC, head and neck cancer; RCC, renal cell carcinoma; HL, Hodgkin's lymphoma; ICI, immune checkpoint inhibitor; irAEs, immune-related adverse events; AChR, acetylcholine receptor; TIF1γ, transcription Intermediary factor 1γ, PSL, prednisolone; IVIG, intravenous immunoglobulin; Bio, biological therapy; MTX, methotrexate; Tac, tacrolimus; AZA, azathioprine; MMF, mycophenolate mofetil; HCQ, hydroxychloroquine. *1, typical cutaneous signs of dermatomyositis; *2, treatment of myasthenia gravis.*

Supplementary Table 2). Third, in terms of myositis treatment, the myocarditis group received more aggressive treatment such as plasmapheresis and biological agents (p=0.002; OR 4.92; 95% CI 1.81–13.35 and p=0.017; OR 10.20; 95% CI 1.17–88.84, respectively). Finally, in terms of prognosis, myositis symptoms including myocarditis were more refractory to treatment and myositis-related deaths were more common in the group with myocarditis (p=0.002; OR 13.75; 95% CI 2.54–74.30), while the group without myocarditis had a better response to treatment for myositis and more deaths because of cancer progression (p=0.005). These data suggest that myocarditis is a serious complication of ICI-related myositis, the onset of which can be predicted by the development of ptosis.

DISCUSSION

Because ICI-related myositis is extremely rare, reported only in individual RCTs and case reports, its incidence and clinical phenotype are poorly understood. Here, we provide the first evidence that ICI treatment significantly increases the incidence of myositis compared with non-ICI treatment. Furthermore, detailed analysis of case reports showed that myocarditis with the poorest prognosis had ocular symptoms as the initial manifestation. These results are expected to be useful for the optimization of ICI use in clinical practice.

We show here that ICI-related myositis occurred in 0.38% of patients treated with ICIs, and was significantly more frequent in patients treated with cytotoxic anti-cancer agents. Both anti-PD-1/PD-L1 and anti-CTLA-4 antibodies can cause myositis, but anti-CTLA-4 antibodies have been reported less frequently and may cause myositis less frequently than treatment with anti-PD-1/PD-L1 antibodies. The present study was is underpowered to determine differences in myositis-inducing effects of anti-CTLA-4 and PD-1/PD-L1 antibodies. Further accumulation of cases, pathological verification, and analysis of combination therapy with these two antibodies will be of benefit.

As shown in the previous (7) and current studies, myositis resulting from ICI treatment can be complicated by myasthenia gravis and myocarditis, indicating that ICI-related myositis is a distinct phenotype from IIM (108). Therefore, prognosis in myositis may also differ from that in IIM. Although rapid diagnosis of fatal conditions—especially myocarditis—is necessary, there is currently no standardized method for diagnosing ICI-related myositis. Applying existing diagnostic criteria for IIM and myasthenia gravis to ICI-related diseases may be inappropriate and too late for diagnosis. We identified particular key features, namely ptosis and respiratory paralysis, as important indicators of myocarditis. Based on the current data, we suggest that these patients are closely monitored for myocarditis.

ICI myositis may have different clinical features from dermatomyositis and polymyositis as illustrated in **Figure 3**. Typical cutaneous signs of dermatomyositis were seen in 16 cases (18%) and anti-TIF1γ antibody was positive in 6 of them. These cases met the classification criteria for dermatomyositis. There were no cases in which anti-TIF1γ antibody was measured before the start of ICI treatment, and it is unclear whether anti-TIF1γ was induced by ICI-treatment or not. The complication rate of interstitial lung disease was low (2%). Although most cases of ICI-related myositis are negative for myositis-specific antibodies, some cases of positive anti-striated muscle antibodies have been reported (**Supplementary Table 1**), and their diagnostic significance needs to be investigated. The fact that myasthenia gravis without thymoma has been reported to be associated with

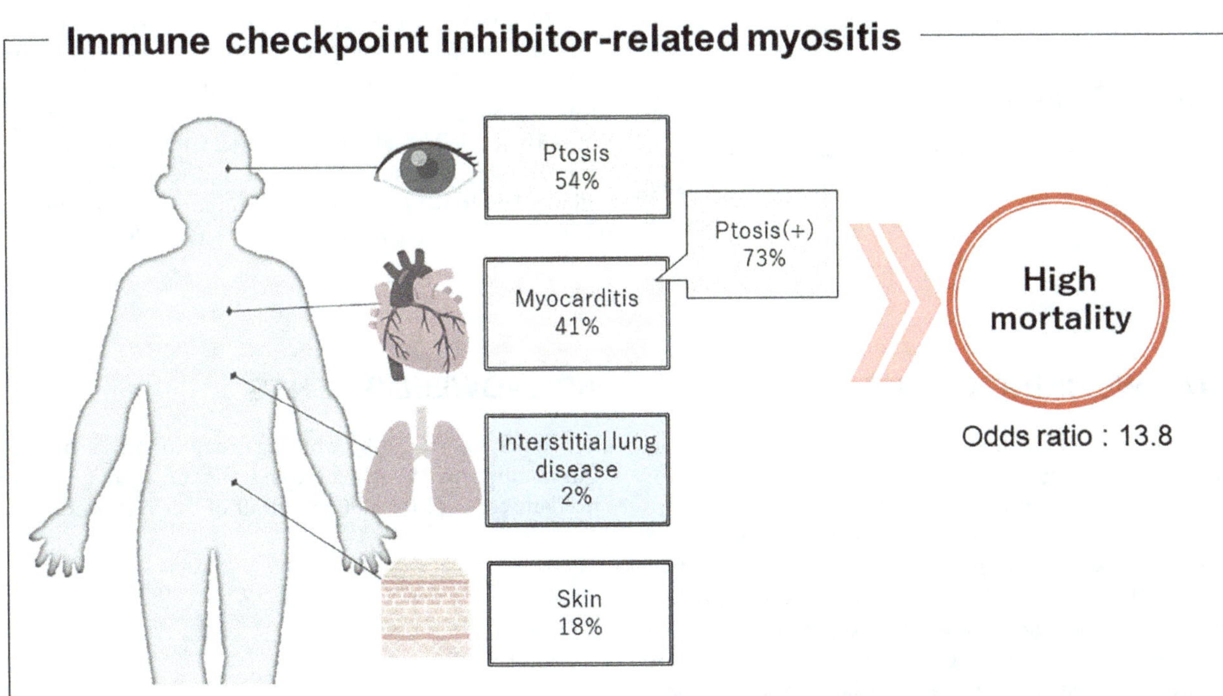

FIGURE 3 | Presumptive clinical features regarding immune checkpoint inhibitor-related myositis. Development of concomitant myocarditis might be predicted by ptosis, therefore, can help prevent the potentially fatal outcome.

a specific human leukocyte antigen suggests that there may be some immunological predisposition, although no association between irAEs and human leukocyte antigen has been identified as yet (109, 110). The time from the initiation of ICI to the onset of myositis and characteristic symptoms that overlap with myasthenia gravis, such as ptosis as reported in this study, may be important in distinguishing between ICI-related myositis and myositis because of malignancy.

A limitation of this study is that ICI-related myositis is a rare complication, and while its incidence can be calculated from RCT data, it was not possible to extract the clinical characteristics of individual cases. Diagnosis of myositis and myasthenia gravis or myocarditis is made by clinicians, and there are no standard criteria for diagnosis. In particular, myasthenia gravis is diagnosed even in cases where anti-acetylcholine receptor antibodies are not detected, and further clarification of phenotypes are needed. Myositis-associated autoantibodies can help define subgroups of patients in terms of the clinical phenotype of IIM, but published case reports did not always provide information on myositis-specific antibodies.

Now that this study has shed light on the clinical characteristics of ICI-related myositis, further accumulation of cases from around the world will enable the development of more detailed algorithms for diagnosis and treatment.

ETHICS STATEMENT

The studies involving human participants were reviewed and approved by the Ethics committee of Yokohama City University. The patients/participants provided their written informed consent to participate in this study.

YCU irAE WORKING GROUP

The following Authors, who are listed in numerical order, contributed to the work of YCU irAE Working Group: Naoki Hamada, Department of Stem Cell and Immune Regulation, Yokohama City University Graduate School of Medicine, Kanazawa-ku, Japan; Yohei Kirino, Department of Stem Cell and Immune Regulation, Yokohama City University Graduate School of Medicine, Kanazawa-ku, Japan; Motohiko Tokuhisa, Department of Oncology, Yokohama City University Graduate School of Medicine, Kanazawa-ku, Japan; Keiichi Kondo, Department of Urology, Yokohama City University Graduate School of Medicine, Kanazawa-ku, Japan; Noboru Nakaigawa, Department of Urology, Yokohama City University Graduate School of Medicine, Kanazawa-ku, Japan; Nobuaki Kobayashi, Department of Pulmonology, Yokohama City University Graduate School of Medicine, Kanazawa-ku, Japan; Daisuke Sano, Department of Otorhinolaryngology, Head and Neck Surgery, Yokohama City University School of Medicine, Kanazawa-ku, Japan; Maki Hagihara, Department of Stem Cell and Immune Regulation, Yokohama City University Graduate School of Medicine, Kanazawa-ku, Japan; Nobuhiko Oridate, Department of Otorhinolaryngology, Head and Neck Surgery, Yokohama City University School of Medicine, Kanazawa-ku, Japan; Takeshi Kaneko, Department of Pulmonology, Yokohama City University Graduate School of Medicine, Kanazawa-ku, Japan; Yukie Yamaguchi, Department of Environmental Immuno-Dermatology, Yokohama City University Graduate School of Medicine, Kanazawa-ku, Japan; Masahiro Yao, Department of Urology, Yokohama City University Graduate School of Medicine, Kanazawa-ku, Japan; Yasushi Ichikawa, Department of Oncology, Yokohama City University Graduate School of Medicine, Kanazawa-ku, Japan; Hideaki Nakajima, Department of Stem Cell and Immune Regulation, Yokohama City University Graduate School of Medicine, Kanazawa-ku, Japan.

AUTHOR CONTRIBUTIONS

NaH, AM, KT-M, and YK designed the research. NaH, AM, KT-M, HoN, and NoH conducted the research, statistical analysis, as well as the interpretation of the data. NaH, AM, KT-M, and YK drafted the manuscript. YS, RY, HoN, and HiN were involved in writing the article or revising it critically for important intellectual content, and all authors approved the final version to be published. NaH, AM and KT-M had full access to all the data in the study and takes responsibility for the integrity of the data and the accuracy of the data analysis.

ACKNOWLEDGMENTS

We thank the YCU irAE working group for advice on preparing this manuscript. We thank Helen Roberton, from Edanz (https://jp.edanz.com/ac) for editing a draft of this manuscript.

REFERENCES

1. Singh S, Hassan D, Aldawsari HM, Molugulu N, Shukla R, Kesharwani P. Immune Checkpoint Inhibitors: A Promising Anticancer Therapy. *Drug Discov Today* (2020) 25(1):223–9. doi: 10.1016/j.drudis.2019.11.003
2. Havel JJ, Chowell D, Chan TA. The Evolving Landscape of Biomarkers for Checkpoint Inhibitor Immunotherapy. *Nat Rev Cancer* (2019) 19(3):133–50. doi: 10.1038/s41568-019-0116-x
3. Nakamura Y. Biomarkers for Immune Checkpoint Inhibitor-Mediated Tumor Response and Adverse Events. *Front Med (Lausanne)* (2019) 6:119. doi: 10.3389/fmed.2019.00119
4. Michot JM, Bigenwald C, Champiat S, Collins M, Carbonnel F, Postel-Vinay S, et al. Immune-Related Adverse Events With Immune Checkpoint Blockade: A Comprehensive Review. *Eur J Cancer* (2016) 54:139–48. doi: 10.1016/j.ejca.2015.11.016
5. Postow MA, Sidlow R, Hellmann MD. Immune-Related Adverse Events Associated With Immune Checkpoint Blockade. *N Engl J Med* (2018) 378 (2):158–68. doi: 10.1056/NEJMra1703481
6. Kostine M, Finckh A, Bingham CO, Visser K, Leipe J, Schulze-Koops H, et al. EULAR Points to Consider for the Diagnosis and Management of Rheumatic Immune-Related Adverse Events Due to Cancer Immunotherapy With Checkpoint Inhibitors. *Ann Rheum Dis* (2021) 80 (1):36–48. doi: 10.1136/annrheumdis-2020-217139
7. Kadota H, Gono T, Shirai Y, Okazaki Y, Takeno M, Kuwana M. Immune Checkpoint Inhibitor-Induced Myositis: A Case Report and Literature Review. *Curr Rheumatol Rep* (2019) 21:10. doi: 10.1007/s11926-019-0811-3
8. Pathak R, Katel A, Massarelli E, Villaflor VM, Sun V, Salgia R. Immune Checkpoint Inhibitor-Induced Myocarditis With Myositis/Myasthenia Gravis Overlap Syndrome: A Systematic Review of Cases. *Oncologist* (2021). doi: 10.1002/onco.13931
9. Liberati A, Altman DG, Tetzlaff J, Mulrow C, Gøtzsche PC, Ioannidis JPA, et al. The PRISMA Statement for Reporting Systematic Reviews and Meta-Analyses of Studies That Evaluate Healthcare Interventions: Explanation and Elaboration. *BMJ* (2009) 339:b2700. doi: 10.1136/bmj.b2700
10. Page MJ, McKenzie JE, Bossuyt PM, Boutron I, Hoffmann TC, Mulrow CD, et al. The PRISMA 2020 Statement: An Updated Guideline for Reporting Systematic Reviews. *BMJ* (2021) 372:n71. doi: 10.1136/bmj.n71
11. UMIN Center. *UMIN Clinical Trials Registry (UMIN-CTR)*. Available at: https://www.umin.ac.jp/ctr/ctr_regist.htm (Accessed September 20, 2021).
12. Higgins JP, Altman DG, Gøtzsche PC, Jüni P, Moher D, Oxman AD, et al. The Cochrane Collaboration's Tool for Assessing Risk of Bias in Randomised Trials. *BMJ* (2011) 343:d5928. doi: 10.1136/bmj.d5928
13. André T, Shiu KK, Kim TW, Jensen BV, Jensen LH, Punt C, et al. Pembrolizumab in Microsatellite-Instability-High Advanced Colorectal Cancer. *N Engl J Med* (2020) 383:2207–18. doi: 10.1056/NEJMoa2017699
14. Eggermont AMM, Blank CU, Mandala M, Long GV, Atkinson V, Dalle S, et al. Adjuvant Pembrolizumab Versus Placebo in Resected Stage III Melanoma. *N Engl J Med* (2018) 378:1789–801. doi: 10.1056/NEJMoa1802357
15. Ferris RL, Blumenschein GJr, Fayette J, Guigay J, Colevas AD, Licitra L, et al. Nivolumab for Recurrent Squamous-Cell Carcinoma of the Head and Neck. *N Engl J Med* (2016) 375:1856–67. doi: 10.1056/NEJMoa1602252
16. Galsky MD, Arija JAA, Bamias A, Davis ID, De Santis M, Kikuchi E, et al. Atezolizumab With or Without Chemotherapy in Metastatic Urothelial Cancer (IMvigor130): A Multicentre, Randomised, Placebo-Controlled Phase 3 Trial. *Lancet* (2020) 395:1547–57. doi: 10.1016/s0140-6736(20) 30230-0
17. Gutzmer R, Stroyakovskiy D, Gogas H, Robert C, Lewis K, Protsenko S, et al. Atezolizumab, Vemurafenib, and Cobimetinib as First-Line Treatment for Unresectable Advanced BRAF V600 Mutation-Positive Melanoma (IMspire150): Primary Analysis of the Randomised, Double-Blind, Placebo-Controlled, Phase 3 Trial. *Lancet* (2020) 395:1835–44. doi: 10.1016/S0140-6736(20)30934-X
18. Kojima T, Shah MA, Muro K, Francois E, Adenis A, Hsu CH, et al. Randomized Phase III KEYNOTE-181 Study of Pembrolizumab Versus Chemotherapy in Advanced Esophageal Cancer. *J Clin Oncol* (2020) 38:4138–48. doi: 10.1200/JCO.20.01888
19. Kuruvilla J, Ramchandren R, Santoro A, Paszkiewicz-Kozik E, Gasiorowski R, Johnson NA, et al. Pembrolizumab Versus Brentuximab Vedotin in Relapsed or Refractory Classical Hodgkin Lymphoma (KEYNOTE-204): An Interim Analysis of a Multicentre, Randomised, Open-Label, Phase 3 Study. *Lancet Oncol* (2021) 22:512–24. doi: 10.1016/S1470-2045(21)00005-X
20. Miles D, Gligorov J, André F, Cameron D, Schneeweiss A, Barrios C, et al. Primary Results From IMpassion131, a Double-Blind, Placebo-Controlled, Randomised Phase III Trial of First-Line Paclitaxel With or Without Atezolizumab for Unresectable Locally Advanced/metastatic Triple-Negative Breast Cancer. *Ann Oncol* (2021) 32:994–1004. doi: 10.1016/j.annonc.2021.05.801
21. Mittendorf EA, Zhang H, Barrios CH, Saji S, Jung KH, Hegg R, et al. Neoadjuvant Atezolizumab in Combination With Sequential Nab-Paclitaxel and Anthracycline-Based Chemotherapy Versus Placebo and Chemotherapy in Patients With Early-Stage Triple-Negative Breast Cancer (IMpassion031): A Randomised, Double-Blind, Phase 3 Trial. *Lancet* (2020) 396:1090–100. doi: 10.1016/S0140-6736(20)31953-X
22. Moore KN, Bookman M, Sehouli J, Miller A, Anderson C, Scambia G, et al. Atezolizumab, Bevacizumab, and Chemotherapy for Newly Diagnosed Stage III or IV Ovarian Cancer: Placebo-Controlled Randomized Phase III Trial (IMagyn050/GOG 3015/ENGOT-Ov39). *J Clin Oncol* (2021) 39:1842–55. doi: 10.1200/JCO.21.00306
23. Powles T, Duran I, van der Heijden MS, Loriot Y, Vogelzang NJ, De Giorgi U, et al. Atezolizumab Versus Chemotherapy in Patients With Platinum-Treated Locally Advanced or Metastatic Urothelial Carcinoma (IMvigor211): A Multicentre, Open-Label, Phase 3 Randomised Controlled Trial. *Lancet* (2018) 391:748–57. doi: 10.1016/s0140-6736(17) 33297-x
24. Powles T, Park SH, Voog E, Caserta C, Valderrama BP, Gurney H, et al. Avelumab Maintenance Therapy for Advanced or Metastatic Urothelial Carcinoma. *N Engl J Med* (2020) 383:1218–30. doi: 10.1056/NEJMoa2002788
25. Reck M, Luft A, Szczesna A, Havel L, Kim SW, Akerley W, et al. Phase III Randomized Trial of Ipilimumab Plus Etoposide and Platinum Versus Placebo Plus Etoposide and Platinum in Extensive-Stage Small-Cell Lung Cancer. *J Clin Oncol* (2016) 34:3740–8. doi: 10.1200/JCO.2016.67.6601
26. Rini BI, Plimack ER, Stus V, Gafanov R, Hawkins R, Nosov D, et al. Pembrolizumab Plus Axitinib Versus Sunitinib for Advanced Renal-Cell Carcinoma. *N Engl J Med* (2019) 380:1116–27. doi: 10.1056/NEJMoa1816714
27. Rini BI, Powles T, Atkins MB, Escudier B, McDermott DF, Suarez C, et al. Atezolizumab Plus Bevacizumab Versus Sunitinib in Patients With Previously Untreated Metastatic Renal Cell Carcinoma (IMmotion151): A Multicentre, Open-Label, Phase 3, Randomised Controlled Trial. *Lancet* (2019) 393:2404–15. doi: 10.1016/S0140-6736(19)30723-8
28. Rudin CM, Awad MM, Navarro A, Gottfried M, Peters S, Csoszi T, et al. Pembrolizumab or Placebo Plus Etoposide and Platinum as First-Line Therapy for Extensive-Stage Small-Cell Lung Cancer: Randomized, Double-Blind, Phase III KEYNOTE-604 Study. *J Clin Oncol* (2020) 38:2369–79. doi: 10.1200/JCO.20.00793
29. Schmid P, Cortes J, Pusztai L, McArthur H, Kümmel S, Bergh J, et al. Pembrolizumab for Early Triple-Negative Breast Cancer. *N Engl J Med* (2020) 382:810–21. doi: 10.1056/NEJMoa1910549
30. Winer EP, Lipatov O, Im SA, Goncalves A, Munoz-Couselo E, Lee KS, et al. Pembrolizumab Versus Investigator-Choice Chemotherapy for Metastatic Triple-Negative Breast Cancer (KEYNOTE-119): A Randomised, Open-Label, Phase 3 Trial. *Lancet Oncol* (2021) 22:499–511. doi: 10.1016/S1470-2045(20)30754-3
31. Allawh T, Quinn A, Joseph V, Khan HH. Pembrolizumab-Induced Necrotizing Polymyositis: A Case Presentation. *J Clin Rheumatol* (2020) 26(7):e268. doi: 10.1097/RHU.0000000000001119
32. Asano R, Shinoda K, Tsuda R, Hounoki H, Kawataka M, Makino T, et al. Anti-Tif1γ Antibody-Positive Dermatomyositis in a 15-Year-Old Boy With Epstein-Barr Virus-Related Nasopharyngeal Cancer Receiving Nivolumab. *Rheumatol (Oxford)* (2021) 60(6):e197–9. doi: 10.1093/rheumatology/keaa832
33. Badovinac S, Korsic M, Zarkovic K, Mursic D, Roglic M, Jakopovic M, et al. Nivolumab-Induced Synchronous Occurrence of Myositis and

Hypothyroidism in a Patient With Squamous Cell Lung Cancer. *Immunotherapy* (2018) 10(6):427–31. doi: 10.2217/imt-2017-0174
34. Behling J, Kaes J, Münzel T, Grabbe S, Loquai C. New-Onset Third-Degree Atrioventricular Block Because of Autoimmune-Induced Myositis Under Treatment With Anti-Programmed Cell Death-1 (Nivolumab) for Metastatic Melanoma. *Melanoma Res* (2017) 27(2):155–8. doi: 10.1097/CMR.0000000000000314
35. Berger M, Legeay AL, Souci S, Streichenberger N, Thomas L, Dalle S. Pembrolizumab-Induced Dermatomyositis in a Patient With Metastatic Melanoma. *Eur J Cancer* (2018) 104:227–30. doi: 10.1016/j.ejca.2018.08.021
36. Bilen MA, Subudhi SK, Gao J, Tannir NM, Tu SM, Sharma P. Acute Rhabdomyolysis With Severe Polymyositis Following Ipilimumab-Nivolumab Treatment in a Cancer Patient With Elevated Anti-Striated Muscle Antibody. *J Immunother Cancer* (2016) 4:36. doi: 10.1186/s40425-016-0139-8
37. Botta C, Agostino RM, Dattola V, Cianci V, Calandruccio ND, Bianco G, et al. Myositis/Myasthenia After Pembrolizumab in a Bladder Cancer Patient With an Autoimmunity-Associated HLA: Immune-Biological Evaluation and Case Report. *Int J Mol Sci* (2021) 22(12). doi: 10.3390/ijms22126246
38. Bourgeois-Vionnet J, Joubert B, Bernard E, Sia MA, Pante V, Fabien N, et al. Nivolumab-Induced Myositis: A Case Report and a Literature Review. *J Neurol Sci* (2018) 387:51–3. doi: 10.1016/j.jns.2018.01.030
39. Chen JH, Lee KY, Hu CJ, Chung CC. Coexisting Myasthenia Gravis, Myositis, and Polyneuropathy Induced by Ipilimumab and Nivolumab in a Patient With Non-Small-Cell Lung Cancer: A Case Report and Literature Review. *Medicine* (2017) 96(50):e9262. doi: 10.1097/MD.0000000000009262
40. Claus J, Van Den Bergh A, Verbeek S, Wauters E, Nackaerts K. Pembrolizumab-Induced Necrotizing Myositis in a Patient With Metastatic Non-Small-Cell Lung Cancer: A Case Report. *Lung Cancer Manag* (2019) 8(2):Lmt10. doi: 10.2217/lmt-2018-0017
41. Diamantopoulos PT, Tsatsou K, Benopoulou O, Anastasopoulou A, Gogas H. Inflammatory Myopathy and Axonal Neuropathy in a Patient With Melanoma Following Pembrolizumab Treatment. *J Immunother* (2017) 40 (6):221–3. doi: 10.1097/CJI.0000000000000172
42. Fazal M, Prentice DA, Kho LK, Fysh E. Nivolumab-Associated Myositis Myocarditis and Myasthenia and Anti-Striated Muscle Antibodies. *Intern Med J* (2020) 50(8):1003–6. doi: 10.1111/imj.14946
43. Fazel M, Jedlowski PM. Severe Myositis, Myocarditis, and Myasthenia Gravis With Elevated Anti-Striated Muscle Antibody Following Single Dose of Ipilimumab-Nivolumab Therapy in a Patient With Metastatic Melanoma. *Case Rep Immunol* (2019) 2019:2539493. doi: 10.1155/2019/2539493
44. Finsterer J. Pembrolizumab-Induced Hypothyroidism Manifesting as Myopathy and Psychosis. *Melanoma Res* (2021) 31(4):405–6. doi: 10.1097/CMR.0000000000000759
45. Fox E, Dabrow M, Ochsner G. A Case of Nivolumab-Induced Myositis. *Oncologist* (2016) 21(12):e3. doi: 10.1634/theoncologist.2016-0170
46. Gandiga PC, Wang AR, Gonzalez-Rivera T, Sreih AG. Pembrolizumab-Associated Inflammatory Myopathy. *Rheumatol (Oxford)* (2018) 57(2):397–8. doi: 10.1093/rheumatology/kex346
47. Haddox CL, Shenoy N, Shah KK, Kao JC, Jain S, Halfdanarson TR, et al. Pembrolizumab Induced Bulbar Myopathy and Respiratory Failure With Necrotizing Myositis of the Diaphragm. *Ann Oncol* (2017) 28(3):673–5. doi: 10.1093/annonc/mdw655
48. Hamada S, Fuseya Y, Tsukino M. Pembrolizumab-Induced Rhabdomyolysis With Myositis in a Patient With Lung Adenocarcinoma. *Arch Bronconeumol* (2018) 54(6):346–8. doi: 10.1016/j.arbres.2018.01.026
49. Hayakawa N, Kikuchi E, Suzuki S, Oya M. Myasthenia Gravis With Myositis Induced by Pembrolizumab Therapy in a Patient With Metastatic Urothelial Carcinoma. *Int Cancer Conf J* (2020) 9(3):123–6. doi: 10.1007/s13691-020-00408-4
50. Hellman JB, Traynis I, Lin LK. Pembrolizumab and Epacadostat Induced Fatal Myocarditis and Myositis Presenting as a Case of Ptosis and Ophthalmoplegia. *Orbit* (2019) 38(3):244–7. doi: 10.1080/01676830.2018.1490439
51. Hibino M, Maeda K, Horiuchi S, Fukuda M, Kondo T. Pembrolizumab-Induced Myasthenia Gravis With Myositis in a Patient With Lung Cancer. *Respirol Case Rep* (2018) 6(7):e00355. doi: 10.1002/rcr2.355
52. Hinogami H, Yamashita C, Tanaka A, Shirai H, Nakano Y, Matsuura Y. Case of Dermatomyositis During Treatment With Pembrolizumab for Lung Cancer. *J Dermatol* (2019) 46(11):e430–2. doi: 10.1111/1346-8138.14993
53. Huh SY, Shin SH, Kim MK, Lee SY, Son KH, Shin HY. Emergence of Myasthenia Gravis With Myositis in a Patient Treated With Pembrolizumab for Thymic Cancer. *J Clin Neurol* (2018) 14(1):115–7. doi: 10.3988/jcn.2018.14.1.115
54. Hunter G, Voll C, Robinson CA. Autoimmune Inflammatory Myopathy After Treatment With Ipilimumab. *Can J Neurol Sci* (2009) 36(4):518–20. doi: 10.1017/s0317167100007939
55. Kamo H, Hatano T, Kanai K, Aoki N, Kamiyama D, Yokoyama K, et al. Pembrolizumab-Related Systemic Myositis Involving Ocular and Hindneck Muscles Resembling Myasthenic Gravis: A Case Report. *BMC Neurol* (2019) 19(1):184. doi: 10.1186/s12883-019-1416-1
56. Kartolo A, Towheed T, Mates M. A Case of Successful Pembrolizumab Rechallenge in a Patient With Non-Small-Cell Lung Cancer and Grade 3 Dermatomyositis. *Immunotherapy* (2021) 13(6):477–81. doi: 10.2217/imt-2020-0309
57. Kim JS, Nam TS, Kim J, Kho BG, Park CK, Oh IJ, et al. Myasthenia Gravis and Myopathy After Nivolumab Treatment for Non-Small Cell Lung Carcinoma: A Case Report. *Thorac Cancer* (2019) 10(10):2045–9. doi: 10.1111/1759-7714.13177
58. Kimura T, Fukushima S, Miyashita A, Aoi J, Jinnin M, Kosaka T, et al. Myasthenic Crisis and Polymyositis Induced by One Dose of Nivolumab. *Cancer Sci* (2016) 107(7):1055–8. doi: 10.1111/cas.12961
59. Kobayashi T, Guo YM, Yamashita T, Nara M, Yoshioka T, Kameoka Y, et al. Relationship Between Clinical Course of Nivolumab-Related Myositis and Immune Status in a Patient With Hodgkin's Lymphoma After Allogeneic Hematopoietic Stem Cell Transplantation. *Int J Hematol* (2019) 109(3):356–60. doi: 10.1007/s12185-018-02584-9
60. Koh B, Tuite K, Khattak A, Dyke JM. Lymphocyte Involvement in Nivolumab-Induced Autoimmune Myositis. *Pathology* (2019) 51(5):555–7. doi: 10.1016/j.pathol.2019.02.006
61. Kosche C, Stout M, Sosman J, Lukas RV, Choi JN. Dermatomyositis in a Patient Undergoing Nivolumab Therapy for Metastatic Melanoma: A Case Report and Review of the Literature. *Melanoma Res* (2020) 30(3):313–6. doi: 10.1097/CMR.0000000000000642
62. Kudo F, Watanabe Y, Iwai Y, Miwa C, Nagai Y, Ota H, et al. Advanced Lung Adenocarcinoma With Nivolumab-Associated Dermatomyositis. *Intern Med* (2018) 57(15):2217–21. doi: 10.2169/internalmedicine.9381-17
63. Lie G, Weickhardt A, Kearney L, Lam Q, John T, Liew D, et al. Nivolumab Resulting in Persistently Elevated Troponin Levels Despite Clinical Remission of Myocarditis and Myositis in a Patient With Malignant Pleural Mesothelioma: Case Report. *Transl Lung Cancer Res* (2020) 9 (2):360–5. doi: 10.21037/tlcr.2020.02.05
64. Liu WK, Naban N, Kaul A, Patel N, Fusi A. Life-Threatening Polymyositis With Spontaneous Hematoma Induced by Nivolumab in a Patient With Previously Resected Melanoma. *Melanoma Res* (2021) 31(1):85–7. doi: 10.1097/CMR.0000000000000706
65. Matsui H, Kawai T, Sato Y, Ishida J, Kadowaki H, Akiyama Y, et al. A Fatal Case of Myocarditis Following Myositis Induced by Pembrolizumab Treatment for Metastatic Upper Urinary Tract Urothelial Carcinoma. *Int Heart J* (2020) 61(5):1070–4. doi: 10.1536/ihj.20-162
66. Messer A, Drozd B, Glitza IC, Lu H, Patel AB. Dermatomyositis Associated With Nivolumab Therapy for Melanoma: A Case Report and Review of the Literature. *Dermatol Online J* (2020) 26(8). doi: 10.5070/D3268049887
67. Nakanishi S, Nishida S, Miyazato M, Goya M, Saito S. A Case Report of Nivolumab-Induced Myasthenia Gravis and Myositis in a Metastatic Renal Cell Carcinoma Patient. *Urol Case Rep* (2020) 29:101105. doi: 10.1016/j.eucr.2019.101105
68. Nosaki Y, Mashimo S, Watanabe M, Yokoi T, Kobayashi Y, Iwai K. Paraspinal Muscle Involvement in Pembrolizumab-Associated Myositis. *Oxf Med Case Rep* (2020) 2020(2):omaa003. doi: 10.1093/omcr/omaa003
69. Okubo N, Kijima T, Nukui A, Kamai T. Immune-Related Myositis Resulting From Combination Therapy of Ipilimumab and Nivolumab in Patient With Metastatic Renal Cell Carcinoma. *BMJ Case Rep* (2020) 13(9). doi: 10.1136/bcr-2020-235199
70. Onda A, Miyagawa S, Takahashi N, Gochi M, Takagi M, Nishino I, et al. Pembrolizumab-Induced Ocular Myasthenia Gravis With Anti-Titin

Antibody and Necrotizing Myopathy. *Intern Med* (2019) 58(11):1635–8. doi: 10.2169/internalmedicine.1956-18

71. Osaki M, Tachikawa R, Ohira J, Hara S, Tomii K. Anti-Transcriptional Intermediary Factor 1-γ Antibody-Positive Dermatomyositis Induced by Nivolumab for Lung Adenocarcinoma: A Case Report. *Invest New Drugs* (2021) 39(1):251–5. doi: 10.1007/s10637-020-00974-7
72. Pagkopoulou E, Simopoulou T, Maragkouli E, Perifanou-Sotiri S, Kotsakis A, Bogdanos DP. Arthritis and Myositis in a Patient Treated With Programmed Cell Death-1 (PD-1) Inhibitor Pembrolizumab for Lung Cancer. *Mediterr J Rheumatol* (2020) 31(3):355–7. doi: 10.31138/mjr.31.3.355
73. Peverelli L, De Rosa A, Domina E, Ciscato P, Sita G, Velardo D, et al. Severe Inflammatory Myopathy in a Pulmonary Carcinoma Patient Treated With Pembrolizumab: An Alert for Myologists. *J Neuromuscul Dis* (2020) 7 (4):511–4. doi: 10.3233/JND-200504
74. Rus T, Kramberger MG, Jakob GB, Leonardis L, Meznaric M. Life-Threatening Myositis After One Dose of Nivolumab in a Patient With Nonmetastatic Completely Resected Cutaneous Melanoma. *Acta Neurol Belg* (2021). doi: 10.1007/s13760-021-01760-9
75. Saini L, Chua N. Severe Inflammatory Myositis in a Patient Receiving Concurrent Nivolumab and Azacitidine. *Leuk Lymphoma* (2017) 58 (8):2011–3. doi: 10.1080/10428194.2016.1265115
76. Sanchez-Sancho P, Selva-O'Callaghan A, Trallero-Araguás E, Ros J, Montoro B. Myositis and Myasteniform Syndrome Related to Pembrolizumab. *BMJ Case Rep* (2021) 14(7). doi: 10.1136/bcr-2021-241766
77. Ali SS, Goddard AL, Luke JJ, Donahue H, Todd DJ, Werchniak A, et al. Drug-Associated Dermatomyositis Following Ipilimumab Therapy: A Novel Immune-Mediated Adverse Event Associated With Cytotoxic T-Lymphocyte Antigen 4 Blockade. *JAMA Dermatol* (2015) 151(2):195–9. doi: 10.1001/jamadermatol.2014.2233
78. Shibata C, Kato J, Toda N, Imai M, Fukumura Y, Arai J, et al. Paraneoplastic Dermatomyositis Appearing After Nivolumab Therapy for Gastric Cancer: A Case Report. *J Med Case Rep* (2019) 13(1):168. doi: 10.1186/s13256-019-2105-9
79. Shikano K, Kaneko K, Kaburaki K, Isobe K, Kawabe K, Homma S, et al. Nivolumab-Induced Anti-Aminoacyl-tRNA Synthetase Antibody-Positive Polymyositis Complicated by Interstitial Pneumonia in a Patient With Lung Adenocarcinoma. *Scand J Rheumatol* (2020) 49(1):82–3. doi: 10.1080/03009742.2019.1596309
80. Sutaria R, Patel P, Danve A. Autoimmune Myositis and Myasthenia Gravis Resulting From a Combination Therapy With Nivolumab and Ipilimumab for Metastatic Melanoma. *Eur J Rheumatol* (2019) 6(3):153–4. doi: 10.5152/eurjrheum.2019.18159
81. Swali R. Pembrolizumab-Induced Myositis in the Setting of Metastatic Melanoma: An Increasingly Common Phenomenon. *J Clin Aesthet Dermatol* (2020) 13(6):44–5.
82. Takahashi S, Mukohara S, Hatachi S, Yamashita M, Kumagai S. A Case of Myositis With Dropped Head Syndrome and Anti-Titin Antibody Positivity Induced by Pembrolizumab. *Scand J Rheumatol* (2020) 49(6):509–11. doi: 10.1080/03009742.2020.1760346
83. Takatsuki K, Yanagihara T, Egashira A, Ogo N, Yoshizawa S, Sunami S, et al. A Rare Case of Pembrolizumab-Induced Dermatomyositis in a Patient With Cancer of Unknown Primary Origin. *Am J Case Rep* (2021) 22:e930286. doi: 10.12659/AJCR.930286
84. Tan RYC, Toh CK, Takano A. Continued Response to One Dose of Nivolumab Complicated by Myasthenic Crisis and Myositis. *J Thorac Oncol* (2017) 12(7):e90–1. doi: 10.1016/j.jtho.2017.02.024
85. Tauber M, Cohen R, Laly P, Josselin L, André T, Mekinian A. Severe Necrotizing Myositis Associated With Long Term Anti-Neoplastic Efficacy Following Nivolumab Plus Ipilimumab Combination Therapy. *Clin Rheumatol* (2019) 38(2):601–2. doi: 10.1007/s10067-018-4373-y
86. Todo M, Kaneko G, Shirotake S, Shimada Y, Nakano S, Okabe T, et al. Pembrolizumab-Induced Myasthenia Gravis With Myositis and Presumable Myocarditis in a Patient With Bladder Cancer. *IJU Case Rep* (2019) 3(1):17–20. doi: 10.1002/iju5.12128
87. Uchio N, Unuma A, Kakumoto T, Osaki M, Zenke Y, Sakuta K, et al. Pembrolizumab on Pre-Existing Inclusion Body Myositis: A Case Report. *BMC Rheumatol* (2020) 4:48. doi: 10.1186/s41927-020-00144-5
88. Valenti-Azcarate R, Vazquez IE, Illan CT, Gastearena MAI, Pérez-Larraya JG. Nivolumab and Ipilimumab-Induced Myositis and Myocarditis Mimicking a Myasthenia Gravis Presentation. *Neuromuscul Disord* (2020) 30(1):67–9. doi: 10.1016/j.nmd.2019.10.006
89. Vallet H, Gaillet A, Weiss N, Vanhaecke C, Saheb S, Touitou V, et al. Pembrolizumab-Induced Necrotic Myositis in a Patient With Metastatic Melanoma. *Ann Oncol* (2016) 27(7):1352–3. doi: 10.1093/annonc/mdw126
90. Veccia A, Kinspergher S, Grego E, Peterlana D, Berti A, Tranquillini E, et al. Myositis and Myasthenia During Nivolumab Administration for Advanced Lung Aancer: A Case Report and Review of the Literature. *Anticancer Drugs* (2020) 31(5):540–4. doi: 10.1097/CAD.0000000000000903
91. Wiggins CJ, Chon SY. Dermatomyositis, Pembrolizumab, and Squamous Cell Carcinoma of the Lung. *Proc (Bayl Univ Med Cent)* (2020) 34(1):120–1. doi: 10.1080/08998280.2020.1811189
92. Yamaguchi Y, Abe R, Haga N, Shimizu H. A Case of Drug-Associated Dermatomyositis Following Ipilimumab Therapy. *Eur J Dermatol* (2016) 26 (3):320–1. doi: 10.1684/ejd.2016.2770
93. Yoshioka M, Kambe N, Yamamoto Y, Suehiro K, Matsue H. Case of Respiratory Discomfort Due to Myositis After Administration of Nivolumab. *J Dermatol* (2015) 42(10):1008–9. doi: 10.1111/1346-8138.12991
94. Johnson ED, Kerrigan K, Butler K, Patel SB. Nivolumab-Induced Hypothyoidism With Consequent Hypothyroid Related Myopathy. *J Oncol Pharm Pract* (2020) 26(1):224–7. doi: 10.1177/1078155219835912
95. Liao B, Shroff S, Kamiya-Matsuoka C, Tummala S. Atypical Neurological Complications of Ipilimumab Therapy in Patients With Metastatic Melanoma. *Neuro Oncol* (2014) 16(4):589–93. doi: 10.1093/neuonc/nou001
96. Fuentes-Antrás J, Peinado P, Guevara-Hoyer K, Arco CDD, Sánchez-Ramón S, Aguado C. Fatal Autoimmune Storm After a Single Cycle of Anti-PD-1 Therapy: A Case of Lethal Toxicity But Pathological Complete Response in Metastatic Lung Adenocarcinoma. *Hematol Oncol Stem Cell Ther* (2020) S1658-3876(20):30098–4. doi: 10.1016/j.hemonc.2020.04.006
97. Imai R, Ono M, Nishimura N, Suzuki K, Komiyama N, Tamura T. Fulminant Myocarditis Caused by an Immune Checkpoint Inhibitor: A Case Report With Pathologic Findings. *J Thorac Oncol* (2019) 14:e36–8. doi: 10.1016/j.jtho.2018.10.156
98. Jeyakumar N, Etchegaray M, Henry J, Lelenwa L, Zhao B, Segura A, et al. The Terrible Triad of Checkpoint Inhibition: A Case Report of Myasthenia Gravis, Myocarditis, and Myositis Induced by Cemiplimab in a Patient With Metastatic Cutaneous Squamous Cell Carcinoma. *Case Rep Immunol* (2020) 2020:5126717. doi: 10.1155/2020/5126717
99. Monge C, Maeng H, Brofferio A, Apolo AB, Sathya B, Arai AE, et al. Myocarditis in a Patient Treated With Nivolumab and PROSTVAC: A Case Report. *J Immunother Cancer* (2018) 6:150. doi: 10.1186/s40425-018-0473-0
100. Nasr F, El Rassy E, Maalouf G, Azar C, Haddad F, Helou J, et al. Severe Ophthalmoplegia and Myocarditis Following the Administration of Pembrolizumab. *Eur J Cancer* (2018) 91:171–3. doi: 10.1016/j.ejca.2017.11.026
101. Sessums M, Yarrarapu S, Guru PK, Sanghavi DK. Atezolizumab-Induced Myositis and Myocarditis in a Patient With Metastatic Urothelial Carcinoma. *BMJ Case Rep* (2020) 13:e236357. doi: 10.1136/bcr-2020-236357
102. Shah M, Tayar JH, Abdel-Wahab N, Suarez-Almazor ME. Myositis as an Adverse Event of Immune Checkpoint Blockade for Cancer Therapy. *Semin Arthritis Rheum* (2019) 48:736–40. doi: 10.1016/j.semarthrit.2018.05.006
103. Shirai T, Kiniwa Y, Sato R, Sano T, Nakamura K, Mikoshiba Y, et al. Presence of Antibodies to Striated Muscle and Acetylcholine Receptor in Association With Occurrence of Myasthenia Gravis With Myositis and Myocarditis in a Patient With Melanoma Treated With an Anti-Programmed Death 1 Antibody. *Eur J Cancer* (2019) 106:193–5. doi: 10.1016/j.ejca.2018.10.025
104. So H, Ikeguchi R, Kobayashi M, Suzuki M, Shimizu Y, Kitagawa K. PD-1 Inhibitor-Associated Severe Myasthenia Gravis With Necrotizing Myopathy and Myocarditis. *J Neurol Sci* (2019) 399:97–100. doi: 10.1016/j.jns.2019.02.023
105. Xing Q, Zhang ZW, Lin QH, Shen LH, Wang PM, Zhang S, et al. Myositis-Myasthenia Gravis Overlap Syndrome Complicated With Myasthenia Crisis and Myocarditis Associated With Anti-Programmed Cell Death-1 (Sintilimab) Therapy for Lung Adenocarcinoma. *Ann Transl Med* (2020) 8:250. doi: 10.21037/atm.2020.01.79

106. Lipe DN, Galvis-Carvajal E, Rajha E, Wechsler AH, Gaeta S. Immune Checkpoint Inhibitor-Associated Myasthenia Gravis, Myositis, and Myocarditis Overlap Syndrome. *Am J Emerg Med* (2021) 46:51–5. doi: 10.1016/j.ajem.2021.03.005
107. Aldrich J, Pundole X, Tummala S, Palaskas N, Andersen CR, Shoukier M, et al. Inflammatory Myositis in Cancer Patients Receiving Immune Checkpoint Inhibitors. *Arthritis Rheumatol* (2021) 73:866–74. doi: 10.1002/art.41604
108. Seki M, Uruha A, Ohnuki Y, Kameda S, Noda T, Suzuki S, et al. Inflammatory Myopathy Associated With PD-1 Inhibitors. *J Autoimmun* (2019) 100:105–13. doi: 10.1016/j.jaut.2019.03.005
109. Ohnuki Y, Suzuki S, Shiina T, Uruha A, Watanabe Y, Suzuki S, et al. HLA-DRB1 Alleles in Immune-Mediated Necrotizing Myopathy. *Neurology* (2016) 87:1954–5. doi: 10.1212/WNL.0000000000003160
110. Suzuki S, Utsugisawa K, Nagane Y, Satoh T, Kuwana M, Suzuki N. Clinical and Immunological Differences Between Early and Late-Onset Myasthenia Gravis in Japan. *J Neuroimmunol* (2011) 230:148–52. doi: 10.1016/j.jneuroim.2010.10.023

11

Different Multivariable Risk Factors for Rapid Progressive Interstitial Lung Disease in Anti-MDA5 Positive Dermatomyositis and Anti-Synthetase Syndrome

Yu Zuo[1], *Lifang Ye*[1,2], *Fang Chen*[1], *Yawen Shen*[3], *Xin Lu*[1], *Guochun Wang*[1,2] *and Xiaoming Shu*[1*]

[1] *Department of Rheumatology, Key Laboratory of Myositis, China-Japan Friendship Hospital, Beijing, China,* [2] *Peking Union Medical College, Chinese Academy of Medical Sciences, Beijing, China,* [3] *Department of Rheumatology, Beijing Shijitan Hospital, Capital Medical University, Beijing, China*

Correspondence:
Xiaoming Shu
sxm992283@hotmail.com

Background: Interstitial lung disease (ILD) is frequently observed in anti-melanoma differentiation-associated protein 5 (MDA5) antibody positive dermatomyositis (DM) and anti-synthetase syndrome (ASS), where they often develop a rapidly progressive ILD (RP-ILD) leading to poor prognosis.

Objective: The aim of this study was to construct multivariable prediction risk factors for rapid progressive ILD (RP-ILD) in anti-MDA5 positive DM ($MDA5^+DM$) and ASS.

Methods: 333 idiopathic inflammatory myopathy (IIM) associated ILD patients were studied retrospectively. Risk factors for RP-ILD in $MDA5^+DM$ and ASS patients were identified by univariate and multivariable logistic regression analysis. The mortality was assessed using Kaplan-Meier analysis.

Results: RP-ILD was more prevalent in $MDA5^+DM$ patients than ASS patients. $MDA5^+DM$ patients with RP-ILD had significantly lower survival rates than those in ASS patients. The independent risk factors for RP-ILD in $MDA5^+DM$ patients were fever (OR 3.67, 95% CI:1.79-7.52), lymphopenia (OR 2.14, 95% CI:1.01-4.53), especially decreased levels of $CD3^+T$ cells (OR 2.56, 95% CI:1.17-5.61), decreased levels of $CD3^+CD4^+$ T cells (OR 2.80, 95% CI:1.37-5.73), $CD3^+CD8^+T$ cells (OR 2.18, 95% CI:1.05-4.50), elevated $CD5^-CD19^+$ B cells (OR 3.17, 95% CI:1.41-7.13), elevated ALT (OR 2.36, 95% CI:1.15-4.81), high lactate dehydrogenase (LDH) (OR 3.08, 95% CI:1.52-6.27), hyper-ferritin (OR 4.97, 95% CI:1.97-12.50), elevated CEA (OR 2.28, 95% CI:1.13-4.59), and elevated CA153 (OR 3.31, 95% CI:1.50-7.27). While the independent risk factors for RP-ILD in ASS patients were elevated CEA (OR 5.25, 95% CI: 1.73-15.93), CA125 (OR 2.79, 95% CI: 1.10-7.11) and NSE (OR 4.86, 95% CI: 1.44-16.37). Importantly, serum ferritin>2200ng/ml predicted patient's death within half a year in $MDA5^+DM$ patients with RP-ILD, but not in ASS patients.

Conclusions: There were significant different mortality and multivariable risk factors for RP-ILD in MDA5$^+$DM patients and ASS patients. Potential clinical benefits of using these different risk factors deserve assessment of severity and prognosis in IIM patients.

Keywords: idiopathic inflammatory myopathy, anti-MDA5 antibody, anti-synthetase syndrome, rapidly progressive interstitial lung disease, hyperferritinemia

INTRODUCTION

IIM comprises a group of systemic autoimmune disorders, including DM, polymyositis, ASS, immune-mediated necrotizing myopathy (IMNM), inclusion body myositis (IBM), affecting skeletal muscles and other organs. In patients with IIM, interstitial lung disease (ILD) is a common extramuscular involvement associated with poor prognosis (1). RP-ILD is defined as a progressive deterioration associated with ILD within 3 months (2).

In the past year, there have been several studies that reported on the risk factor model of amyopathic dermatomyositis combined with ILD, which provides a favorable basis for better clinical assessment of disease progression (3, 4). However, these studies did not separately discuss risk factors and prognosis of RP-ILD in MDA5$^+$DM and ASS patients.

Researches in recent years have shown that myositis-specific antibody (MSA) profiles help IIM classification. Different antibody-positive IIM has different clinical characteristics. Our previous research showed that ILD had different types in patients with different antibodies (5), in addition, RP-ILD was found both in MDA5$^+$DM and ASS patients. Our previous study has reported that anti-MDA5 was an independent risk factor for RP-ILD (6). ASS patients with ILD generally have slower disease progression, however, another research from our study showed that anti-threonyl tRNA synthetase (PL-7), one of the subtypes of anti-aminoacyl-tRNA synthetase (ARS) antibodies, was closely associated with RP-ILD (7). However, there is no report of exact clinical difference between RP-ILD patients with anti-MDA5 and anti-ARS. Additionally, it is still unclear as to the disparity in survival between the two groups. Furthermore, hyperferritinemia has been proven to be the hallmark and a predictor of poor outcome of ILD associated with MDA5$^+$DM, however different studies have different cut-off values of ferritin for prognosis (8, 9) and as far as we know, there is no separate study on ferritin in the RP-ILD population.

Thus, this retrospective study was conducted to elucidate clinical difference and survival rates of RP-ILD in anti-MDA5 positive and anti-ARS positive patients, to analyze the susceptibility factors of RP-ILD in two groups of patients separately. Furthermore, prognostic value of serum ferritin in anti-MDA5 positive patients with RP-ILD was evaluated.

Abbreviations: ALT, alanine transaminase; ARS, aminoacyl-tRNA synthetase; ASS, anti-synthetase syndrome; AST, aspartate transaminase; BALF, bronchoalveolar lavage fluid; CK, creatine kinase; DM, dermatomyositis; EJ, glycyl-tRNA synthetase; FEV1, forced expiratory volume in the first second; FVC, forced vital capacity; IIM, idiopathic inflammatory myopathy; ILD, interstitial lung disease; Jo-1, histidyl tRNA synthetase; LDH, lactate dehydrogenase; MDA5, melanoma differentiation-associated protein 5; MSA, myositis-specific antibody; OJ, isoleucyl-tRNA synthetase; PBL, lymphocytes in the peripheral blood; PL-7, threonyl tRNA synthetase; PL-12, alanyl tRNA synthetase; RP-ILD, rapidly progressive interstitial lung disease.

MATERIALS AND METHODS

Patient Population

A total of 333 patients with IIM associated ILD (IIM-ILD) were enrolled in this study. 175 patients were positive for anti-MDA5 antibody, and 158 patients were positive for anti-ARS antibodies. All patients were treated in China-Japan Friendship Hospital between July 2013 and October 2018. DM was diagnosed on the basis of the Bohan and Peter criteria, and 239th European Neuro Muscular Centre International Workshop guidelines (10, 11). ASS was diagnosed with definitive serology findings of one of anti-ARS antibodies tested, along with at least one triad finding, including myositis, arthritis, and ILD (12). The exclusion criteria were patients with infections, cancers and/or other CTDs. All patient data were used anonymously with written informed consent from all participants. This study was approved by the Human Ethics Board of the China-Japan Friendship Hospital (approval number: 2016-117).

Data Collection

Clinical data collected included demographics, clinical characteristics, laboratory findings containing auto-antibodies, creatine kinase (CK), serum ferritin, and tumor marker levels; pulmonary function test results (forced vital capacity (FVC), forced expiratory volume in the first second (FEV1) and diffusing capacity of the lung for carbon monoxide; BALF analyses mainly included cell types of fluid. All these routine tests were done in all patients at the first visit in our cohort. Among 333 patients, 122 patients had lung function tests. 100 patients had BALF analyses, and mainly performed when ILD worsened. The follow-up time was defined as the time between the first visit for our cohort to the death or the end of 28 February 2019.

ILD was divided into two categories based on clinical manifestations: RP-ILD and chronic ILD. RP-ILD was defined as displaying two or more of the following within 3 months: 1) dyspnea exacerbation; 2) an increase in parenchymal abnormality on high-resolution computed tomography (HRCT) scan; and 3) one of the following physiological changes: >10% decrease in vital capacity (VC) or >1.33 kPa decrease in arterial oxygen tension (PaO_2). The chronic form was defined as a slowly progressive ILD with gradual deterioration over 3 months (2).

Autoantibody Analyses

The autoantibody tests were performed on the patients' first admission. The serum anti-nuclei antibody profiles and MSAs including anti-MDA5, anti-histidyl tRNA synthetase (Jo-1), anti-threonyl tRNA synthetase (PL-7), anti-alanyl tRNA synthetase (PL-12), anti-isoleucyl-tRNA synthetase (OJ), and anti-glycyl-tRNA synthetase (EJ) were tested using commercially available kits (EUROIMMUN, Lübeck, Germany) according to the manufacturer's instructions.

Analysis of Lymphocyte Subsets in Peripheral Blood of Patients With DM

Lymphocyte subsets analyses were underwent in 286 patients at the first visit in our cohort. A part of patients (n=92) did not receive glucocorticoids therapy before, however, there were still a number of patients (n=194) received glucocorticoids therapy for a short time at other hospitals, which may affect the predictive value of lymphocyte subsets. The counts of $CD3^+CD4^+T$ cells, $CD3^+CD8^+T$ cells, $CD3^-CD19^+B$ cells and $CD3^-CD16^+CD56^+$ NK cells in peripheral blood were detected by flow cytometry (Beckman Coulter, USA) using specific monoclonal antibodies (Beckman Coulter, USA), respectively. Data were analyzed using Cytomics FC500 (Beckman Coulter, USA).

Statistical Analysis

Statistical analysis was performed using SPSS version 11.0 (SPSS Inc. Chicago, IL, U.S.A.). For group comparisons involving demographic characteristics, clinical symptoms and laboratory tests, we used χ^2 tests for the categorical data and the Mann–Whitney U test or two-sample t-tests to analyze continuous data. Univariate and multivariate logistic regression analysis were used to determine the predictors of RP-ILD. The prediction was quantified by the odds ratio with its 95% CI and P<0.05 was considered statistically significant. Survival curves were drawn by the Kaplan-Meier method. The log-rank test was used to compare survival rates. In order to compare the predictive performance of serum ferritin, ROC analysis was performed. We calculated alternative cut-off point by the Youden's index.

RESULTS

Clinical Features and Prevalence of RP-ILD of MDA5⁺DM and ASS Patients

The demographics, clinical manifestations, laboratory test results at diagnosis, pulmonary function test results, and BALF analyses of the 333 enrolled patients with IIM-ILD having either anti-MDA5 or anti-ARS antibodies are summarized in **Table 1**. The mean age at disease onset was 49.7 ± 12.3 years. The majority of the patients were women (M: F ratio = 1:2.3). Of the 333 patients, 175 (52.6%) were positive for anti-MDA5 antibody and 158 (47.4%) were positive for anti-ARS (including 79 anti-Jo-1, 35 anti-PL-7, 17 anti-PL-12, 27 anti-EJ respectively) antibodies. We also found that anti-Ro-52 was identified as the most frequent myositis-associated autoantibody in 113 (33.9%) patients.

Among the 333 patients with IIM-ILD, 180 (54.1%) experienced a RP pattern, of whom 110 (61.1%) were anti-MDA5 antibody-positive and 70 (38.9%) were anti-ARS antibody-positive. The percentage of RP-ILD was significantly higher in $MDA5^+DM$ patients than in ASS patients (62.9% *vs.* 44.3%; $p = 0.001$; **Table 2**). The frequencies of RP-ILD varied among the anti-ARS subgroups; however, no statistically significant differences were observed.

Variables Associated With RP-ILD in MDA5⁺DM and ASS Patients

In first, we identified the incidence of typical rash, including the heliotrope, Gottron, V, and Shawl signs, and skin ulcer and the levels of serum alanine transaminase (ALT), aspartate transaminase (AST), and ferritin were significantly higher, whereas CK levels in $MDA5^+$ DM patients with RP-ILD were much lower (all p values < 0.05). The counts of lymphocytes in the peripheral blood (PBL) were also significantly lower in $MDA5^+DM$ patients with RP-ILD. Further the counts of $CD3^+CD4^+$ T cells, $CD3^+CD8^+T$ cells, $CD5^+CD19^+$ B cells, and NK cells were much lower, whereas the proportion of $CD5^-CD19^+$ B cells was higher in $MDA5^+$ DM patients with RP-ILD than in ASS patients (all p values < 0.05) (**Table 3**).

Risk Factors Independently Associated With RP-ILD in MDA5⁺DM and ASS Patients

To determine the independent risk factors for RP-ILD in either $MDA5^+$ DM or ASS patients, we employed univariate and multivariate analyses to identified that fever (OR 3.67, 95% CI:1.79-7.52, p=0.000), lymphopenia (OR 2.14, 95% CI:1.01-4.53, p=0.046), especially decreased levels of $CD3^+T$ cells (OR 2.56, 95% CI:1.17-5.61, p=0.019), decreased levels of $CD3^+CD4^+$ T cells (OR 2.80, 95% CI:1.37-5.73, p=0.005), $CD3^+CD8^+T$ cells (OR 2.18, 95% CI:1.05-4.50, p=0.036), elevated $CD5^-CD19^+$ B cells (OR 3.17, 95% CI:1.41-7.13, p=0.005), elevated ALT (OR 2.36, 95% CI:1.15-4.81, p=0.019), high LDH (OR 3.08, 95% CI:1.52-6.27, p=0.002), hyperferritinemia (OR 4.97, 95% CI:1.97-12.50, p=0.001), elevated CEA (OR 2.28, 95% CI:1.13-4.59, p=0.022), and elevated CA153 (OR 3.31, 95% CI:1.50-7.27, p=0.003) were risk factors for RP-ILD in $MDA5^+DM$ patients. Interestingly, arthralgia was identified as a protective factor for the development of RP-ILD in $MDA5^+DM$ patients (**Figure 1**).

In deviation with $MDA5^+DM$ patients, the age and sex adjusted multivariate analyses showed that fever, increased levels of serum ferritin, ALT, or LDH, lymphocytes subpopulations including $CD3^+T$ cells, $CD3^+CD4^+$ T cells, $CD3^+CD8^+T$ cells were not risk factors for RP-ILD in ASS patients. Of note, elevated tumor marker CEA (OR 5.25, 95% CI: 1.73-15.93, p=0.003), CA125 (OR 2.79, 95% CI: 1.10-7.11, p=0.031) and NSE (OR 4.86, 95% CI: 1.44-16.37, p=0.011) were both significant independent risk factors for RP-ILD in ASS patients (**Figure 2**). Further, the subtypes of anti-ARS antibodies including anti-Jo-1, anti-PL-7, anti-PL-12, and anti-EJ, were not related to high risk for RP-ILD. Similar to that in $MDA5^+DM$,

TABLE 1 | Characteristics of study participants at diagnosis.

	Values	Range
Age on set, years	49.7 ± 12.3	(7-79)
Male/Female	102/231 (1:2.3)	
Fever	158 (47.4%)	
CK, IU/L (Normal 26-200)	433.9 ± 1082.8	(12-10762)
Ferritin, ng/mL (Normal 11-306.8)	793.0 ± 1370.0	(5.7-11871)
Anti-MDA5 antibody	175 (52.6%)	
Anti-ARS antibodies	158 (47.4%)	
Anit-Jo-1 antibody	79 (23.7)	
Anti-PL-7 antibody	35 (10.5)	
Anti-PL-12 antibody	17 (5.1)	
Anti-EJ antibody	27 (8.1)	
Anti-Ro-52 antibody	113 (33.9%)	
FVC%	74.8 ± 19.2	(39-140)
FEV1%	71.8 ± 16.9	(40-112)
DLCO%	54.9 ± 15.5	(29-100)
BALF LYM%	24.4 ± 23.1	(0-97)
BALF NE%	50.7 ± 28.2	(2-99)
BALF Mac%	20.8 ± 15.8	(1-74)
Treatment of MDA5$^+$DM (n, %)		
Glucocorticoids	175 (100%)	
Pulse steroid therapy	8 (4.6%)	
Calcineurin inhibitors	70 (40.0%)	
Cyclophosphamide	42 (24.0%)	
Mycophenolate mofetil	10 (5.7%)	
Treatment of ASS (n, %)		
Glucocorticoids	158 (100%)	
Pulse steroid therapy	2 (1.3%)	
Calcineurin inhibitors	12 (7.6%)	
Cyclophosphamide	64 (40.5%)	
Mycophenolate mofetil	17 (10.8%)	

FVC%, percentage of the predicted forced vital capacity; FEV1%, percent of forced expiratory volume in the first second; DLCO%, percentage of the predicted diffusion capacity for carbon monoxide; BALF LYM%, percentage of lymphocyte in bronchoalveolar lavage fluid; BALF NE%, percentage of neutrophil in bronchoalveolar lavage fluid; BALF Mac%, percentage of macrophage in bronchoalveolar lavage fluid.

arthralgia, myalgia, and muscle weakness appeared to be protective factors for RP-ILD in ASS patients.

Mortality in RP-ILD in MDA5$^+$DM and ASS Patients

The duration of the follow-up period ranged from 1 to 384 months for all patients. The median follow-up time was 32.4 months. Overall, MDA5$^+$DM patients with RP-ILD had significantly lower survival rates than in ASS patients ($p<0.001$, **Figure 3A**). The 1-year survival rates of MDA5$^+$DM patients with RP-ILD and ASS patients with RP-ILD were 53% and 89%, respectively. The 5-year survival rates of MDA5$^+$DM patients with RP-ILD and ASS patients with RP-ILD were 45% and 76%, respectively. These results indicated MDA5$^+$DM patients with RP-ILD had the highest mortality within the first year after disease onset.

Considering serum ferritin as a significant risk factor for RP-ILD in MDA5$^+$DM patients, we next explored the optimal cut-off

TABLE 2 | Frequencies of RP-ILD among patients with different MSAs.

MSAs	Cases	RP-ILD	Chronic ILD	*P* value*
Total	333	180(54.1)	153(45.9)	
Anti-MDA5	175	110(62.9)	65(37.1)	0.001
Anti-ARS	158	70(44.3)	88(55.7)	0.001
Jo-1	79	34(43.0)	45(57.0)	0.024
PL-7	35	19(54.3)	16(45.7)	0.977
PL-12	17	6(35.3)	11(64.7)	0.111
EJ	27	11(40.7)	16(59.3)	0.148

*MSAs, myositis specific autoantibodies. *indicated that the results were certain MSA positive group comparison with negative group.*

TABLE 3 | Clinical difference between anti-MDA5 positive and anti-ARS positive patients with RP-ILD.

Variable	ARS, n=70	MDA5,n=110	*P* value
Heliotrope sign (%)	18.6 (13/70)	73.6 (81/110)	<0.001
Gottron sign (%)	31.4 (22/70)	80.9 (89/110)	<0.001
V sign (%)	14.3 (10/70)	50.9 (56/110)	<0.001
Shawl sign (%)	8.6 (6/70)	34.5 (38/110)	<0.001
Skin ulcer (%)	1.4 (1/70)	24.5 (27/110)	<0.001
CK (IU/L)	541.0 ± 1430.6	250.2 ± 747.3	0.001
ALT (IU/L)	43.4 ± 34.2	87.9 ± 89.7	<0.001
AST (IU/L)	40.3 ± 32.0	111.9 ± 241.8	<0.001
Ferritin (ng/ml)	374.7 ± 461.2	1415.3 ± 1991.1	<0.001
PBL (cell/ul)	1598.0 ± 947.2	770.6 ± 487.4	<0.001
CD3+T	1107.7 ± 655.7	548.9 ± 354.7	<0.001
CD4+T	690.4 ± 546.7	359.4 ± 249.9	<0.001
CD8+T	428.2 ± 357.8	189.2 ± 165.0	<0.001
NK	186.8 ± 189.8	39.6 ± 46.9	<0.001
NK (%)	12.1 ± 7.7	5.5 ± 5.3	<0.001
B1 (CD5+CD19+)	75.4 ± 113.4	23.2 ± 37.2	<0.001
B2 (CD5-CD19+)%	11.9 ± 8.4	19.7 ± 11.7	<0.001
BALF Mac%	14.9 ± 11.5	21.2 ± 15.5	0.090
BALF LYM%	19.3 ± 20.5	27.7 ± 25.0	0.096
BALF NE%	56.7 ± 28.6	47.6 ± 27.3	0.184

BALF Mac%, percentage of macrophage in bronchoalveolar lavage fluid; BALF LYM%, percentage of lymphocyte in bronchoalveolar lavage fluid; BALF NE%, percentage of neutrophil in bronchoalveolar lavage fluid.

levels of serum ferritin in predicting the mortality of $MDA5^{+}DM$ patients. Of the 110 anti-MDA5 antibody-positive patients with RP-ILD, 48 died during follow-up due to exacerbation of ILD or infection. A total of 34 (70.8%) patients died within 6 months from disease onset, and 43 (89.6%) died within 1 year. Because some of the surviving patients had not been followed up for >1 year, we used ROC analysis to study the value of ferritin required to predict patient's mortality within half a year. As shown in **Figure 3B**, the optimal cutoff point for serum ferritin was 2200 ng/mL (AUC, 0.66 (95% CI 0.51–0.80). Using the manufacturer's cutoff value for serum ferritin ≥ 2200 ng/mL, the prognostic sensitivity was 41.7% (95% CI 20.4%–62.9%), whereas the prognostic specificity was 93.2% (95% CI, 86.6%–99.8%). In addition, the positive predictive value for serum ferritin was 71.4% (95% CI 44.4%–98.5%), and the negative predictive value was 79.7% (95% CI 70.0%–89.4%).

DISCUSSION

The present study indicated the following: (1) $MDA5^{+}DM$ was related to a higher frequency of RP-ILD and a worse prognosis

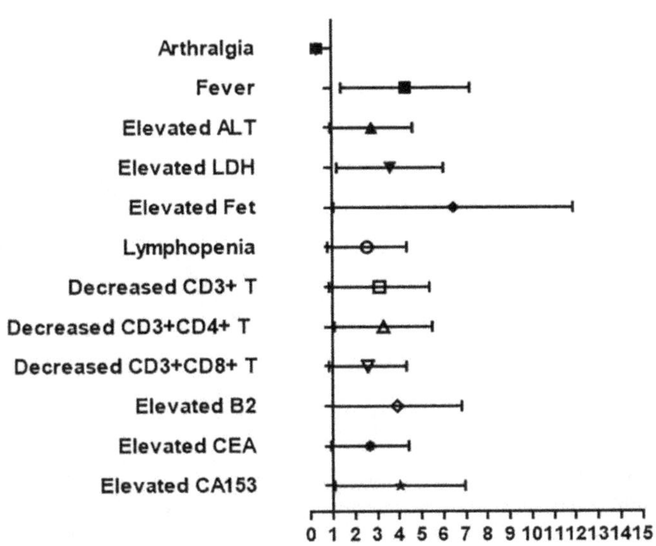

Adjusted OR (95% CI)	p Value
0.281 (0.138-0.570)	<0.001
3.672 (1.794-7.516)	<0.001
2.355 (1.153-4.813)	0.019
3.083 (1.517-6.266)	0.002
4.965 (1.973-12.498)	0.001
2.141 (1.013-4.528)	0.046
2.560 (1.168-5.612)	0.019
2.796 (1.365-5.728)	0.005
2.179 (1.054-4.504)	0.036
3.174 (1.412-7.133)	0.005
2.276 (1.128-4.591)	0.022
3.305 (1.502-7.272)	0.003

FIGURE 1 | Risk factors of RP-ILD in patients with anti-MDA5 antibody.

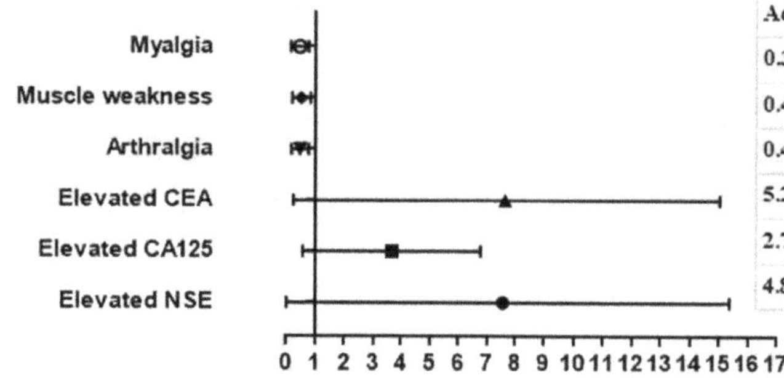

Adjusted OR (95% CI)	p Value
0.397 (0.199-0.793)	0.009
0.454 (0.237-0.872)	0.018
0.411 (0.212-0.797)	0.008
5.254 (1.733-15.932)	0.003
2.792 (1.096-7.110)	0.031
4.861 (1.444-16.366)	0.011

FIGURE 2 | Risk factors of RP-ILD in patients with anti-ARS antibody.

than ASS; (2) There were great different multivariable risk factors for RP-ILD in MDA5$^+$DM and ASS. A more unique result showed serum hyper-ferritin was the risk factor and prognostic value for RP-ILD in MDA5$^+$DM patients but not in ASS patients.

Previous studies had demonstrated that MDA5$^+$DM associated ILD can frequently progress rapidly and have a poor outcome, whereas ASS associated ILD usually responds to therapy. The comparison of the incidence of RP-ILD between the two groups was consistent with observations from literature reports; however, in our cohort, ASS patients could also have RP-ILD, especially in patients with anti-PL-7; however, no statistical difference in incidence compared with that in other subgroups of anti-ARS antibodies was observed.

We further selected patients with RP-ILD and compared the clinical differences between the two groups of patients with different antibodies. MDA5$^+$DM patients were more likely to have typical dermatomyositis rashes, whereas more ASS patients have elevated CK levels. Considering that RNA helicase encoded by MDA5 is a key molecule participating in the innate immune defense against viruses, viral infection may play an important role in the pathogenesis of DM with anti-MDA5 antibody positivity and RP-ILD (13). In our study, MDA5$^+$DM patients with RP-ILD were more likely to have elevated transaminase and ferritin levels and decreased lymphocyte counts, which is consistent with the clinical characteristics of viral infection, and also reflects the difference in pathogenesis of the two groups of patients with RP-ILD having different antibodies.

In addition to the differences in clinical indicators, we also analyzed the survival of the two groups of patients. To our best knowledge, this is the first large sample study showing the difference in survival of patients with RP-ILD having either anti-MDA5 or anti-ARS antibodies. A study on the survival of MDA5$^+$DM patients conducted by Koga T et al. suggested that all of the deaths of MDA5$^+$DM patients occurred within the first six months from the first visit to the hospital (14). Another study on the prognostic significance of ASS patients indicated that the 10-year survival rate was also significantly higher in the ASS group than in the non- ASS group (15). Our research found that patients with RP-ILD having anti-MDA5 antibody had significantly lower survival rates than those having anti-ARS antibody.

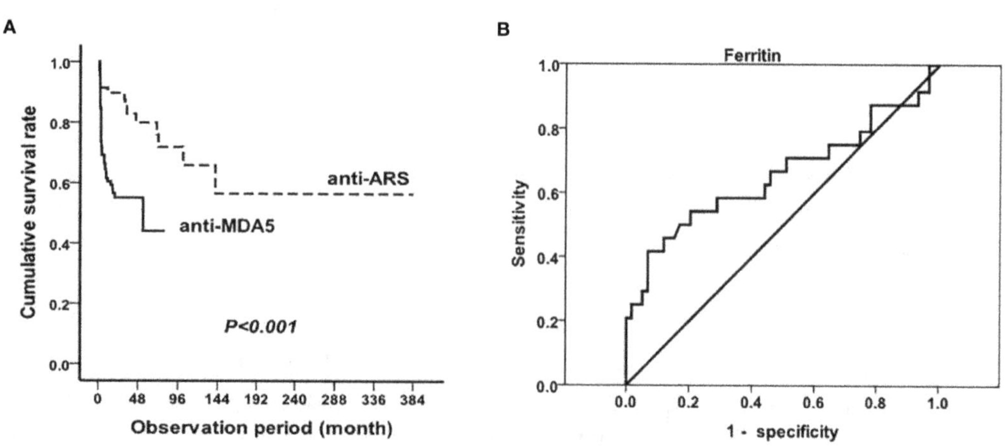

FIGURE 3 | Mortality in RP-ILD in anti-MDA5 and anti-ARS positive DM and prognostic value of serum ferritin Survival analysis in RP-ILD patients with anti-MDA5 or anti-ARS antibodies **(A)** and prognostic value of serum ferritin in MDA5$^+$DM **(B)**.

Furthermore patients with anti-MDA5 antibody had the highest mortality within the first year of disease onset. Thus, for patients with RP-ILD having anti-MDA5 antibody, early and more powerful treatment is critical.

Anti-MDA5 antibody- and anti-ARS antibody-positive patients have some similarities in terms of the risk factors of RP-ILD. Elevated tumor markers indicated an increased risk of RP-ILD in both groups, consistent with our previous observations (5); however, the exact function of tumor-associated markers in IIM-ILD remains unknown. In the present study, arthralgia was identified as a protective factor for the development of RP-ILD in both groups, which was different from the observations of other research teams (16). This may be owing to differences in sample sizes; therefore, further confirmation studies are needed.

Furthermore, for $MDA5^+DM$ patients, we found periphery $CD4^+$ and $CD8^+$ T cells in the RP-ILD group, were significantly lower than in chronic ILD group, confirming previous clinical findings (6, 17), and indicating that T cells play an important role in the development of disease. Knowledge on exactly how the lymphocytes, especially the T cells, work in $MDA5^+DM$ patients requires more research. Previous research has speculated that lymphocytes migrate to the lungs to take part in the local immune response, causing a decrease of periphery blood lymphocytes (17). Because the onset of $MDA5^+DM$ may be associated with a history of pre-infection, we speculate that infection by viruses or other pathogens also causes the depletion of lymphocytes in $MDA5^+DM$ patients. In addition to abnormal T cells, an elevated level of B2 ($CD5^-CD19^+$) cells was also a risk factor for RP-ILD in the $MDA5^+DM$ group. Rituximab is effective in some $MDA5^+DM$ patients with RP-ILD (18). Our results and subsequent further research should provide a trial basis for the application of clinical drugs.

Studies have suggested that serological markers are associated with the prognosis of $MDA5^+DM$ patients, including CRP and KL-6 (3). Nevertheless, our study with a larger sample size showed that serum ferritin was an independent risk factor for poor prognosis, thus providing more parameters for evaluating the prognosis of $MDA5^+DM$ patients, especially those with RP-ILD. Hyperferritinemia has been considered a predictor of poor outcomes for patients with DM having anti-MDA5 antibody; however different researches have different cutoff values of ferritin for prognosis. The research by Gono et al. showed that all patients with a ferritin level of >1600 ng/mL died of respiratory failure (8) while Kurasawa et al. reported that a ferritin level of >1000 ng/mL before treatment was a risk factor for poor outcome in MDA5 DM patients (9). Lian et al. established a mortality risk score model in amyopathic dermatomyositis-associated ILD, identifying a ferritin level of 636 ng/mL as the optimal clinical threshold (4). In this study, we aimed to provide a more accurate cutoff value of ferritin for the prognosis of RP-ILD for $MDA5^+DM$ patients. Through ROC curve analysis, a serum ferritin level of >2200 ng/mL predicted mortality within half a year in $MDA5^+DM$ patients with RP-ILD with a sensitivity of 41.7% and specificity 93.2%. Based on our previous observations, the pathogenesis of DM may be related to the activation of macrophages (5, 19), and in this study, patients with RP-ILD having anti-MDA5 antibodies tended to have hyperferritinemia and lower NK cell counts, supporting previous observations.

CONCLUSION

There were significant different mortality and multivariable risk factors for RP-ILD in $MDA5^+DM$ patients and ASS patients. Potential clinical benefits of using these different risk factors deserve assessment of severity and prognosis in IIM patients. Further studies are required to elucidate any difference in pathogenesis between anti-MDA5 antibody and anti-ARS antibody positive patients.

ETHICS STATEMENT

The studies involving human participants were reviewed and approved by Human Ethics Board of the China-Japan Friendship Hospital (approval number: 2016-117). The patients/participants provided their written informed consent to participate in this study.

AUTHOR CONTRIBUTIONS

YZ, LY, FC, and YS collected and analyzed the data. XL, GW, and XS provided clinical samples and approved the manuscript. All authors contributed to the article and approved the submitted version.

ACKNOWLEDGMENTS

We thank the other members of our department.

REFERENCES

1. Douglas WW, Tazelaar HD, Hartman TE, Hartman RP, Decker PA, Schroeder DR, et al. Polymyositis-Dermatomyositis-Associated Interstitial Lung Disease. *Am J Respir Crit Care Med* (2001) 164(7):1182–5. doi: 10.1164/ajrccm.164.7.2103110
2. Won Huh J, Soon Kim D, Keun Lee C, Yoo B, Bum Seo J, Kitaichi M, et al. Two Distinct Clinical Types of Interstitial Lung Disease Associated With Polymyositis-Dermatomyositis. *Respir Med* (2007) 101(8):1761–9. doi: 10.1016/j.rmed.2007.02.017
3. Gono T, Masui K, Nishina N, Kawaguchi Y, Kawakami A, Ikeda K, et al. Risk Prediction Modeling Based on a Combination of Initial Serum Biomarkers in Myositis-Associated Interstitial Lung Disease. *Arthritis Rheumatol* (2021) 73 (4):677–86. doi: 10.1002/art.41566
4. Lian X, Zou J, Guo Q, Chen S, Lu L, Wang R, et al. Mortality Risk Prediction in Amyopathic Dermatomyositis Associated With Interstitial Lung Disease: The FLAIR Model. *Chest* (2020) 158(4):1535–45. doi: 10.1016/j.chest.2020.04.057
5. Zuo Y, Ye L, Liu M, Li S, Liu W, Chen F, et al. Clinical Significance of Radiological Patterns of HRCT and Their Association With Macrophage

Activation in Dermatomyositis. *Rheumatol (Oxf)* (2020) 59(10):2829–37. doi: 10.1093/rheumatology/keaa034

6. Chen F, Wang D, Shu X, Nakashima R, Wang G. Anti-MDA5 Antibody Is Associated With A/SIP and Decreased T Cells in Peripheral Blood and Predicts Poor Prognosis of ILD in Chinese Patients With Dermatomyositis. *Rheumatol Int* (2012) 32(12):3909–15. doi: 10.1007/s00296-011-2323-y
7. Shi J, Li S, Yang H, Zhang Y, Peng Q, Lu X, et al. Clinical Profiles and Prognosis of Patients With Distinct Antisynthetase Autoantibodies. *J Rheumatol* (2017) 44(7):1051–7. doi: 10.3899/jrheum.161480
8. Gono T, Kawaguchi Y, Satoh T, Kuwana M, Katsumata Y, Takagi K, et al. Clinical Manifestation and Prognostic Factor in Anti-Melanoma Differentiation-Associated Gene 5 Antibody-Associated Interstitial Lung Disease as a Complication of Dermatomyositis. *Rheumatol (Oxf)* (2010) 49 (9):1713–9. doi: 10.1093/rheumatology/keq149
9. Kurasawa K, Arai S, Namiki Y, Tanaka A, Takamura Y, Owada T, et al. Tofacitinib for Refractory Interstitial Lung Diseases in Anti-Melanoma Differentiation-Associated 5 Gene Antibody-Positive Dermatomyositis. *Rheumatol (Oxf)* (2018) 57(12):2114–9. doi: 10.1093/rheumatology/key188
10. Bohan A, Peter JB. Polymyositis and Dermatomyositis (First of Two Parts). *N Engl J Med* (1975) 292(7):344–7. doi: 10.1056/NEJM197502132920706
11. Mammen AL, Allenbach Y, Stenzel W, Benveniste OE.t.W.S. Group. 239th ENMC International Workshop: Classification of Dermatomyositis, Amsterdam, the Netherlands, 14-16 December 2018. *Neuromuscul Disord* (2020) 30(1):70–92. doi: 10.1016/j.nmd.2019.10.005
12. Cavagna L, Trallero-Araguas E, Meloni F, Cavazzana I, Rojas-Serrano J, Feist E, et al. Influence of Antisynthetase Antibodies Specificities on Antisynthetase Syndrome Clinical Spectrum Time Course. *J Clin Med* (2019) 8(11):2013. doi: 10.3390/jcm8112013
13. Sato S, Hoshino K, Satoh T, Fujita T, Kawakami Y, Fujita T, et al. RNA Helicase Encoded by Melanoma Differentiation-Associated Gene 5 Is a Major Autoantigen in Patients With Clinically Amyopathic Dermatomyositis: Association With Rapidly Progressive Interstitial Lung Disease. *Arthritis Rheum* (2009) 60(7):2193–200. doi: 10.1002/art.24621
14. Koga T, Fujikawa K, Horai Y, Okada A, Kawashiri SY, Iwamoto N, et al. The Diagnostic Utility of Anti-Melanoma Differentiation-Associated Gene 5 Antibody Testing for Predicting the Prognosis of Japanese Patients With DM. *Rheumatol (Oxf)* (2012) 51(7):1278–84. doi: 10.1093/rheumatology/ker518
15. Hozumi H, Enomoto N, Kono M, Fujisawa T, Inui N, Nakamura Y, et al. Prognostic Significance of Anti-Aminoacyl-tRNA Synthetase Antibodies in Polymyositis/Dermatomyositis-Associated Interstitial Lung Disease: A Retrospective Case Control Study. *PLoS One* (2015) 10(3):e0120313. doi: 10.1371/journal.pone.0120313
16. Hoa S, Troyanov Y, Fritzler MJ, Targoff IN, Chartrand S, Mansour AM, et al. Describing and Expanding the Clinical Phenotype of Anti-MDA5-Associated Rapidly Progressive Interstitial Lung Disease: Case Series of Nine Canadian Patients and Literature Review. *Scand J Rheumatol* (2018) 47(3):210–24. doi: 10.1080/03009742.2017.1334814
17. Huang W, Ren F, Luo L, Zhou J, Huang D, Pan Z, et al. The Characteristics of Lymphocytes in Patients Positive for Anti-MDA5 Antibodies in Interstitial Lung Disease. *Rheumatol (Oxf)* (2020) 59(12):3886–91. doi: 10.1093/rheumatology/keaa266
18. Ogawa Y, Kishida D, Shimojima Y, Hayashi K, Sekijima Y. Effective Administration of Rituximab in Anti-MDA5 Antibody-Positive Dermatomyositis With Rapidly Progressive Interstitial Lung Disease and Refractory Cutaneous Involvement: A Case Report and Literature Review. *Case Rep Rheumatol* (2017) 2017:5386797. doi: 10.1155/2017/5386797
19. Peng QL, Zhang YL, Shu XM, Yang HB, Zhang L, Chen F, et al. Elevated Serum Levels of Soluble CD163 in Polymyositis and Dermatomyositis: Associated With Macrophage Infiltration in Muscle Tissue. *J Rheumatol* (2015) 42(6):979–87. doi: 10.3899/jrheum.141307

12

Programmed Cell Death Pathways in the Pathogenesis of Idiopathic Inflammatory Myopathies

Jia Shi[1,2]*, Mingwei Tang*[1,2]*, Shuang Zhou*[1,2]*, Dong Xu*[1,2]*, Jiuliang Zhao*[1,2]*,*
Chanyuan Wu[1,2*]*, Qian Wang*[1,2*]*, Xinping Tian*[1,2]*, Mengtao Li*[1,2] *and Xiaofeng Zeng*[1,2]

[1] *Department of Rheumatology and Clinical Immunology, Peking Union Medical College Hospital, Peking Union Medical College & Chinese Academy of Medical Sciences, Key Laboratory of Rheumatology & Clinical Immunology, Ministry of Education, Beijing, China,* [2] *National Clinical Research Center for Dermatologic and Immunologic Diseases (NCRC-DID), Ministry of Science & Technology, Beijing, China*

Correspondence:
Chanyuan Wu
wchypumch@hotmail.com
Qian Wang
wangqian_pumch@126.com

Idiopathic inflammatory myopathy (IIM) is a heterogeneous group of acquired, autoimmune muscle diseases characterized by muscle inflammation and extramuscular involvements. Present literatures have revealed that dysregulated cell death in combination with impaired elimination of dead cells contribute to the release of autoantigens, damage-associated molecular patterns (DAMPs) and inflammatory cytokines, and result in immune responses and tissue damages in autoimmune diseases, including IIMs. This review summarizes the roles of various forms of programmed cell death pathways in the pathogenesis of IIMs and provides evidence for potential therapeutic targets.

Keywords: idiopathic inflammatory myopathy (IIM), programmed cell death (PCD), apoptosis, autophagy, NETosis, pyroptosis

HIGHLIGHTS

- Dysregulated cell death in combination with impaired elimination of dead cells, get involved in the pathogenesis of IIMs.
- Programmed necrosis, such as NETosis and pyroptosis, seems to play a more important role in the pathogenesis of IIMs, which contribute to the release of autoantigens, damage-associated molecular patterns and proinflammatory cytokines.
- The mechanisms of PCD seem to vary among different subtypes of IIM and require even more precise studies according to different myositis-specific antibodies.

INTRODUCTION

Idiopathic inflammatory myopathy (IIM) is a heterogeneous group of acquired, autoimmune muscle diseases characterized by production of a spectrum of autoantibodies [including myositis-specific autoantibodies (MSAs) and myositis-associated autoantibodies (MAAs)], aberrant regulation of inflammatory responses, and tissue damage of different organs. The most common subtypes of IIMs are represented by dermatomyositis (DM), polymyositis (PM), inclusion body myositis (IBM), immune-mediated necrotising myopathy (IMNM), antisynthetase syndrome (ASSD) and overlap myositis (1). The exact pathogenesis of IIMs has not been fully elucidated, but was reported to be related to genetic and environmental factors, abnormal immune responses and non-immune responses (2).

Almost exclusively found in IIM patients, MSAs include antisynthetase autoantibodies (ARS), anti-Mi-2, anti-signal recognition particle (SRP), anti-melanoma differentiation-associated gene 5 (MDA5), anti-nuclear matrix protein 2 (NXP2), anti-transcription intermediary factor 1γ (TIF1γ), anti-small ubiquitin-like modifier activating enzyme (SAE), and anti- 3-Hydroxy-3-methylglutaryl CoA reductase (HMGCR). Their targeting antigens are ubiquitously expressed and are involved in key cellular processes, including gene expression and developmental regulation (3), but how these intracellular components get exposed to the immune system, elicit immune responses and lead to the generation of MSAs, remain unclear. Besides, overexpressed cytokines have been found in the serum and diseased muscle tissues of IIM patients. For instance, the level of type I interferon (IFN) is increased significantly in the muscles of DM patients (4). Therefore, it is reasonable to speculate that abnormal cell death may play a role in the pathogenesis of IIMs. Currently, accumulating evidences have revealed that excessive cell death in combination with impaired elimination of dead cells and debris contribute to the release of autoantigens, danger-associated molecular patterns (DAMPs) and proinflammatory cytokines, and consequently, the over-activated immune and inflammatory responses in IIMs (5). According to functional aspects, cell death can be classified into programmed cell death (PCD) and accidental cell death (ACD) (6). Used to be mistaken for the synonyms of apoptosis, essentially PCD also incorporates autophagy-dependent cell death and programmed necrosis (7) (such as NETosis, pyroptosis, ferroptosis and necroptosis) (**Figure 1**).

In this review, we focus on recent research progression of PCD pathways in the pathogenesis and progression of IIMs to provide evidence for potential therapeutic targets.

APOPTOSIS AND SECONDARY NECROSIS AFTER APOPTOSIS

Apoptosis is a genetically-controlled non-lytic cell death pathway, designed to dismantle and remove senescent and injured cells, thereby preventing unwanted inflammation during development, homeostasis, and infection (8). The main features of apoptosis are cytoplasmic shrinkage, membrane blebbing, chromatin condensation and nuclear fragmentation (6). Two distinct apoptotic signaling pathways, intrinsic (also called the mitochondrial pathway) and extrinsic pathways, have been defined. The extrinsic pathway can be triggered by death factors of the tumor necrosis factor (TNF) family [including Fas ligand (CD95L, FasL), TNF-α, and TNF-related apoptosis-inducing ligand (TRAIL)], while the intrinsic pathway is activated by microenvironmental perturbations including endoplasmic reticulum stress (ERS), reactive oxygen species (ROS), or lack of nutrient support (9). Mitochondrial outer membrane permeabilization (MOMP) is the critical and irreversible step for intrinsic apoptosis, which is regulated by Bcl-2 family members (10). Both apoptotic pathways are mediated by specific sets of caspases which act in cascades, among which caspase-8 and caspase-9 being the initiators for the extrinsic pathway and the intrinsic pathway, respectively. Once activated, either caspase-8 or caspase-9 activates executioner caspase-3 and caspase-7 and leads to apoptosis of the doomed cell (11). Macrophages engulf these dead cells in a process called efferocytosis by recognizing "find me" signals [such as ATP, UTP, sphingosine-1-phosphate (S1P) and CX3CL1 (fractalkine)] and "eat me" molecules (such as phosphatidylserine, oxidized LDL-like molecules and C1q-bound serum proteins) released by these cells (10). However, when apoptotic cells are not engulfed efficiently and timely, they undergo secondary necrosis, which is featured with permeabilization of plasma membranes and release of intracellular contents that may activate the immune system (7).

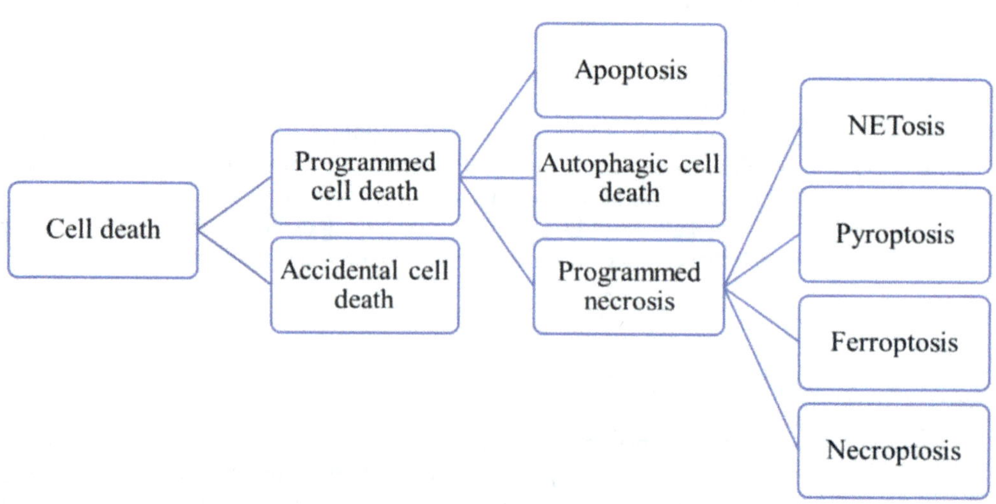

FIGURE 1 | Classification of cell death.

Peripheral T cell lymphopenia has been reported in some patients with DM, which is associated with the increased Fas-mediated apoptosis of T cells. The overexpression of retinoic acid-inducible gene I (RIG-I) could induce T cell apoptosis, but the mechanism is far from clear (12). Also, lymphopenia may be resulted from the decreased autophagy, which is discussed later below (13). Noteworthily, in patients of IIM, T cells infiltrating in the muscles are dominated by $CD28^{null}$ T cells, partly due to chronic antigenic stimulation (14), which show an increased percentage in peripheral blood mononuclear cells (PBMCs) as well (15–18). $CD28^{null}$ T cells infiltrating in IIM muscles are generally regarded as terminally differentiated and apoptosis resistant with properties of replicative senescence (16, 17, 19, 20), because of decreased expression of Fas (21), and increased expression of antiapoptotic molecule Bcl-2 (22), Bcl-x_l and cyclin-dependent kinase inhibitors p16 and p57 (20), upregulation of the phosphoinositide 3-kinase pathway (23) (which inhibits Fas-initiated apoptosis), and upregulation of various inhibitory natural killer cell receptors (iNKRs) (24) (such as CD94/NKG2A). $CD28^{null}$ T cells are not capable of costimulatory interaction with CD80 and CD86, but this does not represent a global loss of costimulatory receptor expression. The upregulation of alternative costimulatory molecules, such as inducible costimulator (ICOS), CD134 and CD137, has been reported in $CD28^{null}$ T cells after CD3 ligation (25). Moreover, this T-cell phenotype is suggested to be treatment-resistant for its persistence in muscle tissue after high doses of glucocorticoids and other immunosuppressive treatment, which is correlated with a poor clinical response (17), and could be due to a significant loss of glucocorticoid receptors (GCRs) (26). Therefore, $CD28^{null}$ T cells are an emerging target of interest for treatment in refractory myositis patients. Existing drugs that could downregulate T cells include calcineurin inhibitors (e.g., tacrolimus and cyclosporine) and abatacept. Calcineurin inhibitors could prevent calcineurin from dephosphorylating nuclear factor of activated T cell (NFAT) proteins and then repress transcription of IL-2, and thereby restraining the differentiation and survival of T cells (27). A single-arm prospective clinical trial revealed that initial combination treatment with tacrolimus and GCs could improve short-term mortality of PM/DM-ILD patients with satisfactory safety (28). Abatacept, an agonist of cytotoxic T-lymphocyte antigen-4 (CTLA-4), could interfere with the activation of T cells by binding CD80/CD86 on the surface of antigen-presenting cells (APCs). A phase IIb, delayed-start clinical trial of abatacept was conducted in 20 refractory DM/PM patients. Decreased disease activity was observed in 42% of the patients, as well as upregulated $Foxp3^+$ regulatory T cells in repeated muscle biopsies (29). There is a phase III, randomized, double-blind trial underway to further evaluate abatacept for myositis treatment (Clinical Trial Identifier NCT02971683).

In PM, $CD28^{null}$ T cells have been demonstrated to be able to exert direct cytotoxicity towards myocytes by polarizing perforin and secreting granzyme B, and indirectly contribute to myotube cell death by releasing proinflammatory cytokines IFN-γ and TNF which could induce surface expression of MHC, rendering the myocytes more sensitive to cytotoxic attacks (30). An *in vitro* study also identified that culturing myoblasts with IFN-γ or TNF alone could upregulate inflammation related transcription factors (NF-κB, nuclear factor-κB) and induce apoptosis (31), implying that extracellular inflammation induces further inflammatory changes and forms a sustained loop of inflammation leading to cell death. One study on IBM showed that the combination of β-amyloid (Aβ) with IFN-γ stimulating pathogenic NO_2^- production *via* induction of iNOS gene expression could induce apoptosis of myocytes (32), while the other found Aβ alone is sufficient for myofiber apoptosis (33). In hereditary IBM, mutations in gene GNE could lead to impaired apoptotic signaling, thus causing degenerative process and muscle loss (34). Moreover, the expressions of Fas and cytoplasmic caspase-8 and -3 of myocytes could be upregulated by proinflammatory cytokines as well (35), but whether myocytes apoptosis mediated by Fas/FasL interaction is involved in the pathogenesis of IIM is controversial. Fas expression in muscle fibers has been reported with very different frequencies (36–39). The presence of myocytes with TUNEL positive nuclei has been reported in IIMs but was very rare. As for this phenomenon, some researchers consider that the frequencies of apoptosis are too low to prove the relevance to pathopoiesis, while others believe that it is attributed to the prompt efferocytosis. These rare apoptotic myocytes were surrounded by $CD8^+$ T cells and granzyme B^+ cells with absence of Fas and upregulating MHC-I, favouring a cytotoxic mode of apoptosis induction rather than a Fas-mediated mechanism (37), which is in line with an earlier study, suggesting Fas expression may be attributed to the new gene expression in regenerating fibers (38). The resistance of myocytes to apoptosis is attributable to anti-apoptotic intracellular proteins, such as Bcl-2 (36), FLICE (Fas-associated death domain-like IL-1-converting enzyme)-inhibitory protein (FLIP) (40) and human IAP-like protein (hILP) (41). Notably, in contrast with previous study, Bcl-2 has been reported to exhibit lower expression in diseased muscle compared with normal muscle (39). Therefore, the mode of myocyte death needs to be further investigated.

Nevertheless, some therapeutic strategies regarding apoptosis have been identified. Resistance exercise (RE) has been demonstrated to reduce Aβ accumulation in chloroquine (CQ)-induced rat model of IBM, thus inhibiting mitochondrial-mediated apoptosis of myofibers and improving mitochondrial function through increased mitochondrial biogenesis, upregulated mitophagy, and activated sirtuin 3 signaling (42). Alemtuzumab, a recombinant DNA-derived humanized monoclonal antibody targeting CD52, was also beneficial for IBM patients, as it lowered the count of peripheral and endomysial T cells with reduced mRNA expression of Fas (43). It could enhance apoptosis in B cells by upregulating the expression of caspase-8 and caspase-3 in chronic lymphocytic leukemia as well (44), which may provide a valuable reference for IIM. Besides, pro-senescent interventions consisting of exercise and AMP-activated protein kinase (AMPK) activation induced apoptosis of fibro-adipogenic progenitors (FAP) and promoted muscle regeneration in a murine chronic inflammatory myopathy (CIM) model, suggesting that the FAP-targeted intervention may be therapeutic (45). In PM/DM, expressions of cathepsin B (CB) and calpain are increased in muscle and lung tissues, which promotes cell apoptosis and inflammation. Calpeptin (calpain inhibitor) ameliorated morphological changes of apoptosis in IFN-γ or TNF-α treated myoblasts through both mitochondrial pathway and ERS pathway (31, 46). Also, the administration of CA-074Me, a specific inhibitor of CB, could attenuate apoptosis of myocytes and lung epithelial cells, and reduce lung interstitial inflammation and fibrosis in the guinea-pig model of PM (47, 48).

AUTOPHAGY AND AUTOPHAGIC CELL DEATH

Autophagy is a highly conserved catabolic and homeostatic process by which subcellular components are secluded and degraded *via* lysosomes under stress conditions, such as ERS, nutritional deprivation, mitochondrial injury, and inflammation (49). It is featured with vacuolization of the cytoplasm and accumulation of double-membraned vacuoles (i.e., autophagosome) in morphology. According to the modes of cargo transferring to the lysosome, autophagy is classified as macroautophagy, microautophagy and chaperone-mediated autophagy (CMA). In addition to elimination of intracellular aggregates and damaged organelles, autophagy plays crucial roles in inflammation and immune-system function, mediating cytoprotective rather than cytotoxic effects. The interplay between autophagy and cytokines is fundamental to modulate inflammatory as well as immune responses. For instance, TNF-α can induce autophagy and in turn, whether autophagy up- or down-regulates TNF-α formation depends on the cellular context (50). Autophagic cell death is a type of PCD that relies upon the autophagic machinery or constituents thereof, with massive autophagic vacuolization of the cytoplasm but without chromatin condensation (51).

Most IIM studies with regard to autophagy focus on IBM. Rare missense variants in autophagy-related genes, such as VCP, HNRPA2B1, BAG3, SQSTM1, FLNC and ZASP have been identified to occur at a higher frequency in IBM patients than in control populations (52). VCP mutations could result in defective myotube formation, increased apoptosis and increased autophagy (53). Moreover, a study based on whole exome sequencing (WES) identified missense variants in FYCO1, which encodes for an LC3-binding protein accumulating at rimmed vacuoles and is implicated in microtubule transport of autophagosomes, were statistically enriched in IBM patients (54). Collectively, these findings revealed a strong tie between IBM susceptibility and autophagy. In IBM muscle tissues, increased formation of vacuolar autophagosomes has been identified along with massive protein aggregation, as indicated by increased levels of p62, LC3, mTOR-mediated phosphorylation of p70SK, α-synuclein and TDP-43 (55–57). These markers could be ancillary tools to differentiate IBM from other IIMs (56). In the inflammatory milieu in muscle, the upregulated proinflammatory cytokines, such as IL-1β (58), TNF-like weak inducer of apoptosis (TWEAK) (59) and TRAIL (60), get involved in stimulating autophagic cell death. Besides, the overexpression of MHC-II in inflamed muscle fibers, partly on account of the increased cytokine TNF-α, could induce autophagy and interact with IFN-γ to translocate intracellular MHC-II to the myocyte surface further (61). Also, defective autophagy could drive increased MHC-I expression because of the weakening ability of MHC-I internalization for degradation (62). All the evidence revealed that dysregulated autophagy might contribute to antigen presentation for MHC-I and II, and maintain the inflammatory response in a vicious circle (63).

The overmuch autophagy reflected by overexpression of autophagic proteins in muscle, and impaired protein degradation, contributing importantly to consequent accumulation of multiprotein aggregates, are key factors in the myofiber degeneration characteristic of IBM (55, 64, 65). Specially, the accumulation of amyloid-β42 oligomers, could cause reduction in muscular peak force and amplitude of Ca^{2+} transients in mouse models of IBM (66), suggesting that their cytotoxicity contribute importantly to IBM pathogenic cascade. Cylindromatosis (CYLD), a deubiquitinating enzyme, co-expressed with autophagy-related proteins in IBM, contributed to muscle damage by attenuating autophagic clearance of protein aggregates (67). Cacciottolo et al. found the upregulation of CMA components in sIBM muscle fibres, which revealed cellular attempts to activate CMA and remove protein aggregates (68). However, this attempted compensation might not fully work because of the decreased activity of proteolytic enzymes in lysosomes (55). Arimoclomol, an inducer of heat shock response, can upregulate chaperone expression, thereby promoting CMA in stressed cells and curbing the formation of protein aggregates. Treatment with arimoclomol ameliorated IBM-like pathology in myoblasts and mutant VCP mice, and it was safe and well tolerated in a proof-of-concept clinical trial of IBM patients (69). To further evaluate the efficacy of this drug in IBM, a multisite phase II clinical trial has been completed (Clinical Trial Identifier NCT02753530). Moreover, RE could facilitate fusion between autophagosomes and lysosomes in IBM animal models, hence improving impaired macroautophagy (70).

In addition to IBM, autophagy activation could also be detected in PM, DM and IMNM muscle tissues, whereas the autophagic activation, modulation and interaction with the immune system, are different in each type of IIM (60, 71, 72). In IBM, lysosomal enzymes Cathepsin B and D, are inhibited, while in PM, their activities were actually increased (55). Dysfunctional CMA (73) and mitophagy (a specific autophagic elimination of mitochondria) (74), were reported to occur in IMNM muscles. The decreased autophagy and increased apoptosis of circulating $CD3^+$ T cells have been demonstrated in PM/DM patients, and this phenomenon could be turned around by the treatment of autophagy inducer rapamycin, hence preventing lymphopenia, which suggested that autophagy may play a potential cytoprotective role in PM/DM *via* inhibition of apoptosis in $CD3^+$ T cells (13). Intravenous immunoglobulin (IVIG) therapy has been demonstrated to induce autophagy in PBMCs and reduce circulation proinflammatory cytokines in IIM by activating AMPK and inhibiting mTOR phosphorylation, thus mediating anti-inflammatory effect (75).

NETS AND NETOSIS

Neutrophils are critical immune cells at the frontline of immune defense, responsible for eliminating pathogens by multiple mechanisms, including phagocytosis, production and release of antimicrobial proteins, and formation of neutrophil extracellular traps (NETs) (76). NETs are web-like structures composed of histones, granular proteins and decondensed chromatin, which could be autoantigens and DAMPs to break immune tolerance in predisposed hosts (77–79). NET-derived mitochondrial DNA could induce type I IFN production through the DNA-sensing cGAS-STING pathway in myeloid cells (80). Antimicrobial peptide LL-37 could activate type I IFN as well (81). Also, the components of NETs are detrimental to vessels and muscles (82–86). Citrullinated histones exerted toxic effect to decrease the viability of myotubes (87). Accompanied by the formation of NETs, neutrophils die, which is called the NETosis. Essentially, the internal environment homeostasis of IIM patients is disrupted with abnormal cytokine levels (88), which may generate unexpected NETs formation. These NETs irritate more production of proinflammatory cytokines, maintaining a vicious circle of sustained NETosis. For instance, this lytic process could promote the production of IL-6 and IL-1β in macrophages (89). If excessive NETs cannot be cleared timely and efficiently by DNase I and macrophages, inflammation and autoimmunity will ensue (90).

IIM patients exhibited significant increased NETs, especially in individuals with ILD, which is resulted from decreased activity of DNase I (91). Low-density granulocytes (LDGs), a unique subset of neutrophils with proinflammatory phenotype, are prone to commit NETosis and secrete proinflammatory cytokines (92). LDGs have been reported to display an increased percentage in PBMCs in DM patients, especially those complicated by ILD, along with increased NETs, which may further contribute to the progression of ILD (93). Abnormal regulation of NETs has been reported to be associated with MSAs. An *in vitro* study showed that anti-MDA5 Ab^+ serum could directly induce NET formation (94). Interestingly, NET levels exhibited a significant rise in patients with anti-MDA5 or anti-TIF1 antibodies, yet not in patients with anti-Jo-1 positive (87). Contradictorily, Zhang et al. found patients with anti-Jo-1 antibodies exhibited lower DNase I activity than those without anti-Jo-1 antibodies (91). Therefore, studies with larger sample sizes are needed to clarify the association between MSAs and NETs. NETosis may be related to prognosis as well. Anti-MDA5 antibody positive and hyperferritinemia have been identified as the poor prognostic factors of DM. The level of serum cfDNA, which is the product of NETosis, was reported to significantly increase in anti-MDA5 Ab^+ subset and hyperferritinemic subset, hence it may be a potential indicator of prognosis (94).

A recent report described the presence of calcium crystal–induced NETosis in JDM. The engulfment of calcium crystals by tissue-infiltrating neutrophils, triggered NETosis which is NADPH oxidase- and complement–dependent (95). Also, circulating immune complexes may contribute to the elevated NET levels in JDM (95). JDM patients can develop atherosclerosis during progression into adulthood. Such IIM-associated cardiovascular disease may be related to the oxidation of high-density lipoprotein (HDL) through NETs-derived MPO (96).

PYROPTOSIS

Pyroptosis is a lytic and proinflammatory form of PCD depending on gasdermin family. Three pathways have been identified, including the caspase-1-mediated canonical pathway stimulated by PAMPs or DAMPs, the noncanonical pathway requiring caspase-4, 5 (for human) or caspase-11 (for murine) triggered by lipopolysaccharide (LPS), and caspase-3-dependent pathway. The best-studied pyroptosis pathway is that mediated by gasdermin D (GSDMD) with downstream of nucleotide-binding and oligomerization domain-like receptor family pyrin-domain containing 3 (NLRP3) inflammasome activation, which can recruit and activate inflammatory caspases. The activated caspase-1 or caspase-4/5/11, cleaves GSDMD and exposes its N-terminal domain, which binds to phosphoinositides in the cell membrane and forms large pores, thus driving cytoplasmic swelling, cytolysis, and release of cellular contents (97). Also, caspase-1 cleaves IL-1β and IL-18 to produce mature cytokines, but whether these cytokines are actively secreted or released *via* pyroptotic membrane rupture remained unclear (98). Other released contents, including cleaved GSDMD, chemokines, ATP and HMGB1, recruit immune cells and expand tissue inflammation (99). Caspase-3, recognized as the apoptotic executioner by convention, has been reported to specifically cleave gasdermin E (GSDME), thereby initiating pyroptosis, and whether cells with caspase-3 activated undergo apoptosis or pyroptosis, depends on the expression level of GSDME (100).

Currently, the three mentioned pathways have all been demonstrated in muscle tissues of IIMs. Liu et al. first reported that the GSDME-dependent pyroptosis got involved in the pathogenesis of perifascicular atrophy (PFA), a pathognomonic histologic feature of DM (101). Soon afterwards, Ma et al. demonstrated the implication of noncanonical pathway in the animal model of experimental autoimmune myositis (EAM) as well, and glyburide and brilliant blue G (BBG) could lower the levels of pyroptotic markers and alleviate symptoms (102). However, these two studies verified pyroptosis by detecting the full length of GSDME or GSDMD, rather than the cleaved forms. Besides, upregulated glycolysis has been reported in the lesioned muscle tissues of DM/PM, which further promoted myocyte pyroptosis by activating the NLRP3 inflammasome and exposing N-GSDMD. Treated IFN-γ-stimulated-myotubes with shikonin, a pyruvate kinase isozyme M2 (PKM2) inhibitor, could mitigate NLRP3 inflammasome activation and suppress pyroptosis (103). Intriguingly, the levels of PKM2 and IL-1β were related to MSAs, and were especially high in patients with anti-SRP autoantibody (103).

OTHER FORMS OF PCD: FERROPTOSIS AND NECROPTOSIS

Ferroptosis

Ferroptosis is a newly proposed cell death with unique morphological structures and biochemical expressions, caused by oxidative damage due to the excessive accumulation of iron-dependent lipid peroxidation products. It usually shows necrosis-like morphological changes with mitochondrial abnormalities, such as condensed membrane and reduced or absent crista (104). Whether a cell will undergo ferroptosis is linked with many factors, such as its level of polyunsaturated fatty acid (PUFA), iron metabolism, and glutathione (GSH) biosynthesis. The inhibition of cystine-glutamate antiporter (system Xc-) and the inactivation of GSH peroxidase-4 (GPX4) lead to the depletion of cellular GSH, and the impaired clearance of ROS, thus causing collapse of cellular redox homeostasis and accumulation of ROS from lipid peroxidation or Fenton reaction, ultimately resulting in lipid membrane damages and cell death (7). Ferroptotic peroxidation products are powerful inducers of autophagy (e.g., reactive aldehydes) (104), and excessive autophagy promotes ferroptosis in turn, by degrading iron-storage protein ferritin and hence increasing cellular iron concentration (105). This specific autophagic process is called ferritinophagy. Of note, hyperferritinemia is frequently accompanied by IIM-ILD, and is associated with disease severity and prognosis (106). Moreover, mitochondria play a proactive role in cysteine-deprivation-induced ferroptosis by fueling metabolism and lipid ROS production (107). Besides, mitochondrial abnormalities and increased level of ROS, have been reported in IIM, proposed to be vital mediators in IIM pathophysiology (108–110). Taken together, it is logical to hypothesize that ferroptosis is implicated in the development of IIM, so further in-depth studies are necessary to elucidate the exact role of ferroptosis in IIMs.

Necroptosis

Necroptosis is an inflammatory form of PCD characterized by receptor-interacting protein kinase 3- (RIPK3-) mediated activation of mixed lineage kinase domain-like protein (MLKL) and permeabilization of the plasma membrane (111). Although apoptosis and necroptosis frequently share common triggers, including death receptors and IFN, downstream signaling pathway of these triggers leading to survival, apoptosis or necroptosis depends on the availability of cellular inhibitor of apoptosis (cIAPs), FLIP, or caspase-8 (112). In the absence of caspase-8, the necrosome (i.e., RIPK1/RIPK3 complex) activates necroptotic pathway, thus promoting the recruitment and phosphorylation of MLKL, and then, the activated MLKL translocates to the cell membrane and damages the integrity, leading to the release of cell contents and generating inflammation (113). In addition, necroptosis regulators RIPK3 and MLKL have been reported to play an independent role in inflammation irrespective of cell death – promoting NLRP3 inflammasome activation and IL-1β secretion (114, 115). Collectively, these results indicated that necroptosis can enhance inflammation and may be implicated in the pathogenesis and progression of autoimmune diseases. For instance, necroptosis has been reported to contribute to B-cell lymphopenia in systemic lupus erythematosus (116). IFN-γ could downregulate necroptosis by inhibiting MLKL and cFLIP, thereby exerting protective effects in autoimmune arthritis (117). GSK2982772 is a highly selective inhibitor of RIPK1, while a latest randomized, placebo-controlled study found GSK2982772 no meaningful clinical improvement of RA compared with placebo (118). No studies investigate the association between IIM and necroptosis currently.

CROSSTALK BETWEEN PCD PATHWAYS

The PCD pathways are tightly connected and the cross regulation between them is complex. In most circumstances, apoptosis and autophagy are mutually inhibited. Autophagy can reduce the abundance of pro-apoptotic proteins in the cytosol (e.g., caspase-8), while activated caspases can degrade essential autophagic proteins (e.g., BECN1) (119). On the contrary, there is a mutual promotion between ferroptosis and autophagy, which is discussed above in the 'Ferroptosis' section.

Different cell death pathways can be activated with the same signal. For example, disturbed redox homeostasis and excessive ROS attributed to sustained activation of ER stress pathway, which is clearly of etiological relevance in IIM (120), could activate all the PCD pathways aforementioned. Moreover, biochemical and cellular consequences of one type of cell death can have profound influence on the activity of another type of cell death (121). GSDMD, the executor of pyroptosis, also plays a crucial role in NETosis. During NETosis, serine proteases released from neutrophil granules could cleave GSDMD, and then activated GSDMD in turn permeabilizes granules to enhance proteases release and promotes nuclear expansion. Further, activated GSDMD forms pores in the plasma membrane, promoting NET release (122).

Various cell death modes can coexist, and cells can switch between one death pathway to another. Caspase-8 is a crucial molecular switch for apoptosis, necroptosis and pyroptosis. It can not only directly cleave caspase-3 to induce extrinsic apoptosis, but also get involved in other cell death pathways. When TGF-β activated kinase-1 (TAK1, cell survival kinase) is inhibited, caspase-8 could cleave GSDMD and induce pyroptosis (123). The loss of caspase-8 or its enzymatic activity could lead to MLKL-dependent necroptosis. If necroptosis is blocked, enzymatic inactive caspase-8 could indirectly activate GSDMD and cause pyroptosis by driving ASC (apoptosis-associated speck-like protein, adaptor protein of NLRP3 inflammasome) speck formation, which leads to caspase-1 activation (124). Overall, increasing evidence points to caspase-8 as a central regulator of cell death, and it promotes apoptosis, necroptosis, or pyroptosis depending on its posttranslational state, the cell type, and the stimuli (125). The intricate crosstalk between pyroptosis, apoptosis, and necroptosis has led to the proposal of PANoptosis. It is regulated by the PANoptosome complex, a molecular scaffold for the contemporaneous engagement of key pyroptotic, apoptotic, and necroptotic machinery (125). PANoptosis has been reported in microbial infection, inflammatory diseases, cancer and cytokine storm. For instance, in COVID-19, increased circulating levels of TNF and IFN-γ synergistically induce PANoptosis characterized by activation of pyroptotic (GSDME), apoptotic (caspase-8/3/7) and necroptotic (pMLKL) molecules, facilitate further pathogenic cytokine release

TABLE 1 | Factors inducing abnormal myocyte death in IIMs.

Factors	Death pathways	Effects	Year	References
Perforin, granzyme B	Apoptosis	Exert direct cytotoxicity	2016	(30)
IFN-γ, TNF	Apoptosis, autophagy	Induce surface expression of MHC	2011, 2016	(30, 31, 61)
Aβ, IFN-γ	Apoptosis	Stimulate NO_2^- production *via* induction of iNOS gene expression	2000, 2001	(32, 33)
Mutations in gene GNE	Apoptosis	Increase caspases-3 and -9 expression	2007	(34)
IFN-γ, TNF, IL-1β	Apoptosis	Increase Fas, caspases-3 and -8 expression	2009	(35)
Mutations in gene VCP	Autophagy, apoptosis	Lead to impaired protein degradation	2009	(53)
Missense variants in gene FYCO1	Autophagy	Lead to impaired microtubule transport of autophagosomes	2017	(54)
IL-1β, IFN-γ	Autophagy	Increase phosphorylation of the mitogen activated protein kinases and induce accumulation of amyloid	2017	(58)
TRAIL	Autophagy	Induce NF-κB activation and autophagic cell death	2011	(60)
MSAs	NETosis	Unclear	2014, 2018, 2020	(87, 91, 94)
Calcium crystal, immune complexes	NETosis	Induce formation of NETs	2020	(95)
PKM2	Pyroptosis	Activate NLRP3 inflammasome	2021	(103)

iNOS, inducible nitric oxide synthase; Aβ, β-amyloid; VCP, valosin containing protein; FYCO1, FYVE and coiled-coil domain containing 1; TRAIL, TNF-related apoptosis-inducing ligand; PKM2, pyruvate kinase isozyme M2.

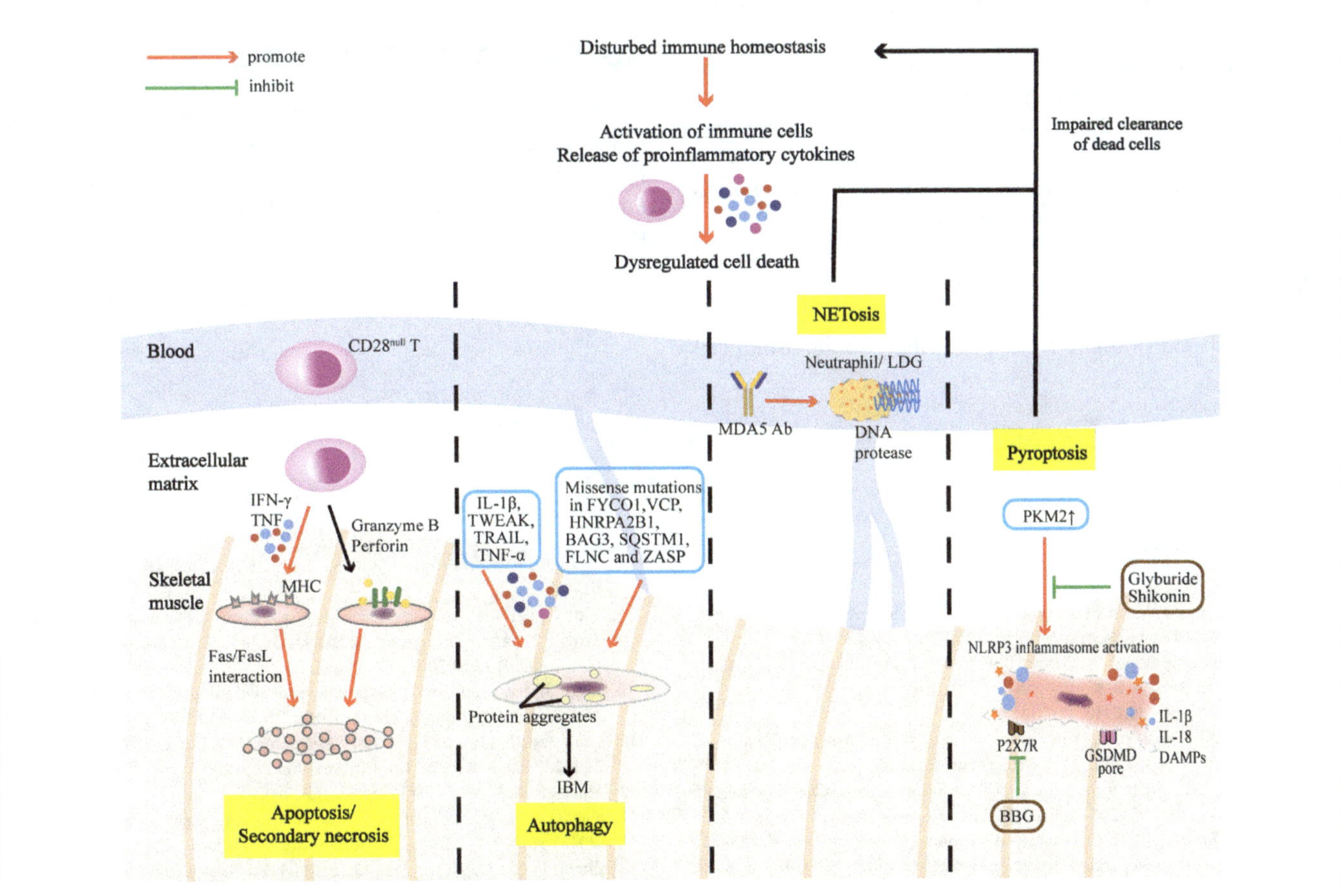

FIGURE 2 | PCD pathways in the pathogenesis and progression of IIMs. The immune homeostasis of IIM patients is disrupted with activation of immune cells and release of proinflammatory cytokines, which could lead to dysregulated cell death. T cells infiltrating in the muscles are dominated by CD28null T cells, which are apoptosis-resistant, and could exert polarize perforin and secrete granzyme B to induce myocyte apoptosis, or release IFN-γ and TNF to induce surface expression of MHC, rendering the myocytes more sensitive to cytotoxic attacks. Overmuch autophagy and impaired protein degradation result in accumulation of multiprotein aggregates, which causes myocyte degeneration characteristic of IBM. Excessive programmed necrosis (such as NETosis and pyroptosis) contribute to the release of proinflammatory cytokines, and DAMPs, and activation of NLRP3 inflammasome, further amplifying immune responses.

TABLE 2 | Possible therapeutic targets for IIMs.

Targets	Interventions	Death pathway	Year	References
Aβ/ macroautophagy	Resistance exercise	Apoptosis, autophagy	2017, 2019	(42, 70)
FAP	Exercise and AMPK	Apoptosis	2020	(45)
Calpain	Calpeptin	Apoptosis	2010, 2011	(31, 46)
Cathepsin B	CA-074Me	Apoptosis	2013, 2015	(47, 48)
mTOR	Rapamycin	Autophagy	2017	(13)
Heat Shock Factor-1	Arimoclomol	Autophagy	2016	(69)
AMPK	IVIG	Autophagy	2018	(74)
NLRP3	Glyburide	Pyroptosis	2021	(102)
P2X7 receptor	Brilliant blue G	Pyroptosis	2021	(102)
PKM2	Shikonin	Pyroptosis	2021	(103)

Aβ, β-amyloid; FAP, fibro-adipogenic progenitor; AMPK, AMP-activated protein kinase; mTOR, mammalian target of rapamycin; IVIG, intravenous immunoglobulin; P2X7, adenosine triphosphate gated cationic channel; PKM2, pyruvate kinase isozyme M2.

through membrane pores and cell lysis, culminating in a life-threatening cytokine storm (126). Whether PANoptosis occurs in anti-MDA5-associated ILD, which is prone to be complicated by cytokine storm, remains uninvestigated.

Therefore, due to the intricacies and connections between each PCD pathways, which death pathway is dominant, and whether there is synergy and the simultaneous activation of multiple pathways in IIM need to be considered. Taking an integral view of cell death in IIM may improve our understanding of pathogenesis and aid in the development of therapeutics.

CONCLUSION

Immune and non-immune factors contribute to abnormal cell death in IIMs (**Table 1**), and dysregulation of PCD further amplifies inflammatory responses, playing an important part in the pathogenesis and progression of IIM (**Figure 2**), although it has not been unveiled clearly. Further in-depth studies on these PCD pathways will extend our knowledge on the pathogenic mechanism of IIMs, and targeting different steps to inhibit PCD processes and promoting the clearance of death materials may be promising therapeutic strategies for IIMs (**Table 2**). In addition, the particularity of autoantibodies is noteworthy, as patients with diverse autoantibodies exhibit different clinical manifestations, prognosis, organ involvements, and treatment responses, suggesting that potential immunopathogenic mechanisms may be different. Besides, targeted antigens by MSAs are intracellular components, so we speculate that their exposure to immune system and followed generation of MSAs are attributed to the dysregulation of PCD. Therefore, it's reasonable to put emphasis on the association of distinct MSAs with PCD pathways in further studies. Also, PCD pathways are intimately linked and interdependent, making it necessary to take a comprehensive approach to investigate PCD pathways.

AUTHOR CONTRIBUTIONS

JS collected materials and wrote the paper. QW, MT, SZ, and CW provided the idea and reviewed the manuscript. DX, JZ, XT, ML, and XZ helped with the final revision of the paper. All authors contributed to the article and approved the submitted version.

REFERENCES

1. Lundberg IE, de Visser M, Werth VP. Classification of Myositis. *Nat Rev Rheumatol* (2018) 14(5):269–78. doi: 10.1038/nrrheum.2018.41
2. Zanframundo G, Tripoli A, Cometi L, Marcucci E, Furini F, Cavagna L, et al. One Year in Review 2020: Idiopathic Inflammatory Myopathies. *Clin Exp Rheumatol* (2020) 39:1–12.
3. McHugh NJ, Tansley SL. Autoantibodies in Myositis. *Nat Rev Rheumatol* (2018) 14(5):290–302. doi: 10.1038/nrrheum.2018.56
4. Greenberg SA. Dermatomyositis and Type 1 Interferons. *Curr Rheumatol Rep* (2010) 12(3):198–203. doi: 10.1007/s11926-010-0101-6
5. Vanden Berghe T, Linkermann A, Jouan-Lanhouet S, Walczak H, Vandenabeele P. Regulated Necrosis: The Expanding Network of non-Apoptotic Cell Death Pathways. *Nat Rev Mol Cell Biol* (2014) 15(2):135–47. doi: 10.1038/nrm3737
6. Kroemer G, Galluzzi L, Vandenabeele P, Abrams J, Alnemri ES, Baehrecke EH, et al. Classification of Cell Death: Recommendations of the Nomenclature Committee on Cell Death 2009. *Cell Death differentiation* (2009) 16(1):3–11. doi: 10.1038/cdd.2008.150
7. Kim EH, Wong SW, Martinez J. Programmed Necrosis and Disease:We Interrupt Your Regular Programming to Bring You Necroinflammation. *Cell Death differentiation* (2019) 26(1):25–40. doi: 10.1038/s41418-018-0179-3
8. Van Opdenbosch N, Lamkanfi M. Caspases in Cell Death, Inflammation, and Disease. *Immunity* (2019) 50(6):1352–64. doi: 10.1016/j.immuni.2019.05.020
9. Riedl SJ, Salvesen GS. The Apoptosome: Signalling Platform of Cell Death. *Nat Rev Mol Cell Biol* (2007) 8(5):405–13. doi: 10.1038/nrm2153
10. Czabotar PE, Lessene G, Strasser A, Adams JM. Control of Apoptosis by the BCL-2 Protein Family: Implications for Physiology and Therapy. *Nat Rev Mol Cell Biol* (2014) 15(1):49–63. doi: 10.1038/nrm3722
11. Nagata S. Apoptosis and Clearance of Apoptotic Cells. *Annu Rev Immunol* (2018) 36:489–517. doi: 10.1146/annurev-immunol-042617-053010
12. Zhang L, Xia Q, Li W, Peng Q, Yang H, Lu X, et al. The RIG-I Pathway is Involved in Peripheral T Cell Lymphopenia in Patients With Dermatomyositis. *Arthritis Res Ther* (2019) 21(1):131. doi: 10.1186/s13075-019-1905-z
13. Shu X, Chen F, Peng Q, Lu X, Tian X, Wang Y, et al. Potential Role of Autophagy in T-cell Survival in Polymyositis and Dermatomyositis. *Mol Med Rep* (2017) 16(2):1180–8. doi: 10.3892/mmr.2017.6693
14. Strioga M, Pasukoniene V, Characiejus D. CD8+ CD28- and CD8+ CD57+ T Cells and Their Role in Health and Disease. *Immunology* (2011) 134 (1):17–32. doi: 10.1111/j.1365-2567.2011.03470.x

15. Espinosa-Ortega F, Gómez-Martin D, Santana-De Anda K, Romo-Tena J, Villaseñor-Ovies P, Alcocer-Varela J. Quantitative T Cell Subsets Profile in Peripheral Blood From Patients With Idiopathic Inflammatory Myopathies: Tilting the Balance Towards Proinflammatory and Pro-Apoptotic Subsets. *Clin Exp Immunol* (2015) 179(3):520–8. doi: 10.1111/cei.12475
16. Fasth AE, Dastmalchi M, Rahbar A, Salomonsson S, Pandya JM, Lindroos E, et al. T Cell Infiltrates in the Muscles of Patients With Dermatomyositis and Polymyositis are Dominated by CD28null T Cells. *J Immunol (Baltimore Md 1950)* (2009) 183(7):4792–9. doi: 10.4049/jimmunol.0803688
17. Pandya JM, Loell I, Hossain MS, Zong M, Alexanderson H, Raghavan S, et al. Effects of Conventional Immunosuppressive Treatment on CD244+ (CD28null) and FOXP3+ T Cells in the Inflamed Muscle of Patients With Polymyositis and Dermatomyositis. *Arthritis Res Ther* (2016) 18:80. doi: 10.1186/s13075-016-0974-5
18. Pandya JM, Fasth AE, Zong M, Arnardottir S, Dani L, Lindroos E, et al. Expanded T Cell Receptor Vβ-Restricted T Cells From Patients With Sporadic Inclusion Body Myositis are Proinflammatory and Cytotoxic CD28null T Cells. *Arthritis Rheumatism* (2010) 62(11):3457–66. doi: 10.1002/art.27665
19. Posnett DN, Edinger JW, Manavalan JS, Irwin C, Marodon G. Differentiation of Human CD8 T Cells: Implications for *In Vivo* Persistence of CD8+ CD28- Cytotoxic Effector Clones. *Int Immunol* (1999) 11(2):229–41. doi: 10.1093/intimm/11.2.229
20. Vattemi G, Tonin P, Filosto M, Spagnolo M, Rizzuto N, Tomelleri G. T-Cell Anti-Apoptotic Mechanisms in Inflammatory Myopathies. *J Neuroimmunology* (2000) 111(1-2):146–51. doi: 10.1016/S0165-5728(00)00381-7
21. Liphaus BL, Sallum AEM, Aikawa NE, Kiss MHB, Carrasco S, Palmeira P, et al. Increased Soluble Cytoplasmic Bcl-2 Protein Serum Levels and Expression and Decreased Fas Expression in Lymphocytes and Monocytes in Juvenile Dermatomyositis. *J Rheumatol* (2018) 45(11):1577–80. doi: 10.3899/jrheum.171248
22. Wood KL, Twigg HL3rd, Doseff AI. Dysregulation of CD8+ Lymphocyte Apoptosis, Chronic Disease, and Immune Regulation. *Front Biosci (Landmark edition)* (2009) 14:3771–81. doi: 10.2741/3487
23. Strauss G, Knape I, Melzner I, Debatin KM. Constitutive Caspase Activation and Impaired Death-Inducing Signaling Complex Formation in CD95-Resistant, Long-Term Activated, Antigen-Specific T Cells. *J Immunol (Baltimore Md 1950)* (2003) 171(3):1172–82. doi: 10.4049/jimmunol.171.3.1172
24. Gunturi A, Berg RE, Forman J. Preferential Survival of CD8 T and NK Cells Expressing High Levels of CD94. *J Immunol (Baltimore Md 1950)* (2003) 170 (4):1737–45. doi: 10.4049/jimmunol.170.4.1737
25. Plunkett FJ, Franzese O, Finney HM, Fletcher JM, Belaramani LL, Salmon M, et al. The Loss of Telomerase Activity in Highly Differentiated CD8 +CD28-CD27- T Cells is Associated With Decreased Akt (Ser473) Phosphorylation. *J Immunol (Baltimore Md 1950)* (2007) 178(12):7710–9. doi: 10.4049/jimmunol.178.12.7710
26. Hodge G, Jersmann H, Tran HB, Holmes M, Reynolds PN, Hodge S. Lymphocyte Senescence in COPD is Associated With Loss of Glucocorticoid Receptor Expression by Pro-Inflammatory/Cytotoxic Lymphocytes. *Respir Res* (2015) 16(1):2. doi: 10.1186/s12931-015-0287-2
27. Barbarino JM, Staatz CE, Venkataramanan R, Klein TE, Altman RB. PharmGKB Summary: Cyclosporine and Tacrolimus Pathways. *Pharmacogenet Genomics* (2013) 23(10):563–85. doi: 10.1097/FPC.0b013e328364db84
28. Takada K, Katada Y, Ito S, Hayashi T, Kishi J, Itoh K, et al. Impact of Adding Tacrolimus to Initial Treatment of Interstitial Pneumonitis in Polymyositis/Dermatomyositis: A Single-Arm Clinical Trial. *Rheumatol (Oxford England)* (2020) 59(5):1084–93. doi: 10.1093/rheumatology/kez394
29. Tjärnlund A, Tang Q, Wick C, Dastmalchi M, Mann H, Tomasová Studýnková J, et al. Abatacept in the Treatment of Adult Dermatomyositis and Polymyositis: A Randomised, Phase IIb Treatment Delayed-Start Trial. *Ann rheumatic Dis* (2018) 77(1):55–62. doi: 10.1136/annrheumdis-2017-211751
30. Pandya JM, Venalis P, Al-Khalili L, Shahadat Hossain M, Stache V, Lundberg IE, et al. CD4+ and CD8+ CD28(null) T Cells Are Cytotoxic to Autologous Muscle Cells in Patients With Polymyositis. *Arthritis Rheumatol (Hoboken NJ)* (2016) 68(8):2016–26. doi: 10.1002/art.39650
31. Nozaki K, Das A, Ray SK, Banik NL. Calpeptin Attenuated Apoptosis and Intracellular Inflammatory Changes in Muscle Cells. *J Neurosci Res* (2011) 89(4):536–43. doi: 10.1002/jnr.22585
32. Baron P, Galimberti D, Meda L, Prat E, Scarpini E, Conti G, et al. Synergistic Effect of Beta-Amyloid Protein and Interferon Gamma on Nitric Oxide Production by C2C12 Muscle Cells. *Brain J Neurol* (2000) 123(Pt 2):374–9. doi: 10.1093/brain/123.2.374
33. Querfurth HW, Suhara T, Rosen KM, McPhie DL, Fujio Y, Tejada G, et al. Beta-Amyloid Peptide Expression is Sufficient for Myotube Death: Implications for Human Inclusion Body Myopathy. *Mol Cell Neurosci* (2001) 17(5):793–810. doi: 10.1006/mcne.2001.0972
34. Amsili S, Shlomai Z, Levitzki R, Krause S, Lochmuller H, Ben-Bassat H, et al. Characterization of Hereditary Inclusion Body Myopathy Myoblasts: Possible Primary Impairment of Apoptotic Events. *Cell Death differentiation* (2007) 14(11):1916–24. doi: 10.1038/sj.cdd.4402208
35. Kondo M, Murakawa Y, Harashima N, Kobayashi S, Yamaguchi S, Harada M. Roles of Proinflammatory Cytokines and the Fas/Fas Ligand Interaction in the Pathogenesis of Inflammatory Myopathies. *Immunology* (2009) 128(1 Suppl):e589–99. doi: 10.1111/j.1365-2567.2008.03039.x
36. Behrens L, Bender A, Johnson MA, Hohlfeld R. Cytotoxic Mechanisms in Inflammatory Myopathies. Co-Expression of Fas and Protective Bcl-2 in Muscle Fibres and Inflammatory Cells. *Brain J Neurol* (1997) 120(Pt 6):929–38. doi: 10.1093/brain/120.6.929
37. Danielsson O, Häggqvist B, Gröntoft L, Öllinger K, Ernerudh J. Apoptosis in Idiopathic Inflammatory Myopathies With Partial Invasion; a Role for CD8+ Cytotoxic T Cells? *PloS One* (2020) 15(9):e0239176. doi: 10.1371/journal.pone.0239176
38. De Bleecker JL, Meire VI, Van Walleghem IE, Groessens IM, Schröder JM. Immunolocalization of FAS and FAS Ligand in Inflammatory Myopathies. *Acta Neuropathol* (2001) 101(6):572–8. doi: 10.1007/s004010000324
39. Danielsson O, Nilsson C, Lindvall B, Ernerudh J. Expression of Apoptosis Related Proteins in Normal and Diseased Muscle: A Possible Role for Bcl-2 in Protection of Striated Muscle. *Neuromuscular Disord NMD* (2009) 19 (6):412–7. doi: 10.1016/j.nmd.2009.03.008
40. Nagaraju K, Casciola-Rosen L, Rosen A, Thompson C, Loeffler L, Parker T, et al. The Inhibition of Apoptosis in Myositis and in Normal Muscle Cells. *J Immunol (Baltimore Md 1950)* (2000) 164(10):5459–65. doi: 10.4049/jimmunol.164.10.5459
41. Li M, Dalakas MC. Expression of Human IAP-Like Protein in Skeletal Muscle: A Possible Explanation for the Rare Incidence of Muscle Fiber Apoptosis in T-Cell Mediated Inflammatory Myopathies. *J Neuroimmunology* (2000) 106(1-2):1–5. doi: 10.1016/S0165-5728(99)00162-9
42. Koo JH, Kang EB, Cho JY. Resistance Exercise Improves Mitochondrial Quality Control in a Rat Model of Sporadic Inclusion Body Myositis. *Gerontology* (2019) 65(3):240–52. doi: 10.1159/000494723
43. Dalakas MC, Rakocevic G, Schmidt J, Salajegheh M, McElroy B, Harris-Love MO, et al. Effect of Alemtuzumab (CAMPATH 1-H) in Patients With Inclusion-Body Myositis. *Brain J Neurol* (2009) 132(Pt 6):1536–44. doi: 10.1093/brain/awp104
44. Nückel H, Frey UH, Röth A, Dührsen U, Siffert W. Alemtuzumab Induces Enhanced Apoptosis *In Vitro* in B-Cells From Patients With Chronic Lymphocytic Leukemia by Antibody-Dependent Cellular Cytotoxicity. *Eur J Pharmacol* (2005) 514(2-3):217–24. doi: 10.1016/j.ejphar.2005.03.024
45. Saito Y, Chikenji TS, Matsumura T, Nakano M, Fujimiya M. Exercise Enhances Skeletal Muscle Regeneration by Promoting Senescence in Fibro-Adipogenic Progenitors. *Nat Commun* (2020) 11(1):889. doi: 10.1038/s41467-020-14734-x
46. Nozaki K, Das A, Ray SK, Banik NL. Calpain Inhibition Attenuates Intracellular Changes in Muscle Cells in Response to Extracellular Inflammatory Stimulation. *Exp Neurol* (2010) 225(2):430–5. doi: 10.1016/j.expneurol.2010.07.021
47. Feng Y, Ni L, Wang Q. Administration of Cathepsin B Inhibitor CA-074Me Reduces Inflammation and Apoptosis in Polymyositis. *J Dermatol Sci* (2013) 72(2):158–67. doi: 10.1016/j.jdermsci.2013.06.014
48. Zhang L, Fu XH, Yu Y, Shui RH, Li C, Zeng HY, et al. Treatment With CA-074Me, a Cathepsin B Inhibitor, Reduces Lung Interstitial Inflammation and Fibrosis in a Rat Model of Polymyositis. *Lab Invest J Tech Methods Pathol* (2015) 95(1):65–77. doi: 10.1038/labinvest.2014.135

49. Choi AM, Ryter SW, Levine B. Autophagy in Human Health and Disease. *New Engl J Med* (2013) 368(7):651–62. doi: 10.1056/NEJMra1205406
50. Ge Y, Huang M, Yao YM. Autophagy and Proinflammatory Cytokines: Interactions and Clinical Implications. *Cytokine Growth factor Rev* (2018) 43:38–46. doi: 10.1016/j.cytogfr.2018.07.001
51. Galluzzi L, Vitale I, Aaronson SA, Abrams JM, Adam D, Agostinis P, et al. Molecular Mechanisms of Cell Death: Recommendations of the Nomenclature Committee on Cell Death 2018. *Cell Death differentiation* (2018) 25(3):486–541. doi: 10.1038/s41418-017-0012-4
52. Britson KA, Yang SY, Lloyd TE. New Developments in the Genetics of Inclusion Body Myositis. *Curr Rheumatol Rep* (2018) 20(5):26. doi: 10.1007/s11926-018-0738-0
53. Vesa J, Su H, Watts GD, Krause S, Walter MC, Martin B, et al. Valosin Containing Protein Associated Inclusion Body Myopathy: Abnormal Vacuolization, Autophagy and Cell Fusion in Myoblasts. *Neuromuscular Disord NMD* (2009) 19(11):766–72. doi: 10.1016/j.nmd.2009.08.003
54. Güttsches AK, Brady S, Krause K, Maerkens A, Uszkoreit J, Eisenacher M, et al. Proteomics of Rimmed Vacuoles Define New Risk Allele in Inclusion Body Myositis. *Ann Neurol* (2017) 81(2):227–39. doi: 10.1002/ana.24847
55. Nogalska A, D'Agostino C, Terracciano C, Engel WK, Askanas V. Impaired Autophagy in Sporadic Inclusion-Body Myositis and in Endoplasmic Reticulum Stress-Provoked Cultured Human Muscle Fibers. *Am J Pathol* (2010) 177(3):1377–87. doi: 10.2353/ajpath.2010.100050
56. de Camargo LV, de Carvalho MS, Shinjo SK, de Oliveira ASB, Zanoteli E. Clinical, Histological, and Immunohistochemical Findings in Inclusion Body Myositis. *BioMed Res Int* (2018) 2018:5069042. doi: 10.1155/2018/5069042
57. Hiniker A, Daniels BH, Lee HS, Margeta M. Comparative Utility of LC3, P62 and TDP-43 Immunohistochemistry in Differentiation of Inclusion Body Myositis From Polymyositis and Related Inflammatory Myopathies. *Acta Neuropathol Commun* (2013) 1:29. doi: 10.1186/2051-5960-1-29
58. Schmidt K, Wienken M, Keller CW, Balcarek P, Münz C, Schmidt J. IL-1β-Induced Accumulation of Amyloid: Macroautophagy in Skeletal Muscle Depends on ERK. *Mediators Inflammation* (2017) 2017:5470831. doi: 10.1155/2017/5470831
59. Bhatnagar S, Mittal A, Gupta SK, Kumar A. TWEAK Causes Myotube Atrophy Through Coordinated Activation of Ubiquitin-Proteasome System, Autophagy, and Caspases. *J Cell Physiol* (2012) 227(3):1042–51. doi: 10.1002/jcp.22821
60. Alger HM, Raben N, Pistilli E, Francia DL, Rawat R, Getnet D, et al. The Role of TRAIL in Mediating Autophagy in Myositis Skeletal Muscle: A Potential Nonimmune Mechanism of Muscle Damage. *Arthritis Rheumatism* (2011) 63(11):3448–57. doi: 10.1002/art.30530
61. Keller CW, Fokken C, Turville SG, Lünemann A, Schmidt J, Münz C, et al. TNF-Alpha Induces Macroautophagy and Regulates MHC Class II Expression in Human Skeletal Muscle Cells. *J Biol Chem* (2011) 286 (5):3970–80. doi: 10.1074/jbc.M110.159392
62. Loi M, Müller A, Steinbach K, Niven J, Barreira da Silva R, Paul P, et al. Macroautophagy Proteins Control MHC Class I Levels on Dendritic Cells and Shape Anti-Viral CD8(+) T Cell Responses. *Cell Rep* (2016) 15(5):1076–87. doi: 10.1016/j.celrep.2016.04.002
63. Lünemann JD, Schmidt J, Schmid D, Barthel K, Wrede A, Dalakas MC, et al. Beta-Amyloid is a Substrate of Autophagy in Sporadic Inclusion Body Myositis. *Ann Neurol* (2007) 61(5):476–83. doi: 10.1002/ana.21115
64. Girolamo F, Lia A, Amati A, Strippoli M, Coppola C, Virgintino D, et al. Overexpression of Autophagic Proteins in the Skeletal Muscle of Sporadic Inclusion Body Myositis. *Neuropathol Appl Neurobiol* (2013) 39(7):736–49. doi: 10.1111/nan.12040
65. Nakano S, Oki M, Kusaka H. The Role of P62/SQSTM1 in Sporadic Inclusion Body Myositis. *Neuromuscular Disord NMD* (2017) 27(4):363–9. doi: 10.1016/j.nmd.2016.12.009
66. Shtifman A, Ward CW, Laver DR, Bannister ML, Lopez JR, Kitazawa M, et al. Amyloid-β Protein Impairs Ca2+ Release and Contractility in Skeletal Muscle. *Neurobiol Aging* (2010) 31(12):2080–90. doi: 10.1016/j.neurobiolaging.2008.11.003
67. Yamashita S, Matsuo Y, Tawara N, Hara K, Yamamoto M, Nishikami T, et al. CYLD Dysregulation in Pathogenesis of Sporadic Inclusion Body Myositis. *Sci Rep* (2019) 9(1):11606. doi: 10.1038/s41598-019-48115-2
68. Cacciottolo M, Nogalska A, D'Agostino C, Engel WK, Askanas V. Chaperone-Mediated Autophagy Components are Upregulated in Sporadic Inclusion-Body Myositis Muscle Fibres. *Neuropathol Appl Neurobiol* (2013) 39(7):750–61. doi: 10.1111/nan.12038
69. Ahmed M, Machado PM, Miller A, Spicer C, Herbelin L, He J, et al. Targeting Protein Homeostasis in Sporadic Inclusion Body Myositis. *Sci Trans Med* (2016) 8(331):331ra41. doi: 10.1126/scitranslmed.aad4583
70. Jeong JH, Yang DS, Koo JH, Hwang DJ, Cho JY, Kang EB. Effect of Resistance Exercise on Muscle Metabolism and Autophagy in sIBM. *Med Sci sports Exercise* (2017) 49(8):1562–71. doi: 10.1249/MSS.0000000000001286
71. Cappelletti C, Galbardi B, Kapetis D, Vattemi G, Guglielmi V, Tonin P, et al. Autophagy, Inflammation and Innate Immunity in Inflammatory Myopathies. *PloS One* (2014) 9(11):e111490. doi: 10.1371/journal.pone.0111490
72. Girolamo F, Lia A, Annese T, Giannini M, Amati A, D'Abbicco D, et al. Autophagy Markers LC3 and P62 Accumulate in Immune-Mediated Necrotizing Myopathy. *Muscle Nerve* (2019) 60(3):315–27. doi: 10.1002/mus.26608
73. Fischer N, Preuße C, Radke J, Pehl D, Allenbach Y, Schneider U, et al. Sequestosome-1 (P62) Expression Reveals Chaperone-Assisted Selective Autophagy in Immune-Mediated Necrotizing Myopathies. *Brain Pathol (Zurich Switzerland)* (2020) 30(2):261–71. doi: 10.1111/bpa.12772
74. Matsubara S, Bokuda K, Asano Y, Morishima R, Sugaya K, Miyamoto K, et al. Mitophagy in Three Cases of Immune-Mediated Necrotizing Myopathy Associated With Anti-3-Hydroxy-3-Methylglutaryl-Coenzyme A Reductase Autoantibodies: Ultrastructural and Immunohistochemical Studies. *Neuromuscular Disord NMD* (2018) 28(3):283–8. doi: 10.1016/j.nmd.2018.01.004
75. Das M, Karnam A, Stephen-Victor E, Gilardin L, Bhatt B, Kumar Sharma V, et al. Intravenous Immunoglobulin Mediates Anti-Inflammatory Effects in Peripheral Blood Mononuclear Cells by Inducing Autophagy. *Cell Death Dis* (2020) 11(1):50. doi: 10.1038/s41419-020-2249-y
76. Kolaczkowska E, Kubes P. Neutrophil Recruitment and Function in Health and Inflammation. *Nat Rev Immunol* (2013) 13(3):159–75. doi: 10.1038/nri3399
77. Knight JS, Carmona-Rivera C, Kaplan MJ. Proteins Derived From Neutrophil Extracellular Traps may Serve as Self-Antigens and Mediate Organ Damage in Autoimmune Diseases. *Front Immunol* (2012) 3:380. doi: 10.3389/fimmu.2012.00380
78. Carmona-Rivera C, Carlucci PM, Moore E, Lingampalli N, Uchtenhagen H, James E, et al. Synovial Fibroblast-Neutrophil Interactions Promote Pathogenic Adaptive Immunity in Rheumatoid Arthritis. *Sci Immunol* (2017) 2(10). doi: 10.1126/sciimmunol.aag3358
79. Khandpur R, Carmona-Rivera C, Vivekanandan-Giri A, Gizinski A, Yalavarthi S, Knight JS, et al. NETs are a Source of Citrullinated Autoantigens and Stimulate Inflammatory Responses in Rheumatoid Arthritis. *Sci Trans Med* (2013) 5(178):178ra40. doi: 10.1126/scitranslmed.3005580
80. Lood C, Blanco LP, Purmalek MM, Carmona-Rivera C, De Ravin SS, Smith CK, et al. Neutrophil Extracellular Traps Enriched in Oxidized Mitochondrial DNA are Interferogenic and Contribute to Lupus-Like Disease. *Nat Med* (2016) 22(2):146–53. doi: 10.1038/nm.4027
81. Lu X, Tang Q, Lindh M, Dastmalchi M, Alexanderson H, Popovic Silwerfeldt K, et al. The Host Defense Peptide LL-37 a Possible Inducer of the Type I Interferon System in Patients With Polymyositis and Dermatomyositis. *J Autoimmun* (2017) 78:46–56. doi: 10.1016/j.jaut.2016.12.003
82. Carmona-Rivera C, Zhao W, Yalavarthi S, Kaplan MJ. Neutrophil Extracellular Traps Induce Endothelial Dysfunction in Systemic Lupus Erythematosus Through the Activation of Matrix Metalloproteinase-2. *Ann rheumatic Dis* (2015) 74(7):1417–24. doi: 10.1136/annrheumdis-2013-204837
83. Saffarzadeh M, Juenemann C, Queisser MA, Lochnit G, Barreto G, Galuska SP, et al. Neutrophil Extracellular Traps Directly Induce Epithelial and Endothelial Cell Death: A Predominant Role of Histones. *PloS One* (2012) 7 (2):e32366. doi: 10.1371/journal.pone.0032366
84. Caudrillier A, Kessenbrock K, Gilliss BM, Nguyen JX, Marques MB, Monestier M, et al. Platelets Induce Neutrophil Extracellular Traps in Transfusion-Related Acute Lung Injury. *J Clin Invest* (2012) 122(7):2661–71. doi: 10.1172/JCI61303

85. Silvestre-Roig C, Braster Q, Wichapong K, Lee EY, Teulon JM, Berrebeh N, et al. Externalized Histone H4 Orchestrates Chronic Inflammation by Inducing Lytic Cell Death. *Nature* (2019) 569(7755):236–40. doi: 10.1038/s41586-019-1167-6
86. Arecco N, Clarke CJ, Jones FK, Simpson DM, Mason D, Beynon RJ, et al. Elastase Levels and Activity are Increased in Dystrophic Muscle and Impair Myoblast Cell Survival, Proliferation and Differentiation. *Sci Rep* (2016) 6:24708. doi: 10.1038/srep24708
87. Seto N, Torres-Ruiz JJ, Carmona-Rivera C, Pinal-Fernandez I, Pak K, Purmalek MM, et al. Neutrophil Dysregulation is Pathogenic in Idiopathic Inflammatory Myopathies. *JCI Insight* (2020) 5(3). doi: 10.1172/jci.insight.134189
88. Dalakas MC. Pathogenesis and Therapies of Immune-Mediated Myopathies. *Autoimmun Rev* (2012) 11(3):203–6. doi: 10.1016/j.autrev.2011.05.013
89. Warnatsch A, Ioannou M, Wang Q, Papayannopoulos V. Inflammation. Neutrophil Extracellular Traps License Macrophages for Cytokine Production in Atherosclerosis. *Sci (New York NY)* (2015) 349(6245):316–20. doi: 10.1126/science.aaa8064
90. Villanueva E, Yalavarthi S, Berthier CC, Hodgin JB, Khandpur R, Lin AM, et al. Netting Neutrophils Induce Endothelial Damage, Infiltrate Tissues, and Expose Immunostimulatory Molecules in Systemic Lupus Erythematosus. *J Immunol (Baltimore Md 1950)* (2011) 187(1):538–52. doi: 10.4049/jimmunol.1100450
91. Zhang S, Shu X, Tian X, Chen F, Lu X, Wang G. Enhanced Formation and Impaired Degradation of Neutrophil Extracellular Traps in Dermatomyositis and Polymyositis: A Potential Contributor to Interstitial Lung Disease Complications. *Clin Exp Immunol* (2014) 177(1):134–41. doi: 10.1111/cei.12319
92. Carmona-Rivera C, Kaplan MJ. Low-Density Granulocytes: A Distinct Class of Neutrophils in Systemic Autoimmunity. *Semin Immunopathol* (2013) 35 (4):455–63. doi: 10.1007/s00281-013-0375-7
93. Zhang S, Shen H, Shu X, Peng Q, Wang G. Abnormally Increased Low-Density Granulocytes in Peripheral Blood Mononuclear Cells are Associated With Interstitial Lung Disease in Dermatomyositis. *Modern Rheumatol* (2017) 27(1):122–9. doi: 10.1080/14397595.2016.1179861
94. Peng Y, Zhang S, Zhao Y, Liu Y, Yan B. Neutrophil Extracellular Traps may Contribute to Interstitial Lung Disease Associated With Anti-MDA5 Autoantibody Positive Dermatomyositis. *Clin Rheumatol* (2018) 37 (1):107–15. doi: 10.1007/s10067-017-3799-y
95. Duvvuri B, Pachman LM, Morgan G, Khojah AM, Klein-Gitelman M, Curran ML, et al. Neutrophil Extracellular Traps in Tissue and Periphery in Juvenile Dermatomyositis. *Arthritis Rheumatol (Hoboken NJ)* (2020) 72 (2):348–58. doi: 10.1002/art.41078
96. Smith CK, Vivekanandan-Giri A, Tang C, Knight JS, Mathew A, Padilla RL, et al. Neutrophil Extracellular Trap-Derived Enzymes Oxidize High-Density Lipoprotein: An Additional Proatherogenic Mechanism in Systemic Lupus Erythematosus. *Arthritis Rheumatol (Hoboken NJ)* (2014) 66(9):2532–44. doi: 10.1002/art.38703
97. Bergsbaken T, Fink SL, Cookson BT. Pyroptosis: Host Cell Death and Inflammation. *Nat Rev Microbiol* (2009) 7(2):99–109. doi: 10.1038/nrmicro2070
98. Kovacs SB, Miao EA. Gasdermins: Effectors of Pyroptosis. *Trends Cell Biol* (2017) 27(9):673–84. doi: 10.1016/j.tcb.2017.05.005
99. Liu X, Xia S, Zhang Z, Wu H, Lieberman J. Channelling Inflammation: Gasdermins in Physiology and Disease. *Nat Rev Drug Discov* (2021) 20:1–22. doi: 10.1038/s41573-021-00154-z
100. Jiang M, Qi L, Li L, Li Y. The Caspase-3/GSDME Signal Pathway as a Switch Between Apoptosis and Pyroptosis in Cancer. *Cell Death Discovery* (2020) 6:112. doi: 10.1038/s41420-020-00349-0
101. Liu M, Li L, Dai T, Hou Y, Li W, Zhao Y, et al. Gasdermine E-Dependent Mitochondrial Pyroptotic Pathway in Dermatomyositis: A Possible Mechanism of Perifascicular Atrophy. *J Neuropathol Exp Neurol* (2020) 79 (5):551–61. doi: 10.1093/jnen/nlaa023
102. Ma M, Chai K, Deng R. Study of the Correlation Between the Noncanonical Pathway of Pyroptosis and Idiopathic Inflammatory Myopathy. *Int Immunopharmacol* (2021) 98:107810. doi: 10.1016/j.intimp.2021.107810
103. Liu D, Xiao Y, Zhou B, Gao S, Li L, Zhao L, et al. PKM2-Dependent Glycolysis Promotes Skeletal Muscle Cell Pyroptosis by Activating the NLRP3 Inflammasome in Dermatomyositis/Polymyositis. *Rheumatol (Oxford England)* (2021) 60(5):2177–89. doi: 10.1093/rheumatology/keaa473
104. Tang D, Chen X, Kang R, Kroemer G. Ferroptosis: Molecular Mechanisms and Health Implications. *Cell Res* (2021) 31(2):107–25. doi: 10.1038/s41422-020-00441-1
105. Gao M, Monian P, Pan Q, Zhang W, Xiang J, Jiang X. Ferroptosis is an Autophagic Cell Death Process. *Cell Res* (2016) 26(9):1021–32. doi: 10.1038/cr.2016.95
106. Gono T, Kawaguchi Y, Hara M, Masuda I, Katsumata Y, Shinozaki M, et al. Increased Ferritin Predicts Development and Severity of Acute Interstitial Lung Disease as a Complication of Dermatomyositis. *Rheumatol (Oxford England)* (2010) 49(7):1354–60. doi: 10.1093/rheumatology/keq073
107. Gao M, Yi J, Zhu J, Minikes AM, Monian P, Thompson CB, et al. Role of Mitochondria in Ferroptosis. *Mol Cell* (2019) 73(2):354–63.e3. doi: 10.1016/j.molcel.2018.10.042
108. Rygiel KA, Miller J, Grady JP, Rocha MC, Taylor RW, Turnbull DM. Mitochondrial and Inflammatory Changes in Sporadic Inclusion Body Myositis. *Neuropathol Appl Neurobiol* (2015) 41(3):288–303. doi: 10.1111/nan.12149
109. Boehler JF, Horn A, Novak JS, Li N, Ghimbovschi S, Lundberg IE, et al. Mitochondrial Dysfunction and Role of Harakiri in the Pathogenesis of Myositis. *J Pathol* (2019) 249(2):215–26. doi: 10.1002/path.5309
110. Meyer A, Laverny G, Allenbach Y, Grelet E, Ueberschlag V, Echaniz-Laguna A, et al. IFN-β-Induced Reactive Oxygen Species and Mitochondrial Damage Contribute to Muscle Impairment and Inflammation Maintenance in Dermatomyositis. *Acta Neuropathol* (2017) 134(4):655–66. doi: 10.1007/s00401-017-1731-9
111. Dhuriya YK, Sharma D. Necroptosis: A Regulated Inflammatory Mode of Cell Death. *J Neuroinflamm* (2018) 15(1):199. doi: 10.1186/s12974-018-1235-0
112. Pasparakis M, Vandenabeele P. Necroptosis and its Role in Inflammation. *Nature* (2015) 517(7534):311–20. doi: 10.1038/nature14191
113. Weinlich R, Oberst A, Beere HM, Green DR. Necroptosis in Development, Inflammation and Disease. *Nat Rev Mol Cell Biol* (2017) 18(2):127–36. doi: 10.1038/nrm.2016.149
114. Lawlor KE, Khan N, Mildenhall A, Gerlic M, Croker BA, D'Cruz AA, et al. RIPK3 Promotes Cell Death and NLRP3 Inflammasome Activation in the Absence of MLKL. *Nat Commun* (2015) 6:6282. doi: 10.1038/ncomms7282
115. Conos SA, Chen KW, De Nardo D, Hara H, Whitehead L, Núñez G, et al. Active MLKL Triggers the NLRP3 Inflammasome in a Cell-Intrinsic Manner. *Proc Natl Acad Sci United States America* (2017) 114(6):E961–e9. doi: 10.1073/pnas.1613305114
116. Fan H, Liu F, Dong G, Ren D, Xu Y, Dou J, et al. Activation-Induced Necroptosis Contributes to B-Cell Lymphopenia in Active Systemic Lupus Erythematosus. *Cell Death Dis* (2014) 5(9):e1416. doi: 10.1038/cddis.2014.375
117. Lee SH, Kwon JY, Kim SY, Jung K, Cho ML. Interferon-Gamma Regulates Inflammatory Cell Death by Targeting Necroptosis in Experimental Autoimmune Arthritis. *Sci Rep* (2017) 7(1):10133. doi: 10.1038/s41598-017-09767-0
118. Weisel K, Berger S, Thorn K, Taylor PC, Peterfy C, Siddall H, et al. A Randomized, Placebo-Controlled Experimental Medicine Study of RIPK1 Inhibitor GSK2982772 in Patients With Moderate to Severe Rheumatoid Arthritis. *Arthritis Res Ther* (2021) 23(1):85. doi: 10.1186/s13075-021-02468-0
119. Mariño G, Niso-Santano M, Baehrecke EH, Kroemer G. Self-Consumption: The Interplay of Autophagy and Apoptosis. *Nat Rev Mol Cell Biol* (2014) 15 (2):81–94. doi: 10.1038/nrm3735
120. Lightfoot AP, Nagaraju K, McArdle A, Cooper RG. Understanding the Origin of non-Immune Cell-Mediated Weakness in the Idiopathic Inflammatory Myopathies - Potential Role of ER Stress Pathways. *Curr Opin Rheumatol* (2015) 27(6):580–5. doi: 10.1097/BOR.0000000000000212
121. Bedoui S, Herold MJ, Strasser A. Emerging Connectivity of Programmed Cell Death Pathways and its Physiological Implications. *Nat Rev Mol Cell Biol* (2020) 21(11):678–95. doi: 10.1038/s41580-020-0270-8
122. Sollberger G, Choidas A, Burn GL, Habenberger P, Di Lucrezia R, Kordes S, et al. Gasdermin D Plays a Vital Role in the Generation of Neutrophil

Extracellular Traps. *Sci Immunol* (2018) 3(26). doi: 10.1126/sciimmunol.aar6689

123. Orning P, Weng D, Starheim K, Ratner D, Best Z, Lee B, et al. Pathogen Blockade of TAK1 Triggers Caspase-8-Dependent Cleavage of Gasdermin D and Cell Death. *Sci (New York NY)* (2018) 362(6418):1064–9. doi: 10.1126/science.aau2818
124. Newton K, Wickliffe KE, Maltzman A, Dugger DL, Reja R, Zhang Y, et al. Activity of Caspase-8 Determines Plasticity Between Cell Death Pathways. *Nature* (2019) 575(7784):679–82. doi: 10.1038/s41586-019-1752-8
125. Wang Y, Kanneganti TD. From Pyroptosis, Apoptosis and Necroptosis to PANoptosis: A Mechanistic Compendium of Programmed Cell Death Pathways. *Comput Struct Biotechnol J* (2021) 19:4641–57. doi: 10.1016/j.csbj.2021.07.038
126. Karki R, Sharma BR, Tuladhar S, Williams EP, Zalduondo L, Samir P, et al. Synergism of TNF-α and IFN-γ Triggers Inflammatory Cell Death, Tissue Damage, and Mortality in SARS-CoV-2 Infection and Cytokine Shock Syndromes. *Cell* (2021) 184(1):149–68.e17. doi: 10.1016/j.cell.2020.11.025

13

Machine Learning Algorithms Identify Clinical Subtypes and Cancer in Anti-TIF1γ+ Myositis: A Longitudinal Study of 87 Patients

Lijuan Zhao [1,2,3], Shuoshan Xie [4], Bin Zhou [5], Chuyu Shen [6], Liya Li [7], Weiwei Pi [8], Zhen Gong [9], Jing Zhao [10], Qi Peng [11], Junyu Zhou [1,2,3], Jiaqi Peng [12], Yan Zhou [13], Lingxiao Zou [14], Liang Song [12], Honglin Zhu [1,2,3] and Hui Luo [1,2,3]**

[1] Department of Rheumatology, Xiangya Hospital of Central South University, Changsha, China, [2] National Clinical Research Center for Geriatric Disorders, Xiangya Hospital of Central South University, Changsha, China, [3] Provincial Clinical Research Center for Rheumatic and Immunologic Diseases, Xiangya Hospital of Central South University, Changsha, China, [4] Department of Nephrology, Hunan Provincial People's Hospital and The First Affiliated Hospital of Hunan Normal University, Changsha, China, [5] Department of Nephrology, The Affiliated Hospital of Qingdao University, Qingdao, China, [6] Department of Rheumatology, The First Affiliated Hospital, Sun Yat-sen University, Guangzhou, China, [7] Department of Rheumatology, The Third Xiangya Hospital of Central South University, Changsha, China, [8] Department of Oncology, The First People's Hospital of Changde City, Changde, China, [9] Department of Rheumatology, Yiyang Central Hospital, Yiyang, China, [10] Department of Rheumatology, The First Affiliated Hospital of Jishou University, Jishou, China, [11] Department of Rheumatology, Yueyang People's Hospital, Yueyang, China, [12] Huaihua No.1 People's Hospital Affiliated to Nanhua University, Huaihua, China, [13] Department of Obstetrics and Gynecology, Zhuzhou Central Hospital, Zhuzhou, China, [14] Department of Obstetrics and Gynecology, The Third Xiangya Hospital of Central South University, Changsha, China

***Correspondence:**
Honglin Zhu
honglinzhu@csu.edu.cn
Hui Luo
luohui@csu.edu.cn

Background: Anti-TIF1γ antibodies are a class of myositis-specific antibodies (MSAs) and are closely associated with adult cancer-associated myositis (CAM). The heterogeneity in anti-TIF1γ+ myositis is poorly explored, and whether anti-TIF1γ+ patients will develop cancer or not is unknown at their first diagnosis. Here, we aimed to explore the subtypes of anti-TIF1γ+ myositis and construct machine learning classifiers to predict cancer in anti-TIF1γ+ patients based on clinical features.

Methods: A cohort of 87 anti-TIF1γ+ patients were enrolled and followed up in Xiangya Hospital from June 2017 to June 2021. Sankey diagrams indicating temporal relationships between anti-TIF1γ+ myositis and cancer were plotted. Elastic net and random forest were used to select and rank the most important variables. Multidimensional scaling (MDS) plot and hierarchical cluster analysis were performed to identify subtypes of anti-TIF1γ+ myositis. The clinical characteristics were compared among subtypes of anti-TIF1γ+ patients. Machine learning classifiers were constructed to predict cancer in anti-TIF1γ+ myositis, the accuracy of which was evaluated by receiver operating characteristic (ROC) curves.

Results: Forty-seven (54.0%) anti-TIF1γ+ patients had cancer, 78.7% of which were diagnosed within 0.5 years of the myositis diagnosis. Fourteen variables contributing most to distinguishing cancer and non-cancer were selected and used for the calculation of the similarities (proximities) of samples and the construction of machine learning classifiers.

The top 10 were disease duration, percentage of lymphocytes (L%), percentage of neutrophils (N%), neutrophil-to-lymphocyte ratio (NLR), sex, C-reactive protein (CRP), shawl sign, arthritis/arthralgia, V-neck sign, and anti-PM-Scl75 antibodies. Anti-TIF1γ+ myositis patients can be clearly separated into three clinical subtypes, which correspond to patients with low, intermediate, and high cancer risk, respectively. Machine learning classifiers [random forest, support vector machines (SVM), extreme gradient boosting (XGBoost), elastic net, and decision tree] had good predictions for cancer in anti-TIF1γ+ myositis patients. In particular, the prediction accuracy of random forest was >90%, and decision tree highlighted disease duration, NLR, and CRP as critical clinical parameters for recognizing cancer patients.

Conclusion: Anti-TIF1γ+ myositis can be separated into three distinct subtypes with low, intermediate, and high risk of cancer. Machine learning classifiers constructed with clinical characteristics have favorable performance in predicting cancer in anti-TIF1γ+ myositis, which can help physicians in choosing appropriate cancer screening programs.

Keywords: myositis, anti-TIF1γ antibody, subtypes, prediction, machine learning algorithms, cancer

INTRODUCTION

Idiopathic inflammatory myopathies (IIMs, collectively called myositis) are a group of highly heterogeneous systemic autoimmune diseases. IIMs have five main subgroups—dermatomyositis (DM), polymyositis (PM), immune-mediated necrotizing myopathy (IMNM), sporadic inclusion body myositis (sIBM), and overlap myositis (including antisynthetase syndrome) (1, 2). An increased cancer risk in adult myositis patients has been observed in numerous large population studies, and the incidences vary from 6.7% to 32.0% (3–5). Most cancers are diagnosed within 3 years of myositis diagnosis, and the time span of cancer-associated myositis (CAM) is accordingly defined (4, 6–8). DM has a stronger association with cancer than other IIM subgroups, and the cancer types are influenced by the geographical and ethnic backgrounds of myositis patients (9).

Autoantibodies are important biomarkers in IIMs. Myositis-specific autoantibodies (MSAs) are specific to IIMs, while myositis-associated autoantibodies (MAAs) are associated with myositis overlap syndromes. MSAs are closely correlated with distinct disease phenotypes; for example, anti-MDA5 antibodies are associated with clinically amyopathic DM and rapidly progressive interstitial lung disease (RP-ILD) (10).

Transcriptional intermediary factor 1γ (TIF1γ) is a protein belonging to the tripartite motif (TRIM) superfamily that plays diverse roles in transcriptional elongation, DNA repair, cell differentiation, mitosis, and embryonic development. Anti-TIF1γ antibodies were first referred to as anti-p155 in the serum of myositis patients, which immunoprecipitated a 155-kDa nuclear protein (11, 12). Anti-TIF1γ antibodies are found in 7% of adult IIMs and are considered as one of the MSAs present in DM (10, 13, 14). Many studies have reported a strong correlation between anti-TIF1γ antibodies and malignancies. Approximately 50% of anti-TIF1γ+ adult myositis patients are diagnosed with cancers within 3 years (12, 15). However, even if the high risk of cancer in anti-TIF1γ+ myositis is known, physicians still cannot exactly predict the anti-TIF1γ+ myositis patients developing cancer or not at the first diagnosis. More extensive cancer screening is needed for the anti-TIF1γ+ patients who will develop cancer, while less effort is needed for those who will not. Thus, earlier identification of anti-TIF1γ+ patients with probable cancers will be clinically important.

In this study, we analyzed 44 clinical characteristics at baseline of 87 anti-TIF1γ+ adult myositis patients and their outcome of cancer during the follow-up time. Fourteen variables most important for distinguishing cancer and non-cancer were selected. Then, multidimensional scaling (MDS) plot and hierarchical cluster analysis divided anti-TIF1γ+ myositis into three clusters based on sample similarities calculated with these variables, which corresponded to patients with low, intermediate, and high cancer risk. Distinct clinical characteristics were found among clusters. In addition, machine learning classifiers for cancer were constructed and verified with excellent performances. Overall, our study highlighted a new strategy to manage anti-TIF1γ+ patients with machine learning algorithms to stratify and predict their cancer risk at their first visit at hospitals.

MATERIALS AND METHODS

Study Design and Participants

This was a longitudinal study conducted at Xiangya Hospital in Hunan Province, south-central China, from June 2017 to June 2021. The inclusion criteria were a clinical diagnosis of myositis in adult patients according to either the 1975 Bohan/Peter (16) or 2017 EULAR/ACR (1) classification for IIMs, with serological positivity for anti-TIF1γ antibodies, and follow-up for three years from the diagnosis of myositis unless cancer was diagnosed earlier. The exclusion criteria were patients who withdrew or failed to finish the follow-up. Myositis overlapping with other connective tissue diseases, such as systemic lupus erythematosus (SLE) and Sjogren's syndrome (SS), was not excluded, because overlap myositis is also recognized as one main subtype of IIMs (2). The antibody repertoire of myositis was detected with serum using commercially available kits (Euroimmun, Germany, and KingMed, China). A flow diagram of the study protocol is shown in **Supplementary File 1**. This study was approved by the Ethics Committee of the Institutional Review Board at Xiangya Hospital (#201212074), and written informed consent was obtained from all patients.

Data Collection

Medical records of patients at the time of enrollment before treatment were reviewed, and data on 44 clinical variables (**Supplementary File 2**) were collected with no missing data. In addition, the cancer categories and time interval from myositis diagnosis to cancer diagnosis were also obtained. In our study, CAM was defined as cancers occurring within 3 years of the myositis diagnosis (before or after) (17).

Variable Selection, Clustering Analysis, and Construction of Machine Learning Classifiers

Machine learning algorithms were performed in R or Python. Elastic net was used to select the most important clinical variables out of all 44 clinical variables for the classification of anti-TIF1γ+ myositis with cancer or not. The importance of selected variables was evaluated by random forest with mean decrease Gini. The similarities (random forest proximities) of samples were calculated with the selected variables, based on which multidimensional scaling (MDS) plot and hierarchical cluster analysis were used to cluster and visualize these samples. Five machine learning classifiers [random forest, support vector machines (SVM), extreme gradient boosting (XGBoost), elastic net, and decision tree] were also constructed with these selected clinical variables to predict cancer probability of anti-TIF1γ+ patients. Stratified 10-fold cross-validation was performed to estimate the accuracy of each model and optimize the models with hyperparameter tuning. Eighty-seven patients were split into a training set containing 70% of the observations and a test set containing the remaining 30%. The training set was used to build the classificatory models, and the testing set was used to evaluate the accuracy of the model. All steps were performed using Python V.3.9.1, scikit-learn V.0.24.2, NumPy V.1.19.5, and pandas V.1.2.1. ROC (receiver operating characteristic) curves were drawn with Matplotlib V.3.3.3.

Statistical Analysis

The statistical analysis of comparisons among anti-TIF1γ+ myositis patients in the three clusters was performed in SPSS v.22 or GraphPad 8.0, and p <0.05 was considered statistically significant. Quantitative data were described as the means (standard deviations) or medians (interquartile ranges) according to data distribution and homoscedasticity. Qualitative data were described as frequencies (percentages). Accordingly, one-way ANOVA or Kruskal–Wallis tests (adjusted with Dunnett T3 or Dunn's test) and Pearson chi-square test or Fisher's exact test (adjusted with Bonferroni test) were performed to compare multiple groups. The heatmap was plotted by ggplot2 in R.

RESULTS

Characteristics of 87 Anti-TIF1γ+ Patients and Their Temporal Relationship Between Myositis and Cancer

Anti-TIF1γ+ myositis patients enrolled in our study were mainly female (64.4%), with an average age of 57 years and a median disease duration of 6 months. Their most common manifestation was typical DM rashes (95.4%), followed by proximal weakness (56.3%), ILD (17.2%), and arthritis/arthralgia (11.5%). Two patients (2.3%) were complicated with another connective tissue disease—Sjogren's syndrome.

Forty-seven (54.0%) of our anti-TIF1γ+ patients in total met the diagnostic criteria of CAM. Their temporal relationships between the diagnosis of myositis and cancer are shown in **Figure 1**. None of the anti-TIF1γ+ patients had cancer until 1.5 years before the myositis diagnosis when two female patients were diagnosed with breast and ovarian carcinomas. From 0.5 to 1.5 years before the myositis diagnosis, six cases of cancer were diagnosed, consisting of five female patients and one male patient. Within 0.5 years before and after the myositis diagnosis, 36 anti-TIF1γ+ patients were diagnosed with cancer, and 72.2% of them had the diagnosis of cancer and myositis simultaneously. Nasopharyngeal carcinoma was the most frequent cancer type, and all cases were developed in males. During the period of 0.5 to 1.5 years after the myositis diagnosis, only three more patients (two male and one female) were reported to have cancer. No cancer was reported in the remaining follow-up time. Overall, cancer was most frequently diagnosed within 0.5 years before and after the myositis diagnosis, especially at the time of myositis diagnosis. A total of 45.0% (9/20) female and 7.4% (2/27) male patients had an earlier diagnosis of cancer before myositis developed. Nasopharyngeal carcinoma, breast cancer, and lung cancer were the top 3 tumor categories with the highest incidence.

Subtypes in Anti-TIF1γ+ Myositis Patients

Anti-TIF1γ+ patients exhibit differences in whether complicated with cancer or not. Using the elastic net and random forest method, 14 variables that contribute most to discriminating between cancer and non-cancer were selected. To identify the heterogeneities among anti-TIF1γ+ myositis, the similarities (random forest proximities) of patients were calculated by these 14 variables. As shown in the MDS plot and hierarchical clustering tree (**Figures 2A, B**), the 87 anti-TIF1γ+ patients can be separated into three distinct clusters. The patient numbers in clusters 1, 2, and 3 were 28 (32.2%), 28 (32.2%), and 31(35.6%), respectively. Twenty-seven (96.4%) patients in cluster 2 developed cancer, which was almost the opposite of cluster 1 with only one (3.6%) cancer patient. Cluster 3 had 19 (61.3%)

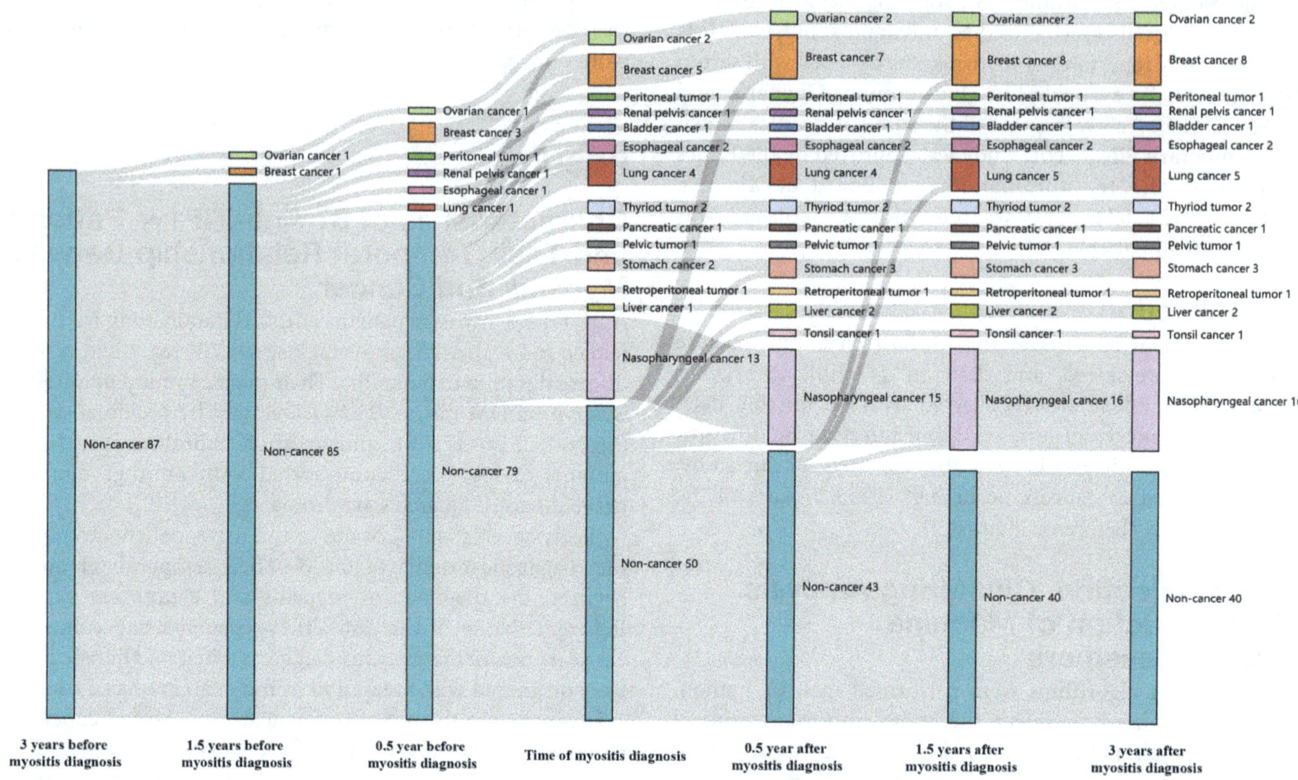

FIGURE 1 | The Sankey diagram showed temporal relationships between the diagnosis of myositis and cancer in 87 anti-TIF1γ+ myositis patients. Seven time points, including 0.5, 1.5, and 3 years before or after myositis diagnosis and the time of the myositis diagnosis, were analyzed.

patients with cancer and were intermediate between clusters 1 and 2. Therefore, we inferred clusters 1, 2, and 3 corresponded to three stratifications with low, high, and intermediate cancer risk. The importance of the 14 selected clinical variables was ranked with random forest algorithm according to mean decrease Gini (**Figure 2C**). The top 10 important variables were disease duration, percentage of lymphocytes (L%), percentage of neutrophils (N%), neutrophil-to-lymphocyte ratio (NLR), sex, C-reactive protein (CRP), shawl sign, arthritis/arthralgia, V-neck sign, and anti-PM-Scl75 antibodies.

Comparison of Clinical Characteristics Among the Three Clusters of Anti-TIF1γ+ Myositis

We then analyzed the clinical characteristics of anti-TIF1γ+ patients in the three clusters (**Table 1**). Significant intergroup differences between cluster 1 (low-risk cancer group) and cluster 2 (high-risk cancer group) were found. For instance, patients in cluster 2 were all male, but most patients in cluster 1 are female ($p < 0.001$). Patients in cluster 2 had an older age ($p = 0.020$); a higher percentage of skin ulcers ($p = 0.008$); a shorter disease duration ($p < 0.001$); higher levels of CRP ($p = 0.005$), lactic dehydrogenase (LDH) ($p < 0.001$), creatine kinase (CK) ($p = 0.005$), N% ($p = 0.013$), and NLR ($p < 0.001$); and a lower level of L% ($p < 0.001$). Clusters 1 and 3 also had significant difference in disease duration ($p < 0.001$), LDH ($p < 0.001$), N% ($p < 0.001$), L% ($p < 0.001$), and NLR ($p < 0.001$). Interestingly, clusters 2 and 3 differed obviously in cancer types: 87.5% patients with breast cancer were in cluster 3 and 100.0% patients with nasopharyngeal carcinoma were in cluster 2 ($p = 0.005$ and $p < 0.001$). Ovarian cancer, peritoneal tumor, renal pelvis cancer, pancreatic cancer, pelvic tumor, and tonsil cancer were all developed in cluster 3. Conversely, bladder cancer, esophageal cancer, retroperitoneal cancer, and liver cancer were all found in cluster 2 (**Figure 2**). The autoantibody profile of myositis in our patients is displayed in **Figure 3A**. A total of 14 (16.1%) anti-TIF1γ+ myositis patients had other MSAs, such as anti-MDA5, anti-Jo1, and anti-PL12. Anti-Ro52 was the most common MAAs. However, there was no difference in the intensities of anti-TIF1γ antibodies or the count of total antibody types among anti-TIF1γ+ myositis patients in the three clusters (**Figures 3B, C**).

Machine Learning Classifiers Predicting Cancer in Anti-TIF1γ+ Patients

Early diagnosis of cancer in anti-TIF1γ+ myositis is crucial for improving prognosis, especially for patients with intermediate and high cancer risk in clusters 2 and 3. We constructed machine learning models with the selected 14 most important variables to predict anti-TIF1γ+ myositis with or without cancer. The ROC curves of machine learning models calculated using the training

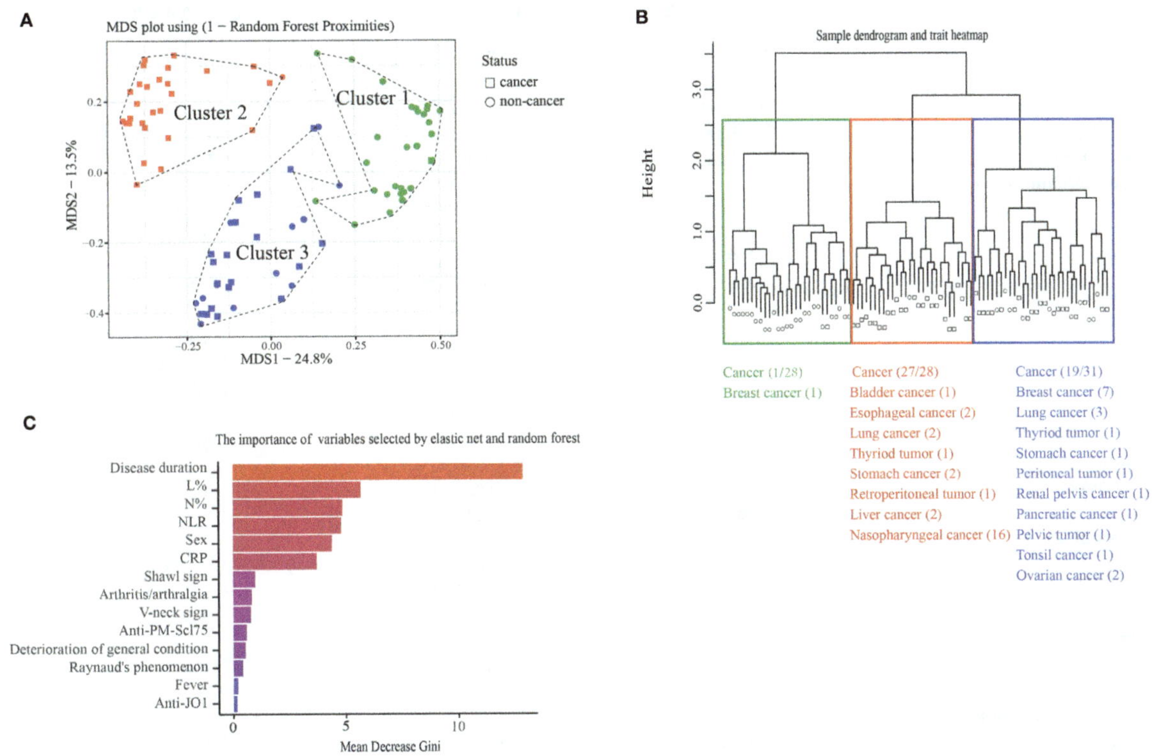

FIGURE 2 | **(A)** The MDS plot and **(B)** hierarchical cluster analysis of 87 anti-TIF1γ+ myositis patients based on random forest proximities that were calculated by 14 clinical variables showed three distinct clusters and the distribution of cancer in each cluster. **(C)** The bar plot represents the importance of clinical variables evaluated by random forest.

and testing sets are shown in **Figure 4**. The SVM model had an AUC (area under the ROC Curve) of 100.0% in the training set and 90.0% in the test set. The elastic net and XGBoost models also had good performance with AUCs higher than 85.0%. In addition, we trained the random forest model with all 87 samples and the AUC was 90.9%. To conveniently predict the cancer risk of anti-TIF1γ+ myositis patients in clinical practice, we built a decision tree model in the training set (**Figure 4C**). This model included three variables—disease duration, NLR, and CRP. Its AUCs in the training set and test set were 95.0% and 70.0% (**Figures 4A, B**), respectively.

DISCUSSION

In this study, anti-TIF1γ+ myositis is separated into three different clinical subtypes. Clusters 1, 2, and 3 correspond to patients with low, high, and intermediate risk of cancer, respectively. Anti-TIF1γ+ patients with low cancer risk have distinct clinical characteristics from those with high and intermediate cancer risk, which enables the construction of models to predict cancer in anti-TIF1γ+ patients. Indeed, machine learning classifiers (random forest, SVM, elastic net, decision trees, and XGBoost) showed good classification in discriminating anti-TIF1γ+ patients with cancer or not. In particular, the prediction accuracy of random forest was >90%. Decision tree can conveniently stratify and manage anti-TIF1γ+ myositis patients with disease duration, NLR, and CRP in clinical practice. It is of great value because myositis patients who are positive for anti-TIF1γ antibodies and predicted to develop cancers by our models should undergo more careful and intensive tumor screening than those predicted with low cancer risk.

Fourteen clinical variables were selected for model construction in our study. The top 10 variables ranked by importance were disease duration, L%, N%, NLR, sex, CRP, shawl sign, arthritis/arthralgia, V-neck sign, and anti-PM-Scl75 antibodies. The disease duration (from myositis onset to visit at our hospital) was shorter in the cluster with intermediate and high cancer risks than in the cluster with low cancer risk. This may be related to the more severe disease state of patients in clusters with higher cancer risk, manifested as more patients with deteriorated general condition and increased CK levels. Anti-TIF1γ+ myositis patients in clusters with intermediate and high cancer risk had a higher N% and NLR but a lower L%. Neutrophil dysregulation is pathogenic in myositis, mainly through neutrophil extracellular traps (NETs) and the subset of low-density granulocytes (LDGs) (18). The underlying mechanisms for decreased L% are uncertain and need further exploration. Our anti-TIF1γ+ myositis patients in cluster 2 with the highest risk of cancer were more often males, had higher CRP levels, and more frequent shawl sign and V-neck sign. These clinical

TABLE 1 | Characteristics of anti-TIF1γ+ myositis patients among three clusters at the time of first visit at our hospital.

	Cluster 1 n = 28	Cluster 2 n = 28	Cluster 3 n = 31	Global p_{adj}
Age (years)	50 ± 18[#]	61 ± 10	58 ± 14	0.018
Sex				
Men	3 (10.7%)[#]	28 (100.0%)	0 (0.0%)[&]	<0.001
Women	25 (89.3%)[#]	0 (0.0%)	31 (100.0%)[&]	
Disease duration (months)	40.5 (49.5)[#*]	3.0 (6.25)	5.0 (10.0)	<0.001
General condition/inflammation				
Fever	1 (3.6%)	2 (7.1%)	1 (3.2%)	0.836
Deterioration of general condition	0 (0.0%)	3 (10.7%)	2 (6.5%)	0.272
ESR (mm/h)	26 (52)	55 (57)	33 (38)	0.127
CRP (mg/L)	2.52 (5.85)[#]	14.25 (17.85)	3.12 (5.00)	0.007
Skin lesions				
Heliotrope rash	24 (85.7%)	26 (92.9%)	27 (87.1%)	0.765
Gottron's sign	12 (42.9%)	16 (57.1%)	16 (51.6%)	0.572
V-neck sign	15 (53.6%)	20 (71.4%)	18 (58.1%)	0.408
Shawl sign	11 (39.3%)	15 (53.6%)	12 (38.7%)	0.451
Holster sign	2 (7.1%)	7 (25.0%)	7 (22.6%)	0.186
Mechanic's hands	1 (3.6%)	0 (0.0%)	3 (9.7%)	0.319
Raynaud phenomenon	0 (0.0%)	0 (0.0%)	2 (6.5%)	0.326
Skin ulcers	0 (0.0%)[#]	6 (21.4%)	1 (3.2%)	0.008
Muscular manifestations				
Proximal weakness	11 (39.3%)	17 (60.7%)	21 (67.7%)	0.076
LDH (U/L)	211.4 (88.9)[#*]	327.5 (209.7)	355.1 (161.0)	<0.001
CK (U/L)	81.1 (161.2)[#]	403.1 (2008.0)	156.0 (355.4)	0.006
Lung manifestations				
ILD	4 (14.3%)	5 (17.9%)	6 (19.4%)	0.938
Lung infection	1 (3.6%)	7 (25.0%)	2 (6.5%)	0.049
Other rheumatologic manifestations				
Arthritis/arthralgia	4 (14.3%)	3 (10.7%)	3 (9.7%)	0.916
Blood cells				
WBC (×10^9/L)	5.5 (1.6)	6.7 (4.4)	6.8 (2.7)	0.090
Hb (g/L)	124 ± 17*	122 ± 15	112 ± 18	0.010
N%	65.4 (14.0)[#*]	72.2 (13.5)	76.7 (13.1)	<0.001
L%	25.3 ± 7.0[#*]	14.5 ± 4.9	15.0 ± 7.3	<0.001
NLR	2.9 (1.9)[#*]	5.1 (3.7)	6.1 (4.6)	<0.001
M%	8.5 (5.2)	9.9 (3.4)	8.0 (3.9)	0.067
Cancer	1 (3.6%)[#*]	27 (96.4%)	19 (61.3%)[&]	<0.001

ESR, erythrocyte sedimentation rate; CRP, C-reactive protein; LDH, lactic dehydrogenase; CK, creatine kinase; ILD, interstitial lung disease; WBC, white blood cells; RBC, red blood cells; N%, percentage of neutrophils; L%, percentage of lymphocytes; NLR, neutrophil-to-lymphocyte ratio; M%, percentage of monocytes.
*[#]$p < 0.05$ for comparison between cluster 1 and cluster 2; *$p < 0.05$ for comparison between cluster 1 and cluster 3; [&]$p < 0.05$ for comparison between cluster 2 and cluster 3.*

characteristics were proven to be related factors for CAM (9, 19–22). For example, a meta-analysis including 69 studies concluded that DM subtype, older age, male gender, dysphagia, cutaneous ulceration, and anti-TIF1γ positivity were associated with increased cancer risk (21). Another large-scale multicenter cohort study found CAM patients had more common older age, heliotrope rash, shawl sign, and V sign (22). In fact, anti-TIF1γ+ myositis patients with cancer account for nearly half of the CAM cases, that is why they exhibit large clinical similarities (15, 17).

There were no differences in anti-TIF1γ intensities (at the time of visit in our hospital) among clusters with different cancer risks. It is still controversial whether the levels of anti-TIF1γ antibodies correlate with the evolution of cancer (23–25). Tests of anti-TIF1γ antibodies at different time points (e.g., after cancer therapy) might be helpful. Although 41 (47.1%) anti-TIF1γ+ patients had more than one type of autoantibody, we found no association between cancer risk and the number of antibody types in our study. All three anti-TIF1γ+ patients with anti-PM-Scl75 antibodies developed cancer in our study. Anti-PM-Scl75 antibodies are usually suggestive of overlapping myositis accompanied by the manifestation of systemic sclerosis (26, 27). The relationship between anti-PM-Scl75 antibodies and CAM is unknown. In another Chinese CAM cohort, a higher positive rate of anti-PM-Scl75 antibodies was also found in cancer patients than in cancer-free patients (4.1% vs. 2.8%) (28). In our study, one anti-TIF1γ+ patient with cancer was positive for another MSA also related to cancer—anti-NXP2 antibody (29, 30). The standardized incidence ratio of anti-TIF1γ antibodies for estimating cancer risk was 17.28, twice that of anti-NXP2 antibodies (17). It is reasonable to believe that anti-TIF1γ antibodies are predominant to link with the presence of cancer in our myositis patient. There are some new potential biomarkers of cancer in myositis: the IgG2 isotype of anti-TIF1γ helps to identify the risk of mortality in anti-TIF1γ+ patients (31); soluble programmed death ligand 1 (sPD-L1), combined with anti-TIF1γ antibodies, yielded greater specificity and positive predictive value in diagnosing cancer, reaching values of 95% and 70%, respectively (32). These indexes show promising values in clinical practice and needed further verification in larger study populations.

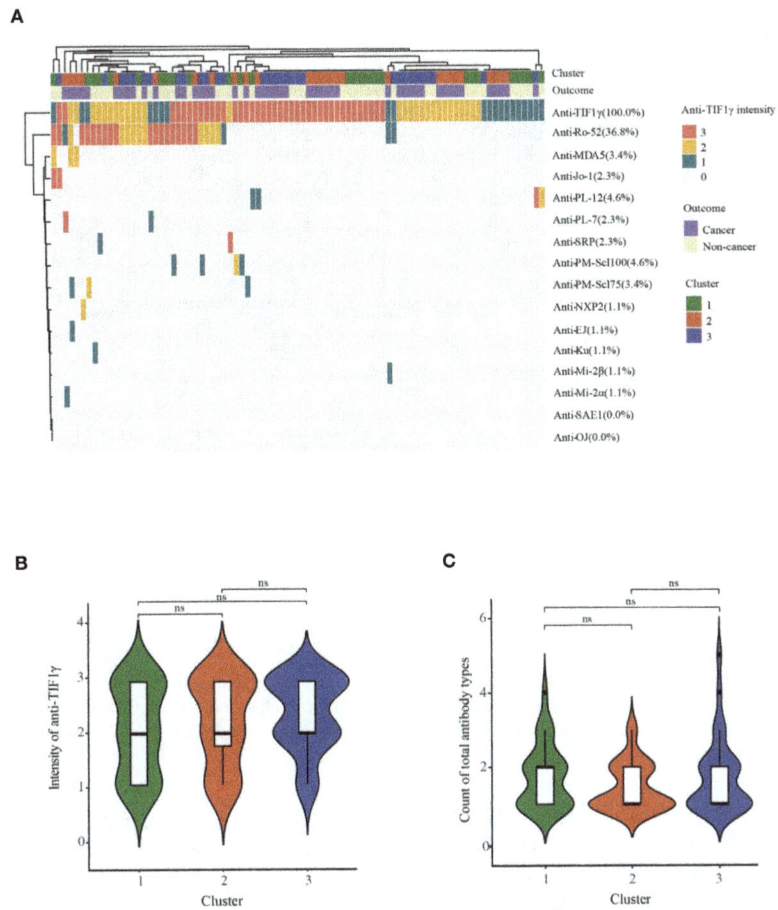

FIGURE 3 | **(A)** The heatmap showed the autoantibody profile of 87 anti-TIF1γ+ myositis patients. **(B)** The comparison of anti-TIF1γ intensities and **(C)** the comparison of count of total antibody types among anti-TIF1γ+ myositis patients in three clusters. n.s. represents no significance.

Our study showed that 78.7% (37/47) of cancers were diagnosed within 0.5 years of the myositis diagnosis. A time span of 3 years before and after myositis diagnosis is emphasized in the definition of CAM (4, 6–8). In fact, most cancers were diagnosed simultaneously with or during the first year after the diagnosis of myositis according to previous studies (7, 33). Anti-TIF1γ was significantly associated with a shorter time between myositis and cancer onset (34–36). In one study with 10-year follow-up, all the detected malignancy cases in the anti-TIF1γ+ cohort occurred between 3 years prior to and 2.5 years after DM onset, whereas cancers were detected in the following 7.5 years in anti-TIF1γ- patients (34). We also found 23.4% (11/47) of cancers diagnosed before the myositis diagnosis; 81.8% (9/11) of these patients were females in cluster 3. This may be partially explained by the theory of paraneoplastic myositis syndrome, which regards manifestations of the skin and skeletal muscle as consequences of underlying malignancy (37). Nasopharyngeal carcinoma (34.0%), breast cancer (17.0%), and lung cancer (10.6%) were the 3 three cancers with the highest incidence in our cohort. The organs where myositis patients are prone to develop a tumor vary in different studies (8, 38–40). This is influenced mainly by genetic background and ethnicity (9). The finding in our study is comparable with the local general population because most patients enrolled in the study live in southeastern China—an area with a high incidence of nasopharyngeal cancer. Interestingly, the nasopharynx and breast were the most common cancer sites in male and female patients, respectively, emphasizing different screening targets in male and female patients.

This is the first study identifying subtypes and predicting cancer in anti-TIF1γ+ myositis by machine learning algorithms, although several limitations exist. First, compared with anti-MDA5 (30%) and anti-JO1 (19%) antibodies, the positive rate of anti-TIF1γ antibodies (7%) among myositis patients is relatively low (41). Thus, multicenter cooperation and a large sample size are needed for further study. Second, the mechanism by which anti-TIF1γ+ myositis patients develop cancer was not explored in our study. We can predict the cancer risk of anti-TIF1γ+ myositis patients and prompt early discovery but cannot prevent the occurrence of cancer from the pathogenesis of the disease.

In conclusion, anti-TIF1γ+ myositis can be divided into three distinct subtypes based on their clinical characteristics, which are corresponding to patients with low, intermediate, and high cancer risk. Machine learning models showed satisfactory

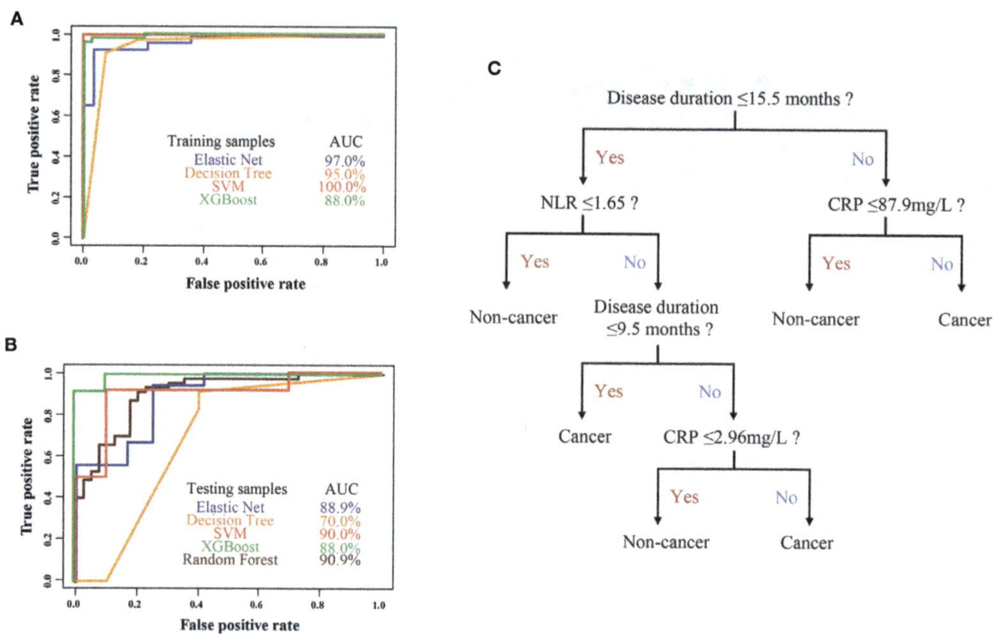

FIGURE 4 | **(A)** The ROC curves of four machine learning models in the anti-TIF1γ+ myositis training samples. **(B)** The ROC curves of four machine learning models (elastic net, decision tree, SVM, XGBoost) in the anti-TIF1γ+ myositis testing samples and random forest model in all patient samples. **(C)** Decision tree model showed disease duration, CRP, and NLR as important clinical features in the prediction of cancer in anti-TIF1γ+ myositis patients.

accuracy in the prediction of cancer in anti-TIF1γ+ myositis patients. These findings suggested that the stratified management of anti-TIF1γ+ myositis patients is necessary to avoid excessive cancer screening examinations in patients with low cancer risk and make the best use of targeted cancer screening in patients predicted to develop cancer.

ETHICS STATEMENT

The studies involving human participants were reviewed and approved by the Ethics Committee of the Institutional Review Board at Xiangya Hospital. The patients/participants provided their written informed consent to participate in this study.

AUTHOR CONTRIBUTIONS

LZ, HZ, and HL designed the study. SX, BZ, CS, ZG, WP, LL, JiZ, QP, JuZ, JP, YZ, LZ, and LS collected the data. LZ and HZ analyzed the results and wrote the draft. HL revised the manuscript for content. All authors contributed to the article and approved the submission for publication.

REFERENCES

1. Lundberg IE, Tjarnlund A, Bottai M, Werth VP, Pilkington C, Visser M, et al. European League Against Rheumatism/American College of Rheumatology Classification Criteria for Adult and Juvenile Idiopathic Inflammatory Myopathies and Their Major Subgroups. *Ann Rheum Dis* (2017) 76 (12):1955–64. doi: 10.1136/annrheumdis-2017-211468
2. Selva-O'Callaghan A, Pinal-Fernandez I, Trallero-Araguas E, Milisenda JC, Grau-Junyent JM, Mammen AL. Classification and Management of Adult Inflammatory Myopathies. *Lancet Neurol* (2018) 17(9):816–28. doi: 10.1016/S1474-4422(18)30254-0
3. Hill CL, Zhang Y, Sigurgeirsson B, Pukkala E, Mellemkjaer L, Airio A, et al. Frequency of Specific Cancer Types in Dermatomyositis and Polymyositis: A Population-Based Study. *Lancet* (2001) 357(9250):96–100. doi: 10.1016/S0140-6736(00)03540-6
4. Sigurgeirsson B, Lindelof B, Edhag O, Allander E. Risk of Cancer in Patients With Dermatomyositis or Polymyositis. A Population-Based Study. *N Engl J Med* (1992) 326(6):363–7. doi: 10.1056/NEJM199202063260602
5. Aussy A, Boyer O, Cordel N. Dermatomyositis and Immune-Mediated Necrotizing Myopathies: A Window on Autoimmunity and Cancer. *Front Immunol* (2017) 8:992. doi: 10.3389/fimmu.2017.00992
6. Buchbinder R, Forbes A, Hall S, Dennett X, Giles G. Incidence of Malignant Disease in Biopsy-Proven Inflammatory Myopathy. A Population-Based Cohort Study. *Ann Intern Med* (2001) 134(12):1087–95. doi: 10.7326/0003-4819-134-12-200106190-00008
7. Stockton D, Doherty VR, Brewster DH. Risk of Cancer in Patients With Dermatomyositis or Polymyositis, and Follow-Up Implications: A Scottish Population-Based Cohort Study. *Br J Cancer* (2001) 85(1):41–5. doi: 10.1054/bjoc.2001.1699
8. Yang Z, Lin F, Qin B, Liang Y, Zhong R. Polymyositis/Dermatomyositis and Malignancy Risk: A Metaanalysis Study. *J Rheumatol* (2015) 42(2):282–91. doi: 10.3899/jrheum.140566
9. Moghadam-Kia S, Oddis CV, Ascherman DP, Aggarwal R. Risk Factors and Cancer Screening in Myositis. *Rheum Dis Clin North Am* (2020) 46(3):565–76. doi: 10.1016/j.rdc.2020.05.006

10. McHugh NJ, Tansley SL. Autoantibodies in Myositis. *Nat Rev Rheumatol* (2018) 14(5):290–302. doi: 10.1038/nrrheum.2018.56
11. Kotobuki Y, Tonomura K, Fujimoto M. Transcriptional Intermediary Factor 1 (TIF1) and Anti-TIF1gamma Antibody-Positive Dermatomyositis. *Immunol Med* (2021) 44(1):23–9. doi: 10.1080/25785826.2020.1791402
12. De Vooght J, Vulsteke JB, De Haes P, Bossuyt X, Lories R, De Langhe E. Anti-TIF1-Gamma Autoantibodies: Warning Lights of a Tumour Autoantigen. *Rheumatol (Oxford)* (2020) 59(3):469–77. doi: 10.1093/rheumatology/kez572
13. Li S, Ge Y, Yang H, Wang T, Zheng X, Peng Q, et al. The Spectrum and Clinical Significance of Myositis-Specific Autoantibodies in Chinese Patients With Idiopathic Inflammatory Myopathies. *Clin Rheumatol* (2019) 38 (8):2171–9. doi: 10.1007/s10067-019-04503-7
14. Mariampillai K, Granger B, Amelin D, Guiguet M, Hachulla E, Maurier F, et al. Development of a New Classification System for Idiopathic Inflammatory Myopathies Based on Clinical Manifestations and Myositis-Specific Autoantibodies. *JAMA Neurol* (2018) 75(12):1528–37. doi: 10.1001/jamaneurol.2018.2598
15. Trallero-Araguas E, Rodrigo-Pendas JA, Selva-O'Callaghan A, Martinez-Gomez X, Bosch X, Labrador-Horrillo M, et al. Usefulness of Anti-P155 Autoantibody for Diagnosing Cancer-Associated Dermatomyositis: A Systematic Review and Meta-Analysis. *Arthritis Rheum* (2012) 64(2):523–32. doi: 10.1002/art.33379
16. Bohan A, Peter JB. Polymyositis and Dermatomyositis (First of Two Parts). *N Engl J Med* (1975) 292(7):344–7. doi: 10.1056/NEJM197502132920706
17. Yang H, Peng Q, Yin L, Li S, Shi J, Zhang Y, et al. Identification of Multiple Cancer-Associated Myositis-Specific Autoantibodies in Idiopathic Inflammatory Myopathies: A Large Longitudinal Cohort Study. *Arthritis Res Ther* (2017) 19(1):259. doi: 10.1186/s13075-017-1469-8
18. Seto N, Torres-Ruiz JJ, Carmona-Rivera C, Pinal-Fernandez I, Pak K, Purmalek MM, et al. Neutrophil Dysregulation Is Pathogenic in Idiopathic Inflammatory Myopathies. *JCI Insight* (2020) 5(3). doi: 10.1172/jci.insight.134189
19. Sparsa A, Liozon E, Herrmann F, Ly K, Lebrun V, Soria P, et al. Routine vs Extensive Malignancy Search for Adult Dermatomyositis and Polymyositis: A Study of 40 Patients. *Arch Dermatol* (2002) 138(7):885–90. doi: 10.1001/archderm.138.7.885
20. Wang J, Guo G, Chen G, Wu B, Lu L, Bao L. Meta-Analysis of the Association of Dermatomyositis and Polymyositis With Cancer. *Br J Dermatol* (2013) 169 (4):838–47. doi: 10.1111/bjd.12564
21. Oldroyd AGS, Allard AB, Callen JP, Chinoy H, Chung L, Fiorentino D, et al. A Systematic Review and Meta-Analysis to Inform Cancer Screening Guidelines in Idiopathic Inflammatory Myopathies. *Rheumatol (Oxford)* (2021) 60 (6):2615–28. doi: 10.1093/rheumatology/keab166
22. Li Y, Jia X, Sun X, Shi L, Lin F, Gan Y, et al. Risk Factors for Cancer-Associated Myositis: A Large-Scale Multicenter Cohort Study. *Int J Rheum Dis* (2021) 24 (2):268–73. doi: 10.1111/1756-185X.14046
23. Abe Y, Ando T, Matsushita M, Tada K, Yamaji K, Tamura N. Changes in Antibody Titres in Patients With Anti-Transcription Intermediary Factor 1-Gamma Antibody-Positive Idiopathic Inflammatory Myositis. *Rheumatol (Oxford)* (2019) 58(1):179–81. doi: 10.1093/rheumatology/key310
24. Ogawa-Momohara M, Muro Y, Mitsuma T, Katayama M, Yanaba K, Nara M, et al. Strong Correlation Between Cancer Progression and Anti-Transcription Intermediary Factor 1gamma Antibodies in Dermatomyositis Patients. *Clin Exp Rheumatol* (2018) 36(6):990 5.
25. Dani L, Holmqvist M, Martinez MA, Trallero-Araguas E, Dastmalchi M, Svensson J, et al. Anti-Transcriptional Intermediary Factor 1 Gamma Antibodies in Cancer-Associated Myositis: A Longitudinal Study. *Clin Exp Rheumatol* (2020) 38(1):67–73.
26. Pakozdi A, Nihtyanova S, Moinzadeh P, Ong VH, Black CM, Denton CP. Clinical and Serological Hallmarks of Systemic Sclerosis Overlap Syndromes. *J Rheumatol* (2011) 38(11):2406–9. doi: 10.3899/jrheum.101248
27. Cruellas MG, Viana Vdos S, Levy-Neto M, Souza FH, Shinjo SK. Myositis-Specific and Myositis-Associated Autoantibody Profiles and Their Clinical Associations in a Large Series of Patients With Polymyositis and Dermatomyositis. *Clinics (Sao Paulo)* (2013) 68(7):909–14. doi: 10.6061/clinics/2013(07)04
28. Li L, Liu C, Wang Q, Wu C, Zhang Y, Cheng L, et al. Analysis of Myositis Autoantibodies in Chinese Patients With Cancer-Associated Myositis. *J Clin Lab Anal* (2020) 34(8):e23307. doi: 10.1002/jcla.23307
29. Fiorentino DF, Chung LS, Christopher-Stine L, Zaba L, Li S, Mammen AL, et al. Most Patients With Cancer-Associated Dermatomyositis Have Antibodies to Nuclear Matrix Protein NXP-2 or Transcription Intermediary Factor 1gamma. *Arthritis Rheum* (2013) 65(11):2954–62. doi: 10.1002/art.38093
30. Ichimura Y, Matsushita T, Hamaguchi Y, Kaji K, Hasegawa M, Tanino Y, et al. Anti-NXP2 Autoantibodies in Adult Patients With Idiopathic Inflammatory Myopathies: Possible Association With Malignancy. *Ann Rheum Dis* (2012) 71(5):710–3. doi: 10.1136/annrheumdis-2011-200697
31. Aussy A, Freret M, Gallay L, Bessis D, Vincent T, Jullien D, et al. The Igg2 Isotype of Anti-Transcription Intermediary Factor 1gamma Autoantibodies Is a Biomarker of Cancer and Mortality in Adult Dermatomyositis. *Arthritis Rheumatol* (2019) 71(8):1360–70. doi: 10.1002/art.40895
32. Chen H, Peng Q, Yang H, Yin L, Shi J, Zhang Y, et al. Increased Levels of Soluble Programmed Death Ligand 1 Associate With Malignancy in Patients With Dermatomyositis. *J Rheumatol* (2018) 45(6):835–40. doi: 10.3899/jrheum.170544
33. Chen YJ, Wu CY, Huang YL, Wang CB, Shen JL, Chang YT. Cancer Risks of Dermatomyositis and Polymyositis: A Nationwide Cohort Study in Taiwan. *Arthritis Res Ther* (2010) 12(2):R70. doi: 10.1186/ar2987
34. Oldroyd A, Sergeant JC, New P, McHugh NJ, Betteridge Z, Lamb JA, et al. The Temporal Relationship Between Cancer and Adult Onset Anti-Transcriptional Intermediary Factor 1 Antibody-Positive Dermatomyositis. *Rheumatol (Oxford)* (2019) 58(4):650–5. doi: 10.1093/rheumatology/key357
35. Hida A, Yamashita T, Hosono Y, Inoue M, Kaida K, Kadoya M, et al. Anti-TIF1-Gamma Antibody and Cancer-Associated Myositis: A Clinicohistopathologic Study. *Neurology* (2016) 87(3):299–308. doi: 10.1212/WNL.0000000000002863
36. Danko K, Ponyi A, Molnar AP, Andras C, Constantin T. Paraneoplastic Myopathy. *Curr Opin Rheumatol* (2009) 21(6):594–8. doi: 10.1097/BOR.0b013e3283317fa5
37. Lu X, Peng Q, Wang G. The Role of Cancer-Associated Autoantibodies as Biomarkers in Paraneoplastic Myositis Syndrome. *Curr Opin Rheumatol* (2019) 31(6):643–9. doi: 10.1097/BOR.0000000000000641
38. Chen D, Yuan S, Wu X, Li H, Qiu Q, Zhan Z, et al. Incidence and Predictive Factors for Malignancies With Dermatomyositis: A Cohort From Southern China. *Clin Exp Rheumatol* (2014) 32(5):615–21.
39. Sung YK, Jung SY, Kim H, Choi S, Im SG, Cha EJ, et al. Temporal Relationship Between Idiopathic Inflammatory Myopathies and Malignancies and Its Mortality: A Nationwide Population-Based Study. *Clin Rheumatol* (2020) 39 (11):3409–16. doi: 10.1007/s10067-019-04782-0
40. Andras C, Bodoki L, Nagy-Vincze M, Griger Z, Csiki E, Danko K. Retrospective Analysis of Cancer-Associated Myositis Patients Over the Past 3 Decades in a Hungarian Myositis Cohort. *Pathol Oncol Res* (2020) 26(3):1749–55. doi: 10.1007/s12253-019-00756-4
41. Satoh M, Tanaka S, Ceribelli A, Calise SJ, Chan EK. A Comprehensive Overview on Myositis-Specific Antibodies: New and Old Biomarkers in Idiopathic Inflammatory Myopathy. *Clin Rev Allergy Immunol* (2017) 52 (1):1–19. doi: 10.1007/s12016-015-8510-y

14

RNA-Containing Immune Complexes Formed by Anti-Melanoma Differentiation Associated Gene 5 Autoantibody Are Potent Inducers of IFN-α

Kaiwen Wang†, Jiangfeng Zhao†, Wanlong Wu, Wenwen Xu, Shuhui Sun, Zhiwei Chen, Yakai Fu, Li Guo, Hui Du and Shuang Ye**

Department of Rheumatology, Renji Hospital, Shanghai Jiao Tong University School of Medicine, Shanghai, China

***Correspondence:**
Shuang Ye
ye_shuang2000@163.com
Hui Du
hui_du1972@126.com*

†These authors have contributed equally to this work

Objective: Anti-melanoma differentiation-associated gene 5 (MDA5) autoantibody is a distinctive serology hallmark of dermatomyositis (DM). As an autoantigen, MDA5 is a cytoplasmic RNA recognition receptor. The aim of this study was to address the question of whether the RNA-containing immune complex (IC) formed by MDA5 and anti-MDA5 could activate type I interferon (IFN) response.

Method: Patients with anti-MDA5$^+$ DM (n = 217), anti-MDA5$^-$ DM (n = 68), anti-synthase syndrome (ASyS, n = 57), systemic lupus erythematosus (SLE, n = 245), rheumatoid arthritis (RA, n = 89), and systemic sclerosis (SSc, n = 30) and healthy donors (HD, n = 94) were enrolled in our studies. Anti-MDA5 antibody was detected by line blotting, enzyme-linked immunosorbent assay (ELISA), immunoprecipitation, and Western blotting. Cytokine profiling was determined by multiplex flow cytometry, and IFN-α was further measured by ELISA. Type I IFN-inducible genes were detected by quantitative PCR (qPCR). RNA–IC binding was analyzed by RNA immunoprecipitation. Plasmacytoid dendritic cells (pDCs) derived from healthy donors were cultivated and stimulated with MDA5 ICs with or without RNase and Toll-like receptor 7 (TLR-7) agonist. The interaction between MDA5 ICs and TLR7 was evaluated by immunoprecipitation and confocal microscopy.

Results: According to our in-house ELISA, the presence of anti-MDA5 antibody in 76.1% of DM patients, along with 14.3% of SLE patients who had a lower titer yet positive anti-MDA5 antibody, was related to the high level of peripheral IFN-α. ICs formed by MDA5 and anti-MDA5 were potent inducers of IFN-α *via* TLR-7 in an RNA-dependent manner *in vitro*.

Conclusion: Our data provided evidence of the mechanistic relevance between the anti-MDA5 antibody and type I IFN pathway.

Keywords: dermatomyositis, anti-MDA5 autoantibody, RNA-containing immune complexes, interferon pathway, IFN-α

INTRODUCTION

Anti-melanoma differentiation-associated gene 5 (MDA5) antibody is considered a specific serological marker in dermatomyositis (DM), which is typically linked to the amyopathic phenotype and rapidly progressive interstitial lung disease (ILD) (1). The pathogenesis of anti-MDA5 antibody-positive (anti-MDA5$^+$) DM is largely unknown; however, possible genetic factors (with East Asian predisposition) and environmental triggers (such as viral infection) have been implicated (2). MDA5, encoded by the *IFIH1* gene, is the key sensor of viral double-strand RNA (dsRNA) and belongs to the retinoic acid-induced gene I (RIG-I)-like receptors (3), which are actively involved in the type I interferon (IFN-α and IFN-β) pathway. Indeed, type I IFN is well conceived to play a crucial role in the pathogenesis of DM and has profound treatment implications (4). It is noteworthy that systemic lupus erythematosus (SLE) is also characterized by the aberrant activation of the type I IFN pathway (5). There is strong genetic evidence for a link between cytoplasmic RNA sensing pathways (RIG-I/MDA5) and SLE (6, 7). The current knowledge suggested that the anti-MDA5 antibody, as a serological marker, is more likely to be a by-product of an "overloaded" type I IFN pathway in DM (8–11). In the present study, however, we are asking the question whether the anti-MDA5 antibody could enhance the type I IFN response.

METHODS

Patients

All DM patients fulfilled the 239th European Neuromuscular Centre (ENMC) criteria (12) with the presence of one of the five DM-specific autoantibodies (anti-MDA5, anti-TIF1γ, anti-SAE1, anti-NXP2, or anti-Mi2), which were determined by EUROLINE Autoimmune Inflammatory Myopathies 16 Ag assays (EUROIMMUN, Lübeck, Germany). Anti-synthase syndrome (ASyS) (12), rheumatoid arthritis (RA), systemic sclerosis (SSc), and SLE patients served as the disease controls, abiding by the respective classification criteria. A Bio-Plex Pro 2200 Luminex LiquiChip immunoassay (Bio-Rad, Hercules, CA, USA) was used to detect autoantibodies against extractable nuclear antigens (ENAs) for all patients. Healthy donor and patient samples were obtained with informed consent. The study protocol was approved by the Ethics Committee of Renji Hospital, Shanghai Jiao Tong University School of Medicine (ethics no. IRB# 2017-041). All participants provided written informed consent.

ELISA for Anti-MDA5 Antibody

ELISA plates were coated overnight at 4°C with 10 µg/well of recombinant full-length MDA5 protein (Shanghai Free Zone Biotechnology Co., Ltd., Shanghai, China). After blocking with 1% bovine serum albumin (BSA), patient sera were used at 1:101 dilution and horseradish peroxidase-labeled anti-human immunoglobulin G (IgG) antibodies (1:60,000; Jackson Laboratory, Bar Harbor, ME, USA) were incubated for 30 min, then stopped by tetramethylbenzidine reagent (Invitrogen, Waltham, MA, USA) and the absorbance read at 450 nm (Sprinter XL, EUROIMMUN, Lübeck, Germany). The cutoff value for this in-house anti-MDA5 antibody ELISA was set as the mean + 3SD of 94 healthy donors. To evaluate the consistency between this in-house and a commercial anti-MDA5 antibody ELISA (MBL, Tokyo, Japan) assay, 92 subjects (DM = 47, HC = 38, and SLE = 7) were tested back to back, with good agreement ($\kappa = 0.847$, $p < 0.001$).

Cytokine Assays

Serum cytokine levels [including IFN-α, IFN-β, IFN-γ, IL-1β, interleukin 2 (IL-2), IL-4, IL-5, IL-6, IL-8, IL-10, IL-12p70, IL-17A, IL-17F, IL-22, tumor necrosis factor alpha (TNF-α), TNF-β, and granulocyte–macrophage colony-stimulating factor (GM-CSF)] were measured with an AimPlex flow cytometer (Tianjin Kuang Bo Tongsheng Biotechnology Co., Ltd., Tianjin, China) and a commercial IFN-α ELISA kit (PBL Biomedical, Piscataway, NJ, USA) following the manufacturers' protocols.

Immunoprecipitation and Western Blotting

Immunoprecipitation (IP) assay using a cell lysate overexpressing Flag-tagged MDA5 was generated using a 293 cell line (Shanghai Free Zone Biotechnology Co., Ltd., Shanghai, China). Of the cell lysate, 100 µg was pre-cleared with protein A beads in NP40 lysis buffer (Thermo Fisher, Waltham, MA, USA) and immunoprecipitated with 5 µl patient serum. The immunoprecipitates were blotted with an anti-Flag antibody (Invitrogen, Waltham, MA, USA) and visualized using enhanced chemiluminescence (Thermo Fisher, Waltham, MA, USA) in a FluorChem M chemiluminescence imager (ProteinSimple, San Jose, CA, USA). Recombinant MDA5 protein (60 µg/lane) was electrophoresed on SDS-PAGE gels and transferred into nitrocellulose membranes for the immunoblotting assays. Sera were used at 1:201 dilution for MDA5 immunoblot.

PBMC Isolation and SYBR Green qRT-PCR

Peripheral blood mononuclear cells (PBMCs) were prepared using Ficoll-Hypaque (TBD, Tianjin, China) density gradient centrifugation from DM and SLE patients. The total RNA extracted from PBMCs using the TRIzol reagent (Invitrogen, Waltham, MA, USA) was reverse transcribed into cDNA with the Superscript II Reverse Transcriptase Kit (Takara, Shiga, Japan). The transcription levels of type I IFN-inducible genes (*LY6E, OAS1, Mx-1, IFIT1*, and *IFIT3*) were measured using SYBR® Premix Ex Taq™ II (Takara, Shiga, Japan) *via* an ABI Prism 7900 system. The primer sequences we have previously reported (13) are as follows: *LY6E*: 5′-CTTACGGTCCAA CATCAGAC-3′, 5′-GCACACATCCCTACTGACAC-3′; *OAS-1*: 5′-GAAGGCAGCTCACGAAAC-3′, 5′-TTCTTAAAGCAT GGGTAATTC-3′; *Mx-1*: 5′-GGGTAGCCACTGGACTGA-3′, 5′-AGGTGGAGCGATTCTGAG-3′; *IFIT1*: 5′-TCAAAGTC AGCAGCCAGTCTCA-3′, 5′-GCCTCCTTGGGTTCGTCTAT AA-3′; *IFIT3*: 5′-AACTACGCCTGGGTCTACTATCACTT-3′, 5′-GCCCTTTCATTTCTTCCACAC-3′; and *GAPDH*: 5′-ATT GCCCTCAACGACCACTTTG-3′, 5′-TTGATGGTACATGA

AAGGTGAGG-3′. The IFN score was calculated as the sum of the five normalized expression levels of the corresponding tar (14):

$$\text{IFN score} = \Sigma \frac{\text{Gene}_{\text{DM or SLE}} - \bar{X}(\text{Gene}_{\text{HD}})}{\text{SD}(\text{Gene}_{\text{HD}})}$$

$\text{Gene}_{(\text{DM or SLE})}$ represents the relative expression of a specific gene in DM or SLE patients. The average value ($\bar{X}$) and the standard deviation (SD) of the expression level of each target gene in healthy donors (HD, $n = 10$) were also presented.

Serum IgG Purification and Immune Complex Formation

IgG from DM and SLE patient sera were purified using a HiTrap Protein G HP column (GE Healthcare, Chicago, IL, USA) and quantified using a BCA Protein Assay Kit (Sigma-Aldrich, St. Louis, MO, USA). The cytosolic protein and nuclear material of 293 cells (2 × 10^6) overexpressing Flag-tagged MDA5 were extracted with the Paris ™ Kit (Invitrogen, Waltham, MA, USA) and the cytosolic protein and RNA concentrations titrated to 2 mg/ml and 400 ng/μl, respectively. One hundred microliters of cytosolic protein, 50 μl purified serum IgG at a concentration of 1 mg/ml, and 10 μL RNA formed the immune complex (IC).

Purification and Activation of pDCs

Healthy donor blood buffy coat was obtained from Shanghai Blood Transfusion Center and fractionated over Ficoll gradients. Plasmacytoid dendritic cells (pDCs) were isolated from PBMCs using the Plasmacytoid Dendritic Cell Isolation Kit II (Miltenyi Biotec, Bergisch Gladbach, Germany). pDCs were cultured at a density of 3 × 10^4 cells/well in 96-well plates in 200 μl complete RPMI supplemented with 10% fetal calf serum (FCS) and stimulated overnight before the levels of IFN-α and CD80 were measured. The ICs, TLR-7 agonist R848 (2 μg/ml), and RNase (5 μg/ml) were added (both from MedChemExpress, Princeton, NJ, USA) when indicated.

RNA-Binding Protein Immunoprecipitation

ICs were lysed with the EZ-Magna RIP™ RNA-Binding Protein Immunoprecipitation Kit (Merck Millipore, Darmstadt, Germany) and incubated with goat anti-human IgG antibody-labeled protein A/G at 4°C overnight. The magnetic beads were washed six times with pre-cooled RIPA buffer. Immunoprecipitates were detected by Western blotting using antibody against MDA5 (1:1,000; Abcam, Cambridge, MA, USA). The purified RNA from immunoprecipitates was measured with 1.5% agarose gel electrophoresis.

Co-Immunoprecipitation Assay

ICs and pDCs were incubated overnight. Thereafter, the pDCs were lysed with RIPA lysis buffer (Thermo Fisher, Waltham, MA, USA) on ice for 4 h. The cell lysates were centrifuged at 13,000 rpm for 15 min. The supernatants were subsequently collected and pre-incubated with ImmunoPure Immobilized Protein A (Pierce, Rockford, IL, USA) with gentle shaking at 4°C for 1 h. Subsequently, the mixture was centrifuged at 13,000 rpm for 15 min and the supernatants (1 mg protein) incubated with 1 μg of goat monoclonal anti-human IgG antibody for 1 h, after which they were incubated with 10 μl of protein A agarose beads with gentle agitation at 4°C overnight. After centrifugation, the pellets were washed with lysis buffer. The target proteins were detected by Western blotting using antibodies against MDA5 (1:1,000) and Toll-like receptor 7 (TLR7) (1:2,000; both from Abcam, Cambridge, MA, USA).

Confocal Microscopy

For lysosome co-localization, pDCs were incubated overnight at 37°C with ICs (Alexa Fluor 488-conjugated serum IgG), cytosolic protein lysate, and nuclear lysate. Then, pDCs were allowed to adhere to poly-L-lysine-coated coverslips for 15 min, fixed with 1% paraformaldehyde in phosphate-buffered saline (PBS), and permeabilized with 0.25% saponin. The samples were stained with Alexa Fluor 647-conjugated anti-LAMP-1 in 0.25% saponin. They were then imaged using a Zeiss LSM510 META confocal microscope and the images analyzed for co-localization using SlideBook software.

Statistics

Student's t-tests, chi-square test, and Spearman's correlation analysis were used as indicated. The clinical variables were only presented without imputation for those with missing data less than 10%. The in-house and commercial anti-MDA5 antibody detection ELISA kits used the kappa test for consistency comparison (15). All statistics were performed using GraphPad Prism 6.0, with $p < 0.05$ considered as statistically significant.

RESULTS

The clinical characteristics of the patients with DM and SLE are shown in **Table 1** (details of this anti-MDA5$^+$ DM patient cohort had been reported previously (16) and data for other disease controls including ASyS, RA, and SSc are in **Table 2**). The titers of the anti-MDA5 antibody according to ELISA for each group are presented in **Figure 1A**. The cutoff value of our in-house ELISA was set at 35 RU/ml, although this study did not include DM-specific antibody-negative DM patients. According to the results of our in-house ELISA, 76.1% of DM patients had anti-MDA5. Anti-MDA5 antibodies were at high titers among line blotting-established anti-MDA5$^+$ DM patients, whereas they were consistently negative across the board among the disease controls, except for SLE. Of the SLE patients, 14.29% (35/245) had low-grade but positive anti-MDA5. Interestingly, anti-MDA5$^+$ SLE was associated with malar rash (with no DM features) and the presence of anti-SmRNP antibody (**Table 1** and **Figure 1B**). This in-house anti-MDA5 ELISA methodology was validated by Flag-tagged MDA5 immunoprecipitation and recombinant MDA5-based Western blotting (**Figure 1C**).

Subsequently, we carried out cytokine profiling (including IFN-α, IFN-β, IFN-γ, IL-1β, IL-2, IL-4, IL-5, IL-6, IL-8, IL-10, IL-12p70, IL-17A, IL-17F, IL-22, TNF-α, TNF-β, and GM-CSF) in sera of DM and SLE patients with or without anti-MDA5. We

TABLE 1 | Clinical and serological characteristics among patients with anti-MDA5$^{+/-}$ dermatomyositis (DM) and systemic lupus erythematosus (SLE).

Index	DM			SLE		
	MDA5⁻ (*N* = 68)	**MDA5⁺ (*N* = 217)**	***p*-value**	**MDA5⁻ (*N* = 210)**	**MDA5⁺ (*N* = 35)**	***p*-value**
Sex, female, *n* (%)	28 (41.18)	84 (38.71)	0.776	192 (91.43)	33 (94.29)	0.747
Age (years), mean (SD)	54.39 (13.14)	49.91 (11.35)	**0.007**	36.05 (11.74)	35.23 (7.00)	0.687
Heliotrope/Gottron's, *n* (%)	61 (89.71)	189 (87.10)	0.675	–	–	–
Malar rash, *n* (%)	–	–	–	43 (20.48)	13 (37.14)	**0.048**
Myositis, *n* (%)	52 (76.47)	27 (12.44)	**<0.001**	4 (1.90)	2 (5.71)	0.206
ILD, *n* (%)	11 (16.18)	217 (100.00)	**<0.001**	14 (6.67)	3 (8.57)	0.718
Fever, *n* (%)	7 (10.29)	139 (64.06)	**<0.001**	11 (5.24)	0 (0.00)	0.373
Arthralgia, *n* (%)	36 (52.94)	97 (44.70)	0.266	71 (33.81)	8 (22.86)	0.243
LN, *n* (%)	–	–	–	55 (26.19)	12 (34.29)	0.314
NPSLE, *n* (%)	–	–	–	5 (2.38)	1 (2.86)	>0.999
WBC (10^3/μl), mean (SD)	7.46 (2.54)	6.92 (3.05)	0.220	5.77 (2.67)	5.29 (1,98)	0.317
HB (g/L), mean (SD)	127.89 (26.29)	124.54 (16.80)	0.244	117.40 (31.10)	120.00 (41.26)	0.665
Lymphopenia (<0.8 × 10^3/μl), *n* (%)	11 (16.18)	128 (58.99)	**<0.001**	55 (26.19)	14 (40.00)	0.106
PLT (10^3/μl), mean (SD)	209.05 (68.76)	196.67 (81.51)	0.298	201.22 (82.82)	201.42 (57.07)	0.453
CK_{max} (U/L), mean (SD)	2450.19 (5349.61)	279.33 (575.59)	**<0.001**	94.23 (60.32)	87.26 (74.21)	0.546
Ferritin (ng/ml), mean (SD)	841.45 (1032.73)	1677.12 (2434.33)	**0.032**	157.43 (177.09)	115.83 (123.12)	0.157
C3 (g/L), mean (SD)	0.95 (0.42)	1.01 (0.22)	0.200	0.83 (0.26)	0.88 (0.21)	0.107
C4 (g/L), mean (SD)	0.25 (0.10)	0.26 (0.08)	0.491	0.19 (0.10)	0.12 (0.06)	0.209
CRP (mg/L), mean (SD)	10.87 (24.36)	11.26 (14.97)	0.891	6.48 (12.86)	4.08 (8.27)	0.287
ESR (mm/h), mean (SD)	28.76 (22.02)	33.24 (20.74)	0.128	21.39 (22.54)	23.06 (17.49)	0.681
IgG (g/L), mean (SD)	14.08 (4.94)	15.29 (5.50)	0.214	14.38 (5.06)	17.17 (5.47)	**0.001**
Anti-dsDNA (IU/ml), *n* (%)	0 (0.00)	0 (0.00)	NA	120 (57.14)	19 (54.29)	0.854
Anti-Sm (AI), *n* (%)	0 (0.00)	0 (0.00)	NA	82 (39.05)	15 (42.86)	0.711
Anti-SmRNP (AI), *n* (%)	0 (0.00)	0 (0.00)	NA	111 (52.86)	25 (71.43)	**0.045**
Anti-Ribo P (AI), *n* (%)	0 (0.00)	0 (0.00)	NA	65 (30.95)	12 (34.29)	0.697
Anti-SS-A52 (AI), *n* (%)	3 (4.41)	139 (64.06)	**<0.001**	83 (39.52)	13 (37.14)	0.853
Anti-SS-A60 (AI), *n* (%)	0.00 (0.00)	0.00 (0.00)	NA	133 (63.33)	23 (65.71)	0.851
Anti-MDA5 titer (RU/ml), mean (SD)	**14.23 (6.37)**	**186.22 (54.98)**	**<0.001**	**20.68 (6.47)**	**51.68 (17.91)**	**<0.001**

Results are depicted as the mean and SD. Student's t-test was used for continuous variables and Fisher's exact test for dichotomous variables. MDA5⁻ DM included patients with anti-Mi-2α/β (n = 13), anti-NXP2 (n = 17), anti-SAE1 (n = 15), and anti-TIF1γ (n = 23).

ILD, interstitial lung disease; CK_{max}, peak plasma CK; LN, lupus nephritis; NPSLE, neuropsychiatric systemic lupus erythematosus; WBC, white blood cell; HB, hemoglobin; PLT, platelet; CRP, C-reactive protein; ESR, erythrocyte sedimentation rate; IgG, immunoglobulin G.

P-value <0.05 is statistically significant in bold text.

TABLE 2 | Clinical and serological characteristics of patients with MDA5⁻ dermatomyositis (DM) and others.

Index	NXP2⁺ (*N* = 17)	TIF1γ⁺ (*N* = 23)	Mi-2α/β⁺ (*N* = 13)	SAE1⁺ (*N* = 15)	ASyS (*N* = 57)	RA (*N* = 89)	SSc (*N* = 30)
Sex, female, *n* (%)	11 (64.71)	10 (43.48)	12 (92.31)	14 (93.33)	35 (61.40)	70 (78.65)	21 (70.00)
Age (years), mean (SD)	48.59 (18.17)	57.00 (9.50)	53.77 (13.65)	58.00 (8.20)	53.03 (13.28)	57.81 (11.20)	52.10 (12.10)
Myositis, *n* (%)	14 (82.35)	17 (73.91)	13 (100.00)	8 (53.33)	22 (38.60)	0 (0.00)	0 (0.00)
ILD, *n* (%)	3 (17.65)	1 (4.35)	2 (15.38)	5 (33.33)	36 (63.16)	11 (12.36)	19 (63.33)
Fever, *n* (%)	4 (23.53)	3 (13.04)	0 (0.00)	0 (0.00)	16 (28.07)	4 (4.49)	0 (0.00)
Arthralgia, *n* (%)	11 (64.71)	13 (56.52)	8 (61.54)	4 (26.67)	14 (24.56)	55 (61.80)	2 (6.67)
WBC (10^3/μl), mean (SD)	9.89 (4.94)	8.82 (3.59)	8.83 (2.75)	7.54 (1.79)	9.83 (4.04)	7.18 (3.01)	6.42 (2.70)
HB (g/L). mean (SD)	111.5 (24.82)	152.52 (28.46)	120.00 (6.97)	129.08 (17.65)	136.23 (12.60)	115.42 (24.18)	137.79 (30.38)
Lymphopenia (<0.8 × 10^3/μl), *n* (%)	4 (23.53)	2 (8.70)	2 (15.38)	4 (26.67)	11 (19.30)	3 (3.37)	1 (3.33)
PLT (10^3/μl), mean (SD)	212.07 (62.60)	244.04 (66.25)	265.00 (64.49)	237.25 (72.78)	242.33 (35.02)	296.57 (124.38)	253.33(77.59)
CKmax (U/L), mean (SD)	5,297.00 (8464.68)	1,312.77 (2479.27)	1,845.17 (1826.54)	306.30 (425.30)	1,164.82 (1904.91)	43.72 (46.63)	53.00 (37.22)
Ferritin (ng/ml), mean (SD)	1,616.22 (1614.39)	558.94 (578.12)	904.54 (829.75)	439.30 (549.87)	487.66 (514.54)	218.65 (243.52)	103.69 (91.17)
CRP (mg/L), mean (SD)	19.22 (38.74)	7.84 (11.74)	12.72 (21.38)	2.82 (0.68)	14.87 (19.03)	19.30 (28.87)	5.59 (7.49)
ESR (mm/h), mean (SD)	20.79 (22.75)	14.89 (13.36)	24.71 (13.47)	13.00 (10.55)	23.85 (19.69)	38.83 (27.67)	15.08 (11.75)
IgG (g/L), mean (SD)	10.55 (3.28)	15.90 (3.72)	15.33 (8.01)	14.00 (6.06)	14.47 (5.83)	22.85 (55.28)	16.36 (3.75)
Anti-SS-A52 (AI), *n* (%)	0 (0.00)	1 (4.35)	0 (0.00)	2 (13.33)	23 (40.35)	15 (16.85)	0 (0.00)
Anti-MDA5 titer (RU/ml), mean (SD)	**18.90 (8.64)**	**13.56 (5.87)**	**12.10 (4.21)**	**11.83 (1.31)**	**16.28 (5.58)**	**13.97 (6.14)**	**14.50 (5.79)**

Anti-MDA5, anti-melanoma differentiation-associated gene 5; ASyS, anti-synthase syndrome; RA, rheumatoid arthritis; ILD, interstitial lung disease; WBC, white blood cell; HB, hemoglobin; PLT, platelet; CRP, C-reactive protein; ESR, erythrocyte sedimentation rate; IgG, immunoglobulin G.

P-value <0.05 is statistically significant in bold text.

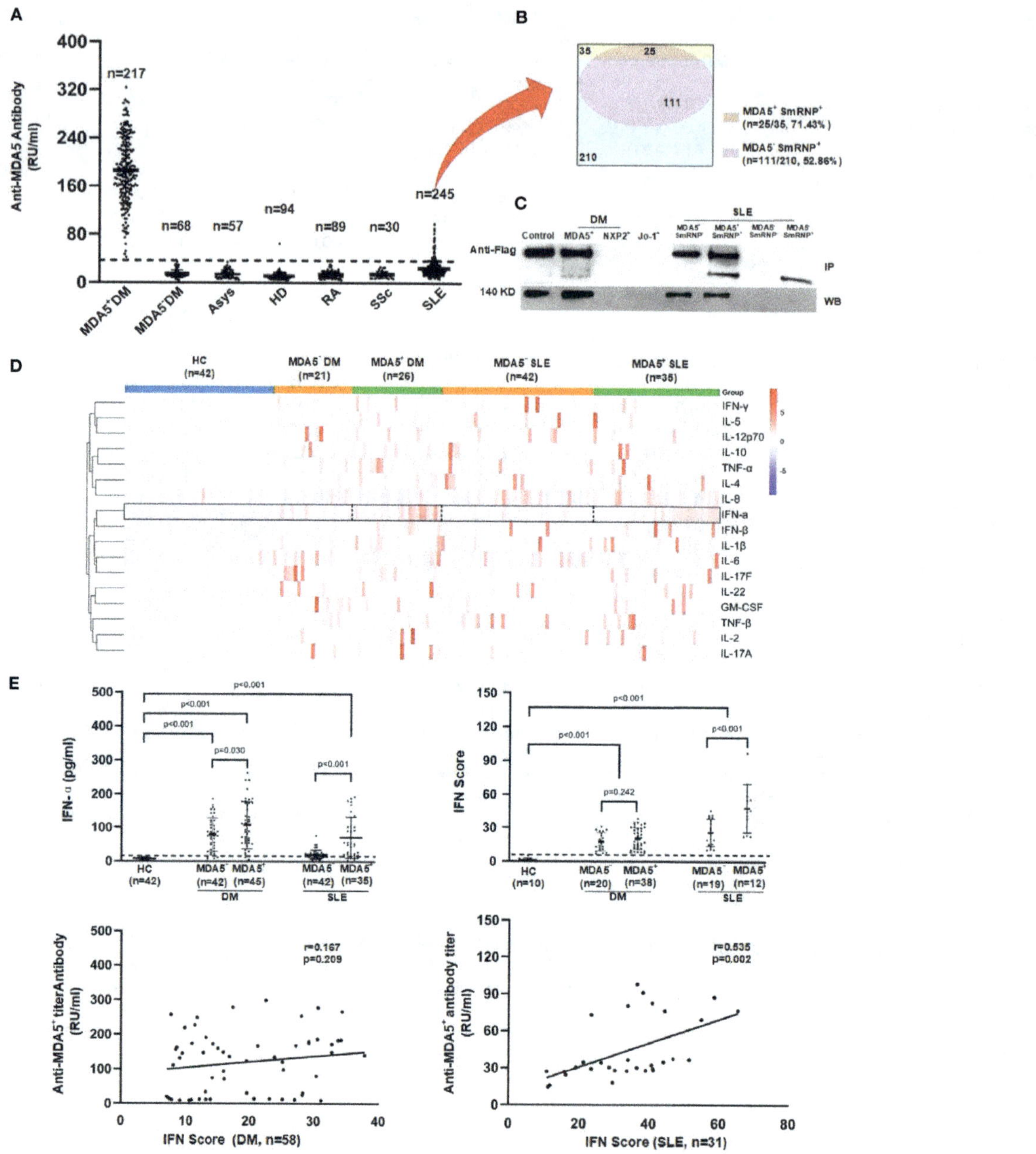

FIGURE 1 | Anti-melanoma differentiation-associated gene 5 (MDA5) autoantibody and cytokine profiling in dermatomyositis (DM) and systemic lupus erythematosus (SLE) patients. **(A)** Quantitative anti-MDA5 measured by ELISA in anti-MDA5$^+$ DM, MDA5$^-$ DM (n = 68, anti-Mi-2α/β = 13, anti-NXP2 = 17, anti-SAE1 = 15, anti-TIF1γ = 23), anti-synthase syndrome (ASyS; n = 57, anti-Jo-1 = 10, anti-PL-7 = 12, anti-PL-12 = 12, anti-EJ = 10, anti-OJ = 13), SLE, systemic sclerosis (SSc), and rheumatoid arthritis (RA) patients and in healthy donors. The *dotted line* represents the cutoff value (35 RU/ml) of the anti-MDA5 antibody titer. **(B)** Overlaps among the anti-MDA5 and anti-SmRNP antibodies in SLE patients. **(C)** Immunoprecipitation (IP, *upper*) and Western blotting (WB, *lower*) were performed to validate the anti-MDA5 ELISA results (representative of more than five independent experiments). **(D)** Heat map of the cytokine expression profiling of DM and SLE patients. **(E)** Serum interferon alpha (IFN-α) and peripheral blood mononuclear cell (PBMC) IFN-inducible genes were measured by ELISA and SYBR green qRT-PCR, respectively. The *dotted line* represents the cutoff value (mean + 3SD of the values of healthy donors) of the serum IFN-α and IFN scores.

found that IFN-α was significantly higher in anti-MDA5$^+$ DM or SLE patients compared to their counterparts (**Figure 1D**). This was independently confirmed by an IFN-α ELISA. Furthermore, the IFN signature genes (*LY6E, OAS1, Mx-1, IFIT1*, and *IFIT3*) were measured and the IFN scores calculated; there was a positive correlation between the anti-MDA5 titer and the IFN scores among SLE patients (p = 0.002). However, this was not the case among DM patients (**Figure 1E**).

Based on the link of anti-MDA5 and IFN-α, we speculated that anti-MDA5 might work just like anti-ribonucleoprotein (anti-RNP), which is a typical IFN-α inducer in the form of RNA-containing ICs (17). We then tested this hypothesis using MDA5 and anti-MDA5 ICs to stimulate pDCs. Anti-RNP ICs were treated as the positive control. Indeed, RNA-containing anti-MDA5 ICs could activate pDCs, as evidenced by the upregulation of CD80 expression (**Figures 2A, B**). The IFN-α production of pDCs was enhanced by the stimulation of RNA-containing ICs, and the effect was more pronounced for the anti-MDA5$^+$ DM-derived ICs. This IFN-α inducer effect apparently required RNA since, in the presence of RNase, the IC-stimulated IFN-α production was significantly inhibited (**Figure 2C**). Further co-immunoprecipitation (co-IP) analysis confirmed the direct interaction between anti-MDA5 ICs and TLR7 (**Figure 2D**) and the indirect co-localization of ICs with TLR7 in lysosome (LAMP-1) in pDCs (**Figure 2E**) (18).

DISCUSSION

Anti-MDA5$^+$ DM is a life-threatening disease when complicated with rapidly progressive ILD. The anti-MDA5 antibody was

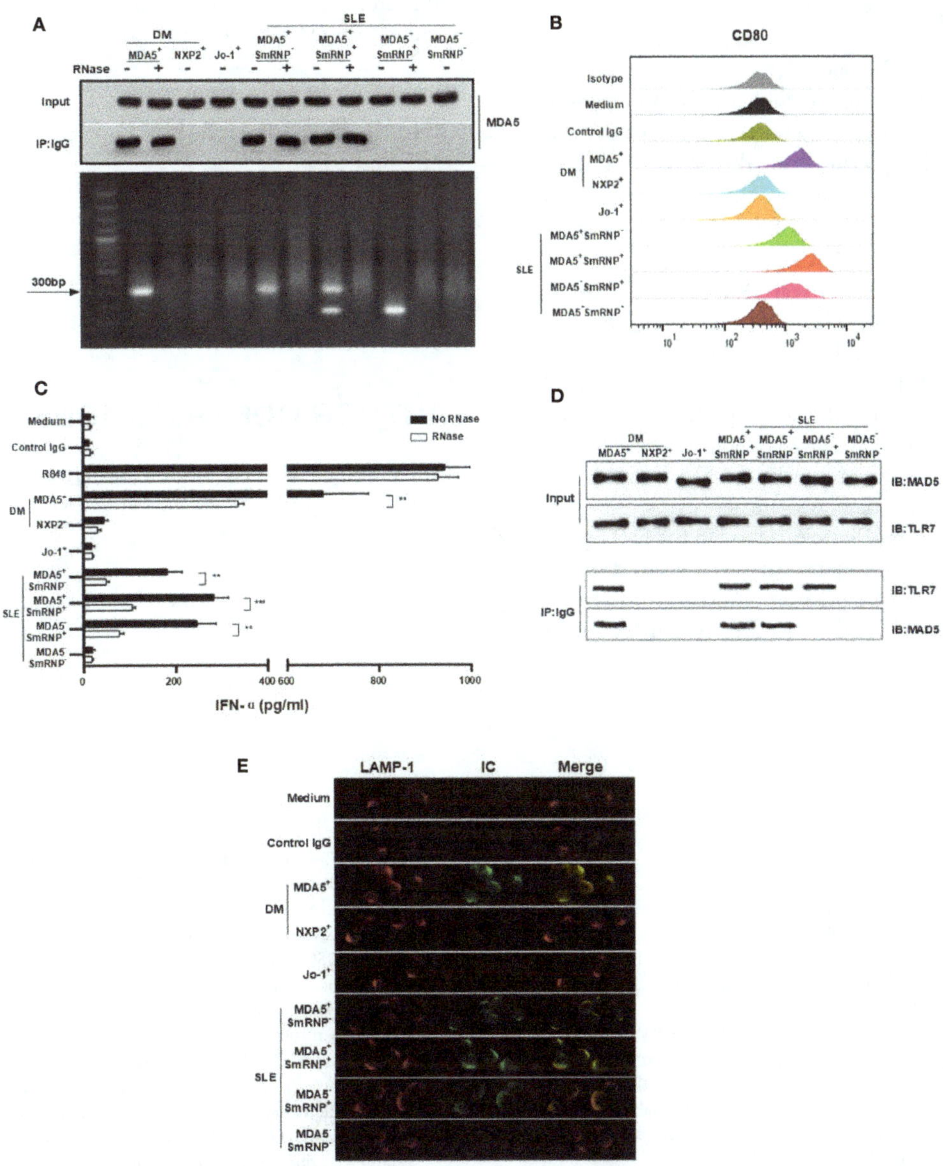

FIGURE 2 | Anti-melanoma differentiation-associated gene 5 (MDA5) immune complexes (ICs) induce interferon alpha (IFN-α) production in plasmacytoid dendritic cells (pDCs). **(A)** MDA5 ICs contain RNA (~300 bp). **(B)** Purified pDCs were cultured with MDA5 ICs overnight and stained for CD80 expression. **(C)** RNA is required for MDA5 ICs to activate pDCs to release IFN-α. **(D)** Co-immunoprecipitation (co-IP) verified protein interaction between Toll-like receptor 7 (TLR7) and MDA5 ICs. **(E)** Confocal images show lysosome-associated membrane protein 1 (LAMP-1) (*red*), ICs (*green*), and the merged image (*yellow*). Results represent at least three biological independent repeats for all experiments **(A–E)**.

considered to be pathognomonic, with little understanding in terms of its relevance to the pathogenesis. In the current study, using our in-house ELISA, we first identified that a small proportion of SLE patients also had autoantibody against MDA5, albeit with lower titer and probably lower affinity compared to that of anti-MDA5^{+} DM patients. It is intriguing that the presence of anti-MDA5 in SLE was not linked to DM features such as myositis or ILD; instead, typical lupus malar rash was more frequently documented. More importantly, these patients had salient peripheral IFN signature. In addition, the presence of anti-MDA5 in SLE was correlated with anti-RNP. It has been well established that SmRNP and anti-SmRNP IgG complexes could induce IFN-α production in pDCs through the TLR7 pathway (17). Thus, we came up with the hypothesis that MDA5, as an RNA sensor, could also exert an IC-mediated IFN-α stimulatory effect through pattern recognition receptors. Subsequently, anti-MDA5^{+} DM patients, along with SLE patients presenting with anti-MDA5 or anti-RNP alone as controls, were subjected to a series of *in vitro* experiments in order to explore the possible antibody-mediated innate immune response.

We confirmed that anti-MDA5^{+} DM, just as in anti-MDA5^{+} SLE, had high levels of peripheral IFN-α. Furthermore, ICs formed by MDA5 and anti-MDA5, either from DM or SLE, are potent IFN-α inducers. The induction of IFN-α is more prominent in the DM-derived anti-MDA5 ICs, which probably reflects a higher affinity effect. As expected, RNA binding is required and interaction with TLR7 is evident in anti-MDA5 ICs. The origin and function of binding RNA will be another intriguing question that deserves further study. Nevertheless, our data implicated a possible vicious loop in the pathogenesis of anti-MDA5^{+} DM, i.e., trigger-activated (viral) type I IFN pathway and subsequent adaptive immune response (including the generation of anti-MDA5^{+} autoantibody). In the meantime, anti-MDA5 and its ICs further enhance IFN-α production. A limitation of this study is that the current analysis was performed without including DM-specific antibody-negative DM patients. Moreover, the anti-MDA5 antibody detection in DM patients enrolled in this study was not performed using the gold standard anti-MDA5 antibody IP assay, but with EUROLINE Autoimmune Inflammatory Myopathies 16 Ag assays.

Our data provided additional evidence to understand the anti-MDA5 autoantibody-mediated, type I IFN-centered mechanism of this disorder. It was made more promising by tackling the IFN pathway [such as through Janus kinase (JAK) inhibitors] as a new treatment approach for anti-MDA5^{+} DM and associated diseases (19, 20).

ETHICS STATEMENT

The studies involving human participants were reviewed and approved by the Ethics Committee of Renji Hospital, Shanghai Jiao Tong University School of Medicine (ethics no. IRB# 2017-041). The patients/participants provided written informed consent to participate in this study.

AUTHOR CONTRIBUTIONS

All authors listed have made a substantial, direct, and intellectual contribution to the work and approved it for publication.

REFERENCES

1. Sato S, Hoshino K, Satoh T, Fujita T, Kawakami Y, Fujita T, et al. RNA Helicase Encoded by Melanoma Differentiation-Associated Gene 5 Is a Major Autoantigen in Patients With Clinically Amyopathic Dermatomyositis: Association With Rapidly Progressive Interstitial Lung Disease. *Arthritis Rheum* (2009) 60(7):2193–200. doi: 10.1002/art.24621
2. Wu WL, Guo L, Fu YK, Wang KW, Zhang DT, Xu WW, et al. Interstitial Lung Disease in Anti-MDA5 Positive Dermatomyositis. *Clin Rev Allergy Immunol* (2021) 60(2):293–304. doi: 10.1007/s12016-020-08822-5
3. Brisse M, Ly H. Comparative Structure and Function Analysis of the RIG-I-Like Receptors: RIG-I and MDA5. *Front Immunol* (2019) 10:1586. doi: 10.3389/fimmu.2019.01586
4. Paik JJ, Livia Casciola-Rosen L, Shin JY, Albayda J, Tiniakou E, Leung DG, et al. Study of Tofacitinib in Refractory Dermatomyositis: An Open-Label Pilot Study of Ten Patients. *Arthritis Rheum* (2021) 73(5):858–65. doi: 10.1002/art.41602
5. Rönnblom L, Alm GV, Eloranta M-L. The Type I Interferon System in the Development of Lupus. *Semin Immunol* (2011) 23:113–21. doi: 10.1016/j.smim.2011.01.009
6. Enevold C, Kjær L, Nielsen CH, Voss A, Jacobsen RS, Hermansen MLF, et al. Genetic Polymorphisms of dsRNA Ligating Pattern Recognition Receptors TLR3, MDA5, and RIG-I. Association With Systemic Lupus Erythematosus and Clinical Phenotypes. *Rheumatol Int* (2014) 34(10):1401–8. doi: 10.1007/s00296-014-3012-4
7. Graham DSC, David L, Morris DL, Bhangale TR, Criswell LA, Syvänen AC, et al. Association of NCF2, IKZF1, IRF8, IFIH1, and TYK2 With Systemic Lupus Erythematosus. *PLoS Genet* (2011) 7(10):e1002341. doi: 10.1371/journal.pgen.1002341
8. Horai Y, Koga T, Fujikawa K, Takatani A, Nishino A, Nakashima Y, et al. Serum Interferon-α Is a Useful Biomarker in Patients With Anti-Melanoma Differentiation-Associated Gene 5 (MDA5) Antibody-Positive Dermatomyositis. *Mod Rheumatol* (2015) 25(1):85–9. doi: 10.3109/14397595.2014.900843
9. Zhang SH, Zhao Y, Xie QB, Jiang Y, Wu YK, Yan B. Aberrant Activation of the Type I Interferon System may Contribute to the Pathogenesis of Anti-Melanoma Differentiation-Associated Gene 5 Dermatomyositis. *Br J Dermatol* (2019) 180(5):1090–8. doi: 10.1111/bjd.16917
10. Dias Junior AG, Sampaio NG, Rehwinkel J. A Balancing Act: MDA5 in Antiviral Immunity and Autoinflammation. *Trends Microbiol* (2019) 27 (1):75–85. doi: 10.1016/j.tim.2018.08.007

11. Muro Y, Sugiura K, Hoshino K, Akiyama M, Tamakoshi K. Epidemiologic Study of Clinically Amyopathic Dermatomyositis and Anti-Melanoma Differentiation-Associated Gene 5 Antibodies in Central Japan. *Arthritis Res Ther* (2011) 13(6):R214. doi: 10.1186/ar3547
12. Mammen AL, Allenbach Y, Stenzel W, Benveniste OENMC 239th Workshop Study Group. 239th ENMC International Workshop: Classification of Dermatomyositis, Amsterdam, the Netherlands, 14-16 December 2018. *Neuromuscul Disord* (2020) 30(1):70–92. doi: 10.1016/j.nmd.2019.10.005
13. Wang H, Li T, Chen S, Gu Y, Ye S. Neutrophil Extracellular Trap Mitochondrial DNA and Its Autoantibody in Systemic Lupus Erythematosus and a Proof-Of-Concept Trial of Metformin. *Arthritis Rheumatol* (2015) 67(12):3190–200. doi: 10.1002/art.39296
14. Feng XB, Wu H, Grossman JM, Hanvivadhanakul P, FitzGerald JD, Park GS, et al. Association of Increased Interferon-Inducible Gene Expression With Disease Activity and Lupus Nephritis in Patients With Systemic Lupus Erythematosus. *Arthritis Rheum* (2006) 54(9):2951–62. doi: 10.1002/art.22044
15. Sato S, Murakami A, Kuwajima A, Takehara K, Mimori T, Kawakami A, et al. Clinical Utility of an Enzyme-Linked Immunosorbent Assay for Detecting Anti-Melanoma Differentiation-Associated Gene 5 Autoantibodies. *PLoS One* (2016) 11(4):e0154285. doi: 10.1371/journal.pone.0154285
16. Wu WL, Xu WW, Sun WJ, Zhang DT, Zhao JF, Luo Q, et al. Forced Vital Capacity Predicts the Survival of Interstitial Lung Disease in Anti-MDA5 Positive Dermatomyositis: A Multi-Centre Cohort Study. *Rheumatol (Oxford)* (2021) keab305. doi: 10.1093/rheumatology/keab305
17. Eloranta M-L, Lövgren T, Finke D, Mathsson L, Rönnelid J, Kastner B, et al. Regulation of the Interferon-Alpha Production Induced by RNA-Containing Immune Complexes in Plasmacytoid Dendritic Cells. *Arthritis Rheum* (2009) 60(8):2418–27. doi: 10.1002/art.24686
18. Mold C, Clos TWD. C-Reactive Protein Inhibits Plasmacytoid Dendritic Cell Interferon Responses to Autoantibody Immune Complexes. *Arthritis Rheum* (2013) 65(7):1891–901. doi: 10.1002/art.37968
19. Chen ZW, Wang XD, Ye S. Tofacitinib in Amyopathic Dermatomyositis-Associated Interstitial Lung Disease. *N Engl J Med* (2019) 381(3):291–3. doi: 10.1056/NEJMc1900045
20. Kurasawa K, Arai S, Namiki Y, Tanaka A, Takamura Y, Owada T, et al. Tofacitinib for Refractory Interstitial Lung Diseases in Anti-Melanoma Differentiation-Associated 5 Gene Antibody-Positive Dermatomyositis. *Rheumatol (Oxford)* (2018) 57(12):2114–9. doi: 10.1093/rheumatology/key188

15

Replacement and Immunomodulatory Activities of 20%Subcutaneous Immunoglobulin Treatment: A Single-Center Retrospective Study in Autoimmune Myositis and CVID Patients

Maria Giovanna Danieli[1,2*], *Jacopo Umberto Verga*[3,4], *Cristina Mezzanotte*[5], *Irene Terrenato*[6], *Silvia Svegliati*[1], *Maria Beatrice Bilo*[1,7] *and Gianluca Moroncini*[1,2]

[1] Department of Clinical and Molecular Sciences, Marche Polytechnic University, Ancona, Italy, [2] Clinica Medica, Department of Internal Medicine, Ospedali Riuniti, Ancona, Italy, [3] Department of Life and Environmental Sciences, Polytechnic University of Marche, Ancona, Italy, [4] The Science Foundation Ireland (SFI) Centre for Research Training in Genomics Data Science, National University of Ireland, Galway, Ireland, [5] Internal Medicine Residency Program, Marche Polytechnic University, Ancona, Italy, [6] Biostatistics and Bioinformatic Unit, Scientific Direction, IRCCS Regina Elena Cancer Institute, Rome, Italy, [7] Allergy Unit, Department of Internal Medicine, Ospedali Riuniti, Ancona, Italy

Correspondence:
Maria Giovanna Danieli
m.g.danieli@univpm.it

Background: Immunoglobulin (Ig) replacement therapy represents a life-saving treatment in primary antibody deficiencies. The introduction of subcutaneous Ig (SCIg) administration brings a major improvement in quality of life for patients, compared to the traditional intravenous administration. In recent years, an additional role has been proposed for Ig therapy for various inflammatory and immune-mediated diseases. Consequently, the use of SCIg has expanded from immunodeficiencies to immune-mediated diseases, such as polymyositis (PM) and dermatomyositis (DM). Given the rarity of these conditions, it is still difficult to evaluate the real impact of SCIg treatment on PM and DM, and additional data are constantly required on this topic, particularly for long-term treatments in real-life settings.

Aim: This study aimed to increase the knowledge about the anti-inflammatory and immunomodulatory effects of SCIg treatment for myositis. To this aim, a long-term evaluation of the effectiveness of 20% human SCIg treatment (20% SCIg, Hizentra®, CSL Behring) was carried out in patients with PM/DM in care at our Center. In addition, an evaluation of the 20% SCIg therapy in CVID patients was provided. This analysis, beside adding knowledge about the use of SCIg therapy in this real-life setting, was intended as a term of comparison, regarding the safety profile.

Results: Results support the beneficial effect and tolerability of long-term 20% SCIg therapy in PM/DM patients, reporting a significant improvement in creatine kinase levels, muscle strength, skin conditions, dysphagia, disease activity (MITAX score) and disability (HAQ-DI score). None of the patients reported systemic reactions. The duration of the reported local reactions was a few hours in 80% of the patients, and all resolved spontaneously. CVID patients reported an improvement in all the considered effectiveness parameters at the end of 20% SCIg therapy. The frequency of the adverse events reported by PM/DM patients was not different from what reported in CVID patients, where the use of SCIg therapy is more consolidated

Conclusions: This study suggests that 20% SCIg treatment represents a viable and safe treatment for PM/DM patients and a valid therapeutic alternative to IVIg, with important advantages for patients' quality of life.

Keywords: common variable immunodeficiency, immunomodulation, intravenous immunoglobulin, polymyositis, dermatomyositis

1 INTRODUCTION

Immunoglobulin (Ig) administered through intravenous injection (IVIg) represented a lifesaving therapy in primary antibody deficiencies (1–5). More recently, subcutaneous Ig (SCIg) administration has become available, bringing a significant improvement in terms of quality of life for patients (6–9). Indeed, SCIg does not require venous access and is associated with more stable serum IgG levels, is able to potentially reduce the "wear-off effect" and presents a lower incidence of systemic adverse events (AEs) (6–13).

In recent years, an additional role for Ig therapy in the treatment of various inflammatory and immune-mediated diseases has been proposed (14, 15). Consequently, although the related mechanisms of action are complex and only partially understood, the use of SCIg treatment has expanded from immunodeficiencies to autoimmune diseases, as polymyositis (PM) and dermatomyositis (DM) (16–19).

PM and DM are idiopathic immune-mediated myopathies characterized by inflammation and weakness of proximal muscles with extra muscular manifestations (20–22). Besides the involvement of skin, high serum creatinine kinase (CK) levels, serum autoantibodies, inflammatory infiltrates in skeletal muscle, and some peculiar features in electromyography and MRI characterize DM and PM patients (21–24).

A correct diagnosis and an early initiation of therapy are essential in these conditions (23). Dalakas firstly reported the efficacy of IVIg in patients with DM (25). Afterward, additional data supported IVIg to control muscular disease activity and improve muscular strength in patients with PM and DM, and an increased survival in patients treated with SCIg compared with older series published in the 1990s also documented (18). Nevertheless, given the rarity of these conditions, it is still difficult to evaluate the real impact of SCIg treatment on PM and DM and additional data are constantly required on this topic, particularly for long-term treatments in real-life settings.

Ours is a referral center for patients affected by autoimmune disorders and immunodeficiency diseases. From November 2011, a 20% human IgG product for subcutaneous administration (Hizentra®, CSL Behring GmbH, Marburg, Germany; hereafter termed 20% SCIg) has been available in Italy and was introduced as reference therapy for patients in care at our center. Compared to other SCIg products, its characteristics of high-level purity (>98% IgG), higher IgG content (20%) and reduced viscosity (14.7 ± 1.2 mPas) enable a low infusion volumes and high infusion rates (26), thus representing an improved SCIg option.

To increase the knowledge about the anti-inflammatory and immunomodulatory effects of SCIg treatment for myositis, we report our experience in a real-life, long-term evaluation of benefit and safety of 20% SCIg treatment in patients with PM/DM. In addition, we provide an evaluation of 20% SCIg therapy in CVID patients. This analysis, beside adding knowledge about the use of SCIg therapy in this real-life setting, was intended as a term of comparison, regarding the safety profile.

2 PATIENTS AND METHODS

2.1 Study Design and Setting

This was a single-center retrospective study, carried out at the Clinica Medica, Ospedali Riuniti Ancona and Marche Polytechnic University (central Italy), which is a member of MyoNet (a global, multicenter, interdisciplinary research project on inflammatory myopathies), a regional referral center for IPINet (Italian Primary Immunodeficiencies Network) and Documenting Centre for European Society for Immunodeficiencies (ESID) (27). All patients' data were analyzed from the dedicated database. Patients who underwent at least one cycle of 20% SCIg treatment and followed-up for more than 1 year were included in the study (cut-off date: June 2021). Patients who initiated a SCIg therapy before 2011 were started on 16% SCIg (Vivaglobin®, CSL Behring GmbH, Marburg, Germany) and then switched to 20% SCIg therapy (28).

The study was notified to the Ethics Committee of Marche Region and was performed in accordance with the International Conference on Harmonization Good Clinical Practice guidelines and the Declaration of Helsinki. All patients previously gave informed consent to demographic, clinical and laboratory data collection and publication (Protocol number: 2012 212024 OR of 02/02/2012; n. 138/DG 20/03/2012 for myositis patients, protocol number: 2016 0561 OR of 27/10/2016; n. 871 DG 7/12/2016 for CVID patients, AOU Ospedali Riuniti, Ancona, Italy).

2.2 PM and DM Patients

The diagnosis of PM/DM was made according to Bohan and Peter's criteria and confirmed in agreement with the new diagnostic criteria of the European League Against Rheumatism/American College of Rheumatology (EULAR/ACR) (29). The 20% SCIg treatment was administered at the weekly dose of 0.2 g/kg, according to the procedures previously described (30).

2.2.1 Study Assessments

All study measures were assessed before (pre-treatment values) and after (post-treatment values) 20% SCIg therapy.

The routine procedure comprises a general physical examination with emphasis on the muscle and the skin. The muscle evaluation was based on the manual muscle test 8 (MMT8), which assesses changes in skeletal muscle strength in six proximal and two distal muscular districts, with a score range of 0–10 for each tested muscle (31). As a biochemical index of muscle damage, we collected data related to CK (normal values <170 U/L). As a working definition, complete skeletal muscle remission was defined in the presence of MMT8 values ≥78 with normal serum CK levels. Partial remission was present when only one of the above criteria was satisfied.

The immunological parameters included antinuclear antibodies and anti-extractable nuclear antigen antibodies by immunoblotting analysis to detect the different patterns. Testing for serum myositis-specific autoantibodies and myositis-associated autoantibodies has been performed by immunoblotting (Alphadia, Belgium).

Lung function was assessed through the diffusing capacity of the lung to carbon monoxide (DLCO) and the forced vital capacity (FVC) evaluations.

All patients underwent a complete cardiologic evaluation, including an echocardiographic examination.

The presence and severity of dysphagia were quantified using the Dysphagia Outcome and Severity Scale (DOSS), a 7-point scale from 1 (severe dysphagia) to 7 (normal in all situations).

In all patients, the presence of underlying malignancies was investigated. We also collected data related to the treatment with glucocorticoids and immunosuppressive agents and side effects.

2.2.1.1 Assessment of Disease Activity

The disease activity, defined as potentially reversible and related only to the myositis disease process, was evaluated with the Myositis Intention to Treat Activities Index (MITAX). MITAX explores the disease activity in seven organ systems (constitutional, cutaneous, skeletal, gastrointestinal, pulmonary, cardiac and muscle). According to the degree of inflammation, each clinical manifestation is calculated from 0 to 4 (not present – new feature). The summed score is then divided by the maximum possible score. Higher scores reflect a more severe activity (32).

2.2.1.2 Assessment of Damage

The myositis damage index (MDI) score was used to evaluate persistent changes in 9 organ systems (muscular, skeletal, cutaneous, gastrointestinal, pulmonary, cardiovascular, peripheral vascular, endocrine, and ocular) plus infections and malignancies. Each scale comprises 2–8 items scored as present (if persisting for at least 6 months) or absent. The scores were summed to provide a total MDI damage score (potential range: 0–38 in adults). The total MDI of each patient was normalized for the number of items considered for the single patient to obtain MDI values comparable to each other (32, 33).

2.2.1.3 Assessment of Disability

The Health Assessment Questionnaire related to physical disability (HAQ-DI) comprises 20 questions investigating eight activities: dressing and grooming, arising, eating, walking, hygiene, reaching, gripping. The HAQ-DI is graded from 0 (no difficulty) to 3 (unable to do). Responses in at least six of the eight categories are necessary. The highest sub-category score determines the value for each category; the HAQ-DI is then computed by dividing the summed component scores by the number of components answered. Disability was classified as moderate to severe with a HAQ-DI score ≥1.0.

2.3 CVID Patients

CVID was diagnosed according to the revised ESID criteria (34), and/or according to the International Consensus Document criteria, for cases preceding ESID 2019 revision (35, 36). The clinical phenotypes of patients were classified according to the work of Chapel and collaborators (37). The 20% SCIg treatment was administered every 7–10 days at a 0.2 g/kg/weekly dose.

2.3.1 Study Assessments

The following parameters were evaluated before and after 20% SCIg treatment: serum IgG trough levels, the number of infection episodes (serious and non-serious), the number of days out of work, the number of days hospitalized due to infections, the duration of antibiotic use for infection prophylaxis and treatment. Safety data were also collected and compared between PM/DM and CVID patients.

2.4 Patients' Satisfaction

All patients were asked to respond to a quick satisfaction survey composed of six questions about their personal experience with 20% SCIg treatment.

2.5 Statistical Analyses

All variables of interest were summarized by descriptive statistics. Categorical data were presented as frequencies and percentage values while continuous variables as median values and their relative range. The Wilcoxon and McNemar non-parametric tests were applied to test efficacy indicators before and after SCIg therapy administration, when appropriate. The Mann-Whitney non-parametric test was used to compare independent groups. A $p<0.05$ was considered statistically significant. All Analyses were carried out with SPSS (SPSS version 21.0, IBM, Armonk, NY, USA).

3 RESULTS

3.1 PM and DM Patients

Overall, data from 30 PM/DM patients were analyzed. **Table 1** summarizes the baseline characteristics of these patients.

The median duration of 20% SCIg treatment was 42 months (min–max: 7–112 months).

Five out of 30 patients received two distinct cycles of SCIg at 3–5 years between one cycle and another. Five out of 30 patients were still on SCIg therapy at the end of the study period, of whom two were in their second cycle.

3.1.1 Effectiveness Parameters

Overall, serum CK levels were significantly reduced after 20% SCIg treatment ($p<0.001$). The muscle strength was improved, with the median MMT8 score significantly increased after the treatment ($p<0.001$). The four patients suffering from dropped head syndrome due to severe weakness of neck extensor muscles improved dramatically after treatment.

Complete and partial skeletal muscle remission was documented in 12 and 18 patients, respectively, with no differences among PM and DM.

Before the initiation of 20% SCIg treatment, all the enrolled DM patients showed multiple skin events as heliotrope rash, periungual erythema, and skin psoriasis. Of them, 10 reported an improvement of skin condition after the treatment, one reported a worsening, whereas two patients remained stable.

The parameters related to the pulmonary function were comparable between the pre- and post-treatment evaluations (pre-treatment mean DLCO: 44% [range: 29–75%]; post-treatment mean DLCO: 48% [range: 28–68%], n=11. Pre-treatment mean FVC: 74% [range: 60–98%]; post-treatment mean FVC: 79% [range: 62–110%], n=11).

High-resolution chest CT documented interstitial lung disease in nine patients, which improved in two of them after combined treatment with glucocorticoid, 20% SCIg and immunosuppressant (methotrexate and rituximab respectively).

Clinically overt cardiac involvement was documented in 11 (36%) patients, ranging from arrhythmic disorders (n=1, 3%) and myopericarditis (n=3, 10%) to non-ischemic cardiomyopathy (n=7, 23%). Heart disease progressed in six patients (20%), with exitus in two of them, despite aggressive treatment. Finally, four patients (13%) had pulmonary arterial hypertension.

A significant improvement in dysphagia was reported after 20% SCIg treatment in nine out of 15 patients. Pre-treatment mean DOSS increased from 5.0 (range: 3.0–5.0) to post-treatment mean DOSS 6.0 (range: 5.0–7.0, $p=0.002$).

Nine patients (30%) presented with arthritis before the treatment. We documented stable, improved or worsened disease in 5 (16%), 2 (6%) and 2 (6%) patients, respectively. Three DM female patients (10%) had associated neoplasia (thyroid, breast, and vulvar cancers).

Table 2 shows mean MITAX values at the start of SCIg treatment, which improved significantly, as documented at the last evaluation visit ($p=0.022$). Even if no significant changes were reported for mean MDI scores, HAQ-DI scores significantly improved after treatment ($p=0.002$).

As for glucocorticoid therapy, the median prednisone-equivalent dose after the treatment was 3.8 mg/day (range 0–

TABLE 1 | Baseline characteristics of PM and DM patients (n = 30).

	n		%
Age at diagnosis (years), median (min–max)		**58 (18–77)**	
Gender: Females	24		80
Type of myositis			
PM	16		54
DM	14		46
Autoantibodies positivity:			
Antinuclear antibodies	13		43
Anti-SRP	3		10
Anti-Jo1	3		10
Anti-Mi-2	3		10
Anti-MDA-5	1		3
Anti-myositis-associated autoantibodies (SSA, SSB, RNP)	6		20
Previous IVIg treatment	19		63
Other therapies			
Oral prednisone/methylprednisolone	29		100
Hydroxychloroquine	6		20
Immunosuppressant (CsA, MTX, MMF)	23		77
Rituximab	2		6
Organ involvement			
Interstitial lung disease	9		30
Clinically overt heart involvement	11		37
Dysphagia	15		50
Arthritis	9		30
Median follow-up period (min–max) (From 20% SCIg start to the last visit; months)		87 (12–148)	

CsA, Cyclosporin A; MTX, Methotrexate; MMF, Mycophenolate mofetil; SCIg, Subcutaneous Immunoglobulin.

TABLE 2 | Selected parameters before and after 20% SCIg treatment in patients with PM and DM.

Parameters	n	Pre-treatment; median (min-max)	Post-treatment; median (min-max)	p-value
CK levels	30	884 (33–1,525)	104 (24–800)	<0.001
MMT8	29	67 (46–78)	78 (48–80)	<0.001
PDN, mg*	30	25 (5–100)	4 (0–25)	<0.001**
Disease activity				
MITAX	26	0.11 (0–0.52)	0.09 (0–0.32)	0.022
Assessment of damage				
MDI	28	0.09 (0–1.04)	0.14 (0–0.90)	0.100
Assessment of disability				
HAQ-DI	15	0.31 (0–3.0)	0.66 (0–3.0)	0.002

*Mean previous versus current daily prednisone-equivalent dose.
**Wilcoxon non-parametric test.*

25 mg/day), which is significantly lower than the mean prednisone-equivalent dose before the treatment (25 mg/day; range: 5–100 mg/day; **Table 2**, p<0.001). Seven patients (23%) withdraw prednisone after 20% SCIg therapy.

Fourteen patients (60%) withdrew from the immunosuppressant at the end of the 20% SCIg therapy; this reduction was significant (p<0.001).

The selected parameters were compared between patients previously treated with IVIg (n=19) versus patients who started Ig therapy with 20% SCIg therapy (n=11). For any indicator, we did not detect any difference between the two groups at the end of 20% SCIg therapy.

3.1.2 Safety Data

Three death events unrelated to SCIg therapy were reported during the study period (10% of patients). These were caused by cardiovascular complications in two cases and COVID-19 in one case. None of the remaining patients reported systemic reactions to the 20% SCIg preparation, and none discontinued the treatment. Local reactions were evaluated on 27 patients and were erythema (n=16, 53%), swelling (n=9, 30%) and nodule (n=2, 6%) (**Table 3**). In most cases, the duration of local reactions was less than 30 minutes after injection (n=14, 47%). The duration was a few hours for 10 patients (33%) and 1 day for three patients (10%). All the local reactions resolved spontaneously.

Patient Satisfaction

Table 4 shows the results of the satisfaction questionnaire related to the use of 20% SCIg. Overall, most DM/PM patients reported a well-tolerated use of the 20% SCIg treatment.

TABLE 3 | Comparison between local adverse events in PM/DM and CVID patients.

	PM/DM, n (%)	CVID, n (%)	p-value
			0.275
Erythema	16 (53)	9 (31)	
Erythema + swelling	0 (0)	6 (7)	
Swelling	9 (30)	10 (35)	
Erythema + swelling + subcutaneous nodules	0 (0)	1 (3)	
Subcutaneous nodules	2 (6)	1 (3)	
None	3 (10)	6 (21)	

3.2 CVID Patients

Data of 29 CVID patients were evaluated. All the baseline characteristics of CVID patients are reported in **Supplementary Table 1**. Recurrent respiratory infections, including upper respiratory infection (URI), lower respiratory infection (LRI) and sinusitis, were present in almost all patients (28/29, 96%). In 15 (51%) patients, URI or LRI were the only features of the CVID, while in 13 (44%) patients, at least two concomitant respiratory infections were present (**Supplementary Table 1**). Fourteen patients (48%) had chronic lung disease with bronchiectasis. Ten patients (34%) had infections only ("not complicated" phenotype), whereas the remaining patients presented with a "complicated phenotype". Autoimmune diseases were present in 11 patients (38%), mostly immune thrombocytopenia (ITP; n= 6, 20%) and polyautoimmunity (n=5, 17%). Finally, 12 patients (41%) had polyclonal lymphoproliferation, 7 (24%) enteropathy, and 6 (21%) a neoplasm.

Nine (31%) CVID patients were treated with 20% SCIg as the first Ig treatment, whereas 20 patients (69%) switched to 20% SCIg after IVIg treatment.

The median duration of 20% SCIg treatment was 56 months (min-max: 12–150 months) at a weekly dose of 8 g in 72% of patients (n=21) and 6 g in the remaining patients (n=8, 28%).

TABLE 4 | Satisfaction data in the 27 PM/DM surviving patients.

Satisfaction data	n=27; n (%)
Opinion about the experience with the 20% SCIg treatment:	
• Good	14 (47)
• Very good	13 (43)
Opinion about the training period:	
• Good	14 (47)
• Very good	13 (43)
Difficulty in preparing the infusion:	
• No difficulty	23 (77)
• NA	4 (15)
Support from the healthcare staff:	
• Yes	24 (80)
• No	2 (7)
• NA	1 (4)
During the infusion, patients reported:	
• To stay still	14 (47)
• To walk	7 (23)
• To do small jobs	6 (20)

NA, not available. All patients receive the infusion in the abdomen.

The standard treatment was followed by 16 patients (55%), whereas 8 (28%) patients followed a seasonal modified regimen, which extends the dosing interval in summer months. Due to severe enteropathy, one patient (3%) underwent a combination treatment (20% SCIg + IVIg). Twenty-two (76%) patients were still on SCIg therapy at the study cut-off date.

3.2.1 Effectiveness Parameters

After 20% SCIg therapy, a significant improvement was observed for all the investigated parameters (**Table 5**).

Considering the infection status, after 20% SCIg therapy, three out of 29 patients (10%) no longer have infections. In eleven patients (38%), the severity of infections decreased, as seven patients (24%) went from a URI + LRI diagnosis to a URI-only diagnosis, and four patients (14%) went from LRI to URI diagnosis.

The diagnostic delay, categorized as ≤10 years versus >10 years, did not affect any of the indicators mentioned in **Table 5**.

The selected parameters were compared between patients previously treated with IVIg (n=20) versus patients treated with 20% SCIg as the first Ig treatment (n=9). For any indicator, no significant differences were found between the two groups at the end of the 20% SCIg therapy.

An additional analysis was performed comparing CVID patients with a "not complicated" phenotype (n=10, 34%) to those with a "complicated phenotype" (n=19, 66%), In this subgroup of patients, a significant improvement was observed for all the investigated parameters except for the number of hospitalized patients, which reduction was not statistically significant after the therapy (**Supplementary Table 2**). The complementary analysis performed on patients with "not complicated" phenotype showed that the hospitalized patients, the days in hospital and absences from work were not significantly reduced after the treatment (**Supplementary Table 3**).

3.2.2 Safety Data

Table 3 summarizes the adverse events (AEs) observed in CVID patients after the treatment with 20% SCIg. All AEs were of a mild entity and self-limiting. Of note, two patients received 20% SCIg therapy (tolerated) after a not tolerated IVIg therapy. Four patients stopped SCIg therapy and switched to IVIg therapy (one for aesthetic reasons, three for poor compliance). Three death events unrelated to the SCIg therapy were reported during the study period (10% of patients). In one case, these were caused by a cerebral hemorrhage and were related to a gastric and a pancreatic cancer in the other two cases.

3.2.3 Patient Satisfaction

Results of the satisfaction questionnaire related to the treatment with 20% SCIg are summarized in **Table 6**. Overall, a well-tolerated use of 20% SCIg treatment was reported by the majority of CVID patients.

4 DISCUSSION

The experience of our center shows the beneficial effects in terms of immunomodulatory and anti-inflammatory activities and the safety of long-term 20% SCIg administration in PM and DM patients.

Overall, after a median follow-up of 87 months, the CK levels were significantly reduced in these patients after the treatment, compared with before the initiation of therapy (p<0.001). The biological reduction of serum CK levels is mirrored by the clinical improvement in muscle strength and the resolution of dysphagia, as documented by the significant increase in MMT8

TABLE 6 | Satisfaction data in CVID patients.

Satisfaction data	n=27, n (%)
Opinion about the experience with the 20% SCIg treatment:	
• Very good	18 (62)
• Good	7 (24)
• Sufficient	2 (7)
Opinion about the training period:	
• Very good	11 (38)
• Good	16 (55)
Difficulty in preparing the infusion:	
• No difficulty	27 (93)
Support from the healthcare staff:	
• Yes	27 (93)
During the infusion, patients reported:	
• To stay still	10 (34)
• To walk	2 (7)
• To do small jobs	15 (52)

All patients receive the infusion in the abdomen.

TABLE 5 | Selected parameters before and after 20% SCIg treatment in patients with CVID (n=29).

	Pre-treatment; median (min–max)	Post-treatment; median (min–max)	p-value*
IgG	347 (24–618)	875 (326–1250)	**<0.001**
No. of infections	5.5 (2–9)	0.5 (0–3.5)	**<0.001**
Patients with serious infections, n (%)	21 (72)	3 (10)	**<0.001****
No. of serious infections	1 (0–6)	0 (0–2)	**<0.001**
No. of antibiotics administration per year	4.5 (1–8)	0.5 (0–2.5)	**<0.001**
Hospitalizations (per year)	1 (1–4)	1 (0-1)	**0.001**
Hospitalized patients, n (%)	13 (43)	6 (21)	**0.050**
Days in hospital	7 (2–30)	4 (0–30)	**0.002**
Absence from work (days)	7 (2–30)	4 (3–5)	**0.010**

**Wilcoxon non-parametric test; **McNemar non-parametric test.*
Statistically significant p-value are reported in bold.

and in the DOSS scale ($p<0.001$ and $p=0.002$, respectively) and in line with previous data that related SCIg therapy with an improvement in dysphagia (38). Of note, our study reports the first evaluation of MITAX, MDI and HAQ-DI parameters after 20% SCIg treatment.

Although the mechanism of action is still to be clarified, different hypotheses have been formulated to explain the immunomodulatory activity of Ig in autoimmune diseases, such as the anti-idiotype regulation, modifications in cytokine production, inhibition of complement activation, neutralization of autoantibodies, killing of target cells by antibody-dependent cytotoxicity and the blockade of cell–cell interaction. Part of these mechanisms is mediated by the Fc-dependent pathways, which comprise the accelerated clearance of pathogenic antibodies by the saturation of the neonatal Fc receptor, the expansion of regulatory T cells, and the blockade of immune complexes (39–41). In particular, the therapeutic benefits of SCIg therapy in myositis patients could be linked to the administration route with Ig used at low dosages (<1 g/kg/monthly), that guarantees serum IgG steady-state levels which in turn probably influence chronic mechanisms of damage, such as regulation of T regulatory activity and dendritic cells functions (30, 42). As reported in previous studies, the role of T-regulatory cells in autoimmune diseases can be linked to their action in suppressing the activity of self-reactive T cells, contributing to the prevention of autoimmune phenomena (30). This hypothesis could be supported by the long-term evaluation of disability (as reflected by the improvement in HAQ-DI scores). In contrast, the index reflecting the activity of the disease is less impacted by 20%SCIg treatment (less reduction in MITAX scores). Therefore, in the active phase of the disease, it is better to use a more aggressive induction therapy based on glucocorticoid, immunosuppressant and IVIg, whereas the remission could be successfully maintained by the chronic use of 20% SCIg (42, 43).

The use of 20% SCIg in our study was also associated with an important steroid and immunosuppressant sparing effect, further explaining the improvement in HAQ-DI scores. None of the patients reported systemic reactions to the therapy. The duration of the reported local reactions was less than 30 minutes, and all resolved spontaneously. For instance, the frequency of the adverse events reported by PM/DM patients was not different from what reported in CVID patients, where the use SCIg therapy is more consolidated. The results of the satisfaction questionnaire administered to PM/DM patients suggest a good tolerability profile of 20% SCIg therapy.

Within this study, the long-term effectiveness of 20% SCIg therapy was also evaluated in a cohort of CVID patients. A significant improvement was observed for all the considered parameters at the end of the treatment. In these patients, the treatment was effective even in the case of modified therapeutic regimens (e.g., the seasonal regimen), underlining the versatility of 20% SCIg (44, 45). Of note, the analysis of the effectiveness parameters in a subgroup of CVID patients with a complicated phenotype suggested the relevant impact of the 20% SCIg therapy in these patients, with a consequent improvement in their quality of life.

Our data show that serum IgG levels have more than doubled at the end of 20% SCIg treatment in CVID patients. In line with previous data, the achievement of a sustained IgG serum level after 20% SCIg therapy shows to protect patients from recurrent infections, as supported by the significant reduction of days of hospitalization and work absence (9, 46). This also suggests a good adherence to effective dosing and administration in these patients.

The effect of the Ig therapy at replacement dosage on non-infectious concomitant co-morbidities (autoimmunity, polyclonal lymphoproliferation, and enteropathy) are not fully elucidated. All our CVID patients presented with autoimmune disease before the initiation of 20% SCIg therapy, and therefore it was not possible to evaluate the immunomodulatory effect of SCIg treatment in this setting. No patient showed relapses of autoimmune disease during 20% SCIg therapy, except for a patient with recurrence of myelitis and one with the onset of ex novo hepatic granulomatosis (considered as a form of polyclonal lymphoproliferation).

For instance, literature suggests that in patients with specific co-morbidities, such as protein-losing enteropathy, the treatment with SCIg may result in more stable IgG levels compared to IVIg therapy (47).

In our experience, cancer represents the first cause of death in CVID patients. A role for IVIg therapy in the treatment of cancer and its metastases has been suggested in previous studies (48, 49), while no evidence is available on SCIg. It has been suggested that the administration of IVIg supplemented with SCIg can support the cancer treatment, but more evidence is needed to confirm this preliminary observation (50).

Long-term tolerability is a fundamental issue to those with chronic diseases, such as CVID, as treatment is expected to extend throughout a patient's lifetime. None of our patients reported systemic reactions, and none of them discontinued the treatment. Only local self-limiting AEs were reported, mainly swelling and erythema. It is noteworthy that various reports described the safe use of SCIg in patients with previous serious systemic AEs to IVIg, along with a better-tolerated profile of SCIg (51, 52). In line with this observation, two patients in our cohort of CVID patients tolerated the 20% SCIg therapy after not tolerating IVIg.

Previous studies evaluated the treatment satisfaction with 20% SCIg therapy, showing a significant improvement in the domain 'Convenience' in patients switching from IVIg and sustained treatment satisfaction in patients switching from another SCIg regimen, suggesting favorable effects on patients' quality of life (9, 53). Within this study, the results of the satisfaction questionnaire administered to CVID patients support this evidence.

Even if this study presents some limitations, as the observational nature in a single-center context and the small population, it suggests the feasibility, effectiveness, and tolerability of 20% SCIg therapy in patients with DM/PM offering a valid therapeutic alternative to IVIg with important advantages for the quality of life of patients, especially those with difficult venous access, with unsatisfactory clinical response, and in patients preferring home care administration. Moreover, this study suggests that 20% SCIg therapy represents an important therapeutic alternative to the use of immunosuppressants: therapy with SCIg is, in fact, linked to a lower risk of infections, leading to a global improvement in the quality of life of patients.

ETHICS STATEMENT

The studies involving human participants were reviewed and approved by Comitato Etico Regione Marche (CERM). The patients/participants provided their written informed consent to participate in this study.

AUTHOR CONTRIBUTIONS

Study conception and design: MGD. Data collection: JUV and CM. Statistical analysis: IT. Interpretation of data: MGD, JUV, CM, SS, and MBB. Manuscript drafting and editing: MGD. Manuscript approval to submit: MGD, JUV, CM, IT, SS, MBB, and GM. All authors contributed to the article and approved the submitted version.

ACKNOWLEDGMENTS

Editorial assistance was provided by Simonetta Papa, PhD, and Aashni Shah (Polistudium SRL, Milan, Italy). This assistance was supported by CSL Behring Spa (Milan, Italy).

REFERENCES

1. Perez EE, Orange JS, Bonilla F, Chinen J, Chinn IK, Dorsey M, et al. Update on the Use of Immunoglobulin in Human Disease: A Review of Evidence. *J Allergy Clin Immunol* (2017) 139:S1–46. doi: 10.1016/j.jaci.2016.09.023
2. Kerr J, Quinti I, Eibl M, Chapel H, Späth PJ, Sewell WAC, et al. Is Dosing of Therapeutic Immunoglobulins Optimal? A Review of a Three-Decade Long Debate in Europe. *Front Immunol* (2014) 5:629. doi: 10.3389/fimmu.2014.00629
3. Quinti I, Soresina A, Guerra A, Rondelli R, Spadaro G, Agostini C, et al. Effectiveness of Immunoglobulin Replacement Therapy on Clinical Outcome in Patients With Primary Antibody Deficiencies: Results From a Multicenter Prospective Cohort Study. *J Clin Immunol* (2011) 31:315–22. doi: 10.1007/s10875-011-9511-0
4. Berger M. Principles of and Advances in Immunoglobulin Replacement Therapy for Primary Immunodeficiency. *Immunol Allergy Clin N Am* (2008) 28:413–37. doi: 10.1016/j.iac.2008.01.008
5. Demirdag YY, Gupta S. Update on Infections in Primary Antibody Deficiencies. *Front Immunol* (2021) 12:634181. doi: 10.3389/fimmu.2021.634181
6. Rojavin MA, Hubsch A, Lawo J-P. Quantitative Evidence of Wear-Off Effect at the End of the Intravenous IgG (IVIG) Dosing Cycle in Primary Immunodeficiency. *J Clin Immunol* (2016) 36:210–9. doi: 10.1007/s10875-016-0243-z
7. Vultaggio A, Azzari C, Milito C, Finocchi A, Toppino C, Spadaro G, et al. Subcutaneous Immunoglobulin Replacement Therapy in Patients With Primary Immunodeficiency in Routine Clinical Practice: The VISPO Prospective Multicenter Study. *Clin Drug Investig* (2015) 35(3):179–85. doi: 10.1007/s40261-015-0270-1
8. Jolles S, Borte M, Nelson RPJr, Rojavin M, Bexon M, Lawo JP, et al. Long-Term Efficacy, Safety, and Tolerability of Hizentra® for Treatment of Primary Immunodeficiency Disease. *Clin Immunol* (2014) 150(2):161–9. doi: 10.1016/j.clim.2013.10.008
9. Jolles S, Bernatowska E, de Gracia J, Borte M, Cristea V, Peter HH, et al. Efficacy and Safety of Hizentra in Patients With Primary Immunodeficiency After a Dose-Equivalent Switch From Intravenous or Subcutaneous Replacement Therapy. *Clin Immunol* (2011) 141(1):90–102. doi: 10.1016/j.clim.2011.06.002
10. Wasserman RL, Melamed I, Nelson RP, Knutsen AP, Fasano MB, Stein MR, et al. Pharmacokinetics of Subcutaneous IgPro20 in Patients With Primary Immunodeficiency. *Clin Pharmacokinet* (2011) 50:405–14. doi: 10.2165/11587030-000000000-00000
11. Misbah S, Sturzenegger MH, Borte M, Shapiro RS, Wasserman RL, Berger M, et al. Subcutaneous Immunoglobulin: Opportunities and Outlook. *Clin Exp Immunol* (2009) 158(Suppl 1):51–9. doi: 10.1111/j.1365-2249.2009.04027.x
12. Chapel HM, Spickett GP, Ericson D, Engl W, Eibl MM, Bjorkander J. The Comparison of the Efficacy and Safety of Intravenous Versus Subcutaneous Immunoglobulin Replacement Therapy. *J Clin Immunol* (2000) 20:94–100. doi: 10.1023/A:1006678312925
13. Shrestha P, Karmacharya P, Wang Z, Donato A, Joshi AY. Impact of IVIG vs. SCIG on IgG Trough Level and Infection Incidence in Primary Immunodeficiency Diseases: A Systematic Review and Meta-Analysis of Clinical Studies. *World Allergy Organ J* (2019) 12(10):100068. doi: 10.1016/j.waojou.2019
14. Matucci A, Maggi E, Vultaggio A. Mechanisms of Action of Ig Preparations: Immunomodulatory and Anti-Inflammatory Effects. *Front Immunol* (2015) 5:690. doi: 10.3389/fimmu.2014.00690
15. Gilardin L, Bayry J, Kaveri SV. Intravenous Immunoglobulin as Clinical Immune-Modulating Therapy. *CMAJ* (2015) 187(4):257–64. doi: 10.1503/cmaj.130375
16. Farini A, Villa C, Tripodi L, Legato M, Torrente Y. Role of Immunoglobulins in Muscular Dystrophies and Inflammatory Myopathies. *Front Immunol* (2021) 12:666879. doi: 10.3389/fimmu.2021.666879
17. Danieli MG, Gelardi C, Pedini V, Menghini D, Benfaremo D, Gabrielli A. Subcutaneous Immunoglobulin in Inflammatory Myopathies: Efficacy in Different Organ Systems. *Autoimmun Rev* (2020) 19(1):102426. doi: 10.1016/j.autrev.2019.102426
18. Danieli MG, Gambini S, Pettinari L, Logullo F, Veronesi G, Gabrielli A. Impact of Treatment on Survival in Polymyositis and Dermatomyositis. A Single-Centre Long-Term Follow-Up Study. *Autoimmun Rev* (2014) 13(10):1048–54. doi: 10.1016/j.autrev.2014.08.023
19. Dalakas MC, Illa I, Dambrosia JM, Soueidan SA, Stein DP, Otero C, et al. A Controlled Trial of High-Dose Intravenous Immune Globulin Infusions as Treatment for Dermatomyositis. *N Engl J Med* (1993) 329(27):1993–2000. doi: 10.1056/NEJM199312303292704
20. Lilleker JB, Vencovsky J, Wang G, Wedderburn LR, Diederichsen LP, Schmidt J, et al. The EuroMyositis Registry: An International Collaborative Tool to Facilitate Myositis Research. *Ann Rheum Dis* (2018) 77(1):30–9. doi: 10.1136/annrheumdis-2017-211868
21. Lundberg IE, de Visser M, Werth VP. Classification of Myositis. *Nat Rev Rheumatol* (2018) 14(5):269–78. doi: 10.1038/nrrheum.2018.41
22. Dalakas MC. Inflammatory Muscle Diseases. *N Engl J Med* (2015) 372(18):1734–47. doi: 10.1056/NEJMra1402225
23. Yang SH, Chang C, Lian ZX. Polymyositis and Dermatomyositis - Challenges in Diagnosis and Management. *J Transl Autoimmun* (2019) 2:100018. doi: 10.1016/j.jtauto.2019.100018
24. Iaccarino L, Pegoraro E, Bello L, Bettio S, Borella E, Nalotto L, et al. Assessment of Patients With Idiopathic Inflammatory Myopathies and Isolated Creatin-Kinase Elevation. *Autoimmun Highlights* (2014) 5:87–94. doi: 10.1007/s13317-014-0063-1
25. Dalakas MC. Immunopathogenesis of Inflammatory Myopathies. *Ann Neurol* (1995) 37 Suppl 1:S74–86. doi: 10.1002/ana.410370709
26. Berger M. L-Proline-Stabilized Human IgG: Privigen® 10% for Intravenous Use and Hizentra® 20% for Subcutaneous Use. *Immunotherapy* (2011) 3(2):163–76. doi: 10.2217/imt.10.108
27. Registry Working Party Documenting Centers. Available at: https://esid.org/Working-Parties/Registry-Working-Party/Documenting-centers.
28. Canessa C, Iacopelli J, Pecoraro A, Spadaro G, Matucci A, Milito C, et al. Shift From Intravenous or 16% Subcutaneous Replacement Therapy to 20% Subcutaneous Immunoglobulin in Patients With Primary Antibody Deficiencies. *Int J Immunopathol Pharmacol* (2017) 30(1):73–82. doi: 10.1177/0394632016681577

29. Lundberg IE, Tjärnlund A, Bottai M, Werth VP, Pilkington C, Visser M, et al. 2017 European League Against Rheumatism/American College of Rheumatology Classification Criteria for Adult and Juvenile Idiopathic Inflammatory Myopathies and Their Major Subgroups. *Ann Rheum Dis* (2017) 76(12):1955–64. doi: 10.1136/annrheumdis-2017-211468
30. Danieli MG, Pettinari L, Moretti R, Logullo F, Gabrielli A. Subcutaneous Immunoglobulin in Polymyositis and Dermatomyositis: A Novel Application. *Autoimmun Rev* (2011) 10(3):144–9. doi: 10.1016/j.autrev.2010.09.004
31. Rider LG, Werth VP, Huber AM, Alexanderson H, Rao AP, Ruperto N, et al. Measures of Adult and Juvenile Dermatomyositis, Polymyositis, and Inclusion Body Myositis: Physician and Patient/Parent Global Activity, Manual Muscle Testing (MMT), Health Assessment Questionnaire (HAQ)/Childhood Health Assessment Questionnaire (C-HAQ), Childhood Myositis Assessment Scale (CMAS), Myositis Disease Activity Assessment Tool (MDAAT), Disease Activity Score (DAS), Short Form 36 (SF-36), Child Health Questionnaire (CHQ), Physician Global Damage, Myositis Damage Index (MDI), Quantitative Muscle Testing (QMT), Myositis Functional Index-2 (FI-2), Myositis Activities Profile (MAP), Inclusion Body Myositis Functional Rating Scale (IBMFRS), Cutaneous Dermatomyositis Disease Area and Severity Index (CDASI), Cutaneous Assessment Tool (CAT), Dermatomyositis Skin Severity Index (DSSI), Skindex, and Dermatology Life Quality Index (DLQI). *Arthritis Care Res (Hoboken)* (2011) 63 Suppl 11(0 11):S118–57. doi: 10.1002/acr.20532
32. Isenberg DA, Allen E, Farewell V, Ehrenstein MR, Hanna MG, Lundberg IE, et al. International Myositis and Clinical Studies Group (IMACS). International Consensus Outcome Measures for Patients With Idiopathic Inflammatory Myopathies. Development and Initial Validation of Myositis Activity and Damage Indices in Patients With Adult Onset Disease. *Rheumatol (Oxf)* (2004) 43:49–54. doi: 10.1093/rheumatology/keg427
33. Sultan SM, Allen E, Cooper RG, Agarwal S, Kiely P, Oddis CV, et al. Interrater Reliability and Aspects of Validity of the Myositis Damage Index. *Ann Rheum Dis* (2011) 70(7):1272–6. doi: 10.1136/ard.2010.142117
34. Available at: https://esid.org/Education/Diagnostic-Criteria-PID.
35. Bonilla FA, Barlan I, Chapel H, Costa-Carvalho BT, Cunningham-Rundles C, de la Morena MT, et al. International Consensus Document (ICON): Common Variable Immunodeficiency Disorders. *J Allergy Clin Immunol Pract* (2016) 4(1):38–59. doi: 10.1016/j.jaip.2015.07.025
36. European Society for immunodeficiencies (ESID). *Common Variable Immunodeficiency Diagnostic Criteria*. Available at: https://esid.org/Working-Parties/Clinical-Working-Party/Resources/Diagnostic-criteria-for-PID2#Q3.
37. Chapel H, Lucas M, Lee M, Bjorkander J, Webster D, Grimbacher B, et al. Common Variable Immunodeficiency Disorders: Division Into Distinct Clinical Phenotypes. *Blood* (2008) J112(2):277–86. doi: 10.1182/blood-2007-11-124545
38. Cherin P, Delain JC, de Jaeger C, Crave JC. Subcutaneous Immunoglobulin Use in Inclusion Body Myositis: A Review of 6 Cases. *Case Rep Neurol* (2015) 7(3):227–32. doi: 10.1159/000441490
39. Shemer A, Kivity S, Shoenfeld Y. Clinical Indications for Intravenous Immunoglobulin Utilization in a Tertiary Medical Center: A 9-Year Retrospective Study. *Transfusion* (2018) 58:430–35. doi: 10.1111/trf.14427
40. Cousens LP, Tassone R, Mazer BD, Ramachandiran V, Scott DW, DeGroot AS. Tregitope Update: Mechanism of Action Parallels IVIg. *Autoimmun Rev* (2013) 12(3):436–43. doi: 10.1016/j.autrev.2012.08.017
41. Zandman-Goddard G, Krauthammer A, Levy Y, Langevitz P, Shoenfeld Y. Long-Term Therapy With Intravenous Immunoglobulin Is Beneficial in Patients With Autoimmune Diseases. *Clin Rev Allergy Immunol* (2012) 42:247–55. doi: 10.1007/s12016-011-8278-7
42. Danieli MG, Gelardi C, Pedini V, Moretti R, Gabrielli A, Logullo F. Subcutaneous IgG in Immune-Mediate Diseases: Proposed Mechanisms of Action and Literature Review. *Autoimmun Rev* (2014) 13(12):1182–8. doi: 10.1016/j.autrev.2014.08.018
43. Cherin P, Belizna C, Cartry O, Lascu-Dubos G, de Jaeger C, Delain JC, et al. Long-Term Subcutaneous Immunoglobulin Use in Inflammatory Myopathies: A Retrospective Review of 19 Cases. *Autoimmun Rev* (2016) 15:281–6. doi: 10.1016/j.autrev.2015.12.003
44. Rojavin MA, Chapdelaine H, Tortorici MA, Praus M, Baheti G, Zhang Y, et al. Pharmacokinetic Analysis of Weekly Versus Biweekly Igpro20 Dosing in Patients With Primary Immunodeficiency. *Clin Pharmacol Drug Dev* (2020) 9 (6):664–70. doi: 10.1002/cpdd.753
45. Sidhu J, Rojavin M, Pfister M, Edelman J. Enhancing Patient Flexibility of Subcutaneous Immunoglobulin G Dosing: Pharmacokinetic Outcomes of Various Maintenance and Loading Regimens in the Treatment of Primary Immunodeficiency. *Biol Ther* (2014) 4(1-2):41–55. doi: 10.1007/s13554-014-0018-0
46. Jolles S, Rojavin MA, Lawo JP, Nelson RJr, Wasserman RL, Borte M, et al. Long-Term Efficacy and Safety of Hizentra® in Patients With Primary Immunodeficiency in Japan, Europe, and the United States: A Review of 7 Phase 3 Trials. *J Clin Immunol* (2018) 38(8):864–75. doi: 10.1007/s10875-018-0560-5
47. Shah SN, Todoric K, Tarrant TK. Improved Outcomes on Subcutaneous IgG in Patients With Humoral Immunodeficiency and Co-Morbid Bowel Disease. *Clin Case Rep Rev* (2015) 1(7):151–2. doi: 10.15761/CCRR.1000149
48. Corbí AL, Sánchez-Ramón S, Domínguez-Soto A. The Potential of Intravenous Immunoglobulins for Cancer Therapy: A Road That is Worth Taking? *Immunotherapy* (2016) 8:601–12. doi: 10.2217/imt.16.9
49. Sapir T, Shoenfeld Y. Uncovering the Hidden Potential of Intravenous Immunoglobulin as an Anticancer Therapy. *Clin Rev Allergy Immunol* (2005) 29:307–10. doi: 10.1385/CRIAI:29:3:307
50. Danieli MG, Gelardi C, Pedini V, Gabrielli A. Potential Anti-Tumor Activity of Intravenous and Subcutaneous Immunoglobulin. *Isr Med Assoc J* (2018) 20(12):782–3.
51. Cherin P, Marie I, Michallet M, Pelus E, Dantal J, Crave JC, et al. Management of Adverse Events in the Treatment of Patients With Immunoglobulin Therapy: A Review of Evidence. *Autoimmun Rev* (2016) 15(1):71–81. doi: 10.1016/j.autrev.2015.09.002
52. Quinti I, Soresina A, Agostini C, Spadaro G, Matucci A, Sfika I, et al. Prospective Study on CVID Patients With Adverse Reactions to Intravenous or Subcutaneous IgG Administration. *J Clin Immunol* (2008) 28(3):263–7. doi: 10.1007/s10875-007-9169-9
53. Danieli MG, Moretti R, Gambini S, Paolini L, Gabrielli A. Open-Label Study on Treatment With 20% Subcutaneous IgG Administration in Polymyositis and Dermatomyositis. *Clin Rheumatol* (2014) 33(4):531–6. doi: 10.1007/s10067-013-2478-x

16

Single-Cell Transcriptomics Reveals Peripheral Immune Responses in Anti-Synthetase Syndrome-Associated Interstitial Lung Disease

Lili Zhu[1,2,3†], Zhong Cao[4†], Shiyao Wang[1,2,3], Changshui Zhang[4], Lei Fang[5], Yanhong Ren[1,2,3], Bingbing Xie[1,2,3], Jing Geng[1,2,3], Sheng Xie[6], Ling Zhao[7], Li Ma[8], Huaping Dai[1,2,3*] and Chen Wang[1,2,3*]*

[1] Department of Pulmonary and Critical Care Medicine, China-Japan Friendship Hospital, Capital Medical University, Beijing, China, [2] National Center for Respiratory Medicine, Beijing, China, [3] National Clinical Research Center for Respiratory Diseases, Institute of Respiratory Medicine, Chinese Academy of Medical Sciences, Peking Union Medical College, Beijing, China, [4] Institute for Artificial Intelligence, Tsinghua University (THUAI), State Key Lab of Intelligent Technologies and Systems, Beijing National Research Center for Information Science and Technology (BNRist), Beijing, China, [5] DataCanvas Technology Co., Ltd, Beijing, China, [6] Department of Radiology, China-Japan Friendship Hospital, Beijing, China, [7] Department of Pathology, China-Japan Friendship Hospital, Beijing, China, [8] Department of Rheumatology, China-Japan Friendship Hospital, Beijing, China

***Correspondence:**
Huaping Dai
daihuaping@ccmu.edu.cn
Chen Wang
wangchen@pumc.edu.cn
Changshui Zhang
zcs@mail.tsinghua.edu.cn

[†]These authors have contributed equally to this work

Objective: Interstitial lung diseases (ILDs) secondary to anti-synthetase syndrome (ASS) greatly influence the prognoses of patients with ASS. Here we aimed to investigate the peripheral immune responses to understand the pathogenesis of this condition.

Methods: We performed single-cell RNA sequencing (scRNA-seq) of peripheral blood mononuclear cells (PBMCs) from 5 patients with ASS-ILD and 3 healthy donors (HDs). Flow cytometry of PBMCs was performed to replenish the results of scRNA-seq.

Results: We used scRNA-seq to depict a high-resolution visualization of cellular landscape in PBMCs from patients with ASS-ILD. Patients showed upregulated interferon responses among NK cells, monocytes, T cells, and B cells. And the ratio of effector memory CD8 T cells to naïve CD8 T cells was significantly higher in patients than that in HDs. Additionally, Th1, Th2, and Th17 cell differentiation signaling pathways were enriched in T cells. Flow cytometry analyses showed increased proportions of Th17 cells and Th2 cells, and decreased proportion of Th1 cells in patients with ASS-ILD when compared with HDs, evaluated by the expression patterns of chemokine receptors.

Conclusions: The scRNA-seq data analyses reveal that ASS-ILD is characterized by upregulated interferon responses, altered CD8 T cell homeostasis, and involvement of differentiation signaling pathways of CD4 T cells. The flow cytometry analyses show that the proportions of Th17 cells and Th2 cells are increased and the proportion of Th1 cells is decreased in patients with ASS-ILD. These findings may provide foundations of novel therapeutic targets for patients with this condition.

Keywords: interstitial lung disease, anti-synthetase syndrome, scRNA-seq, immune responses, differentiation of CD4 T cells

INTRODUCTION

Interstitial lung diseases (ILDs), which encompass a large spectrum of distinct etiologies, can be idiopathic or manifest as a pulmonary complication of a connective tissue disease (CTD), such as idiopathic inflammatory myositis (IIM) (1, 2). With the discovery of myositis specific antibodies (MSAs) and development of more commercially available assays for MSAs, anti-synthetase syndrome (ASS) has been recognized as an important cause of ILDs (3). ASS is characterized by myositis, ILD, "mechanic's hands", fever, arthritis, and Raynaud's phenomenon (4). The hallmark in the diagnosis of ASS is detecting an anti-synthetase antibody in the serum of patients. Up to now, there are 8 anti-synthetase antibodies, including anti-histidyl (Jo-1), anti-threonyl (PL-7), anti-alanyl (PL-12), anti-isoleucyl (OJ), anti-glycyl (EJ), anti-asparaginyl (KS), anti-phenylalanyl (Zo), and anti-tyrosyl (Ha)-tRNA-synthetase antibody (5). ILD is an increasingly recognized complication of ASS, and it is reported that 67-100% of ASS patients develop ILD (6). Besides, ILD is the leading cause of deaths related to ASS (7). The most frequent high-resolution computed tomography (HRCT) pattern of ASS-associated ILD (ASS-ILD) is non-specific interstitial pneumonia (NSIP), followed by organizing pneumonia (OP); usual interstitial pneumonia (UIP), and concomitant NSIP and OP are less common HRCT patterns (8). ILD may occur alone without signs of muscle or skin involvement, to differentiate ASS-ILD from other types of ILD is not easy but of great significance (9). Early diagnosis, timely intervention, regular screening, and referral to promising clinical trials might help to improve the prognoses of patients with ASS-ILD.

Although great advances have been made in the pathogenesis of this condition, there remain substantial gaps in our knowledge of ASS-ILD. A prospective Pittsburgh ASS cohort study reported that 33% (66/202) of patients died and 6% (12/202) of patients received lung transplantation from 1985 to 2009. The 5-year and 10-year unadjusted cumulative survival rate was 84% and 61%, respectively. ILD is associated with high mortality, 49% of mortality was attributed to pulmonary fibrosis in the cohort study (7). The mainstay of treatment regimens for ASS is glucocorticoids combined with immunosuppressant or biological agents, including azathioprine, calcineurin inhibitors, methotrexate, cyclophosphamide, mycophenolate mofetil, and rituximab (10, 11). Options for ASS-ILD patients who are refractory to conventional therapies are lacking, further investigations into the pathogenesis of this condition may help to target specific pathogenic pathways.

Dysregulated immune equilibriums contribute to the development of CTDs (12). The pathogenic roles of autoantigen and auto-reactive CD4 T cells in ASS have been proposed (13, 14). However, a global visualization of the pathogenic immune responses has not been reported. Here, we used single-cell RNA sequencing (scRNA-seq) technology to depict a high-resolution visualization of cellular landscape in peripheral blood mononuclear cells (PBMCs) from patients with ASS-ILD, which will facilitate a better understanding of the pathogenesis of this condition.

MATERIALS AND METHODS

Subjects and Sample Collection

This study was approved by the ethics committee of the China-Japan Friendship Hospital, China (2019-123-K85), and each donor signed written informed consent. All patients who were hospitalized at the department of pulmonary and critical care medicine, China-Japan Friendship Hospital, China, were consecutively enrolled after the successful screening. The patients were divided into two cohorts, one is the single-cell RNA sequencing (scRNA-seq) cohort, and the other is the flow cytometry cohort. In our scRNA-seq cohort, five patients with anti-synthetase syndrome-associated interstitial lung disease (ASS-ILD) and three healthy donors (HDs) were recruited. There are overlapping chest radiological manifestations between ASS-ILD and idiopathic interstitial pneumonia (IIP), and clues for differential diagnoses are of great significance. So we enrolled patients with IIP as disease controls in the flow cytometry cohort. In our flow cytometry cohort, sixteen patients with ASS-ILD, ten patients with idiopathic non-specific interstitial pneumonia (iNSIP), ten patients with idiopathic pulmonary fibrosis (IPF), five patients with cryptogenic organizing pneumonia (COP), and ten HDs were recruited. To be included in this study, ASS-ILD and IIP (including iNSIP, COP, and IPF) must be diagnosed by a multi-disciplinary team (MDT), including at least two pulmonologists, a radiologist, a pathologist, and a rheumatologist. ASS was defined according to Connors GR's diagnostic criteria, which included strong positive testing for an anti-synthetase antibody (identified by immunoblotting assays) and one or more of the following conditions: myositis, ILD, arthritis, unexplained and persistent fever, Raynaud phenomenon, and "Mechanic's hands" (15). In both cohorts, all patients received no immunosuppressive therapies prior to our enrollment. And patients vaccinated within 3 months, with malignancy, infection, or other autoimmune diseases were all excluded. Chest high-resolution computed tomography (HRCT) pattern was categorized as usual interstitial pneumonia (UIP), NSIP, organizing pneumonia (OP), and NSIP/OP pattern according to the 2013 American Thoracic Society (ATS) classification of IIP independently by at least a radiologist and two pulmonologists. The classification of different entities of IIP was also determined according to ATS classification criteria (16, 17). In the scRNA-seq cohort, 10 ml of peripheral venous blood was collected from each sample, and peripheral blood mononuclear cells (PBMCs) were immediately isolated using density-gradient centrifugation with Ficoll-Hypaque according to the manufacturer's protocol. For each sample, cell viability exceeded 90%. In the flow cytometry cohort, 6 ml of peripheral venous blood was collected from each sample, and PBMCs were isolated using density-gradient centrifugation with Ficoll-Paque Plus (GE Healthcare) according to the manufacturer's protocol; then cells were frozen in fetal bovine serum (FBS) with 10% dimethyl sulfoxide (DMSO) for storage in liquid nitrogen until use.

Single-Cell RNA Sequencing

Using a Chromium Next GEM Single Cell 5' Library and Gel Bead Kit v1.1 (10X Genomics, 1000165) and Chromium Next GEM Chip G Single Cell Kit (10X Genomics, 1000127), we loaded the fresh cell suspension (300 to 600 living cells per microliter counted by Count Star) onto a Chromium single cell controller (10X Genomics) to generate single-cell gel beads in the emulsion (GEMs) in accordance with the manufacturer's protocol. Briefly, we suspended single cells in phosphate-buffered saline (PBS) containing 0.04% bovine serum albumin (BSA). And about 10,000 cells were added to the individual channel and approximately 5,000 target cells were recovered. Captured cells were then lysed and the released RNA was barcoded through the process of reverse transcription (RT) in each GEM. RT was conducted on a S1000TM Touch Thermal Cycler (Bio Rad) at 53°C for 45 min, followed by 85°C for 5 min and held at 4°C. The complementary DNA (cDNA) was generated and amplified, after that, quality assessment was performed using an Agilent 4200 (performed by CapitalBio Technology, Beijing). According to the manufacturer's introduction, scRNA-seq libraries were constructed using a Single Cell 5′ Library and Gel Bead kit. The libraries were then sequenced using an Illumina Novaseq6000 sequencer with a sequencing depth of at least 100,000 reads per cell with a pair-end 150-bp (PE150) reading strategy (performed by CapitalBio Technology, Beijing).

Single-Cell RNA Sequencing Transcriptome Analysis

Raw gene expression matrices of each sample were aggregated using Cell Ranger (v.6.0.0) Pipeline coupled with human reference version GRCh38. The merged matrices were transferred to the R statistical environment for further analyses using the Seurat package (v.4.0.3). And genes expressed at more than 0.1% of the cells and cells with more than 200 genes detected were selected for further analyses. Cells with >10% mitochondrial unique molecular identifiers (UMIs), >12000 UMIs, or over 3000 or below 500 genes were removed as low-quality cells (**Supplementary Figure 1A**). After removal of low-quality cells, gene expression metrices were normalized using the SCTtransform normalization, and 3,000 highly variable genes (HVGs) were identified by the FindVariableFeatures function. Batch effects were corrected by SCT Integration (**Supplementary Figure 1B**). In order to reduce the dimension of the datasets, principal component analysis (PCA) was performed with HVGs by the ScaleData function. Cells were then clustered using the FindNeighbors and FindClusters functions with a resolution of 0.4. After that, clusters were projected into a two-dimensional plot for visualization using the RunUMAP function.

Cell-Type Annotation and Cluster Marker Identification

Cells were clustered using the FindNeighbors and FindClusters functions in Seurat, and non-linear dimensional reduction was conducted with the RunUMAP function. Cells were clustered together according to common transcriptome features, and FindAllMarkers function was performed to find marker genes for each cluster. Clusters were then identified and annotated according to the expression of canonical markers. Cells expressing more than one canonical cell-type markers were regarded as doublets and excluded for further analysis. Naïve T cells, central memory T cells, effector memory T cells, $\gamma\delta$ T cells, and proliferative T cells were combined. After integration, PCA and sub-clustering were performed as described above. PCA and sub-clustering were also conducted in B cells.

DEG Identification and Functional Enrichment

Differentially expressed genes (DEGs) were analyzed using the FindMarkers function with parameter 'test. use = Wilcox' by default. The false discovery rate (FDR) adjusted p-value was calculated by the Bonferroni correction method. DEGs were calculated using a minimum log (fold change) of 0.3 and a maximum FDR adjusted p-value of 0.05. Then the upregulated expressed genes were mapped to terms in the Geno Ontology (GO) database. Only GO Biological Process was used in this study. Kyoto Encyclopedia of Genes and Genomes (KEGG) pathway analysis was performed in the same way as GO.

Antibodies and Flow Cytometry Analysis

Cells recovered from liquid nitrogen were incubated with human Fc Block (BD Pharmingen) after being washed by Dulbecco's PBS (D-PBS). BD Horizon™ Fixable Viability Stain 510 (FVS510) was used for the exclusion of dead cells. Each sample was then stained for expressions of cell surface markers, including CD3 (BUV 395), CD4 (BUV496), CD45RA (BV711), CCR6 (BB515), CCR4 (BV421), CXCR3 (PE), and intracellular marker of Foxp3 (Alexa Fluor 647). Prior to intracellular staining, Transcription Factor Buffer Set (BD Pharmingen) was used for cell fixing and permeabilization. Fluorescence minus one (FMO) controls for CD3, CD4, CD45RA, CCR6, CCR4, CXCR3, and Foxp3 were used. Single-stained Comp Beads (Anti-Mouse Ig, κ/Negative Control Compensation Particles Set, BD) were applied for compensation controls. Each T cell subset was defined as follows: CD3+CD4+ T cells were selected according to CD3 and CD4 expressions in lymphocytes. Five CD3+CD4+ T cell subsets were defined according to CD45RA and Foxp3 expressions, including a naïve T cell subset (CD45RA$^+$Foxp3$^-$), a memory T cell subset (CD45RA$^-$Foxp3$^-$), an activated T cell subset (CD45RA$^-$Foxp3^{int}), a naïve Treg cell subset (CD45RA$^+$Foxp3^{int}), and an activated Treg cell subset

(CD45RA⁻Foxp3^{high}). The total memory CD4 T cells included the memory T cell subset and activated T cell subset. Distinct Th cell subsets of total memory T cells were defined according to chemokine-receptor expressions. CCR6- total memory T cells were divided into two subsets, including a Th1 cell subset (CXCR3+CCR4-), and a Th2 cell subset (CXCR3-CCR4+). CCR6+ total memory T cells were divided into three subsets, including a Th17 subset (CXCR3-CCR4+), a Th17.1 cell subset (CXCR3+CCR4-), and a double positive cell subset (CXCR3+CCR4+) (18). Monoclonal antibodies were purchased from BD Pharmingen, and we processed PBMCs in accordance with the manufacturer's protocol. Cells were analyzed using FlowJo software version 10.8 or Becton Dickenson FACS DIVA software version 7.0.

Statistical Analysis

We used the Mann-Whitney test to compare differences between ASS-ILD group and different control groups (iNSIP group, COP group, IPF group, and HD group) for continuous variables, respectively. Analyses were determined using GraphPad Prism version 9. The results were regarded as statistically significant when a two-sided p-value was <0.05.

RESULTS

Single-Cell Transcriptomic Profiles of PBMCs

To characterize the immunological features of patients with ASS-ILD, we performed scRNA-seq (10X Genomics) on PBMCs from 5 patients with ASS-ILD (ASS-ILD 1-5) and 3 healthy donors (HD 1-3) (**Figure 1** and **Supplementary Figure 2A**). The clinical manifestations, laboratory features, chest HRCT patterns, and pulmonary function test (PFT) parameters of recruited patients and HDs were detailed in **Supplementary Tables 1** and **2**. We analyzed a whole of 52973 PBMCs from 5 ASS-ILD and 3 HD samples. Poor-quality cells were filtered out, we integrated all high-quality cells into an unbiased and comparable dataset. Using uniform manifold approximation and projection (UMAP), we identified the transcriptomes of 14 clusters, and 2 of them were identified as doublets (**Supplementary Figures 2B, C**). Thus 12 major cell types were clustered and annotated based on the expressions of canonical marker genes (**Figures 2A, B**). These cells included naïve T lymphocytes (Naïve T, CD3D+CCR7+), central memory T lymphocytes (TCM, CD3D+CCR7+S100A4+), effector memory T lymphocytes (TEM, CD3D+ S100A4+ GZMA+), γδ T cells (gdT, TRDC+), proliferative T cells (pro T, CD3D+MKI67+), natural killer cells (NK, KLRF1+FCGR3A+), CD14+ monocytes (CD14 mono, LYZ+CD14+), CD16+ monocytes (CD16 mono, LYZ +FCGR3A+), B cells (CD19+MS4A1+), dendritic cells (DC, CD1C +CLEC10A+), plasmacytoid DCs (pDC; LILRA4+CLEC4C+), and platelets (PPBP+GP9+) (**Figures 2C, D**). In downstream analyses, platelets were excluded. To reveal cell compositions between patients with ASS-ILD and HDs, we compared the relative percentages of the 12 cell types between them. No significant differences in cell compositions were found (**Supplementary Figures 3A, B**).

Features of NK Cells and Monocytes in Patients With ASS-ILD

Among innate immune cells, CD14 mono, CD16 mono, and NK cells were the most three prevalent subsets, and next, we further

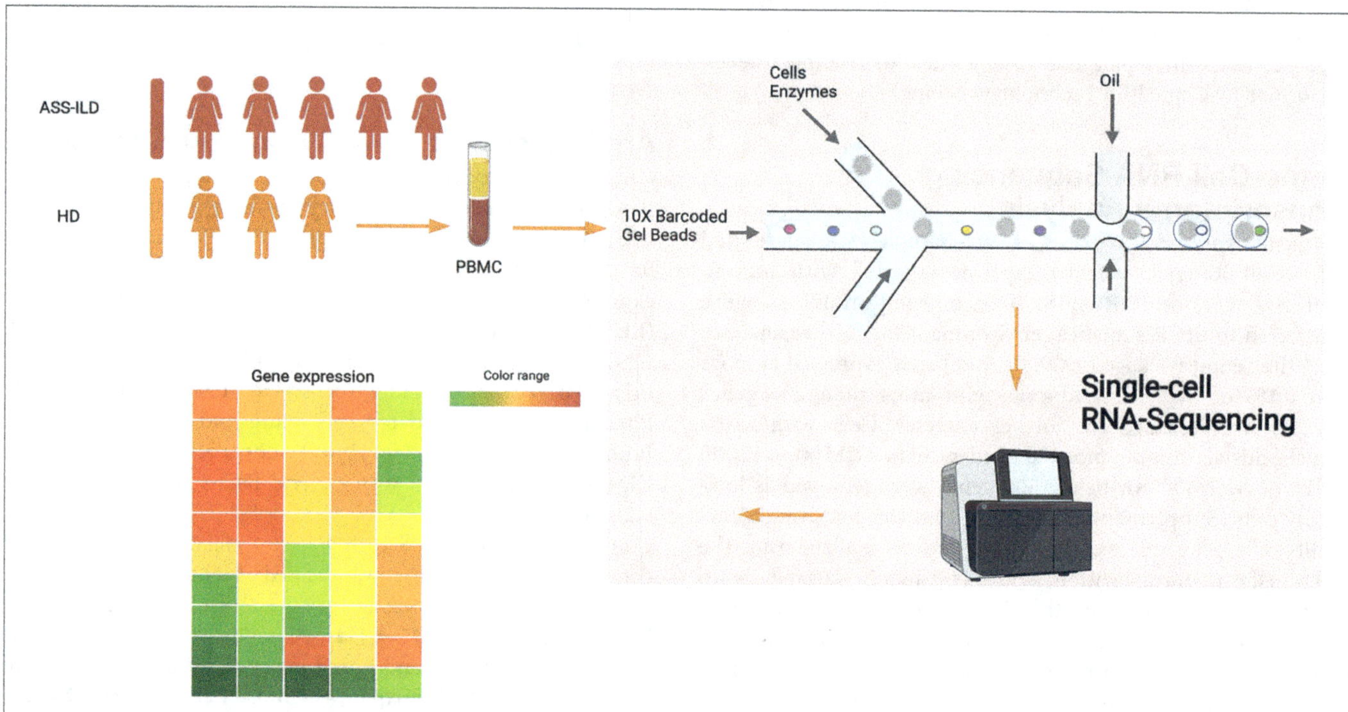

FIGURE 1 | Schematic of overall experimental workflow.

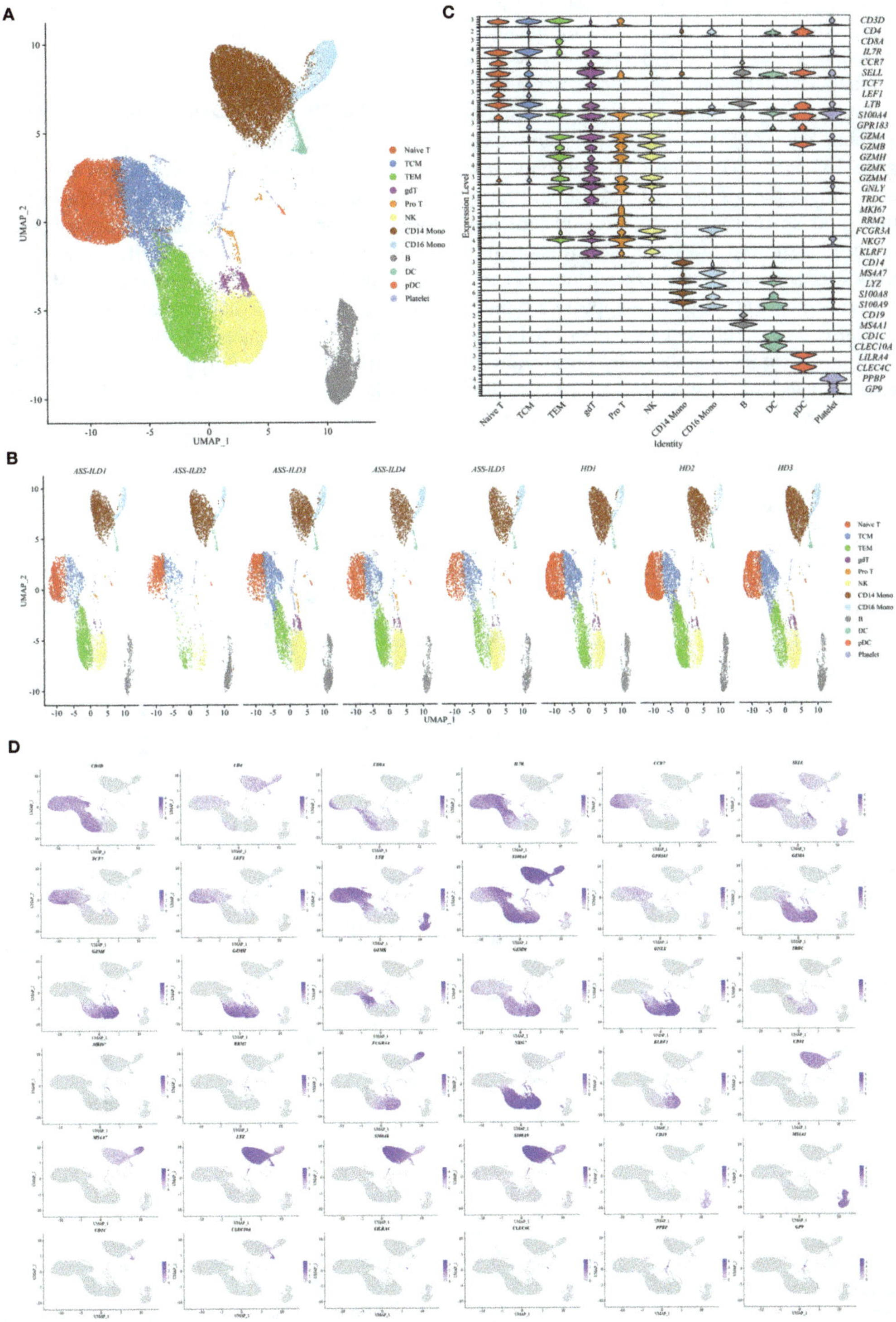

FIGURE 2 | Single-cell RNA sequencing of PBMCs from patients with ASS-ILD and HDs. **(A)** A two-dimensional UMAP plot for visualization of 52973 cells from patients with ASS-ILD (n=5) and HDs (n=3). **(B)** Annotating condition of each patient with ASS-ILD and HD. **(C)** Violin plot depicting the expression distribution of selected marker genes in the 12 clusters. The rows represent selected marker genes and the columns represent clusters with the same color as in **(A)**. **(D)** Expressions of canonical marker genes for 12 major cell types as represented in the UMAP plot. Data are colored according to expression levels and the legend is labeled in log scale. PBMC, peripheral blood mononuclear cell; ASS-ILD, anti-synthetase syndrome-associated interstitial lung disease; HD, healthy donor; UMAP, uniform manifold approximation and projection; TCM, central memory T lymphocyte; TEM, effector memory T lymphocyte; pro T, proliferative T cell; NK, natural killer cell; mono, monocyte; DC, dendritic cell; pDC, plasmacytoid DC.

characterized the transcriptomic features of these three subsets. We first compared the expression patterns of the patients with those of the HDs in NK cells. We found that significantly differentially expressed genes (DEGs) were involved in responses to type I and II interferons, neutrophil activation, and antigen processing and presentation of peptide antigen *via* MHC class II in patients with ASS-ILD using Geno Ontology (GO) analysis (**Figure 3A**). For CD14+ and CD16+ monocytes, DEGs were associated with responses to type I and II interferons, neutrophil activation, and chemokine or cytokine production (**Figures 3B, C**). A dot plot showed the average expression and percentage of expressed cells of selected marker genes in each labeled cell subset (**Figure 3D**). IFN-signature appears a typical feature of IIM, and it varies among different subtypes (19). In our study, we found that monocytes and NK cells both showed upregulated responses to type I and II interferons. These results suggest that innate immune cell types in patients with ASS-ILD show consistent inflammatory responses, like upregulated responses to interferons.

Features of T Cell Subsets in Patients With ASS-ILD

To trace the transcriptomic changes of different T subtypes, we sub-clustered T cells into 18 subsets and those with similar T cell markers were categorized together (**Supplementary Figures 4A–H**). Then we identified 11 subsets of T cells based on the expressions of canonical T cell markers: 4 subsets of CD4+ T lymphocytes (CD3D+CD4+), 2 subsets of CD8+ T lymphocytes (CD3D +CD8A+), and 5 subsets of other T cells (**Figures 4A, B**). The 4 subsets of CD4+ T lymphocytes included naïve CD4+ T lymphocytes (CD4 Naïve, CCR7+SELL+), and central memory

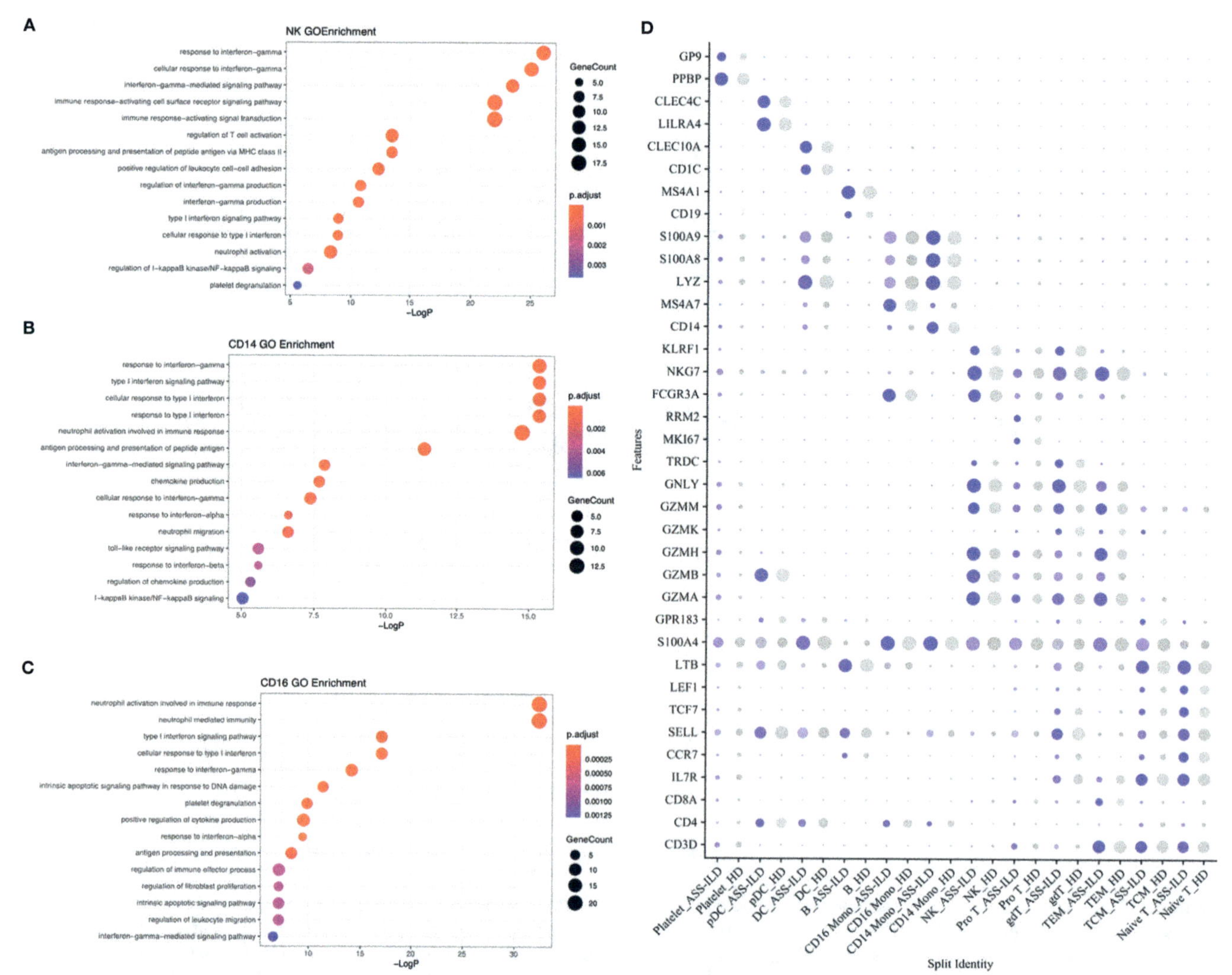

FIGURE 3 | GO enrichment analyses of the upregulated genes in patients with ASS-ILD. **(A)** GO enrichment analysis for NK cells. **(B)** GO enrichment analysis for CD14 monocytes. **(C)** GO enrichment analysis for CD16 monocytes. **(D)** Dot plot depicting average expression and percentage of expressed cells of selected marker genes in each labeled cell subset. GO, Geno Ontology; ASS-ILD, anti-synthetase syndrome-associated interstitial lung disease; NK, natural killer.

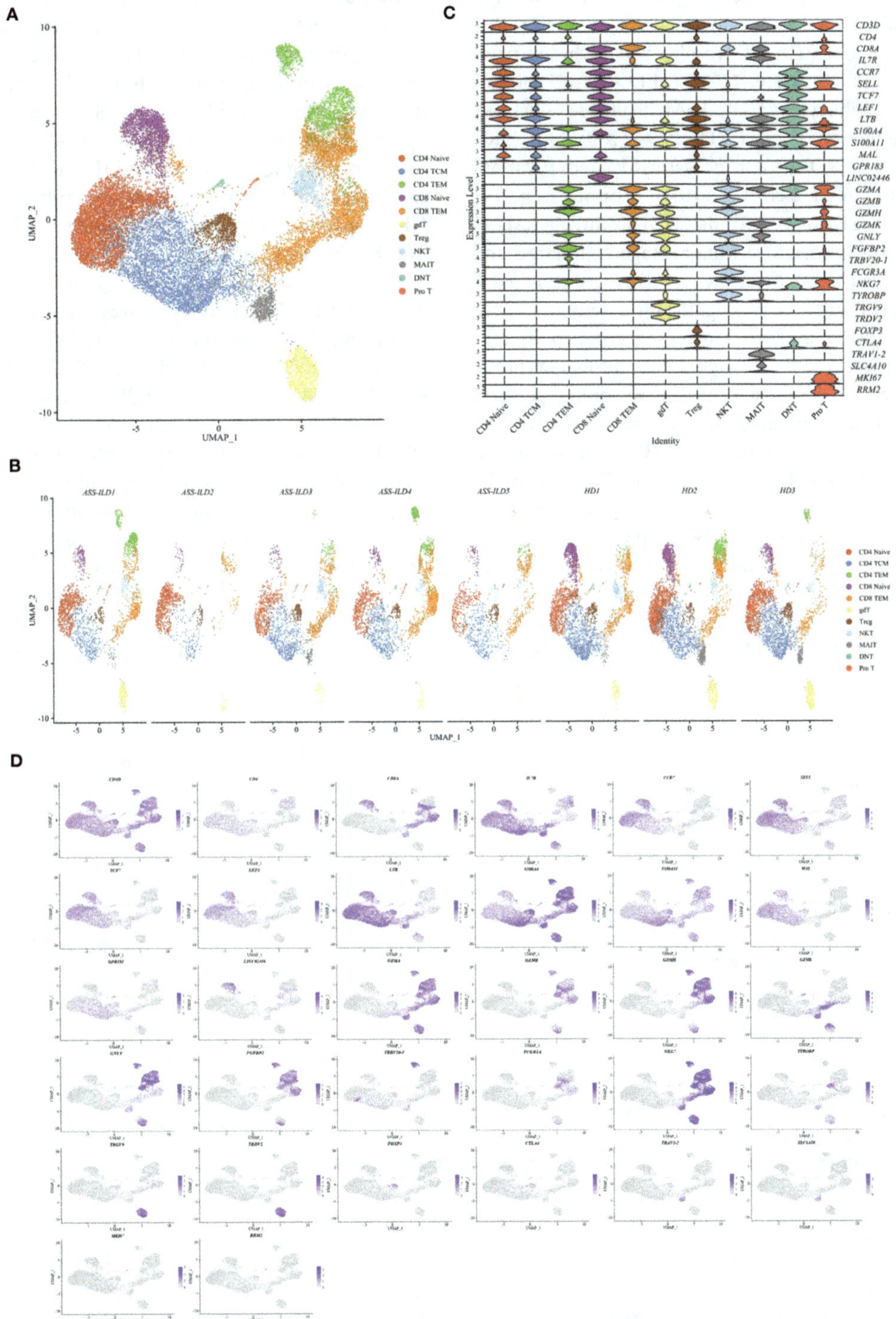

FIGURE 4 | Immunological features of T cell subsets. **(A)** UMAP visualization of 26843 T cells, including 4 CD4+ T cell subsets, 2 CD8+ T cell subsets, and 5 other T cell subsets. **(B)** Annotating condition of each patient with ASS-ILD and HD. **(C)** Violin plot depicting the expression distribution of selected marker genes in the 11 T cell subsets. The rows represent selected marker genes and the columns represent clusters with the same color as in **(A)**. **(D)** Expression of canonical marker genes for 11 T cell subsets as represented in the UMAP plot. Data are colored according to expression levels and the legend is labeled in log scale. UMAP, uniform manifold approximation and projection; ASS-ILD, anti-synthetase syndrome-associated interstitial lung disease; HD, healthy donor; TCM, central memory T lymphocyte; TEM, effector memory T lymphocyte; Treg, regulatory CD4 T lymphocyte; NKT, natural killer T cell; MAIT, mucosal-associated invariant T cell; DNT, double negative T cell; pro T, proliferative T cell.

CD4+ T lymphocytes (CD4 TCM, CCR7+SELL+S100A4+), effector memory CD4+ T lymphocytes (CD4 TEM, S100A4+ GZMA+), and regulatory CD4 T lymphocytes (Treg, FOXP3+ CTLA4+); the 2 subsets of CD8+ T lymphocytes included naïve CD8 T lymphocytes (CD8 Naïve, CCR7+SELL+), and effector memory CD8+ T lymphocytes (CD8 TEM, S100A4+GZMA+); other T cells included $\gamma\delta$ T cells (TRGV9+TRDV2+), NKT cells (CD3D+NKG7+TYROBP+), mucosal-associated invariant T (MAIT) cells (TRAV1-2+SLC4A10+), double-negative T cells (DNT, CD4-CD8A-), and pro T (MKI67+RRM2+) (**Figures 4C, D**). A dot plot showed the average expression and percentage of expressed cells of selected marker genes in each labeled T cell subset (**Figure 5A**). No significant differences in cell compositions were found in each cluster except pro T cells (**Supplementary Figures 5A, B**). However, the number of pro T cells was too small to get a robust result, so we didn't perform further analysis. Next, we compared the expression of CD4 and CD8 between patients with ASS-ILD and HDs, no significant differences were found (**Supplementary Figure 5C**). Then the ratios of CD4 TCM to CD4 Naïve, CD4 TEM to CD4 Naïve, CD8 TEM to CD8 Naïve were compared between patients with ASS-ILD and HDs, respectively. Only the differences in the ratio of CD8 TEM to CD8 Naïve were statistically significant (**Figure 5B**). After that, we further compared the ratios of CD8 TEM GZMK, CD8 TEM GNLY, and CD8 TEM TRAV27 to CD8 Naïve between patients with ASS-ILD and HDs, respectively; only the differences in the ratio of CD8 TEM GNLY to CD8 Naïve were statistically significant between patients and HDs (**Figure 5C**).

To gain insights into the differential transcriptomic changes in T cells between patients with ASS-ILD and HDs, we compared their expression profiles of T cells. We observed that DEGs upregulated in patients with ASS-ILD were involved in processes including responses to type I and II interferons, cellular response to interleukin-1, cellular response to tumor necrosis factor, and NF-kappaB signaling using GO analysis (**Figure 6A**). We also did Kyoto Encyclopedia of Genes and Genomes (KEGG) pathway analysis. Of note, Th1, Th2, and Th17 cell differentiation signaling pathways were enriched in T cells, indicating the involvement of Th1, Th2, and Th17 cells in the pathogenesis of ASS-ILD (**Figure 6B**). Enriched genes associated with Th1, Th2, and Th17 cell differentiation signaling pathways included HLA-DRB5, HLA-DQA1, IL2RG, HLA-DPA1, HLA-DPB1, HLA-DRB1, and HLA-DRA. The expressions of genes associated with the differentiation of CD4 T cells were mapped (**Figures 6C, D**). To validate these findings, we performed flow cytometry experiments to compare the differences in Th1 proportions, Th2 proportions, Th17 cell proportions, Th17.1 proportions, and ratios of Th17 cells to Th1 cells between patients with ASS-ILD and patients with idiopathic interstitial pneumonia (IIP, including iNSIP, COP, and IPF), and HDs,

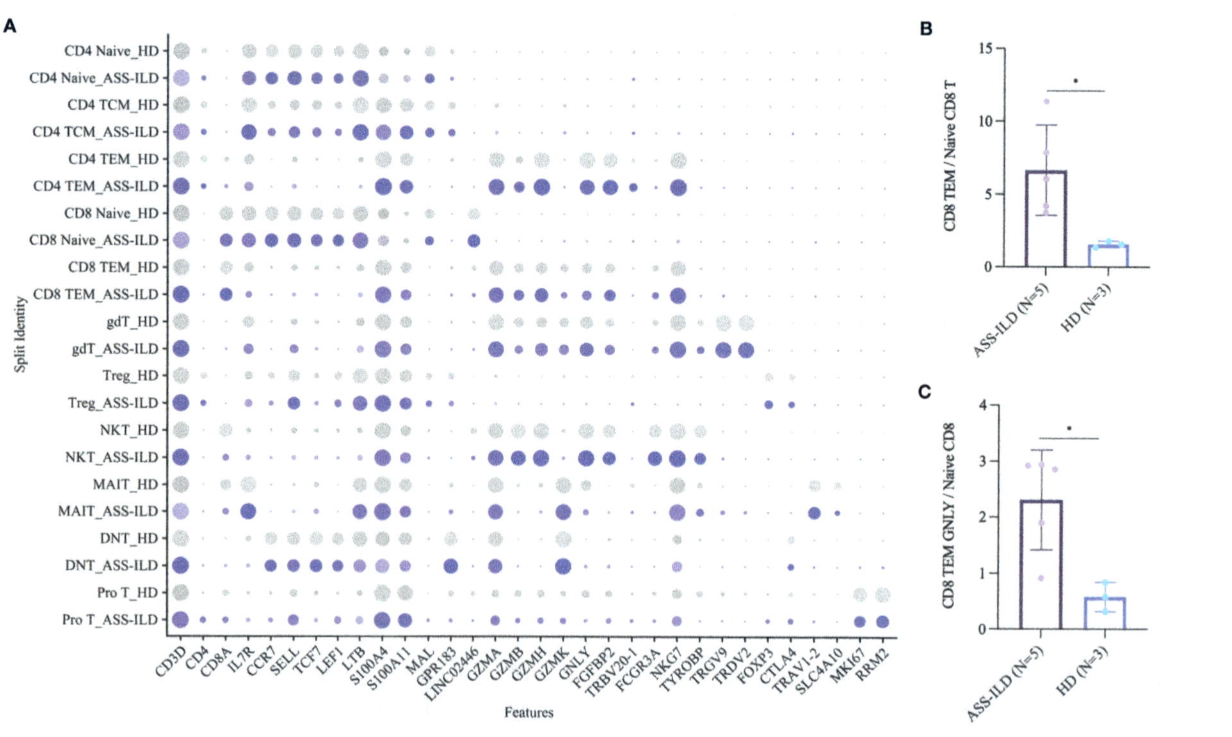

FIGURE 5 | Comparisons of T cell subsets between patients with ASS-ILD and HDs. **(A)** Dot plot depicting the average expression and percentage of expressed cells of selected marker genes in each labeled T cell subset. **(B)** Box plot of the ratios of CD8 TEM cells to CD8 Naïve T cells in patients with ASS-ILD and HDs, the result calculated by the Mann-Whitney test. The result was considered significant when a two-sided p-value was <0.05. **(C)** Box plot of the ratios of CD8 TEM GNLY cells to CD8 Naïve T cells, analysis similar to **(B)** ASS-ILD, anti-synthetase syndrome-associated interstitial lung disease; HD, healthy donor; TEM, effector memory T. $^*p < 0.05$.

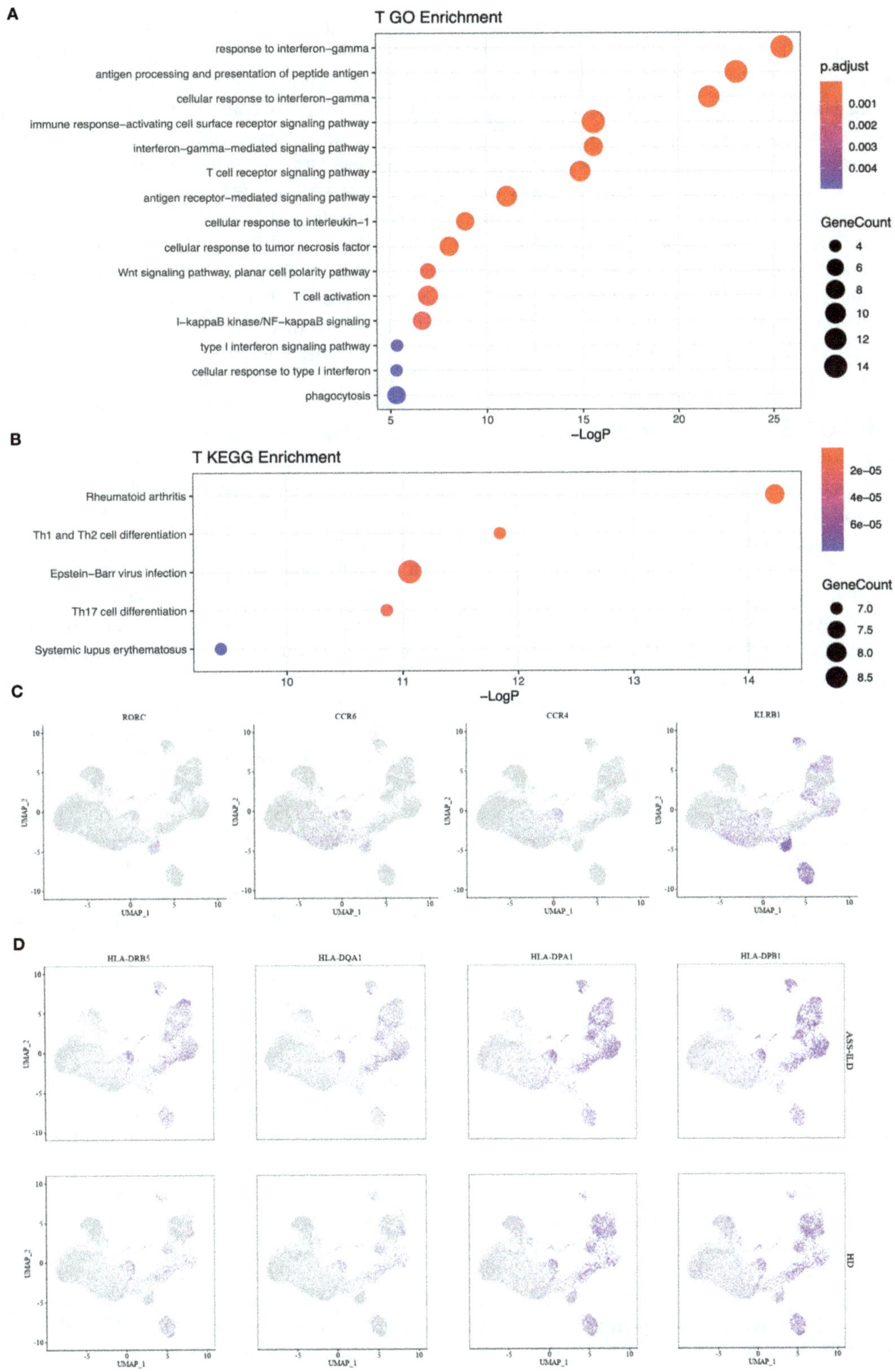

FIGURE 6 | Enrichment analyses for T cells. **(A)** GO enrichment analysis of upregulated genes for T cells. **(B)** KEGG pathway enrichment analysis of upregulated genes for T cells. **(C)** Th17 cell-related gene expressions in the UMAP plot. **(D)** Enriched genes associated with Th1, Th2, and Th17 cell differentiation signaling pathways. GO, Geno Ontology; KEGG, Kyoto Encyclopedia of Genes and Genomes; UMAP, uniform manifold approximation and projection.

respectively. The clinical manifestations, laboratory features, chest HRCT patterns, and PFT parameters of recruited patients and HDs were detailed in **Supplementary Tables 3** and **4**. The results indicated that the proportion of Th1 cells among total memory CD4 T cells was lower in patients with ASS-ILD than that in HDs; the proportion of Th2 cells among total memory CD4 T cells was higher in patients with ASS-ILD than that in patients with IPF, and HDs, respectively; the proportion of Th17 cells among total memory CD4 T cells was higher in patients with ASS-ILD than that in HDs, patients with iNSIP, patients with COP, and patients with IPF, respectively; the proportions of Th17.1 cells among total memory CD4 T cells were similar in patients with ASS-ILD and HDs; the ratio of Th17 cells to Th1 cells was higher in patients with ASS-ILD than that in patients with iNSIP, patients with IPF, and HDs, respectively (**Figures 7A, B**).

Features of B Cell Subsets in Patients With ASS-ILD

To characterize changes of different B subsets, we sub-clustered B cells into 8 subsets and those with similar B cell markers were categorized together (**Supplementary Figures 6A–H**). Then we identified 4 subsets of B cells based on the expression of canonical B cell markers (**Figures 8A, B**). We identified naïve B lymphocytes (CD79A+CD19+IGHD+), IgM+ memory B lymphocytes (CD79A+CD19+CD27+IGHM+), IgM- memory B lymphocytes (CD79A+CD19+CD27+IGHM-), and plasma (CD38+MZB1+) (**Figures 8C, D**). No significant differences in cell proportions were seen in B cells (**Supplementary Figures 7A, B**).

To investigate the differential transcriptomic changes in B cells between patients with ASS-ILD and HDs, we then compared their expression profiles of B cells. We observed that DEGs upregulated in patients with ASS-ILD were involved in processes including responses to type I and II interferons, regulation of viral life cycle, and response to reactive oxygen species (**Figure 9A**). We also performed KEGG pathway analysis, Influenza A, Measles, antigen processing and presentation were enriched in B cells (**Figure 9B**). A dot plot showed the average expression and percentage of expressed cells of selected marker genes in each labeled B cell subset (**Figure 9C**).

DISCUSSION

Currently, the management of patients with ASS-ILD relies on glucocorticoids combined with immunosuppressant or biological agents (10, 11). However, the pathogenesis of ASS remains to be clearly elucidated and specific target therapies are still lacking. Several studies have shown the features of innate and adaptive immune responses, which have helped us understand the pathogenic immune responses of ASS-ILD (13, 20, 21). It is evident that both the innate and adaptive immune responses contribute to the breakdown of immune tolerance to self-antigen in autoimmune diseases, and adaptive immune cells including T and B cells are primary contributors. In this study, we aimed to profile the immunological landscape in PBMCs from patients with ASS-ILD at single-cell resolution and investigate the roles of different CD4 T cells in this condition.

First, patients with ASS-ILD showed upregulated interferon responses among NK cells, monocytes, T cells, and B cells in PBMCs, which is consistent with previous studies (19, 21). In autoimmune diseases, the presence of persistent production of both type I and type II interferons has been well established (22). The most well-defined type I interferons are interferon α and interferon β, and type II interferon only includes interferon γ (23). Interferon α, β, and γ induce the expression of transcription factors, especially canonical interferon-stimulating genes (ISGs), by activating different JAK-STAT pathways (23). Targeting therapies against JAK-STAT pathways have been developed and some of them were used in clinics as an alternative to biological therapies. Tofacitinib is an oral small molecule targeting all JAKs but preferentially inhibits JAK1 and JAK3, and it is the first approved JAK inhibitor for rheumatic arthritis (24). Two prospective clinical trials reported that tofacitinib is effective in treating amyopathic dermatomyositis-associated ILD (25, 26). The efficacy and safety of tofacitinib in patient with ASS-ILD have only been reported in a case report (27). There are more small-molecule compounds targeting JAKs in development and different JAK inhibitors show different specificities (28, 29). Tofacitinib and other JAK inhibitors may be of benefit in treating ASS-ILD, but further investigations are still warranted to evaluate their efficacy and safety profiles.

Second, the proportion of naïve CD8 T cells in patients with ASS-ILD measured by scRNA-seq seemed lower than that in HDs, while the proportion of CD8 TEM cells seemed higher, but no significant differences were detected. We further compared the ratio of CD8 TEM to CD8 Naïve, patients with ASS-ILD showed a significantly higher proportion than that in HDs. CD8 TEM could be categorized into 3 subsets according to specific transcriptional features in this study: CD8 TEM GZMK, CD8 TEM GNLY, CD8 TEM TRAV 27. GZMK, GNLY, TRAV 27 was specifically up-regulated in these three subsets, respectively. GZMK and GNLY are different lytic granules (30), TRAV 27 gene encodes V region of the variable domain of T cell receptor α chain to participate in antigen recognition (31). We only found significant differences in the ratio CD8 TEM GNLY to CD8 Naïve between patients with ASS-ILD and HDs. Current researches have reported the correlations between GNLY or CD8 T cells and several autoimmune diseases, such as differential expressions of GNLY in rheumatic arthritis and healthy state, an association of GNLY expressions in CD8 cells and steroid resistance in polymyositis, an association of disease flares and proportions of activated CD8 T cells in systemic lupus erythematosus (32–34). Our study showed that CD8 T cells in the blood of patients with ASS-ILD were skewed towards an activated phenotype characterized by high expression of GNLY. Further investigations into whether CD8 T cells infiltrate and mediate damages in target organs might help to better illustrate the role of CD8 T cells in ASS-ILD. And the role of GNLY and other cytolytic granules in CD8 T cells is worth exploring to disclose various functions of CD8 T cells.

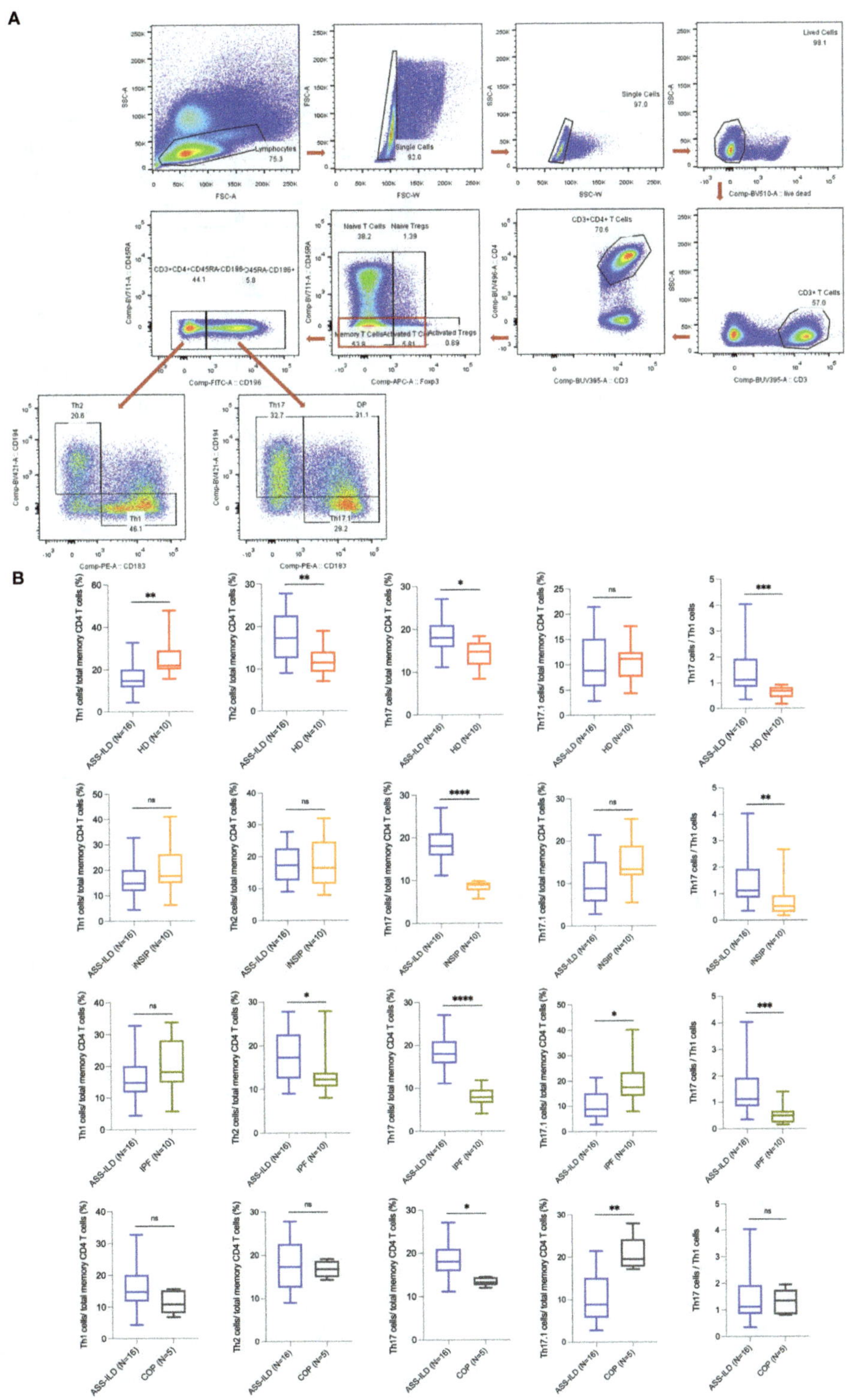

FIGURE 7 | Flow cytometry experiments. **(A)** Representative flow cytometry analyses of PBMCs from one patient with ASS-ILD. **(B)** Percentages of Th1, Th2, Th17, and Th17.1 cells in total memory CD4 T cells among PBMCs of 16 patients with ASS-ILD, 10 patients with iNSIP, 10 patients with IPF, 5 patients with COP, and 10 HDs, respectively. And the ratio of Th17 cells to Th1 cells. The results were calculated by the Mann-Whitney test, respectively. The results were considered significant when a two-sided p-value was <0.05. PBMC, peripheral blood mononuclear cell; ASS-ILD, anti-synthetase syndrome-associated interstitial lung disease; iNSIP, idiopathic non-specific interstitial pneumonia; IPF, idiopathic pulmonary fibrosis; COP, cryptogenic organizing pneumonia; HD, healthy donor. *$p < 0.05$; **$p < 0.01$; ***$p < 0.001$; ****$p < 0.0001$; ns, not statistically significant.

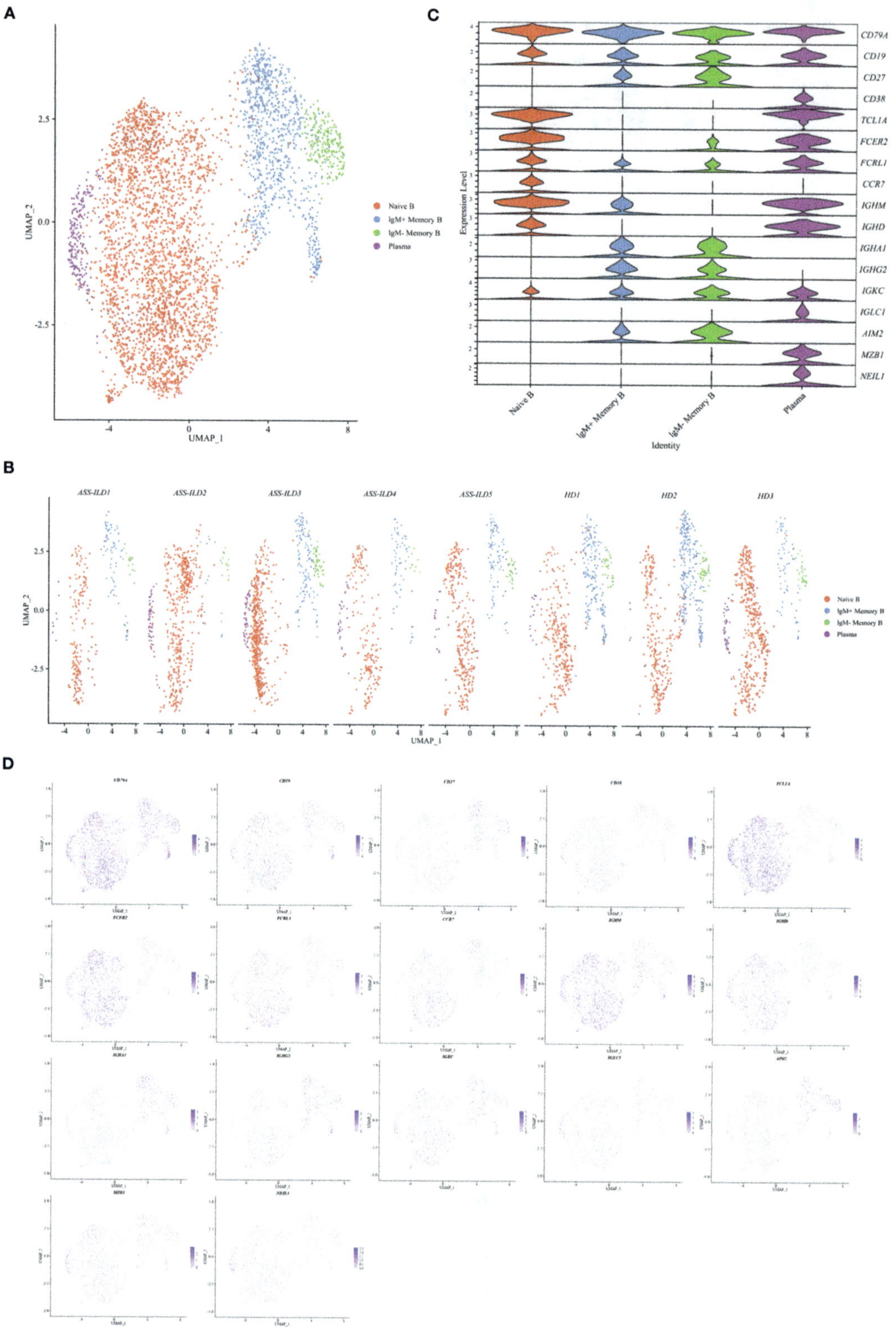

FIGURE 8 | Immunological features of B cell subsets. **(A)** UMAP visualization of 4709 B cells. **(B)** Annotating condition of each patient with ASS-ILD and HD. **(C)** Violin plot showing the expression distribution of selected marker genes in the 4 B cell subsets. The rows represent selected marker genes and the columns represent clusters with the same color as in **(A)**. **(D)** Expression of canonical marker genes for 4 B cell subsets as represented in the UMAP plot. Data are colored according to expression levels and the legend is labeled in log scale. UMAP, uniform manifold approximation and projection; ASS-ILD, anti-synthetase syndrome-associated interstitial lung disease; HD, healthy donor.

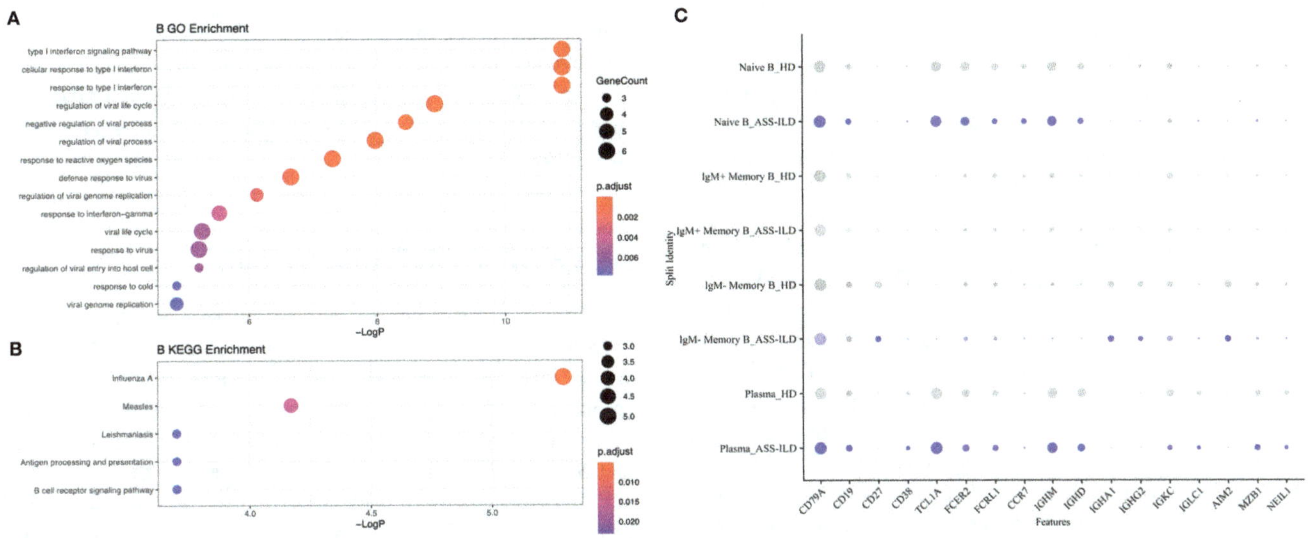

FIGURE 9 | Enrichment analyses for B cells. **(A)** GO enrichment analysis of upregulated genes for B cells. **(B)** KEGG pathway enrichment analysis of upregulated genes for B cells. **(C)** Dot plot depicting average expression and percentage of expressed cells of selected marker genes in each labeled B cell subset. GO, Geno Ontology; KEGG, Kyoto Encyclopedia of Genes and Genomes.

Third, Th1, Th2, and Th17 cell differentiation signaling pathways were enriched in T cells in this study. Using scRNA-seq here was unable to directly compare the differences in the compositions of Th1, Th2, and Th17 cells between patients with ASS-ILD and HDs. We performed validation experiments using flow cytometry, which was consistent with our scRNA-seq results. In consideration for overlapping chest radiological manifestations between ASS-ILD and IIP (especially NSIP, COP, and IPF), we enrolled patients with IIP as disease controls in validation experiments. The proportions of Th2 cells and Th17 cells were higher in patients with ASS-ILD, and the proportion of Th1 cells was lower. Although hallmark pathogenic conditions associated with Th2 cells are allergy and asthma (35), it is worth mentioning that Th2 dominant autoimmune diseases are present, like multiple sclerosis (36). Besides a shift to a predominant Th2 response has been reported to lead to chronic inflammation and pulmonary fibrosis in sarcoidosis and hypersensitivity pneumonitis, as well as airway fibrosis induced by asthma (37–39). It is worth thinking whether the dynamic changes of Th2 cells are related with the fibrotic evolution of ILD in ASS. Establishing the risk factors for fibrotic ASS-ILD could provide us with the opportunity to early identify and intervene the progression of pulmonary fibrosis. Th17 cells have been demonstrated to play important roles in several autoimmune diseases and chronic respiratory diseases, such as rheumatic arthritis, psoriasis, multiple sclerosis, asthma, and sarcoidosis (18, 40, 41).Th17 cells are characterized by the hallmark cytokine of IL-17A, and have a critically important role in the induction of multiple autoimmune disorders (40). Th17 cells display remarkable plasticity, which is also closely associated with their pathogenicity (42, 43). Here we used chemokine receptors to define different subsets of CD4 T cells and found the increased numbers of Th17 cells in this study. It remains uncertain how Th17 cells with a high grade of plasticity function in this condition. It is not only important to evaluate Th17 cell frequency in this condition, but also to explore the proinflammatory capacity of Th17 cells. Thus how Th17 cells function in this condition is worthy of exploration.

Fourth, GO analysis for NK cells showed the enrichment of antigen processing and presentation of peptide antigen *via* MHC II, which needs to be interpreted carefully. NK cells are not professional antigen-presenting cells (APCs), and they are important members of the innate immune system to directly eliminate virus-infected cells and tumor cells through their natural cytotoxic capacity without prior priming (44). Genes enriched for antigen processing and presentation mainly included human leukocyte antigen (HLA) -DPB1, HLA-DPA1, HLA-DQA1, HLA-DRB1, and HLA-DRB5, all these enriched genes are classical HLA II molecules. HLA-DR-expressing NK cells have been reported to be detected in the blood and tissues in healthy individuals, and their functions are associated with enhanced production of proinflammatory cytokines, degranulation, and proliferation upon stimuli (44). *In vitro*, HLA-DR-expressing NK cells pre-activated with cytokines have been reported to induce nonspecific activation and partial differentiation of CD4 T cells in previous publications (45, 46). However, how NK cells process and present antigen is unclear and *in vivo* validation experiments are still lacking. The ability of antigen processing and presentation remains to be determined for NK cells. Type I interferons are well-known powerful regulators of NK cell activation (47), and HLA-DR expressing NK cells are reported to display profound ability to induce secretion of interferon γ (48). Functional divergence of NK cells from patients with ASS-ILD and HDs exists based on our analysis. We speculate that DEGs associated with classical HLA II molecules could be the effect of interferons in this condition. Nevertheless, more analyses are needed to verify the enriched functions profiled by scRNA-seq analyses.

There are several limitations in our study. First, the sample size is comparatively small. Second, we don't have tissue samples, limiting our interpretation of cellular interchange between target organs and peripheral compartments. Third, longitudinal follow-up studies are needed to further elucidate the pathogenic roles of upregulated interferon responses, altered CD8 T cell homeostasis, and involvement of differentiation signaling pathways of CD4 T cells in the pathogenesis of ASS-ILD. Fourth, scRNA-seq of PBMCs is a powerful tool for visualization of peripheral cellular landscape, but it remains to be interpreted carefully owing to technical limitations and heterogeneity of algorithms for data analyses in different researches. Nevertheless, our research reveals peripheral immune responses in patients with ASS-ILD, and may provide foundations for further exploration into the pathogenesis of this condition.

In conclusion, our study reveals that patients with ASS-ILD are characterized by upregulated interferon responses, altered CD8 T cell homeostasis, and involvement of differentiation pathways for different subsets of CD4+ T cells. And the proportions of Th17 cells and Th2 cells are increased in patients with ASS-ILD than those in HDs based on the expression patterns of chemokine receptors through flow cytometry, while the proportion of Th1 cells is decreased. Further studies with longitudinal samples from more patients and investigations into cellular interchange between target organs and peripheral immune cells are still warranted to advance our understanding of the pathogenesis, which may pave the way for novel therapeutic interventions against ASS-ILD.

ETHICS STATEMENT

The studies involving human participants were reviewed and approved by the ethics committee of the China-Japan Friendship Hospital, China (2019-123-K85). The patients/participants provided their written informed consent to participate in this study.

AUTHOR CONTRIBUTIONS

CZ, HD, and CW contributed equally to this article and are joint corresponding authors. LilZ, ZC, SW, HD, and CW designed the study. LilZ was responsible for the data collection. ZC was responsible for the data analysis, with support from CZ and LF. LilZ and ZC interpreted the data and prepared the first draft. LilZ, ZC, SW, CZ, LF, YR, BX, JG, HD, CW revised the draft. SX, LZ, and LM were involved in identification of patients with ASS-ILD or IIP. LilZ, ZC, HD, and CW had full access to all of the data in the study and took responsibility for the integrity of the data and the accuracy of the data analyses. The corresponding authors attest that all listed authors meet authorship criteria and that no others meeting the criteria have been omitted. All authors contributed to the article and approved the submitted version.

ACKNOWLEDGMENTS

Figure 1 was created with Biorender.com.

REFERENCES

1. American Thoracic Society and European Respiratory Society. American Thoracic Society/European Respiratory Society International Multidisciplinary Consensus Classification of the Idiopathic Interstitial Pneumonias. This Joint Statement of the American Thoracic Society (ATS), and the European Respiratory Society (ERS) was Adopted by the ATS Board of Directors, June 2001 and by the ERS Executive Committee, June 2001. *Am J Respir Crit Care Med* (2002) 165(2):277–304. doi: 10.1164/ajrccm.165.2.ats01
2. Lega J-C, Reynaud Q, Belot A, Fabien N, Durieu I, Cottin V. Idiopathic Inflammatory Myopathies and the Lung. *Eur Respir Rev* (2015) 24(137):216–38. doi: 10.1183/16000617.00002015
3. McHugh NJ, Tansley SL. Autoantibodies in Myositis. *Nat Rev Rheumatol* (2018) 14(5):290–302. doi: 10.1038/nrrheum.2018.56
4. Dalakas MC. Inflammatory Muscle Diseases. *N Engl J Med* (2015) 372 (18):1734–47. doi: 10.1056/NEJMra1402225
5. Noguchi E, Uruha A, Suzuki S, Hamanaka K, Ohnuki Y, Tsugawa J, et al. Skeletal Muscle Involvement in Antisynthetase Syndrome. *JAMA Neurol* (2017) 74(8):992–99. doi: 10.1001/jamaneurol.2017.0934
6. Gasparotto M, Gatto M, Saccon F, Ghirardello A, Iaccarino L, Doria A. Pulmonary Involvement in Antisynthetase Syndrome. *Curr Opin Rheumatol* (2019) 31(6):603–10. doi: 10.1097/BOR.0000000000000663
7. Aggarwal R, Cassidy E, Fertig N, Koontz DC, Lucas M, Ascherman DP, et al. Patients With Non-Jo-1 Anti-tRNA-Synthetase Autoantibodies Have Worse Survival Than Jo-1 Positive Patients. *Ann Rheum Dis* (2014) 73(1):227–32. doi: 10.1136/annrheumdis-2012-201800
8. Liu H, Xie S, Liang T, Ma L, Sun H, Dai H, et al. Prognostic Factors of Interstitial Lung Disease Progression at Sequential HRCT in Anti-Synthetase Syndrome. *Eur Radiol* (2019) 29(10):5349–57. doi: 10.1007/s00330-019-06152-5
9. Trallero-Araguas E, Grau-Junyent JM, Labirua-Iturburu A, Garcia-Hernandez FJ, Monteagudo-Jimenez M, Fraile-Rodriguez G, et al. Clinical Manifestations and Long-Term Outcome of Anti-Jo1 Antisynthetase Patients in a Large Cohort of Spanish Patients From the GEAS-IIM Group. *Semin Arthritis Rheum* (2016) 46(2):225–31. doi: 10.1016/j.semarthrit.2016.03.011
10. Oddis CV, Aggarwal R. Treatment in Myositis. *Nat Rev Rheumatol* (2018) 14 (5):279–89. doi: 10.1038/nrrheum.2018.42
11. Andersson H, Sem M, Lund MB, Aalokken TM, Gunther A, Walle-Hansen R, et al. Long-Term Experience With Rituximab in Anti-Synthetase Syndrome-Related Interstitial Lung Disease. *Rheumatol (Oxf)* (2015) 54(8):1420–8. doi: 10.1093/rheumatology/kev004
12. Horwitz DA, Fahmy TM, Piccirillo CA, La Cava A. Rebalancing Immune Homeostasis to Treat Autoimmune Diseases. *Trends Immunol* (2019) 40 (10):888–908. doi: 10.1016/j.it.2019.08.003
13. Galindo-Feria AS, Albrecht I, Fernandes-Cerqueira C, Notarnicola A, James EA, Herrath J, et al. Proinflammatory Histidyl-Transfer RNA Synthetase-Specific CD4+ T Cells in the Blood and Lungs of Patients With Idiopathic Inflammatory Myopathies. *Arthritis Rheumatol* (2020) 72(1):179–91. doi: 10.1002/art.41075
14. Howard OM, Dong HF, Yang D, Raben N, Nagaraju K, Rosen A, et al. Histidyl-tRNA Synthetase and asparaginyl-tRNA Synthetase, Autoantigens in Myositis, Activate Chemokine Receptors on T Lymphocytes and Immature Dendritic Cells. *J Exp Med* (2002) 196(6):781 91. doi: 10.1084/jem.20020186
15. Connors GR, Christopher-Stine L, Oddis CV, Danoff SK. Interstitial Lung Disease Associated With the Idiopathic Inflammatory Myopathies. *Chest* (2010) 138(6):1464–74. doi: 10.1378/chest.10-0180

16. Travis WD, Costabel U, Hansell DM, King TE, Lynch DA, Nicholson AG, et al. An Official American Thoracic Society/European Respiratory Society Statement: Update of the International Multidisciplinary Classification of the Idiopathic Interstitial Pneumonias. *Am J Respir Crit Care Med* (2013) 188 (6):733–48. doi: 10.1164/rccm.201308-1483ST
17. Raghu G, Remy-Jardin M, Myers JL, Richeldi L, Ryerson CJ, Lederer DJ, et al. Diagnosis of Idiopathic Pulmonary Fibrosis. An Official ATS/ERS/JRS/ALAT Clinical Practice Guideline. *Am J Respir Crit Care Med* (2018) 198(5):e44–68. doi: 10.1164/rccm.201807-1255ST
18. Broos CE, Koth LL, van Nimwegen M, In 't Veen J, Paulissen SMJ, van Hamburg JP, et al. Increased T-Helper 17.1 Cells in Sarcoidosis Mediastinal Lymph Nodes. *Eur Respir J* (2018) 51(3). doi: 10.1183/13993003.01124-2017
19. Gallay L, Mouchiroud G, Chazaud B. Interferon-Signature in Idiopathic Inflammatory Myopathies. *Curr Opin Rheumatol* (2019) 31(6):634–42. doi: 10.1097/BOR.0000000000000653
20. Nie A, Sun B, Fu Z, Yu D. Roles of aminoacyl-tRNA Synthetases in Immune Regulation and Immune Diseases. *Cell Death Dis* (2019) 10(12):901. doi: 10.1038/s41419-019-2145-5
21. Pinal-Fernandez I, Casal-Dominguez M, Derfoul A, Pak K, Miller FW, Milisenda JC, et al. Machine Learning Algorithms Reveal Unique Gene Expression Profiles in Muscle Biopsies From Patients With Different Types of Myositis. *Ann Rheum Dis* (2020) 79(9):1234–42. doi: 10.1136/annrheumdis-2019-216599
22. Barrat FJ, Crow MK, Ivashkiv LB. Interferon Target-Gene Expression and Epigenomic Signatures in Health and Disease. *Nat Immunol* (2019) 20 (12):1574–83. doi: 10.1038/s41590-019-0466-2
23. Schoggins JW. Interferon-Stimulated Genes: What Do They All do? *Annu Rev Virol* (2019) 6(1):567–84. doi: 10.1146/annurev-virology-092818-015756
24. Dhillon S. Tofacitinib: A Review in Rheumatoid Arthritis. *Drugs* (2017) 77 (18):1987–2001. doi: 10.1007/s40265-017-0835-9
25. Paik JJ, Casciola-Rosen L, Shin JY, Albayda J, Tiniakou E, Leung DG, et al. Study of Tofacitinib in Refractory Dermatomyositis: An Open-Label Pilot Study of Ten Patients. *Arthritis Rheumatol* (2021) 73(5):858–65. doi: 10.1002/art.41602
26. Chen Z, Wang X, Ye S. Tofacitinib in Amyopathic Dermatomyositis-Associated Interstitial Lung Disease. *N Engl J Med* (2019) 381(3):291–93. doi: 10.1056/NEJMc1900045
27. Pineton de Chambrun M, Hervier B, Chauveau S, Tandjaoui-Lambiotte Y, Combes A, Uzunhan Y. Tofacitinib in Antisynthetase Syndrome-Related Rapidly Progressive Interstitial Lung Disease. *Rheumatol (Oxf)* (2020) 59 (12):e142–3. doi: 10.1093/rheumatology/keaa323
28. Fragoulis GE, McInnes IB, Siebert S. JAK-Inhibitors. New Players in the Field of Immune-Mediated Diseases, Beyond Rheumatoid Arthritis. *Rheumatol (Oxf)* (2019) 58(Suppl 1):i43–54. doi: 10.1093/rheumatology/key276
29. Winthrop KL. The Emerging Safety Profile of JAK Inhibitors in Rheumatic Disease. *Nat Rev Rheumatol* (2017) 13(4):234–43. doi: 10.1038/nrrheum.2017.23
30. Chavez-Galan L, Arenas-Del Angel MC, Zenteno E, Chavez R, Lascurain R. Cell Death Mechanisms Induced by Cytotoxic Lymphocytes. *Cell Mol Immunol* (2009) 6(1):15–25. doi: 10.1038/cmi.2009.3
31. Rossjohn J, Gras S, Miles JJ, Turner SJ, Godfrey DI, McCluskey J. T Cell Antigen Receptor Recognition of Antigen-Presenting Molecules. *Annu Rev Immunol* (2015) 33(1):169–200. doi: 10.1146/annurev-immunol-032414-112334
32. Yu R, Zhang J, Zhuo Y, Hong X, Ye J, Tang S, et al. Identification of Diagnostic Signatures and Immune Cell Infiltration Characteristics in Rheumatoid Arthritis by Integrating Bioinformatic Analysis and Machine-Learning Strategies. *Front Immunol* (2021) 12:724934. doi: 10.3389/fimmu.2021.724934
33. Ikezoe K, Ohshima S, Osoegawa M, Tanaka M, Ogawa K, Nagata K, et al. Expression of Granulysin in Polymyositis and Inclusion-Body Myositis. *J Neurol Neurosurg Psychiatry* (2006) 77(10):1187–90. doi: 10.1136/jnnp.2005.081810
34. Blanco P, Pitard V, Viallard JF, Taupin JL, Pellegrin JL, Moreau JF. Increase in Activated CD8+ T Lymphocytes Expressing Perforin and Granzyme B Correlates With Disease Activity in Patients With Systemic Lupus Erythematosus. *Arthritis Rheum* (2005) 52(1):201–11. doi: 10.1002/art.20745
35. Annunziato F, Romagnani C, Romagnani S. The 3 Major Types of Innate and Adaptive Cell-Mediated Effector Immunity. *J Allergy Clin Immunol* (2015) 135(3):626–35. doi: 10.1016/j.jaci.2014.11.001
36. Costanza M. Type 2 Inflammatory Responses in Autoimmune Demyelination of the Central Nervous System: Recent Advances. *J Immunol Res* (2019) 2019:4204512. doi: 10.1155/2019/4204512
37. Barrera L, Mendoza F, Zuñiga J, Estrada A, Zamora AC, Melendro EI, et al. Functional Diversity of T-Cell Subpopulations in Subacute and Chronic Hypersensitivity Pneumonitis. *Am J Respir Crit Care Med* (2008) 177(1):44–55. doi: 10.1164/rccm.200701-093OC
38. Patterson KC, Hogarth K, Husain AN, Sperling AI, Niewold TB. The Clinical and Immunologic Features of Pulmonary Fibrosis in Sarcoidosis. *Trans Res* (2012) 160(5):321–31. doi: 10.1016/j.trsl.2012.03.005
39. Morimoto Y, Hirahara K, Kiuchi M, Wada T, Ichikawa T, Kanno T, et al. Amphiregulin-Producing Pathogenic Memory T Helper 2 Cells Instruct Eosinophils to Secrete Osteopontin and Facilitate Airway Fibrosis. *Immunity* (2018) 49(1):134–50.e6. doi: 10.1016/j.immuni.2018.04.023
40. Patel DD, Kuchroo VK. Th17 Cell Pathway in Human Immunity: Lessons From Genetics and Therapeutic Interventions. *Immunity* (2015) 43(6):1040–51. doi: 10.1016/j.immuni.2015.12.003
41. Ten Berge B, Paats MS, Bergen IM, van den Blink B, Hoogsteden HC, Lambrecht BN, et al. Increased IL-17A Expression in Granulomas and in Circulating Memory T Cells in Sarcoidosis. *Rheumatol (Oxf)* (2012) 51(1):37–46. doi: 10.1093/rheumatology/ker316
42. Lee YK, Turner H, Maynard CL, Oliver JR, Chen D, Elson CO, et al. Late Developmental Plasticity in the T Helper 17 Lineage. *Immunity* (2009) 30 (1):92–107. doi: 10.1016/j.immuni.2008.11.005
43. Hirota K, Turner JE, Villa M, Duarte JH, Demengeot J, Steinmetz OM, et al. Plasticity of Th17 Cells in Peyer's Patches is Responsible for the Induction of T Cell-Dependent IgA Responses. *Nat Immunol* (2013) 14(4):372–9. doi: 10.1038/ni.2552
44. Erokhina SA, Streltsova MA, Kanevskiy LM, Grechikhina MV, Sapozhnikov AM, Kovalenko EI. HLA-DR-Expressing NK Cells: Effective Killers Suspected for Antigen Presentation. *J Leukoc Biol* (2021) 109(2):327–37. doi: 10.1002/JLB.3RU0420-668RR
45. Loyon R, Picard E, Mauvais O, Queiroz L, Mougey V, Pallandre JR, et al. IL-21-Induced MHC Class II+ NK Cells Promote the Expansion of Human Uncommitted CD4+ Central Memory T Cells in a Macrophage Migration Inhibitory Factor-Dependent Manner. *J Immunol* (2016) 197(1):85–96. doi: 10.4049/jimmunol.1501147
46. Zingoni A, Sornasse T, Cocks BG, Tanaka Y, Santoni A, Lanier LL. Cross-Talk Between Activated Human NK Cells and CD4+ T Cells *via* OX40-OX40 Ligand Interactions. *J Immunol* (2004) 173(6):3716–24. doi: 10.4049/jimmunol.173.6.3716
47. Biron CA, Nguyen KB, Pien GC, Cousens LP, Salazar-Mather TP. Natural Killer Cells in Antiviral Defense: Function and Regulation by Innate Cytokines. *Annu Rev Immunol* (1999) 17:189–220. doi: 10.1146/annurev.immunol.17.1.189
48. Evans JH, Horowitz A, Mehrabi M, Wise EL, Pease JE, Riley EM, et al. A Distinct Subset of Human NK Cells Expressing HLA-DR Expand in Response to IL-2 and Can Aid Immune Responses to BCG. *Eur J Immunol* (2011) 41 (7):1924–33. doi: 10.1002/eji.201041180

17

Description and Analysis of a Novel Subtype of the Anti-Synthetase Syndrome Characterized by Frequent Attacks of Fever and Systemic Inflammation in a Single-Center Cohort Study

*Shuhui Sun, Zhiwei Chen, Danting Zhang, Wenwen Xu, Wanlong Wu, Fangfang Sun, Liyang Gu, Jie Chen, Jiajie Li, Ting Li, Xiaodong Wang and Shuang Ye**

Department of Rheumatology, Renji Hospital, Shanghai Jiaotong University School of Medicine, Shanghai, China

Correspondence:
Shuang Ye
ye_shuang2000@163.com

Objectives: The aim of this study was to investigate anti-synthetase syndrome (ASyS) patients who presented with recurrent episodes of fever and systemic inflammation.

Methods: A retrospective cohort of Chinese ASyS patients (n=126) in our center (between January 2013 and January 2020) was included. Patients presenting with concomitant autoimmune rheumatic diseases or malignancies were subsequently excluded. The number of non-infectious fever attacks and attack frequency were recorded and calculated. Patients with two or more attacks and within the upper three quartiles of attack frequency were defined as high-inflammation group. Univariate and multivariate analyses were carried out to characterize the high-inflammation subtype.

Results: Out of 113 eligible patients with an average of 5 years follow up, 25 patients were defined as the high-inflammation group (16 for anti-Jo1, 9 for anti-PL7), with an average of 1.12 attack/patient-year. Compared to low-inflammation group (0–1 attack only and a frequency lower than 0.5 attack/patient-year), the high-inflammation group had higher occurrence of fever and rapid progressive interstitial lung disease (RPILD) as the first presentation (84% *vs.* 21% and 40% *vs.* 9%, respectively, both p<0.01). Anti-PL-7 was related to the more inflammatory phenotype (p=0.014). Cumulative disease-modifying agent exposures (>=3) were much higher in the high-inflammation group (60% *vs.* 26%), while biological agents, i.e., rituximab and tocilizumab, showed better "drug survival" for Jo-1+ and PL-7+ ASyS patients with high inflammation, respectively, in our cohort.

Conclusions: ASyS with recurrent systemic inflammatory episodes reflects a subtype of more aggressive and refractory disease in the spectrum of ASyS. Increased awareness of this subtype might lead to more appropriate management.

Keywords: idiopathic inflammatory myopathies, anti-synthetase syndrome, fever, inflammation, anti-PL-7

INTRODUCTION

Anti-synthetase syndrome (ASyS) is one of the most common forms of idiopathic inflammatory myopathies (IIMs) in adults. Although ASyS shares many features with dermatomyositis (DM) and polymyositis, it has distinctive serological and clinical patterns (1). Serological hallmarks, i.e., anti-tRNA-synthetase antibodies (ARSs), have been identified, with anti-Jo-1 (histidyl-) ARS being the most common, followed by anti-PL-7 (threonyl-), anti-PL-12 (alanyl-), anti-EJ (glycyl-), and anti-OJ (isoleucyl-) antibodies, which are tested routinely in clinical practice. ASyS encompasses a cluster of clinical features, including myositis, interstitial lung disease (ILD), arthralgia or arthritis, Raynaud's phenomenon, fever, and cutaneous manifestations such as mechanic's hands and DM-like rashes, forming a constellation under the name ASyS (2). A meta-analysis including 27 idiopathic inflammatory myopathy studies (n=3,487) (3) found that patients positive for ARSs presented significantly more ILD (70%, CI 63–73), arthralgia (62%, CI 59–65), fever (43%, CI 43–47), and Raynaud's phenomenon (47%, CI 43–51) than patients with other myositis-specific autoantibodies (mainly anti-Mi2 and anti-SRP) (4).

It is noteworthy that fever is a common and prominent clinical manifestation of ASyS, which is different from other IIMs, with a reported incidence varying from 26% to 61% (5, 6). Although most disease courses of ASyS are chronic with good-to-moderate response to conventional immunosuppressive treatments, patients who presented with recurrent episodes of fever and elevated acute phase reactants due to systemic inflammation were deemed to be more aggressive and difficult to treat.

In the current study, by analyzing a retrospective ASyS cohort, we focused on a subgroup of patients who presented with recurrent non-infectious fever and systemic inflammation. Our aim was to delineate the clinical characteristics of this special subtype in the spectrum of ASyS in a real-world setting.

METHODS

Study Cohort

A retrospective cohort was established with consecutive patients diagnosed with ASyS referred to the Department of Rheumatology, Renji Hospital South Campus, Shanghai Jiao Tong University School of Medicine, from January 2013 to January 2020. The inclusion criteria were a clinical diagnosis of ASyS, with definitive serology findings of one of the five ARSs (Jo-1, PL-7, PL-12, EJ, and OJ) tested, along with at least one triad finding, encompassing myositis, arthritis, and ILD (1). The exclusion criteria were patients with malignancy within 3 years before or after the ASyS diagnosis and overlapping with other connective tissue diseases, such as systemic lupus erythematosus (SLE) and systemic sclerosis (SSc). Erosive or non-erosive arthritis with or without the presence of rheumatoid factor (RF) and anti-citrullinated protein antibody (ACPA) in ASyS patients had been demonstrated (7, 8). Thus, rheumatoid arthritis classification criteria were not implemented as exclusion criteria. This study protocol was approved by the internal ethics committee with informed consent for desensitized clinical data collection obtained from all patients.

Patient demographic information, clinical manifestations, laboratory tests, radiographic findings, and treatments were all retrospectively collected and evaluated. All eligible patients were ranked by the total number of systemic inflammation attacks.

Terminologies

An *attack* of systemic inflammation was defined as acute episode of fever (with a documented temperature of 38°C or higher) during the disease course with elevated acute phase reactant (ESR >20 mm/h and/or CRP>8 mg/L), not otherwise explained, such as infection or drug fever, and was controlled only by enhanced immunosuppression (glucocorticoids and/or immunosuppressants). Recurrent fever within 1 month was only counted once.

Fever at disease onset referred to fever attack within 3 months from the onset of disease.

Interstitial lung disease (ILD) was identified by chest high-resolution CT (HRCT) with or without a consistent pulmonary function test. Radiological patterns of ILD were predominantly classified as usual interstitial pneumonia (UIP), non-specific interstitial pneumonia (NSIP), or organizing pneumonia (OP) according to the 2002 American Thoracic Society/European Respiratory Society classification criteria (9). All HRCT images were independently evaluated by two experienced investigators who were blinded to the clinical information.

Rapid progressive ILD (RPILD) including acute/subacute interstitial pneumonia was defined as the deterioration of the radiological interstitial changes with progressive dyspnea and hypoxemia associated with ILD within 3 months (10), which was attributed to ASyS *per se* rather than other causes such as infection, heart failure, or pulmonary embolism.

Myositis was defined as proximal muscle weakness and/or pain along with creatinine kinase elevation, with a compatible muscle magnetic resonance or electromyography or muscle biopsy findings.

Refractory disease was defined as exposure to at least three disease-modifying antirheumatic drugs (DMARDs), including methotrexate, azathioprine, cyclophosphamide, mycophenolate mofetil, cyclosporine, tacrolimus, leflunomide, and biological DMARDs (bDMARDs), namely, rituximab or tocilizumab, as the DMARDs used in our cohort, given sequentially or concomitantly.

A good response to a given DMARD was defined as clinical improvement without fever, active arthritis or myositis, or worsening pulmonary function test results and/or chest HRCT images and allowed glucocorticoids to be tapered to a maintenance prednisone dose of 5 to 10 mg per day or equivalent dosage (11); otherwise, the patient was categorized as a poor responder. *Undetermined response* was for patients still under follow-up and glucocorticoid tapering but not reaching a maintenance dosage.

Detection of Myositis-Specific Autoantibodies

The identification of the anti-synthetase autoantibodies (anti-Jo-1, anti-PL-7, anti-PL-12, anti-OJ, anti-EJ) was determined by the

Euroline Autoimmune Inflammatory Myopathies 16 Ag kit (Euroimmun, Luebeck, Germany). Simultaneously, a Bio-Plex Pro 2200 (Bio-Rad, USA) immunoassay system for Luminex-liquichip was used to detect autoantibodies against extractable nuclear antigens (ENA, anti-Jo1 included) and ACPA.

Statistical Analysis

Categorical variables were compared using Fisher's exact test or Pearson Chi-square test, while continuous variables were compared for two groups using independent sample Student's t test or Mann-Whitney U test, as appropriate. One-way ANOVA or Kruskal–Wallis rank sum tests were performed for multiple comparisons. Multivariate logistic regression analysis was performed to assess the independent risk factors and presented as odds ratios [ORs with 95% confidence intervals (CIs)]. All analyses were performed using SPSS V.19 (Armonk, NY, USA) or GraphPad 5.0 (San Diego, CA, USA) software. The difference was considered statistically significant when the p-value was less than 0.05.

RESULTS

Study Cohort

We initially included 126 ASyS patients between January 2013 and January 2020 (**Figure 1**). Concomitant malignancies within 3 years (n=5, one pancreatic cancer, one lung cancer, one colon cancer, one breast cancer, and one for high clinical suspicion of cancer with bloody pericardial effusion/tamponade who deceased rapidly after being complicated with pulmonary embolism, for whom cytological or pathological evidence of malignancy was not established) and overlap syndrome (SLE, n=6; SSc, n=1; ankylosing spondylitis, n=1) were excluded. Ultimately, 113 patients were eligible, with 55 patients positive for anti-Jo1 (49%), 22 for anti-EJ (20%), 19 for anti-PL7 (17%), 11 for anti-PL12 (10%), and 6 for anti-OJ (5%). The average age at disease onset was 50 years, with a female predominance (76%), and the mean follow-up time was 58 ± 56 months. Myositis and ILD were present in 64% and 89% of patients, respectively. Seven patients died during follow-up and had a 6% 5-year mortality rate in this cohort. The profile is consistent with other ASyS cohorts reported (12).

Fever Attacks

Overall, 67 patients (59%) experienced fever attacks during the observed follow-up time; of those, 31 (27%) had one, 18 (16%) had two, and 18 (16%) had three or more attacks. As shown in **Table 1**, significant intergroup differences (according to the numbers of attacks) were revealed for fever at disease onset (p<0.001) and RPILD (p=0.002), which favored patients with two or more attacks. There were no significant intergroup differences in myositis, arthralgia, Raynaud's phenomenon, mechanic's hands, or DM-like rashes. The most common radiological pattern of ILD associated with ASyS was NSIP (73%); meanwhile, patients also presented OP (3%), UIP (4%), or NSIP/OP overlap radiological patterns (11%). Of the 12 patients described as a radiological NSIP/OP overlap pattern, up to eight patients presented as RPILD, which was in line with the predisposition of this NSIP/OP overlap pattern among patients with more attacks. Regarding ARSs, 53% of PL-7 patients presented two or more attacks. Stacked column plots

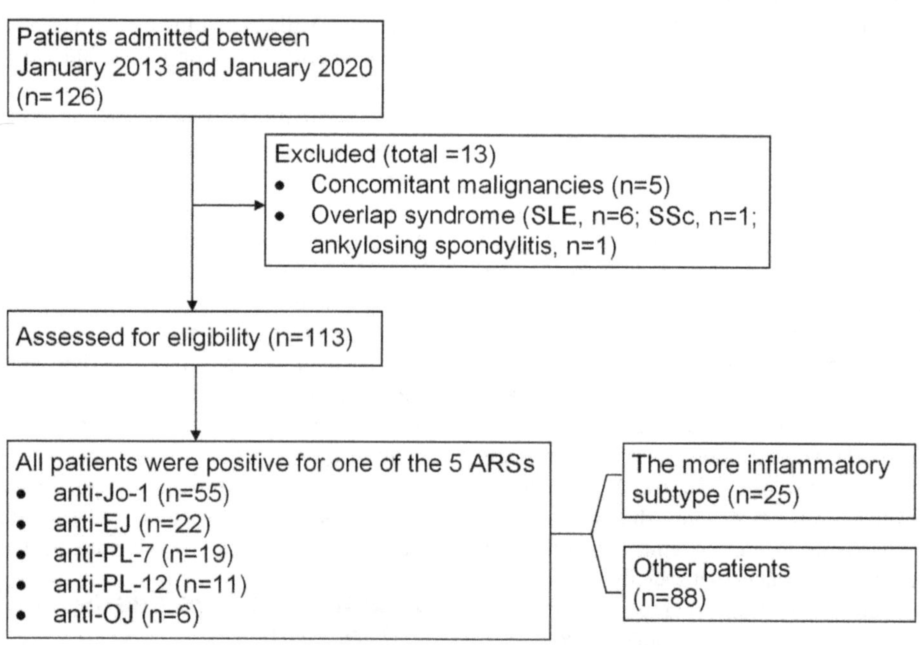

FIGURE 1 | Flowchart of patients with ASyS.

TABLE 1 | Clinical manifestations regarding the numbers of attacks of systemic inflammation in an ASyS Chinese cohort.

	Attacks				≥3	*Global P value*
	Total cohort	**0**	**1**	**2**		
No. of patients	113	46 (41%)	31 (27%)	18 (16%)	18 (16%)	
Age at onset, years	50 ± 14	51 ± 13	51 ± 15	52 ± 14	47 ± 14	0.632
Female	86 (76%)	37 (80%)	20 (65%)	15 (83%)	14 (78%)	0.378
Disease duration, months	58 ± 56	51 ± 65	45 ± 34	74 ± 60	73 ± 33	0.129
Attacks per patient-year*	0.39 ± 0.54	0	0.43 ± 0.39	0.73 ± 0.72	1.00 ± 0.42	0.000
Fever at disease onset*	44 (39%)	0 (0%)	19 (61%)	12 (67%)	13 (72%)	0.000
Clinical findings						
Myositis	72 (64%)	26 (57%)	22 (71%)	10 (56%)	14 (78%)	0.285
Arthralgia	55 (49%)	17 (37%)	17 (55%)	11 (61%)	10 (56%)	0.216
ILD	102 (90%)	40 (87%)	28 (90%)	18 (100%)	16 (89%)	0.466
HRCT pattern of ILD						
NSIP	82 (73%)	35 (76%)	23 (74%)	10 (56%)	14 (78%)	0.363
OP	3 (3%)	1 (2%)	1 (3%)	1 (6%)	0 (0%)	0.763
NSIP/OP overlap*	12 (11%)	2 (4%)	3 (10%)	7 (39%)	0 (0%)	0.000
UIP	5 (4%)	2 (4%)	1 (3%)	0 (0%)	2 (11%)	0.417
RPILD*	17 (16%)	3 (7%)	4 (13%)	8 (44%)	2 (11%)	0.002
DM-like rashes	64 (57%)	24 (52%)	24 (77%)	8 (44%)	8 (44%)	0.051
Mechanic's hand	27 (24%)	11 (24%)	10 (32%)	2 (11%)	4 (22%)	0.431
Raynaud's phenomenon	15 (13%)	8 (17%)	3 (10%)	1 (6%)	3 (17%)	0.611
Serositis	42 (39%)	15 (36%)	10 (32%)	11 (65%)	6 (33%)	0.124
Antibodies						
Subtypes of ARS						
Anti-Jo-1	55 (49%)	20 (44%)	13 (42%)	12 (67%)	10 (56%)	0.292
Anti-EJ*	22 (20%)	14 (30%)	5 (16%)	3 (17%)	0 (0%)	0.031
Anti-PL-7*	19 (17%)	3 (7%)	6 (19%)	2 (11%)	8 (44%)	0.005
Anti-PL-12	11 (10%)	4 (9%)	6 (19%)	1 (6%)	0 (0%)	0.159
Anti-OJ	6 (5%)	5 (11%)	1 (3%)	0 (0%)	0 (0%)	0.303
Anti-Ro52	79 (73%)	34 (77%)	20 (67%)	13 (81%)	12 (67%)	0.611
Anti-Ro60	27 (25%)	9 (21%)	6 (19%)	4 (25%)	8 (47%)	0.169
Anti-La	14 (13%)	4 (9%)	2 (7%)	2 (11%)	6 (33%)	0.060
Anti-Pm-scl	6 (5%)	1 (2%)	1 (3%)	1 (6%)	3 (17%)	0.111
ACPA	12 (11%)	4 (9%)	2 (7%)	3 (17%)	3 (18%)	0.523
Treatments						
Maintenance GC, mg/d	10.2 ± 6.1	8.5 ± 5.1	7.4 ± 5.2	10.6 ± 5.8	11.0 ± 5.4	0.062
cDMARDs						
Methotrexate	24 (21%)	7 (15%)	6 (19%)	7 (39%)	4 (22%)	0.219
Azathioprine	52 (46%)	20 (44%)	13 (42%)	10 (56%)	9 (50%)	0.777
Cyclophosphamide	47 (42%)	17 (37%)	13 (42%)	8 (44%)	9 (50%)	0.803
Mycophenolate mofetil	45 (40%)	22 (48%)	9 (29%)	4 (22%)	10 (56%)	0.074
Cyclosporine	17 (15%)	6 (13%)	7 (23%)	1 (6%)	3 (17%)	0.419
Tacrolimus	21 (19%)	8 (17%)	4 (13%)	2 (11%)	7 (39%)	0.099
Leflunomide	4 (4%)	2 (4%)	0 (0%)	0 (0%)	2 (11%)	0.179
bDMARDs						
Rituximab*	28 (25%)	8 (17%)	6 (19%)	5 (28%)	9 (50%)	0.045
Tocilizumab*	5 (4%)	0 (0%)	1 (3%)	1 (6%)	3 (17%)	0.004
Cumulative DMARDs exposure ≥3*	34 (30%)	10 (22%)	5 (16%)	5 (28%)	14 (78%)	0.000
Use of bDMARDs*	33 (29%)	8 (17%)	7 (22%)	6 (33%)	12 (67%)	0.003
Deaths	7 (6%)	4 (9%)	2 (7%)	0 (0%)	1 (6%)	0.430

Data are presented as mean ± SD for continuous variables and number (frequency) for categorical variables. Missing data<5%.
**global p value < 0.05.*
ILD, interstitial lung disease; RPILD, Rapidly Progressive Interstitial Lung Disease; DM, dermatomyositis; ARS, aminoacyl tRNA synthetase; ACPA, anti-citrullinated protein antibody; GC, glucocorticoids, expressed as the daily dose of prednisone equivalent; cDMARDs, Conventional disease modifying antirheumatic drugs; bDMARDs, Biologic disease-modifying antirheumatic drugs; DMARDs, disease-modifying antirheumatic drugs (including cDMARDs and bDMARDs).

displayed discordance of the distribution of such attacks in different ARS subtypes, with a higher cumulative number of attacks among Jo-1+ and PL-7+ ASyS patients (**Figure 2A**). No significant difference was observed in anti-Ro52, anti-Ro60, anti-La, ACPA, and anti-Pm-Scl. The treatment difference was prominent, with more DMARD (biologics included) exposure among patients with more attacks ($p<0.001$).

Definition and Characterization of High-Inflammation Subtype in ASyS Patients

We next calculated the frequency of attacks (per patient-year) for all eligible patients. The mean frequency of such attacks in our cohort was 0.39 per patient-year. For the ASyS patients manifested by recurrent (two or more) attacks (n=36), the median frequency was 0.77 (IQR 0.40, 1.26) attacks/patient-

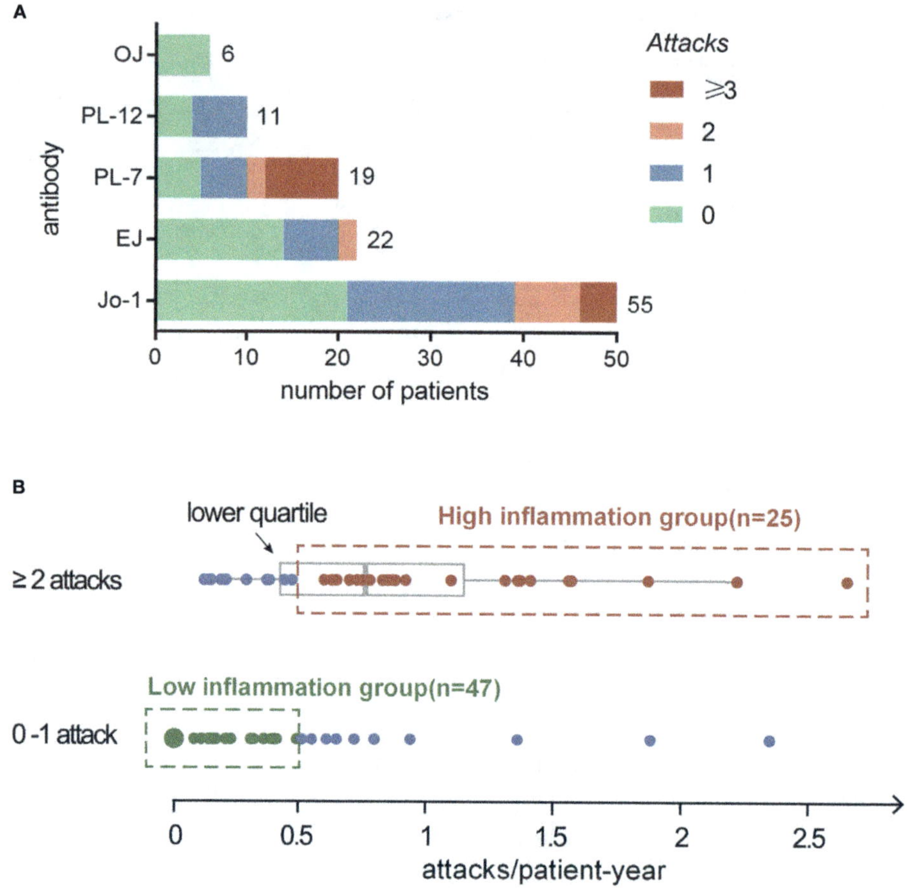

FIGURE 2 | **(A)** Distribution analysis of systemic inflammation attacks in different ARS+ ASyS. **(B)** High-inflammation group is determined as the patients with ≥2 attacks and higher than 0.5 attacks per year during the follow up. Low-inflammation group is determined as patients with no more than one attack and a frequency <0.5 attack/patient-year.

year. The lower quartile rounding to 0.5 attack/patient-year was set as the cutoff, and patients with higher frequency attacks and had at least two attacks were defined as high-inflammation group (n=25). For comparison, low-inflammation group was defined as patients who had only 0–1 attacks and no additional attack after at least 2 years of follow-up (<0.5 attack/patient-year, n=47) (**Figure 2B**). Of note, the rest of the patients who met neither definition were categorized as undetermined (n=41). Comparison analyses between undetermined *vs.* high-inflammation group and low-inflammation group were presented as **Supplementary Table 1**. The attack frequencies in the high-inflammation and low-inflammation groups were 1.12 ± 0.53 and 0.07 ± 0.13 (attacks/patient-year), respectively.

Univariate analysis comparing high-inflammation group *versus* low-inflammation group suggested that the more inflammatory subtype of ASyS patients was more likely to have fever and RPILD as the first presentation (84% *vs.* 21%, p<0.001 and 40% *vs.* 9%, p=0.003, respectively, both p<0.01). Importantly, anti-PL-7 (p=0.014) was significantly correlated with high-inflammation subtype compared to other ARSs. These three baseline parameters were subjected to multivariate logistic regression. Finally, fever at disease onset and RPILD remained independent risk factors for the high-inflammation group (p<0.001 and p=0.016, respectively) (**Table 2**). To further characterize the high-inflammation subtype, the 25 patients were divided into anti-Jo-1+ and Anti-PL-7+ ASyS patients (**Table 3**). Anti-PL-7+ ASyS patients with high inflammation showed higher CRP/ESR/Ferritin/IL-6 levels during attack compared with Anti-Jo-1+ ASyS patients, but only ESR reached the statistical significance (p<0.01). To evaluate the hyper-inflammation status, HScore were calculated (13), and the median HScore of high-inflammation subtype was around 70 (the probability of having Macrophage Activation Syndrome (MAS) <1%). In addition, PL-7+ ASyS patients with high inflammation had a higher positive rate of ACPA (p=0.028), although no difference in terms of the presence of arthralgia/ arthritis compared to Jo-1+ ASyS patients.

Response to Treatment

The more inflammatory subtype of ASyS patients was more refractory to treatments, as evidenced by higher (>=3) cumulative DMARD exposures (60% *vs.* 26%) and more

TABLE 2 | Univariate and multivariate analyses in ASyS patients with high inflammation and low inflammation.

	Low-inflammation group (n=47)	High-inflammation group (n=25)	*P-value*	Multivariate analysis		
				OR	95% CI	*P-value*
Baseline characteristics						
Age, years	50 ± 14	49 ± 15	*0.923*			
Gender, female	38 (81%)	19 (76%)	*0.629*			
Fever at disease onset	10 (21%)	21 (84%)	*0.000**	20.62	5.05, 84.14	*0.000**
RPILD	4 (9%)	10 (40%)	*0.003**	8.03	1.48, 43.52	*0.016**
Anti-Jo-1	20 (43%)	16 (64%)	*0.083*			
Anti-PL-7	5 (11%)	9 (36%)	*0.014**			
Follow-up characteristics						
Attacks per patient-year	0.07 ± 0.13	1.12 ± 0.53	*0.000**			
Maintenance GC, mg/d	8.5 ± 5.3	11.1 ± 6.1	*0.069*			
Cumulative DMARDs exposure≥3	12 (26%)	15 (60%)	*0.004**			
Use of bDMARDs	9 (19%)	18 (72%)	*0.000**			
Deaths	3 (6%)[a]	1 (4%)[b]	*1.000*			

Data are presented as mean ± SD for continuous variables and number (frequency) for categorical variables.
*OR, Odds Ratio, *p < 0.05.*
[a]*Two patients died from opportunistic infection. Another death was family members reported with definitive cause of death unavailable.*
[b]*The only patient in high-inflammation group died from gastrointestinal (GI) bleeding.*

TABLE 3 | Characterization of the high-inflammation group in ASyS patients (Anti-Jo-1+ *vs.* Anti-PL-7+).

	High-inflammation group (n=25)		P value
	Anti-Jo-1 (n=16)	Anti-PL-7 (n=9)	
Age at onset, years	51 ± 16	46 ± 13	*0.462*
Female	12 (75%)	7 (78%)	*1.000*
Disease duration, months	48 ± 35	63 ± 28	*0.283*
Fever at disease onset	13 (81%)	8 (89%)	*1.000*
Attacks per patient-year	1.14 ± 0.56	1.09 ± 0.50	*0.820*
Clinical findings			
Myositis	11 (69%)	4 (44%)	*0.397*
Arthralgia	11 (69%)	5 (56%)	*0.671*
ILD	14 (88%)	9 (100.0%)	*0.520*
RPILD	6 (38%)	3 (33%)	*1.000*
DM-like rashes	5 (31%)	6 (67%)	*0.115*
Mechanic's hand	2 (13%)	3 (33%)	*0.312*
Raynaud's phenomenon	1 (6%)	1 (11%)	*1.000*
Laboratory values			
Anti-Ro52	12 (75%)	6 (67%)	*0.635*
Anti-Ro60	4 (25%)	5 (56%)	*0.383*
Anti-La	4 (25%)	2 (22%)	*1.000*
ACPA[†]	1 (6%)	4 (50%)	*0.028*
CRP*, mg/L	24.1 ± 26.5	33.6 ± 17.3	*0.346*
ESR*, mm/h	19.6 ± 11.6	55.1 ± 27.7	*0.002*
Ferritin*, ng/ml	300.6 ± 219.5	438.9 ± 532.7	*0.910*
IL-6*[†], pg/ml	6.5 ± 6.8	9.8 ± 9.9	*0.365*
HScore*	68 ± 30	72 ± 30	*0.778*
Treatments			
Maintenance GC, mg/d	12.6 ± 6.4	8.5 ± 4.8	*0.107*
Cumulative DMARDs exposure ≥3	8 (50%)	6 (67%)	*0.691*
Use of bDMARDs	11 (69%)	7 (78%)	*1.000*
Response rate of RTX	9/11 (82%)	1/3 (33%)	*0.176*
Response rate of TCZ	–	4/4 (100%)	-

Data are presented as mean ± SD for continuous variables and number (frequency) for categorical variables.
**Collected or calculated during the fever attack phase.*
[†]*Valid cases for variables with missing data: ACPA (n= 24), IL-6 (n=21).*

bDMARD exposures (72% *vs.* 19%). The responsiveness to specific DMARDs is presented by a heat map with green, red, and yellow colors, representing good, poor, and undetermined responses, respectively (**Figure 3**). The overall responsiveness to conventional DMARDs among ASyS patients with high inflammation was poor. Notably, among 11 out of the 16 Jo-1+ ASyS patients with high inflammation receiving rituximab, nine patients had a good response. Conversely, among three out of nine PL-7+ ASyS patients with high inflammation treated with rituximab, two failed treatment; whereas tocilizumab exposure (intravenous standard dose at 8 mg/kg every 4 weeks) in another four PL-7+ ASyS patients achieved a good response.

DISCUSSION

Currently, there is no international consensus for the classification of ASyS. However, according to the largest ASyS cohort AENEAS (American and European NEtwork of Antisynthetase Syndrome) (1), a combination of ARS and any manifestation of the "triad" (myositis, ILD, and arthritis) might be a legitimate ASyS. By using our single-center cohort, we focused on fever attacks beyond the classic triad among Chinese ASyS patients. We have found that ~60% of patients experienced one or more febrile attacks during an average 5-year follow-up. In addition, ~30% of the patients had recurrent attacks (>=2). We took those with more than two febrile attacks and combined with the time-adjusted frequency of attacks to further define this subpopulation.

These patients, represented ~20% of our ASyS cohort and had three distinctive features. First, these patients experienced more RPILD (40%) and tended to present fever (84%) within 3 months from disease onset, providing important clues for early recognition of the more inflammatory phenotype. Indeed, RPILD has been reported in 7.8–29.2% of ASyS patients (14). The link between recurrent fever attacks and RPILD suggests

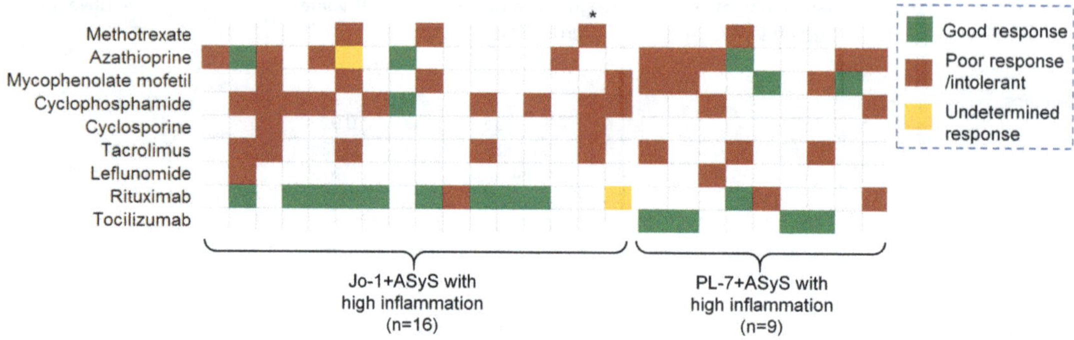

FIGURE 3 | Treatment response in the high-inflammation group of ASyS patients. Each column represents one individual patient. * Deceased due to GI bleeding.

that RPILD may be a component of profound systemic inflammation. It is noteworthy that this hyper-inflammation status in ASyS is quite different from the classic macrophage activation syndrome, according to our data.

Second, the correlation between PL-7 and the more inflammatory phenotype was informative. The ARS serology of high-inflammation subtype in our cohort was exclusively either PL-7+ or Jo-1+. Nearly ~50% of PL-7 patients in our cohort were labeled as high-inflammation subtype, which might "ring-a-bell" for clinical judgment when PL-7 was encountered. On the other hand, ~30% of Jo-1 patients were classified as high-inflammation group. Therefore, the number of Jo-1+ ASyS patients with high inflammation was more attributed to the high prevalence of Jo-1 in the ASyS cohort. Likewise, none of the EJ+, PL-12, or OJ+ ASyS patients in our cohort fulfilled the high-inflammation subtype definition, which might simply be because of the small number of patients. As an example, in a larger single-center Chinese ASyS cohort (n=234), the authors reported 46 EJ+ patients who had similar occurrences of fever (60.9%) and RPILD (21.7%) (6). Some patients might well be labeled as high-inflammation subtype. And there is no explicit relationship between high-inflammation phenotype and the ARS antibodies that are not routinely measured.

Third, high-inflammation subtype of ASyS patients was more refractory to conventional immunosuppressive therapies. In this descriptive study, we observed a good response to rituximab for most Jo-1+ ASyS patients with high inflammation. The rituximab in myositis (RIM) study and subanalysis suggested that Jo-1+ patients were better responders to rituximab (15, 16). The observation in our study probably reflects evidence-driven decision-making processes. More interestingly, for PL-7+ ASyS patients with high inflammation, this is the first anecdotal report of a promising response to tocilizumab. As an interleukin-6-receptor inhibitor, tocilizumab has been extensively tried out in various hyperinflammatory status. The underlying physiopathology in high-inflammation subtype of ASyS patients might turn out to be a good rationale to justify using tocilizumab instead of conventional treatment. Subsequent clinical trials in PL-7+ ASyS patients are needed to fully address its possible efficacy.

The disease spectrum of ASyS is likely to be continuum, and the high-inflammation subtype of ASyS definition we used in the current study is somewhat arbitrary; however, the terminology reflects the endeavor to understand the systemic inflammatory aspect of ASyS. Another major limitation of this study is the retrospective single-center design and limited number of patients. Larger, independent, multicenter studies ideally covering different ethnic populations are mandatory to thoroughly evaluate this intriguing subtype of ASyS. This will be the only way to surpass the possible "auto-analysis" issue. Finally, the treatment options in the current study were highly investigator-dependent; nevertheless, the data might reflect "drug survival" during "trial-and-error" selection in a real-world setting.

ETHICS STATEMENT

The studies involving human participants were reviewed and approved by Renji Hospital, Shanghai Jiaotong University School of Medicine. The patients/participants provided their written informed consent to participate in this study. Written informed consent was obtained from the individual(s) for the publication of any potentially identifiable images or data included in this article.

AUTHOR CONTRIBUTIONS

Study conception and design: SY, SS. Acquisition of data: SS, ZC, DZ, LG, FS, WW, WX, JC, and JL. Analysis and interpretation of data: SY, SS, DZ, XW, TL. Drafting the article: SS and DZ. Revising the article: SY, ZC, XW, and TL. All authors contributed to the article and approved the submitted version.

REFERENCES

1. Cavagna L, Trallero-Araguás E, Meloni F, Cavazzana I, Rojas-Serrano J, Feist E, et al. Influence of Antisynthetase Antibodies Specificities on Antisynthetase Syndrome Clinical Spectrum Time Course. *J Clin Med* (2019) 8(11). doi: 10.3390/jcm8112013
2. Monti S, Montecucco C, Cavagna L. Clinical Spectrum of Anti-Jo-1-Associated Disease. *Curr Opin Rheumatol* (2017) 29(6):612–7. doi: 10.1097/BOR.0000000000000434
3. Lega J-C, Fabien N, Reynaud Q, Durieu I, Durupt S, Dutertre M, et al. The Clinical Phenotype Associated With Myositis-Specific and Associated Autoantibodies: A Meta-Analysis Revisiting the So-Called Antisynthetase Syndrome. *Autoimmun Rev* (2014) 13(9):883–91. doi: 10.1016/j.autrev.2014.03.004
4. Pinal-Fernandez I, Casal-Dominguez M, Huapaya JA, Albayda J, Paik JJ, Johnson C, et al. A Longitudinal Cohort Study of the Anti-Synthetase Syndrome: Increased Severity of Interstitial Lung Disease in Black Patients and Patients With Anti-PL7 and Anti-PL12 Autoantibodies. *Rheumatology* (2017) 56(6):999–1007. doi: 10.1093/rheumatology/kex021
5. Masiak A, Marzec M, Kulczycka J, Zdrojewski Z. The Clinical Phenotype Associated With Antisynthetase Autoantibodies. *Reumatologia/Rheumatology* (2020) 58(1):4–8. doi: 10.5114/reum.2020.93505
6. Zhang Y, Ge Y, Yang H, Chen H, Tian X, Huang Z, et al. Clinical Features and Outcomes of the Patients With Anti-Glycyl tRNA Synthetase Syndrome. *Clin Rheumatol* (2020) 39(8):2417–24. doi: 10.1007/s10067-020-04979-8
7. Meyer A, Lefevre G, Bierry G, Duval A, Ottaviani S, Meyer O, et al. In Antisynthetase Syndrome, ACPA Are Associated With Severe and Erosive Arthritis. *Medicine* (2015) 94(20):e523. doi: 10.1097/MD.0000000000000523
8. Miller JB, Danoff SK, Bingham CO 3rd, Paik JJ, Mecoli CA, Tiniakou E, et al. Sonographic Findings From Inflammatory Arthritis Due to Antisynthetase Syndrome. *Clin Rheumatol* (2019) 38(5):1477–83. doi: 10.1007/s10067-019-04471-y
9. American Thoracic Society, European Respiratory Society and American Thoracic Society/European Respiratory Society International Multidisciplinary Consensus Classification of the Idiopathic Interstitial Pneumonias. This Joint Statement of the American Thoracic Society (ATS), and the European Respiratory Society (ERS) was Adopted by the ATS Board of Directors, June 2001 and by the ERS Executive Committee, June 2001. *Am J Respir Crit Care Med* (2002) 165:277–304.
10. American Thoracic Society. Idiopathic Pulmonary Fibrosis: Diagnosis and Treatment. International Consensus Statement. American Thoracic Society (ATS), and the European Respiratory Society (ERS). *Am J Respir Crit Care Med* (2000) 161(2 Pt 1):646–64. doi: 10.1164/ajrccm.161.2.ats3-00
11. Moghadam-Kia S, Aggarwal R, Oddis CV. Treatment of Inflammatory Myopathy: Emerging Therapies and Therapeutic Targets. *Expert Rev Clin Immunol* (2015) 11(11):1265–75. doi: 10.1586/1744666X.2015.1082908
12. Aggarwal R, Cassidy E, Fertig N, Koontz DC, Lucas M, Ascherman DP, et al. Patients With non-Jo-1 anti-tRNA-Synthetase Autoantibodies Have Worse Survival Than Jo-1 Positive Patients. *Ann Rheum Dis* (2014) 73(1):227–32. doi: 10.1136/annrheumdis-2012-201800
13. Fardet L, Galicier L, Lambotte O, Marzac C, Aumont C, Chahwan D, et al. Development and Validation of the HScore, a Score for the Diagnosis of Reactive Hemophagocytic Syndrome. *Arthritis Rheumatol* (2014) 66(9):2613–20. doi: 10.1002/art.38690
14. Yanagihara T, Suzuki K, Egashira A, Ogo N, Asoh T, Nara T, et al. Nintedanib and Intensive Immunosuppressive Therapy to Treat Rapidly Progressive Interstitial Lung Disease Presenting Anti-ARS Antibodies. *Respir Med Case Rep* (2020) 31:101272. doi: 10.1016/j.rmcr.2020.101272
15. Oddis CV, Reed AM, Aggarwal R, Rider LG, Ascherman DP, Levesque MC, et al. Rituximab in the Treatment of Refractory Adult and Juvenile Dermatomyositis and Adult Polymyositis: A Randomized, Placebo-Phase Trial. *Arthritis Rheum* (2013) 65(2):314–24. doi: 10.1002/art.37754
16. Aggarwal R, Bandos A, Reed AM, Ascherman DP, Barohn RJ, Feldman BM, et al. Predictors of Clinical Improvement in Rituximab-Treated Refractory Adult and Juvenile Dermatomyositis and Adult Polymyositis. *Arthritis Rheumatol* (2014) 66(3):740–9. doi: 10.1002/art.38270

18

Case Report: IgA Nephropathy in a Patient With Anti-Transcription Intermediary Factor-1γ Antibody-Positive Dermatomyositis

Suo Zhang [1,2†], Yu-Lan Chen [1†], Cui-Lian Liu [1], Jing-Yi Xie [1], Bao-Dong Sun [1] and Dong-Zhou Liu [1]*

[1] Department of Rheumatology and Immunology, Shenzhen People's Hospital (The Second Clinical Medical College, Jinan University, The First Affiliated Hospital, Southern University of Science and Technology), Shenzhen, China, [2] Department of Rheumatology and Immunology, Shenzhen Second People's Hospital, Shenzhen, China

***Correspondence:**
Dong-Zhou Liu
liu_dz2001@sina.com

†These authors have contributed equally to this work

Immunoglobulin A nephropathy (IgAN) is the most common primary glomerulonephritis characterized by IgA deposits in the mesangial area of glomeruli. Connective tissue disorders are some of the most frequent causes of secondary IgAN. Nevertheless, IgAN rarely occurs in systemic autoimmune myopathies (SAMs). The present case study reports on a 58-year-old patient with dermatomyositis with positive anti-transcription intermediary factor (TIF)-1γ antibodies who was diagnosed with IgAN during standard immunosuppressive therapy. Moreover, we have made a systematic review regarding the association of SAMs and IgAN. To the best of the authors' knowledge, this is the first case study describing a patient with anti-TIF1γ antibody-positive dermatomyositis who developed IgAN, which demonstrates a potential relationship between anti-TIF1γ-positive dermatomyositis and IgAN. It is important for clinicians to be aware of the possibility of renal involvement in patients with SAMs, even in those with anti-TIF1γ-positive dermatomyositis.

Keywords: IgA nephropathy, systemic autoimmune myopathies, dermatomyositis, anti- transcription intermediary factor-1γ antibody, dermatomyositis-specific antibodies

INTRODUCTION

Systemic autoimmune myopathies (SAMs) are a complex heterogeneous group of diseases characterized by muscle inflammation and involve extramuscular organs, including the skin, joints, lungs, heart, and gastrointestinal tract (1, 2). Dermatomyositis (DM) and polymyositis (PM) are two main types of SAMs. Unlike respiratory and gastrointestinal involvement, renal involvement rarely occurs in SAMs compared with other autoimmune diseases, such as systemic lupus erythematosus and scleroderma (3). Immunoglobulin A nephropathy (IgAN) is the most common primary glomerulonephritis characterized by IgA deposits in the mesangial area of glomeruli. Connective tissue disorders are some of the most frequent causes of secondary IgAN (4). Nevertheless, SAM-associated IgAN has rarely been reported. Here, to the best of our knowledge, we describe for the first time a 58-year-old patient with DM with positive anti-transcription intermediary factor (TIF)-1γ antibodies who developed IgAN during standard immunosuppressive therapy.

CASE PRESENTATION

A 58-year-old Chinese man was admitted to our hospital in June 2020 due to a six-year history of a recurrent rash and a new onset of haematuria and proteinuria. In June 2014, the patient was diagnosed with DM based on the presence of a heliotrope rash and Gottron's papules, progressive proximal muscle weakness with a significant elevation in creatine kinase (CK 1867 U/L, reference range 25-192), and proximal myopathic changes indicated by electromyography (5). The routine urinalysis was normal. Methylprednisolone (80 mg/day), methotrexate (12.5 mg/week) and cyclophosphamide (400 mg/week) were initiated. However, the patient developed a pulmonary cytomegalovirus infection within a month (July 2014) and therefore was changed from methotrexate and cyclophosphamide to tacrolimus (4 mg/day). His DM was stable without any rash or muscle weakness for five years with low-dose prednisolone (5 mg/day) and tacrolimus (2 mg/day) for maintenance therapy.

In May 2019, the patient again developed a heliotrope rash and proximal muscle weakness, with a mild elevation in CK (362 U/L). His routine urinalysis was normal. Further tests revealed that his anti-TIF1γ antibodies were positive based on an immune blotting assay. A positron emission tomography-computer tomography (PET-CT) was unremarkable. There was no evidence to suggest infection or malignancy. Therefore, the methylprednisolone dosage was increased to 40 mg/day and the tacrolimus dosage was increased to 3 mg/day, resulting in gradual improvement of his rash. In April 2020, the methylprednisolone was gradually tapered until it was discontinued, and tacrolimus (3 mg/day) was continued for maintenance therapy. In June 2020, the patient's rash reoccurred, and there was a new onset of haematuria (3+) and proteinuria (2+) on the urinalysis. He denied other past medical history, including diabetes mellitus, hypertension, and nephropathies.

Physical examination on admission revealed the presence of a heliotrope rash and Gottron's papules (**Supplementary Figures 1A, C**) without any signs of muscle weakness or pain. Laboratory tests revealed the following metabolic levels: CK at 171 U/L, lactate dehydrogenase (LDH; reference range 110-240) at 281 U/L, alanine aminotransferase (ALT; reference range 0-40) at 85 U/L, aspartate transaminase (AST; reference range 0-40) at 59 U/L, C-reactive protein (CRP; reference range <5) at 3.46 mg/L, erythrocyte sedimentation rate (ESR; reference range 0-20) at 30 mm/h, ferritin (reference range 11.0-306.8) at 708.7 ng/mL, immunoglobulin A (reference range 0.7-4.5) at 6.25 g/L, serum urea nitrogen (BUN; reference range 2.5-7.5) at 3.99 mmol/L, and creatinine (Cr; reference range 44-133) at 58 μmol/L. A urinalysis revealed a proteinuria (0.3 g/L) with a strongly positive haematuria with a 24-hour urine protein (reference range 0.028-0.141) of 0.94 g. Further assessment of urinary red blood cell morphology by phase-contrast microscopy showed that the urinary red blood cell count was 35854/ml, with only 22% normal urinary red blood cells, and there was no evidence of malignancy, diabetes, hypertension or urolithiasis. The main laboratory results are shown in **Supplementary Table 1**.

A percutaneous renal biopsy was performed to confirm nephropathy. The renal biopsy revealed that one was globally sclerotic among 30 glomeruli sampled. The remainder had mild to moderate mesangial hypercellularity, accompanied by excessive intracapillary cells (**Figures 1A, B**). Segmental sclerosis, interstitial fibrosis or tubular atrophy, or cellular or fibrocellular crescent could not be found in the renal biopsy. Immunofluorescence staining demonstrated proliferative mesangial deposits of IgA (3+) (**Figure 1C**), C3 (2+), IgM (1+), kappa (1+), and lambda (2+). In addition, electron-dense deposits in the mesangium and matrix were also detected by electron microscopy (**Figure 1D**). The Oxford MEST-C score (M: mesangial hypercellularity; E: endocapillary hypercellularity; S: segmental sclerosis; T: percentage of interstitial fibrosis or tubular atrophy; C: active cellular or fibrocellular crescent) was M1E1S0T0C0 according to the Oxford classification of IgAN (6). These findings led to the diagnosis of a DM flare complicated by IgAN. Therefore, methylprednisolone (40 mg/day) and methotrexate (10 mg/week) with valsartan were initiated for the patient, and tacrolimus was discontinued. During the follow-up, the patient's rash gradually improved. After 3 months of immunosuppressive treatment, the patient's rash substantially improved (**Supplementary Figures 1B, D**), with normal levels of CK, LDH, ALT, and AST. His 24-hour urine protein decreased to 0.640 g, but red blood cells were still found on the urinalysis. At the time of writing this report, the patient was being treated with 6 mg/day methylprednisolone, 15 mg/week methotrexate and valsartan, and his DM was stable with a minimal rash on his face and neck. The clinical course of the patient is shown in **Table 1**.

DISCUSSION

SAMs consist of five main forms: DM, PM, anti-synthetase syndrome, immune-mediated necrotizing myopathy and inclusion body myositis (2). Over the last few decades, several DM-specific autoantibodies have been discovered, such as anti-Mi2, anti-nuclear matrix protein (NXP)2, anti-TIF1γ, anti-small ubiquitin-like modifier activating enzyme (SAE) and anti-melanoma differentiation-associated protein (MDA)5 antibodies (7). Approximately 70% of patients with DM have DM-specific autoantibodies, and each of these has been associated with a unique clinical phenotype (8). TIF1γ, encoded by the tripartite motif containing (TRIM) 33 gene, is involved in various biological pathways, such as transforming growth factor (TGF)-β signaling pathway and Wnt/β-catenin pathway (9). The relationship between anti-TIF1γ antibodies and cancer in patients with DM has been well established. As many as 50% of anti-TIF1γ-positive DM patients have developed cancers within 3 years from the onset of myositis (7). The pathogenic mechanism of the anti-TIF1γ antibody is not yet clear and may

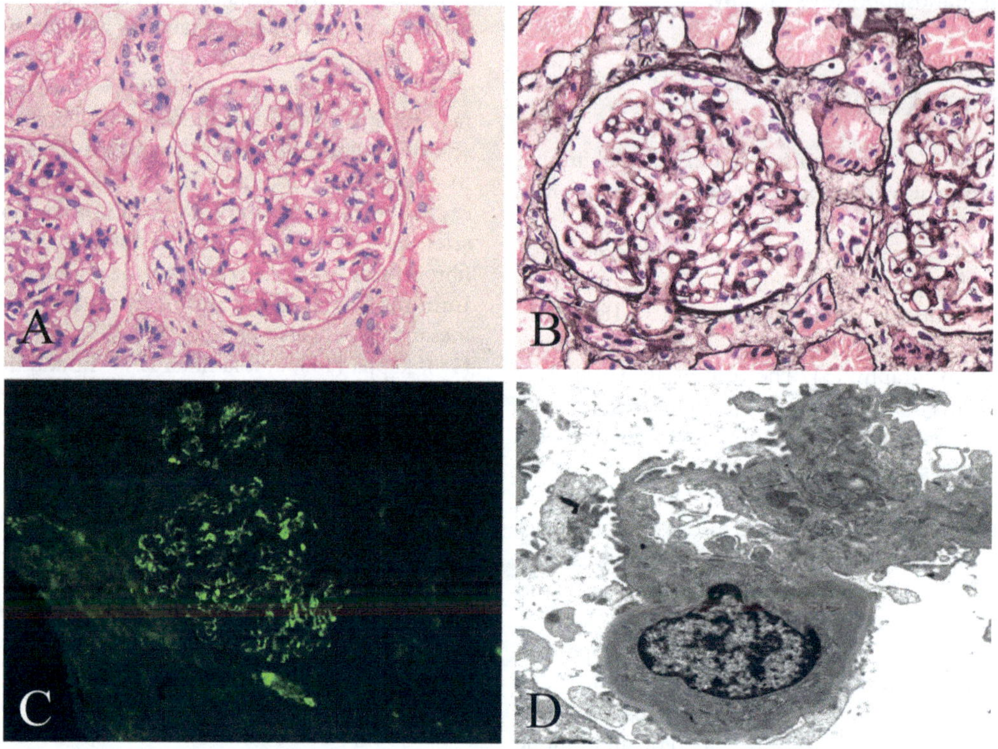

FIGURE 1 | Histopathological changes of renal biopsy in the patient. **(A, B)** Light microscopy shows a glomerulus with mild to moderate mesangial hypercellularity and endocapillary hypercellularity. **(A)** Periodic acid-Schiff staining; original magnification ×400. **(B)** Periodic acid-silver methenamine staining; original magnification ×400. **(C)** IgA deposits along the glomerular mesangial area by immunofluorescence. original magnification ×400. **(D)** Deposits along the mesangium and matrix by electron microscopy. original magnification ×5000.

be related to the tumorigenic role of the TIF1 family proteins (10). In this study, a diagnosis of anti-TIF1γ antibody-positive DM was established in our patient. However, there was no evidence of malignancies in the patient during the six-year follow-up. Intriguingly, a new onset of IgAN was found in the patient. To the best of our knowledge, we describe for the first time that a DM patient with anti-TIF1γ antibodies developed IgAN during standard immunosuppressive therapy. Our case study highlights a potential association between anti-TIF1γ-positive DM and IgAN, suggesting the need for close monitoring of new-onset IgAN during the course of the preexisting DM for an early diagnosis and management of IgAN. Renal biopsy is advisable in patients who manifest with persistent renal abnormalities during the follow-up. It is important for clinicians to be aware of the possibility of renal involvement in patients with SAMs, even in those with anti-

TABLE 1 | Timeline of the disease and treatment.

Timeline	Symptoms/diagnosis	Treatment	Outcome
June 2014	Heliotrope rash, Gottron's papules, muscle weakness with elevated creatine kinase, and myopathic changes indicated by electromyography; normal urinalysis	mPSL (80 mg/day), MTX (12.5 mg/week) and CTX (400 mg/week) as initial therapy	Improved
July 2014	Pulmonary cytomegalovirus infection; normal urinalysis	Changed MTX and CTX to tacrolimus (4 mg/day); low-dose prednisolone (5 mg/day) and tacrolimus (2 mg/day) for maintenance therapy	Improved and stable for 5 years
May 2019	Heliotrope rash and muscle weakness with elevated CK, positive anti-TIF1γ antibodies; normal urinalysis	mPSL (40 mg/day) and tacrolimus (3mg/day); mPSL was tapered until discontinued, and tacrolimus (3 mg/day) was remained for maintenance therapy	Improved
June 2020	Heliotrope rash and Gottron's papules without muscle weakness; new-onset of hematuria and proteinuria, and biopsy-proven IgAN	Tacrolimus was stopped; mPSL (40 mg/day), MTX (10 mg/week) and valsartan as initial therapy; mPSL (gradually tapered to 6 mg/day), MTX (15 mg/week) and valsartan at the time of writing this report	Rash improved, 24-hour urine protein decreased, but urine red blood cells could still be found

IgAN, IgA nephropathy; anti-TIF1γ, anti-transcription intermediary factor; mPSL, methylprednisolone; MTX, methotrexate; CTX, cyclophosphamide.

TIF1γ-positive DM rather than only considering the association with malignancy.

Renal involvement is rare in SAMs. The most common renal involvement includes acute tubular necrosis and chronic glomerulonephritis (11, 12). A multicentre study including 150 patients with SAMs (DM, PM, or anti-synthetase syndrome) showed that renal involvement occurred in 35 patients (23.3%): acute kidney injury in 16 patients (10.7%) and chronic kidney disease in 31 patients (20.7%). The main cause of acute kidney injury was acute tubular necrosis caused by drugs or myoglobinuria (11). Yen et al. (12) reported that 14 out of 65 patients with PM/DM had renal involvement. Takizawa et al. (13) reported 21 cases of PM/DM-associated glomerulonephritis confirmed by biopsy. The diagnosis included 12 cases of glomerular proliferative glomerulonephritis, six cases of membranous glomerulonephritis, one case of minimal change glomerulonephritis and two cases of crescentic glomerulonephritis. A common finding of PM is mesangial proliferative glomerulonephritis, while that of DM is membranous glomerulonephritis. However, IgAN is rarely reported in SAMs according to the previously published literature, which was confirmed in our patient based on the biopsy.

IgAN is the most common primary glomerulonephritis in the world. Renal histopathology has shown that IgA was the major immunoglobulin in glomeruli, usually accompanied by complement C3, and often accompanied by IgG and IgM (4). Abnormal glycosylation of the IgA1 molecule has been reported to be the key cause of IgAN. Abnormal IgA1 molecules polymerize or bind with IgG or IgA1 antibodies *in vivo* as autoantigens to form immune complexes, which promote inflammatory reactions and complement activation. Complement activation can also increase the direct damage to podocytes caused by various cytokines or chemokines. Notably, an *in vitro* study has revealed a decreased activity of β-1,3-galactosyltransferase that is essential in IgA1 glycosylation in IgA1-producing cells, which contributes to hypoglycosylation of IgA1 in patients with IgAN (14). Secondary IgAN is mainly reported in IgA vasculitis, liver diseases, chronic infections, and tumors (4, 15). In addition, IgAN may also be associated with a variety of rheumatic diseases, including inflammatory bowel disease (IBD) (16), spondyloarthritis (17), systemic lupus erythematosus (18), Sjögren syndrome (19) and rheumatoid arthritis (RA) (20). Case reports of PM/DM complicated with IgAN are not common. To date, 11 cases of SAMs with IgAN have been reported previously: two cases of juvenile DM (21, 22), two DM (23, 24), three PM (25–27), and four anti-synthetase syndrome (11, 13, 28). The details of the reported 11 cases are shown in **Table 2**. Current studies have revealed a similar galactose-deficient IgA1-mediated pathogenesis in secondary IgAN (15). Furthermore, the pathogenesis of IgAN in Sjögren syndrome is probably attributed to the deposition of IgA-containing circulating immune complexes that are secreted by activated monoclonal B lymphocytes and the dysregulation of polymeric IgA (19). However, the relationship between IgAN and DM is still unclear. It is more likely that the two immune diseases may have similar immune pathogenic mechanisms (21), both of which are mainly mediated by humoral immune system. Nevertheless, the relationship between IgAN and PM seems to be unclear, in which cellular immunity is considered to be the dominant mechanism (26).

Intriguingly, our patient developed IgAN during standard immunosuppressive therapy, which is the first case report describing the development of IgAN in a DM patient with anti-TIF1γ antibodies. However, IgAN is known as a "multi-hit hypothesis" of pathogenesis (29), and the mechanism by which TIF1γ may be associated with the development of IgAN is still unclear. TIF1γ, as a member of TRIM family, has E3 ubiquitinprotein ligase activity (9), which may be involved in

TABLE 2 | Case reports regarding systemic autoimmune myopathies with IgA nephropathy.

Ref	Sex/age	Myopathy	Concomitant disease	Time#	Antibody	Treatment	Outcome
(21)	F/14	JDM	None	0	Negative	GCs, MTX	Improved
(22)	M/10	JDM	None	0	Negative	GCs, MTX	Improved
(23)	F/26	DM	None	1.5 years	NA	GCs, AZA	NA
(25)	M/32	PM	Scleroderma, adult coeliac disease and diabetes mellitus	1 year	RF, anti-nucleolus, anti-reticulin	GCs	Improved
(24)	M/49	DM	Pulmonary fibrosis and lung cancer	0	Negative	GCs	Dead
(26)	M/35	PM	Acute lung injury	6 months	Negative	GCs, AZA, CYC	Improved
(27)	F/56	PM	Thyroid papillary carcinoma	0	ANA (speckled pattern, 1:320)	GCs, CYC, IVIG, total thyroidectomy	Improved
(13)	M/58	ASS	Interstitial lung disease	0	Anti-Jo-1	GCs, IVIg, CSA	Improved
(28)	F/65	ASS	Lung cancer	0	Anti-Jo-1	Surgical treatment of lung cancer	Improved
(11)	F/38	ASS	None	0	Anti-Jo-1, anti-SSA, anti-SSB,	GCs, MTX, IVIg, TNF-i	Improved
(11)	M/43	ASS	None	18 years	Anti-Jo-1, anti-SSA	GCs, MTX	Improved

Ref, reference; NA, not available; JDM, juvenile dermatomyositis; DM, dermatomyositis; PM, polymyositis; ASS, anti-synthetase syndrome; GCs, glucocorticosteroids; MTX, methotrexate; AZA, azathioprine; CYC, cyclophosphamide; CyA, cyclosporine A; MMF, mycophenolate mofetil; RF, rheumatoid factor; IVIg, intravenous immunoglobulin; TNF-i, TNF-α inhibitor; M, male; F, female.

#Time between myositis onset and IgA nephropathy.

the degradation of the specific glycosyltransferases in IgA1 glycosylation, such as β-1,3-galactosyltransferase mentioned above. Moreover, anti-TIF1-γ antibodies have been reported to be specially associated with human leucocyte antigen (HLA)-DQB1*02 in adult-onset patients (30). Genome-wide association analyses of IgAN identified HLA-DQB1 as one of the loci with high susceptibility (31, 32). Therefore, a similar genetic predisposition may partially explain the relationship between anti-TIF1γ antibody and IgAN. In addition, an active immune response could directly or indirectly contribute to inducing the excessive production of galactose-deficient IgA1 and subsequent heightened immune responses (33, 34). Of note, the new onset of haematuria and proteinuria was found simultaneously with a flare of DM in this patient. Therefore, the development of IgAN may also be attributed to a systemic active immune response in the patient. Additional studies are required to determine the pathogenetic mechanisms of IgAN underlying anti-TIF1-γ antibody-positive DM. On the other hand, the prevalence of IgAN varies largely according to geography and ethnicity, and IgAN is more common among Asians than in Caucasians (35). Importantly, IgAN has been reported to account for 54.3% of primary glomerular diseases in China (36). In this respect, this case study might simply reflect the higher prevalence of IgAN in China. The possibility of a coincidence finding between IgAN and anti-TIF1-γ antibody-positive DM in this patient cannot be completely ruled out. Additionally, although time intervals between the occurrence of SAMs and IgAN reported previously can be as long as 18 years (11), it might be, to some extent, more likely to be coincidental rather than causative relationship between these two diseases due to the relatively long time interval (six years) in this patient.

There are currently no guidelines for the treatment of secondary IgAN. According to the different clinical conditions of the patients, the standard treatment for primary IgAN is the use of angiotensin-converting enzyme inhibitors and steroids or even immunosuppressants. However, recent studies have shown that adding immunosuppressive therapy to the intensive supportive treatment of patients with high-risk IgAN does not significantly improve the prognosis, because the estimated glomerular filtration rate does not change and more adverse reactions have been observed (37). Accordingly, a single angiotensin receptor blocker was added to treat the IgAN in our patient due to having no crescent formation found in the kidney biopsy and a normal renal function. Compared with patients with primary IgAN, patients with secondary IgAN were older, had more complications and had higher levels of haematuria but lower levels of proteinuria. The pathological changes and clinical outcomes of secondary IgAN were similar to those in primary IgAN (38). The conclusion of this retrospective study may not be robust enough and should be interpreted with caution, due to the fact that only 16 patients with systemic autoimmune diseases were included. Intriguingly, several recent studies have demonstrated that secondary IgAN, such as spondyloarthritis-associated and IBD-associated IgAN, is related with a poor renal outcome, with an elevated risk of progression to end-stage kidney disease (17, 39). Compared with those without renal involvement, an increased risk of cardiovascular diseases was observed in RA patients with renal abnormalities (40). Taken together, it could be reasonable to postulate that IgAN secondary to systemic autoimmune diseases may have a worse prognosis than primary IgAN, probably due to the underlying systemic diseases. Therefore, careful monitoring of urinalysis and renal function should be performed routinely in patients with systemic autoimmune diseases, such as DM, for the purpose of early diagnosis of IgAN and avoiding nephrotoxic immunosuppressants. However, more studies are needed to investigate the prognosis of patients with DM and concurrent IgAN.

The main limitation of the current study is that this is a case report. Although several cases of IgAN developing in SAMs have been previously described, to the best of our knowledge, this is the first case study depicting an anti-TIF1γ antibody-positive DM patient complicated with IgAN, which indicates that IgAN may be secondary to DM with positive anti-TIF1γ antibodies. Further studies are needed to explore the relationship between SAMs and IgAN, as well as the underlying mechanisms.

CONCLUSION

We describe the first case of a patient with DM with positive anti-TIF-1γ antibodies who was diagnosed with IgAN during standard immunosuppressive therapy, which adds to the small body of existing evidence on the possible association of SAMs and IgAN. Urinalysis and renal function tests should be performed routinely in patients with SAMs, even in those with anti-TIF1γ-positive DM, for an early diagnosis and management of IgAN. Further studies are needed to explore the relationship between SAMs and IgAN.

ETHICS STATEMENT

The studies involving human participants were reviewed and approved by Medical Ethics Committee of Shenzhen People's Hospital. The patients/participants provided their written informed consent to participate in this study. Written informed consent was obtained from the individual(s) for the publication of any potentially identifiable images or data included in this article.

AUTHOR CONTRIBUTIONS

SZ and Y-LC summarized the case, reviewed the literature, and drafted the manuscript. C-LL gathered the clinical data. J-YX and

B-DS helped draft the manuscript. D-ZL reviewed and summarized the case. All authors have read and approved the submitted version of the manuscript.

ACKNOWLEDGMENTS

The authors wish to thank the patient in this study.

SUPPLEMENTARY MATERIAL

Supplementary Figure 1 | Clinical presentation of the patient. **(A)** Heliotrope rash over the face and neck. **(C)** Gottron's papules over the extensor surfaces of the dorsal interphalangeal and metacarpophalangeal joints. **(B, D)** Three months after treatment.

REFERENCES

1. Rgm A, Ibpb A, Amds A, Lg B, Sks A. Effect of Exercise Training on Fatigue and Pain in Patients With Systemic Autoimmune Myopathies: A Systematic Review. *Autoimmun Rev* (2021) 20:102897. doi: 10.1016/j.autrev.2021.102897
2. Mcgrath ER, Doughty CT, Amato AA. Autoimmune Myopathies: Updates on Evaluation and Treatment. *Neurotherapeutics* (2018) 15:976–94. doi: 10.1007/s13311-018-00676-2
3. Cucchiari D, Angelini C. Renal Involvement in Idiopathic Inflammatory Myopathies. *Clin Rev Allergy Immunol* (2017) 52:99–107. doi: 10.1007/s12016-015-8524-5
4. Saha M, Julian B, Novak J, Rizk D. Secondary IgA Nephropathy. *Kidney Int* (2018) 94:674–81. doi: 10.1016/j.kint.2018.02.030
5. Bohan A, Peter J. Polymyositis and Dermatomyositis (First of Two Parts). *N Engl J Med* (1975) 292:344–7. doi: 10.1056/NEJM197502132920706
6. Roberts IS, Cook HT, Troyanov S, Alpers CE, Amore A, Barratt J, et al. The Oxford Classification of IgA Nephropathy: Pathology Definitions, Correlations, and Reproducibility. *Kidney Int* (2009) 76:546–56. doi: 10.1038/ki.2009.168
7. Riddell V, Bagby S, Mchugh N. Myositis Autoantibodies: Recent Perspectives. *Curr Opin Rheumatol* (2020) 32:548–52. doi: 10.1097/BOR.0000000000000742
8. Mammen A, Allenbach Y, Stenzel W, Benveniste O. 239th ENMC International Workshop: Classification of Dermatomyositis, Amsterdam, The Netherlands, 14-16 December 2018. *Neuromuscul Disord* (2019) 30:70–92. doi: 10.1016/j.nmd.2019.10.005
9. De Vooght J, Vulsteke JB, De Haes P, Bossuyt X, Lories R, De Langhe E. Anti-TIF1-Gamma Autoantibodies: Warning Lights of a Tumour Autoantigen. *Rheumatol (Oxf)* (2020) 59:469–77. doi: 10.1093/rheumatology/kez572
10. Fiorentino D, Casciola-Rosen L. Autoantibodies to Transcription Intermediary Factor 1 in Dermatomyositis Shed Insight Into the Cancer-Myositis Connection. *Arthritis Rheum* (2012) 64:346–9. doi: 10.1002/art.33402
11. Couvrat-Desvergnes G, Masseau A, Benveniste O, Bruel A, Hervier B, Mussini JM, et al. The Spectrum of Renal Involvement in Patients With Inflammatory Myopathies. *Med (Baltimore)* (2014) 93:33–41. doi: 10.1097/MD.0000000000000015
12. Yen T, Lai P, Chen C, Hsueh S, Huang J. Renal Involvement in Patients With Polymyositis and Dermatomyositis. *Int J Clin Pract* (2005) 59:188–93. doi: 10.1111/j.1742-1241.2004.00248.x
13. Takizawa Y, Kanda H, Sato K, Kawahata K, Yamaguchi A, Uozaki H, et al. Polymyositis Associated With Focal Mesangial Proliferative Glomerulonephritis With Depositions of Immune Complexes. *Clin Rheumatol* (2007) 26:792–6. doi: 10.1007/s10067-006-0200-y
14. Suzuki H, Moldoveanu Z, Hall S, Brown R, Novak J. IgA1-Secreting Cell Lines From Patients With IgA Nephropathy Produce Aberrantly Glycosylated Iga1. *J Clin Invest* (2008) 118:629–39. doi: 10.1172/JCI33189
15. Wang M, Lv J, Zhang X, Chen P, Zhao M, Zhang H. Secondary IgA Nephropathy Shares the Same Immune Features With Primary IgA Nephropathy. *Kidney Int Rep* (2020) 5:165–72. doi: 10.1016/j.ekir.2019.10.012
16. Ambruzs J, Walker P, Larsen C. The Histopathologic Spectrum of Kidney Biopsies in Patients With Inflammatory Bowel Disease. *Clin J Am Soc Nephrol* (2014) 9:265–70. doi: 10.2215/CJN.04660513
17. Champtiaux N, Liote F, El Karoui K, Vigneau C, Miceli C, Cornec-Le Gall E, et al. Spondyloarthritis-Associated IgA Nephropathy. *Kidney Int Rep* (2020) 5:813–20. doi: 10.1016/j.ekir.2020.03.012
18. Horino T, Takao T, Terada Y. IgA Nephropathy in a Patient With Systemic Lupus Erythematosus. *Lupus* (2010) 19:650–4. doi: 10.1177/0961203309349384
19. Chen Y, Zhao X, Tang D, Xu C, Sun L, Sun L, et al. IgA Nephropathy in Two Patients With Sjögren's Syndrome : One With Concomitant Autoimmune Hepatitis. *Intern Med* (2010) 49:37–43. doi: 10.2169/internalmedicine.49.2722
20. Zhang T, Liang S, Feng X, Li M, Zhou H, Zeng C, et al. Spectrum and Prognosis of Renal Histopathological Lesions in 56 Chinese Patients With Rheumatoid Arthritis With Renal Involvement. *Clin Exp Med* (2020) 20:191 97. doi: 10.1007/s10238-019-00602-6
21. Civilibal M, Selcuk Duru N, Ozagari A, Durali K, Elevli M. Immunoglobulin A Nephropathy Associated With Juvenile Dermatomyositis. *Pediatr Nephrol* (2009) 24:2073–5. doi: 10.1007/s00467-009-1178-x
22. Mantoo M, Tripathy S, Phulware R, Bagri N, Hari P, Barwad A. Juvenile Dermatomyositis With IgA Nephropathy: Case-Based Review. *Rheumatol Int* (2019) 39:577–81. doi: 10.1007/s00296-018-4229-4
23. Yen T, Huang J, Chen C. Unexpected IgA Nephropathy During the Treatment of a Young Woman With Idiopathic Dermatomyositis: Case Report and Review of the Literature. *J Nephrol* (2003) 16:148–53.
24. Kaneoka H, Sasatomi Y, Miyagi K, Kiyoshi Y, Saito T. A Rare Case of Dermatomyositis Associated With Immune-Complex Type Glomerulonephritis, Idiopathic Thrombopenic Purpura, Pulmonary Fibrosis and Lung Cancer. *Clin Exp Rheumatol* (2003) 21:801–2.
25. Vilppula A, Aine R. Polymyositis Associated With Several Immunological Disorders. *Clin Rheumatol* (1984) 3:533–39. doi: 10.1007/BF02031278
26. Barros T, de Souza F, Malheiros D, Levy-Neto M, Shinjo S. IgA Nephropathy and Polymyositis: A Rare Association. *Rev Bras Reumatol* (2014) 54:231–33. doi: 10.1016/j.rbre.2012.11.001
27. Oh Y-J, Park ES, Jang M, Kang EW, Kie J-H, Lee S-W, et al. A Case of Polymyositis Associated With Immunoglobulin A Nephropathy. *J Rheum Dis* (2017) 24:241–45. doi: 10.4078/jrd.2017.24.4.241
28. Chiu K, Tsai T, Lin W, Lee W, Su C, Chen C. Paraneoplastic Polymyositis Associated With Crescentic Glomerulonephritis. *Ren Fail* (2008) 30:939–42. doi: 10.1080/08860220802353918
29. Pattrapornpisut P, Avila-Casado C, Reich HN. IgA Nephropathy: Core Curriculum 2021. *Am J Kidney Dis: Off J Natl Kidney Found* (2021) 78:429 41. doi: 10.1053/j.ajkd.2021.01.024
30. Rothwell S, Chinoy H, Lamb JA, Miller FW, Rider LG, Wedderburn LR, et al. Focused HLA Analysis in Caucasians With Myositis Identifies Significant Associations With Autoantibody Subgroups. *Ann Rheum Dis* (2019) 78:996 1002. doi: 10.1136/annrheumdis-2019-215046
31. Kiryluk K, Li Y, Scolari F, Sanna-Cherchi S, Choi M, Verbitsky M, et al. Discovery of New Risk Loci for IgA Nephropathy Implicates Genes Involved in Immunity Against Intestinal Pathogens. *Nat Genet* (2014) 46:1187–96. doi: 10.1038/ng.3118
32. Gharavi AG, Kiryluk K, Choi M, Li Y, Hou P, Xie J, et al. Genome-Wide Association Study Identifies Susceptibility Loci for IgA Nephropathy. *Nat Genet* (2011) 43:321–7. doi: 10.1038/ng.787
33. Makita Y, Suzuki H, Kano T, Takahata A, Julian BA, Novak J, et al. TLR9 Activation Induces Aberrant IgA Glycosylation *via* APRIL- and IL-6-

Mediated Pathways in IgA Nephropathy. *Kidney Int* (2020) 97:340–9. doi: 10.1016/j.kint.2019.08.022

34. Chang S, Li XK. The Role of Immune Modulation in Pathogenesis of IgA Nephropathy. *Front Med* (2020) 7:92. doi: 10.3389/fmed.2020.00092
35. Schena FP, Nistor I. Epidemiology of IgA Nephropathy: A Global Perspective. *Semin Nephrol* (2018) 38:435–42. doi: 10.1016/j.semnephrol.2018.05.013
36. Zhou FD, Zhao MH, Zou WZ, Liu G, Wang H. The Changing Spectrum of Primary Glomerular Diseases Within 15 Years: A Survey of 3331 Patients in a Single Chinese Centre. *Nephrol Dialysis Transplant: Off Publ Eur Dialysis Transplant Assoc - Eur Renal Assoc* (2009) 24:870–6. doi: 10.1093/ndt/gfn554
37. Rauen T, Eitner F, Fitzner C, Sommerer C, Zeier M, Otte B, et al. Intensive Supportive Care Plus Immunosuppression in IgA Nephropathy. *N Engl J Med* (2015) 373:2225–36. doi: 10.1056/NEJMoa1415463
38. Obrisca B, Stefan G, Gherghiceanu M, Mandache E, Ismail G, Stancu S, et al. “Associated” or “Secondary” IgA Nephropathy? An Outcome Analysis. *PloS One* (2019) 14:e0221014. doi: 10.1371/journal.pone.0221014
39. Rehnberg J, Symreng A, Ludvigsson J, Emilsson L. Inflammatory Bowel Disease Is More Common in Patients With IgA Nephropathy and Predicts Progression of ESKD: A Swedish Population-Based Cohort Study. *J Am Soc Nephrol* (2020) 32:411–23. doi: 10.1681/ASN.2020060848
40. Kochi M, Kohagura K, Shiohira Y, Iseki K, Ohya Y. Chronic Kidney Disease, Inflammation, and Cardiovascular Disease Risk in Rheumatoid Arthritis. *J Cardiol* (2018) 71:277–83. doi: 10.1016/j.jjcc.2017.08.008

19

High-Dimensional Analysis Reveals Distinct Endotypes in Patients With Idiopathic Inflammatory Myopathies

Erin M. Wilfong[1,2,3,4], Todd Bartkowiak[5,6], Katherine N. Vowell[1], Camille S. Westlake[1], Jonathan M. Irish[3,4,5,6,7], Peggy L. Kendall[2,3,7,8], Leslie J. Crofford[1,3,4,7] and Rachel H. Bonami[1,3,4,6,7] on behalf of the MYSTIC Investigators*

[1] Division of Rheumatology and Immunology, Vanderbilt University Medical Center, Nashville, TN, United States, [2] Division of Allergy, Pulmonary, and Critical Care Medicine, Vanderbilt University Medical Center, Nashville, TN, United States, [3] Vanderbilt Institute for Infection, Immunology, and Inflammation, Vanderbilt University Medical Center, Nashville, TN, United States, [4] Human Immunology Discovery Initiative and Vanderbilt Center for Immunobiology, Vanderbilt University Medical Center, Nashville, TN, United States, [5] Department of Cell and Developmental Biology, Vanderbilt University, Nashville, TN, United States, [6] Vanderbilt-Ingram Cancer Center, Vanderbilt University Medical Center, Nashville, TN, United States, [7] Deparment of Pathology, Microbiology, and Immunology, Vanderbilt University Medical Center, Nashville, TN, United States, [8] Department of Medicine, Division of Allergy and Immunology, Washington University School of Medicine St. Louis, MO, United States

***Correspondence:**
Erin M. Wilfong
erin.m.wilfong@vumc.org

The idiopathic inflammatory myopathies (IIM) are a rare clinically heterogeneous group of conditions affecting the skin, muscle, joint, and lung in various combinations. While myositis specific autoantibodies are well described, we postulate that broader immune endotypes exist in IIM spanning B cell, T cell, and monocyte compartments. This study aims to identify immune endotypes through detailed immunophenotyping of peripheral blood mononuclear cells (PBMCs) in IIM patients compared to healthy controls. We collected PBMCs from 17 patients with a clinical diagnosis of inflammatory myositis and characterized the B, T, and myeloid cell subsets using mass cytometry by time of flight (CyTOF). Data were analyzed using a combination of the dimensionality reduction algorithm t-distributed stochastic neighbor embedding (t-SNE), cluster identification, characterization, and regression (CITRUS), and marker enrichment modeling (MEM); supervised biaxial gating validated populations identified by these methods to be differentially abundant between groups. Using these approaches, we identified shared immunologic features across all IIM patients, despite different clinical features, as well as two distinct immune endotypes. All IIM patients had decreased surface expression of RP105/CD180 on B cells and a reduction in circulating CD3+CXCR3+ subsets relative to healthy controls. One IIM endotype featured CXCR4 upregulation across all cellular compartments. The second endotype was hallmarked by an increased frequency of CD19+CD21loCD11c+ and CD3+CD4+PD1+ subsets. The experimental and analytical methods we describe here are broadly applicable to studying other immune-mediated diseases (e.g., autoimmunity, immunodeficiency) or protective immune responses (e.g., infection, vaccination).

Keywords: idiopathic inflammatory myopathies (IIM), dermatomyositis (DM), polymyositis (PM), mass cytometry (CyTOF), immunophenotype

INTRODUCTION

The idiopathic inflammatory myopathies (IIM) are a family of autoimmune diseases afflicting 2.4 to 33.8 per 100,000 individuals. IIM are associated with significant morbidity and mortality (1). IIM patients have a three-fold increased risk of death (2), and 14% cannot dress independently (3). Clinically, IIM are quite heterogenous and causes varying degrees of skin rash, proximal muscle weakness, esophageal dysmotility, and interstitial lung disease (ILD). The presence of different autoantibodies is associated with specific clinical phenotypes (4–15). For example, Mi-2 positive patients frequently manifest with classical rashes, mild to moderate muscle involvement, and rarely have ILD (15), whereas MDA5 positive patients have cutaneous ulcerations, arthritis, and progressive lung disease that can rapidly lead to death (14). Immune subsets interact and influence each other (16–23). B cells, T cells, dendritic cells, and monocytes have been independently characterized in IIM patients (24–29), but all compartments have not been immunophenotyped in tandem from the same patient. Recent technical and analytical advances create an opportunity to probe relational changes in all of these subsets simultaneously to build a more complete picture of immune dysfunction in IIM.

Cryopreserved PBMC samples enable longitudinal studies of the same donor as one batch. Aliquots of the same sample can also be run in different assays. Several groups have shown that cryopreserved lymphocytes approximate fresh *ex vivo* results (30–33). To improve our understanding of IIM immunophenotypes across all PBMC compartments, we performed detailed immunophenotyping using mass cytometry by time of flight (CyTOF) to analyze cryopreserved PBMC samples isolated from a cohort of IIM patients with active disease compared to healthy controls. A challenge in analyzing mass cytometric data is the number of parameters analyzed simultaneously. While canonical immune subsets (34) and previously described autoimmune-prone subsets (35–40) can be analyzed using traditional biaxial gating, dimensionality reduction tools, such as t-SNE and UMAP, facilitate discovery of non-canonical immune subsets that may otherwise be missed by manual biaxial gating approaches that require *a priori* knowledge to identify subsets. Dimensionality reduction tools convert plots of cells in multi-dimensional space into a two-dimensional map for manual review by scientists (41). In contrast, clustering algorithms, such as CITRUS (42) and FlowSOM (43), use automated approaches to detect and define cell populations for downstream analyses, including manual biaxial gating. While FlowSOM stands out compared to other unsupervised clustering tools due to its fast and accurate grouping of cells by phenotype, FlowSOM does not analyze external categories as part of finding cell clusters (44). In contrast, CITRUS is a statistically robust tool for supervised analysis, meaning that it allows the user to guide the analysis using an external categorization of comparison groups and incorporates key statistical concepts like false discovery rate. Additional algorithms, such as marker enrichment modeling (45), can further characterize these clusters and facilitate the development of biaxial gating schemes for cluster validation. We therefore elected to use t-SNE, as well as CITRUS and MEM to identify immune perturbations that distinguished groups and manual biaxial gating to validate proportional differences in these putative populations between groups.

Previously, CD21lo/neg (46) and CD180lo (37) B cell subsets were found to be increased in IIM. We hypothesized that machine learning would identify additional atypical B cell populations. Therefore, in addition to measuring perturbation of canonical PBMC (34) and autoimmune prone B cell subsets (35–37, 39, 40) in IIM patients *via* biaxial gating, we employed t-SNE to visualize the B cell immunophenotypes in IIM and identify additional atypical populations. We then grouped patients by the presence of atypical B cell subsets and exploited the statistical robustness of CITRUS to identify other PBMC subsets associated with the t-SNE identified B cell subsets, which would support the hypotheses that immune endotypes exist within IIM. Such immune endotypes may have important clinical correlates such as disease severity, end-organ involvement, or treatment response.

MATERIALS AND METHODS

Patients

Institutional Review Board approval was obtained (VUMC IRB 141415). Patients clinically diagnosed with IIM were enrolled into the Myositis and Scleroderma Treatment Initiative Center (MYSTIC) Cohort in either the outpatient clinic or inpatient setting at Vanderbilt University Medical Center between 9/17/2017 and 9/30/2018. Individuals enrolling as healthy controls completed a health questionnaire to verify a negative review of systems and no personal or family history of autoimmunity in a first degree relative. We performed clinical phenotyping by chart abstraction to estimate the date of symptom onset and collected serologic data, including anti-nuclear antibodies (ANA), rheumatoid factor (RF), cyclic citrullinated peptide (CCP), and an extended myositis panel obtained through ARUP (Salt Lake City, UT), which included Jo-1, PL-7, PL-12, EJ, OJ, Ro52, Ro60, Ku, MDA5, Mi-2, NXP-2, P155/140, Pm/Scl 100, SAE-1/SUMO, SRP, Tif-1γ, U1RNP, and U3RNP. We defined patients as having ILD if a radiologist determined that fibrosis was present on a CT scan. If the treating clinician escalated immunosuppression, the patient was defined as having active disease. Clinical data are reported as the mean ± standard deviation unless otherwise indicated. We isolated peripheral blood mononuclear cells (PBMCs) from blood collected in sodium heparin CPT tubes (BD Biosciences, San Jose CA) per manufacturer's directions and cryopreserved for future study.

Mass Cytometry

Seventeen IIM patients with active disease and eighteen healthy controls were included for CyTOF analysis. For CyTOF acquisition, we thawed 3-5 million PBMCs per individual,

Abbreviations: ARS, anti-tRNA synthetase syndrome; BCR, B cell receptor; CITRUS, cluster identification, characterization, and regression; ILD, interstitial lung disease; CyTOF, mass cytometry by time of flight; IIM, idiopathic inflammatory myopathies; MEM, marker enrichment modeling; MHCII, major histocompatibility complex class II; MMI, Median Mass Intensities; MFI, mean fluorescence intensity; PMBCs, peripheral blood mononuclear cells; t-SNE, t-distributed stochastic neighbor embedding.

viability stained with cisplatin, and stained for surface and intracellular markers (see **Supplemental Methods** and **Tables S1, S2**). Data were acquired using a CyTOF Helios 3.0 (Fluidigm Sciences, Sunnyvale, CA) and CyTOF software (version 6.7.1014) at the Vanderbilt University Medical Center Mass Cytometry Center of Excellence. Dual count calibration and noise reduction were applied prior to acquisition; 100,000-400,000 events were collected per sample.

Flow Cytometry

We selected six representative IIM patients and six healthy controls for flow cytometric studies of CD180 expression, for which 4-5 million cells per individual were thawed and stained (see **Supplemental Methods** and **Table S3**). We measured intracellular and extracellular CD180 levels simultaneously on the same day. All data were acquired on a BD LSRII Fortessa instrument.

Data Analysis

Mass cytometry FCS files underwent Fluidigm bead normalization and analysis using Cytobank software per established methods (47). Dimensionality reduction (t-SNE (41) and UMAP (48)), clustering (CITRUS (42)), or supervised (traditional biaxial gating) analyses were conducted using CytoBank (Santa Clara, CA). Marker enrichment modeling (MEM) labels (45) aided in determining biaxial gating schemes for CITRUS-identified populations. Details of mass cytometric data analysis are included in the **Supplemental Methods** and **Tables S4, S5**. Fluorescence cytometry data was analyzed using FlowJo version 9.9.6.

Statistical Methods

Population statistics were exported from CytoBank or FlowJo as appropriate and analyzed with Prism software (GraphPad, La Jolla, CA) to calculate descriptive statistics. Data are expressed as mean ± standard deviation unless otherwise indicated. If multiple groups were compared, we performed a Kruskal-Wallis ANOVA and, if $p<0.05$, *post-hoc* Mann-Whitney U-tests were performed. For comparison of two continuous variables, we utilized Mann-Whitney U-tests. For comparison of two dichotomous variables, a Fisher's exact test was performed. Spearman's correlation coefficients were utilized to identify the presence of a statistical correlation between populations.

RESULTS

Patient Characteristics

We studied 17 patients clinically diagnosed with IIM and 18 healthy controls. Basic demographics and clinical information are shown in **Table 1**. Detailed clinical phenotyping is shown in **Supplemental Table S6**. IIM patients were slightly older than healthy controls (56.8 ± 12.0 v. 46.4 ± 12.0 years, $p=0.01$). Seven patients were receiving corticosteroids at the time of enrollment; one patient was taking methotrexate at the time of enrollment with active skin, lung, and joint involvement. Eleven patients met the 2017 classification criteria for probable or definite IIM. Those not meeting classification criteria all had interstitial lung disease and myositis-specific autoantibodies.

Lymphoid and Myeloid Subsets Are Altered in IIM Patients Compared to Healthy Controls

We evaluated common myeloid, T, and B cell subsets based on standardized immunophenotypic markers (34) using traditional biaxial gating (**Supplemental Figure S1**). Regions for each subset are pseudocolored on a t-SNE plot including all donors concatenated (**Figure 1A**) or divided into concatenated healthy control or IIM t-SNE plots, in which major subset regions are indicated by shading (**Figure 1B**). **Figure 1C** shows a heatmap of all markers for each population to ensure all populations were correctly identified. **Table 2** shows the average, standard deviation, and p value comparing all populations between IIM and healthy controls based on manually-defined populations on t-SNE plots. Complete blood count with differential was available for 14 IIM patients and 14 healthy controls. There was no difference between the number of circulating PBMCs between IIM patients and healthy controls (**Figure 1D**). There was no difference in the percent of live cells for healthy controls compared to IIM patients (92.2 ± 5.1% v. 94.2 ± 2.7%, $p=0.27$). As shown in **Figure 1E**, IIM patients had a decreased frequency of class-switched (CD19+CD27+IgM-) and non-class-switched (CD19+CD27+IgM+) memory B cells compared to healthy controls; there was no difference in the frequency of naïve (CD19+CD27-IgD+) or total B cells. While there was no statistically significant difference in CD8+ T cells, there was a decrease in CD4+, CD4-CD8- and CD4+CXCR5+PD1+ T cells. Classical monocytes (CD14+CD16-CD19-CD3-) were increased in IIM patients compared to healthy controls, but there was no difference in the frequency of natural killer cells (CD16+CD19-CD3-CD14-) or non-classical monocytes (CD14+CD16+CD19-CD3-).

Autoimmune-Prone CD21lo and DN B Cell Subsets Are Increased in IIM Compared to Healthy Controls

Next, we used manual biaxial gating to investigate the previously described autoreactive CD24hiCD38hi transitional B cell (40), CD21lo/negative B cell (36), CD27-IgD- DN B cell (50), and B_{ND} cell (35) subsets as shown in **Figure 2A**. There was no difference in the frequency of CD24hiCD38hi transitional B cells or B_{ND} cells in IIM patients compared to healthy controls. However, IIM patients had increased CD21lo/neg and DN B cells compared to healthy controls (**Figure 2B**). CD21lo/negative cells were previously shown to be autoreactive and/or anergic (36). The frequency of CD21lo/negative cells can be increased in systemic lupus erythematosus (51), rheumatoid arthritis (36), juvenile idiopathic arthritis (52), and systemic sclerosis (53, 54).

Kikuchi et al. reported an RP105/CD180 lo B cell population that was increased in dermatomyositis (37). Examination of CD180 median mass intensity (MMI) revealed decreased expression on naïve, class-switched memory, and non-class switched memory B cells in IIM patients compared to healthy

TABLE 1 | Patient demographics.

	IIM Patients (n = 17)	Healthy Controls (n = 18)
Average Age	56.8 ± 11.7	46.4 ± 11.7
Female Gender	8 (44.4%)	14 (82%)
Race		
Caucasian	13 (76.4%)	16 (88.8%)
African American	4 (23.5%)	1 (5.6%)
Other	0 (0%)	1 (5.6%)
Average Disease Duration in Months (median, IQR)	10.8 (8.4,15.6)	
Clinical Categorization		
Dermatomyositis	6 (35.3%)	
Polymyositis	4 (23.5%)	
Anti-synthetase syndrome	7 (41.2%)	
Interstitial Lung Disease	14 (82.3%)	
Average % predicted FVC (n=11)	56.9 ± 11.9%	
Average % predicted DLCO (n=9)	49.1 ± 15.1%	
Supplemental oxygen use at enrollment	6 (42.9%)	
History of elevated creatinine kinase	9 (52.9%)	
Serologic Status		
+ANA	8 (47.0%)	
+Rheumatoid factor (n=14)	5 (35.6%)	
+Ro52	6 (35.3%)	
+Myositis specific or associated autoantibody	16 (94.1%)	
Probable or definite idiopathic inflammatory myositis according to 2017 classification criteria (49)	11 (64.7%)	

Data reported as mean ± standard deviation unless otherwise noted.
FVC, forced vital capacity; DLCO, diffusing capacity of the lung for carbon monoxide; ANA, anti-nuclear antibodies.

donors (**Figure 2C**). There was no difference in the CD180 MMI on CD19+ cells of patients taking or not taking prednisone (41.7 ± 3.7% v. 54.2 ± 17.5%, p=0.14). To evaluate whether surface CD180 expression was decreased due to global protein downregulation, fluorescence cytometry was performed on IIM patients and healthy controls to quantify extracellular versus intracellular protein. Extracellular CD180 median fluorescent intensity was decreased in IIM patients compared to healthy controls, whereas intracellular CD180 expression was not different (**Figures 2D–F**). These data are consistent with surface downregulation, rather than reduced expression of CD180 in IIM B cells.

Circulating Subsets of CXCR3+ T Cells Are Decreased in IIM

We used previously defined biaxial gating schemes (34, 55) to evaluate CD4+ T cell subsets (**Figures 3A, B** and **Supplemental Figure S2A**) as defined in **Table 2**. There were no differences in CD4+ naïve, central memory, effector memory, or effector cells between IIM patients and healthy controls (**Supplemental Figure S2B**). IIM patients had an increased frequency of CD8+ effector cells but not CD8+ naïve, central memory or effector memory cells (**Supplemental Figure S2C**). However, as shown in **Figure 3C**, all CXCR3+ Th subsets, including Th1, Th1Th17, CXCR3+Th2, and CXCR3+Th17 cells, were strikingly decreased in IIM compared to healthy controls. There was no difference in the CXCR3- subsets Th0, Th2, and Th17. We additionally determined that the CXCR3+ subsets of CD8+ and CD4-CD8- T cells were decreased in IIM compared to healthy controls, but there was again no difference in the CXCR3- subsets (**Figures 3D, E**). There was no difference in the global frequency of CXCR3+ T cells in IIM patients taking prednisone compared to those not on prednisone (2.6 ± 3.2% v. 2.6 ± 1.7% of live PBMCs, p=0.37).

Dimensionality Reduction Algorithms Reveal Two Abnormal CD19+ Cell Populations in IIM

Population identification using biaxial gating strategies relies on prior phenotypic marker knowledge. However, t-SNE plots represent multidimensional cellular information in 2D space, allowing for unbiased population identification and manual visual comparison (41). The t-SNE plots in **Figure 4A** and heatmap in **Figure 4B** show two atypical CD19+ cell subsets with varying frequencies in IIM patients as well as the previously seen decrease in class-switched and non-class switched memory CD19+ cell subsets (46) (**Figure 4C**). The CD19+CXCR4hiCCR7hi subset was increased in IIM patients compared to healthy controls. The second CD19+CD21loCD11c+ subset did not reach statistical significance but was increased in some IIM patients. The atypical populations identified *via* manual gating of t-SNE plots could also be found using biaxial gating (**Supplemental Figure 3**) and UMAP (**Supplemental Figure 4**). Thus, dimensionality reduction visualization of resulting data identified perturbed CD19+ cell subsets that were not captured by previous IIM studies.

High Frequencies of Abnormal CD19+ Populations Predict the Presence of Altered Circulating CD4+ Populations

CITRUS is a fully automated machine learning algorithm that identifies cell populations correlated with a particular biologic or clinical feature (42). CITRUS also incorporates regularized

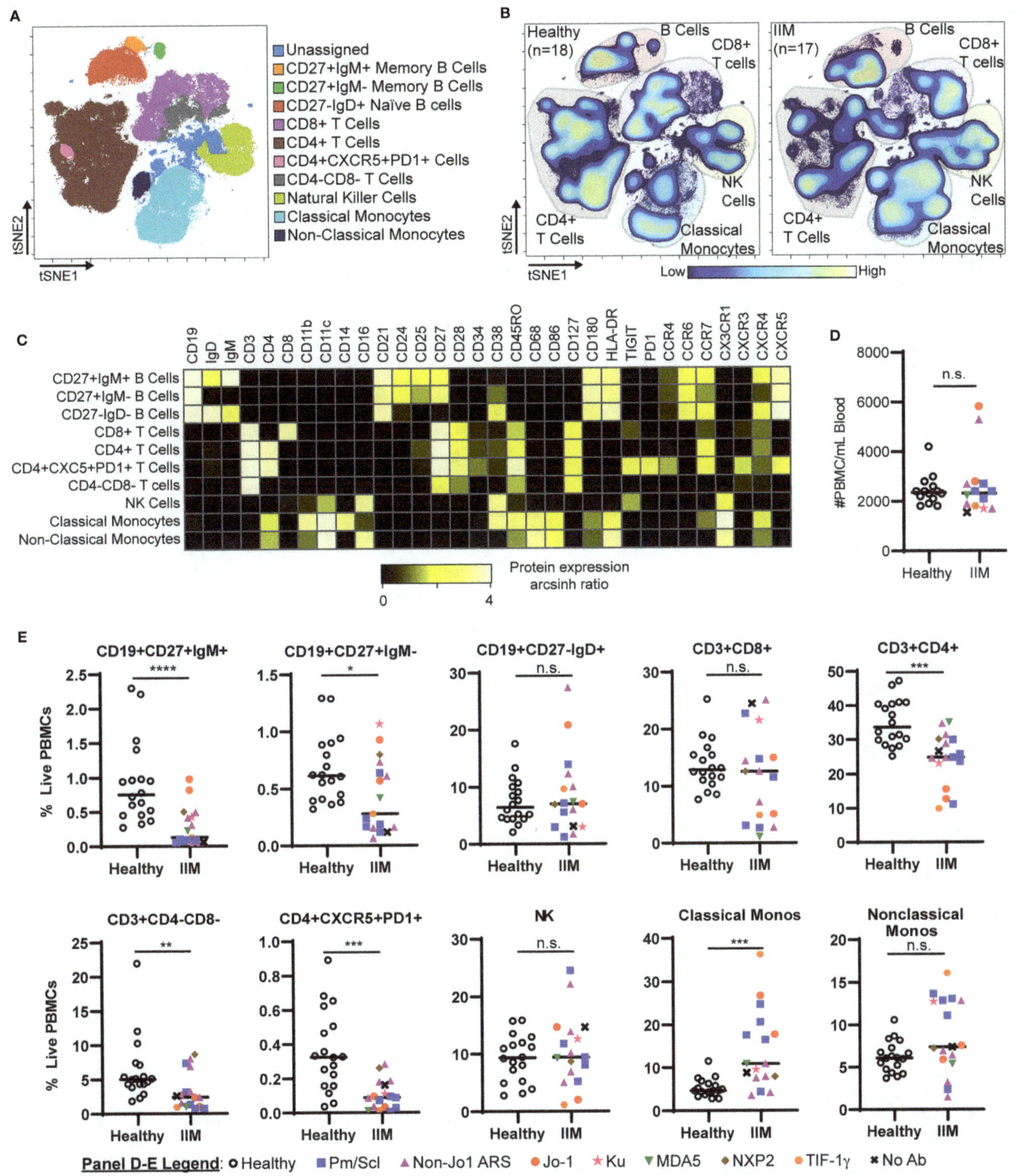

FIGURE 1 | IIM patients show differences in peripheral blood immune subsets from healthy controls. **(A)** Live PBMCs from healthy controls (n=18) and IIM patients (n=17) were visualized using t-SNE and manually assigned to traditional immune cell populations (indicated by color). **(B)** Density contour maps of concatenated healthy controls versus IIM patients. **(C)** Expression heatmaps of representative markers for t-SNE islands displaying the arcsinh ratio by table's minimum. **(D, E)** Clinical seropositivity for the indicated autoantibodies is shown by legend symbols at the bottom of Panel **(E)**. Individual donors are plotted. **(D)** Absolute number of circulating PBMCs for healthy controls (n=14) and IIM patients (n=14) for whom count data were available. **(E)** Comparison of major circulating PBMC subsets between healthy controls and IIM patients using t-SNE visualization and manual gating from panel **(A)**. Statistical comparisons were performed using Mann-Whitney U tests. *p < 0.05, **p < 0.01, ***p < 0.001, ****p < 0.0001, not significant (n.s.).

TABLE 2 | Peripheral blood mononuclear cell (PBMC) subsets and median mass intensities (MMI) in healthy controls and idiopathic inflammatory myopathy (IIM) patients.

Population	Healthy (n = 18)	IIM (n = 17)	P value
Total number of circulating PBMCs (cells/mL)	2443 ± 614	2649 ± 1301	0.72
CD19+			
Total CD19+[†]	10.3 ± 4.3%	10.8 ± 7.8	0.61
CD19+CD27- (naïve) [‡]	7.5 ± 4.0%	8.6 ± 6.9%	0.96
CD19+CD27+IgM+ (non-class switched memory) [‡]	0.9 ± 0.6%	0.3 ± 0.3%	<0.0001
CD19+CD27+IgM- (class switched memory) [‡]	0.7 ± 0.3%	0.4 ± 0.3%	0.03
CD19+CD24hiCD38hi[‡]	3.8 ± 1.7%	4.9 ± 5.1%	0.66
CD19+CD21lo[‡]	5.8 ± 2.2%	11.7 ± 7.2%	0.001
CD19+CD27-IgD- (DN B cells) [‡]	7.4 ± 2.9%	12.7 ± 5.8%	0.002
CD19+CD27-IgD+IgM- (BND cells) [‡]	2.7 ± 1.0%	2.6 ± 1.7%	0.33
CD19+ CD180 MMI	60.9 ± 20.8	39.8 ± 16.0	0.002
CD19+CD27- CD180 MMI	58.3 ± 22.5	38.5 ± 16.3	0.009
CD19+CD27+IgM+ CD180 MMI	80.9 ± 19.1	58.5 ± 15.2	0.0005
CD19+CD27+IgM- CD180 MMI	73.5 ± 19.0	38.2 ± 28.5	<0.0001
CD19+CXCR4hiCCR7hiCD21lo (t-SNE) [‡]	0.1 ± 0.1%	6.1 ± 19.1%	0.0001
CD19+CD21loCD11c+ (t-SNE) [‡]	2.3 ± 1.2%	4.1 ± 3.8%	0.09
CD3+			
CD3+CXCR3+[†]	9.6 ± 8.1%	2.6 ± 2.4%	0.0004
CD3+CXCR3-[†]	45.6 ± 9.8%	37.1 ± 13.4%	0.08
CD3+CD4+			
Total CD3+CD4+[†]	35.1 ± 6.6%	24.3 ± 7.8%	0.0001
CD3+CD4+CD45RO-CCR7+ (CD4+ Naive)[§]	27.7 ± 9.0%	31.8 ± 17.8%	0.89
CD3+CD4+CD45RO+CCR7+ (CD4+ Central Memory)[§]	18.5 ± 4.9%	15.7 ± 5.9%	0.23
CD3+CD4+CD45RO+CCR7- (CD4+ Effector Memory)[§]	13.5 ± 3.9%	11.3 ± 6.9%	0.13
CD3+CD4+CD45RO-CCR7- (CD4+ Effector)[§]	2.2 ± 1.2%	3.4 ± 3.0%	0.19
CD4+CD45RO-CCR4-CCR6-CXCR3- (Th0)[§]	27.9 ± 8.8%	31.9 ± 16.1%	0.64
CD4+CD45RO+CCR4-CCR6-CXCR3+ (Th1)[§]	2.8 ± 2.0%	0.8 ± 0.8%	0.0002
CD4+CD45RO+CCR4-CCR6+CXCR3+ (Th1Th17)[§]	1.1 ± 2.1%	0.1 ± 0.1%	0.01
CD4+CD45RO+CCR4+CCR6-CXCR3- (Th2)[§]	10.1 ± 4.6%	11.1 ± 4.7%	0.66
CD4+CD45RO+CCR4+CCR6-CXCR3+ (Th2CXCR3+)[§]	1.9 ± 1.3%	0.8 ± 0.6%	0.003
CD4+CD45RO+CCR4+CCR6+CXCR3- (Th17)[§]	1.5 ± 1.4%	1.3 ± 1.2%	0.57
CD4+CD45RO+CCR4+CCR6+CXCR3+ (Th17CXCR3+)[§]	0.6 ± 0.8%	0.1 ± 0.1%	0.03
CD3+CD4+CXCR5+PD1+ (T follicular helper) [§]	0.4 ± 0.2%	0.1 ± 0.09%	0.0001
CD3+CD4+CCR4+CD25+CD127- (Treg) [§]	2.2 ± 0.8	2.7 ± 2.0	0.88
CD3+CD4+CXCR4hiCD38- (Cluster "A")[§]	0.3 ± 0.3%	5.5 ± 8.6	<0.0001
CD3+CD4+CD27-PD1+ (Cluster "B")[§]	1.5 ± 1.6%	3.2 ± 3.3%	0.25
CD3+CD8+			
Total CD3+CD8+[†]	13.7 ± 4.3%	11.9 ± 8.1%	0.40
CD3+CD8+CXCR3+[§]	7.6 ± 5.6%	4.2 ± 4.6%	0.03
CD3+CD8+CXCR3-[§]	16.1 ± 6.9%	22.5 ± 11.5%	0.06
CD3+CD8+CD45RO-CCR7+ (CD8+ Naïve)[§]	5.5 ± 2.3%	4.5 ± 3.5%	0.26
CD3+CD8+CD45RO+CCR7+ (CD8+ Central Memory)[§]	3.3 ± 1.3%	1.8 ± 1.4%	0.002
CD3+CD8+CD45RO+CCR7- (CD8+ Effector Memory)[§]	8.9 ± 4.1%	8.8 ± 8.3%	0.42
CD3+CD8+CD45RO-CCR7- (CD8+ Effector)[§]	2.6 ± 2.7%	7.1 ± 6.8%	0.02
CD3-CD4-CD8-			
Total CD3+CD4-CD8-[†]	6.3 ± 4.7%	3.2 ± 2.7%	0.006
CD3-CD4-CD8-CXCR3+[§]	4.7 ± 6.5%	1.0 ± 0.7%	0.0002
CD3-CD4-CD8-CXCR3-[§]	5.7 ± 3.2%	6.0 ± 4.0%	0.71
CD19-CD3-			
CD3-CD19-CD14+ Classical Monocytes[†]	5.3 ± 2.1%	13.9 ± 9.1%	0.0003
CD3-CD19-CD14+CD16+ Non-classical monocytes[†]	6.2 ± 1.8%	8.6 ± 4.4%	0.10
CD3-CD19-CD14-CD16+ NK cells[†]	9.2 ± 4.1%	10.6 ± 6.3%	0.66
Biaxial "Cluster C" [‡‡]	2.3 ± 1.4%	6.3 ± 5.3%	0.0029
Biaxial "Cluster D" [‡‡]	1.9 ± 1.2%	3.9 ± 2.0%	0.0001

Values reported as average ± standard deviation. Statistical comparisons performed using Mann-Whitney U-test.
[†]Frequency of all PBMCs, [‡]frequency of all CD19+ cells, [§]frequency of all CD3+ cells, [‡‡]frequency of all CD3-CD19- cells.

regression modeling to make statistically robust comparisons between groups, which was highly valued given the cohort heterogeneity. As specific B cell subsets can affect T cell phenotype (19, 20, 23), we used CITRUS to investigate correlations between CD19+CXCR4hiCCR7hi and CD19+CD21loCD11c+ cell subsets with T cell subsets. We created three mutually exclusive groups of IIM patients with high expression of CD19+CXCR4hiCCR7hi, CD19+CD21loCD11c+, or neither compared to healthy controls (**Table S7**). IIM patients assigned to the CD19+CXCR4hiCCR7hi group had ten-fold more cells in that population than the average for

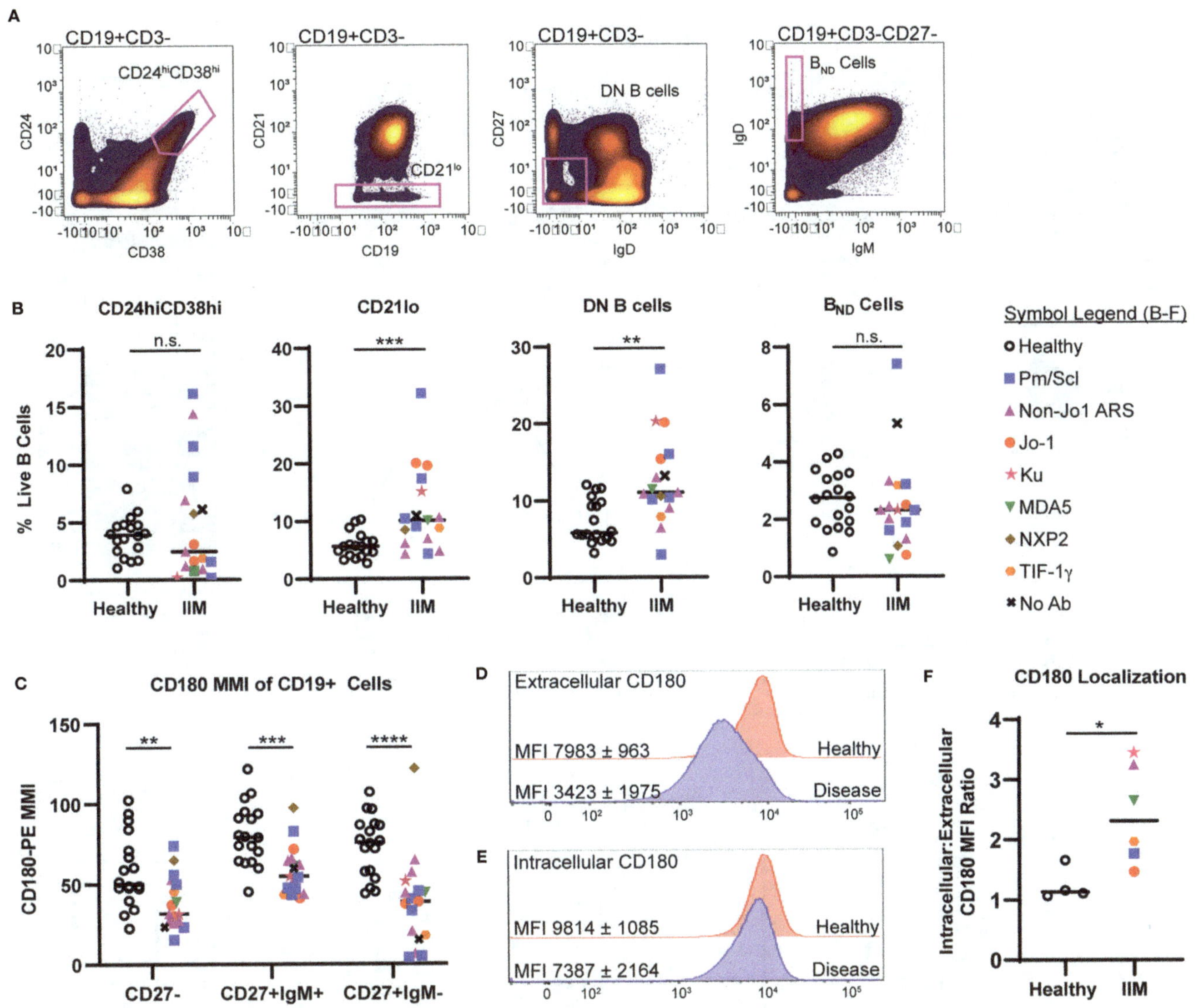

FIGURE 2 | Autoreactive-prone CD21lo and DN B cells and CD180 surface expression are reduced in IIM patients. **(A)** Mass cytometry gating scheme to identify CD19+CD24hiCD38hi transitional B cells, CD19+CD21lo cells, CD19+CD27-IgD- (DN B) cells, and CD27-IgD+IgM- (BND) cells in healthy controls (n=18) and IIM patients (n=17). **(B)** Population frequencies for panel A subsets are shown for each donor; symbols represent clinical autoantibody status as in **Figure 1**. **(C)** CD180/RP105 mean mass intensity (MMI) for naive and memory CD19+ populations. **(D)** Fluorescent cytometry data quantifying CD180 expression on the cell surface and **(E)** intracellularly for four heathy controls and six IIM patients. Data are expressed as the mean ± standard deviation. **(F)** Ratio of intracellular to extracellular CD180 mean fluorescence intensity (MFI). Statistical comparisons were performed using Mann-Whitney U tests, *$p < 0.05$, **$p < 0.01$, ***$p < 0.001$, ****$p < 0.0001$, not significant (n.s.).

healthy controls. IIM patients assigned to CD19+CD21loCD11c+ group had two-fold more cells in that population than the average for healthy controls. As shown in **Figure 5A**, CITRUS identified increased abundance of CD4+CXCR4hiCD38hi naïve cells (Cluster A) in IIM patients defined by increased CD19+CXCR4hiCCR7hi cell frequency. CD4+CD27-PD1+ effector memory cells (Cluster B) were increased in the group with a high frequency of CD19+CD21loCD11c+ cells. To further characterize the phenotype of CD4+ cells in Clusters A and B, a heatmap of surface marker expression is shown for both populations. **Figure 5B** shows that Cluster A is comprised of a CD4+ naïve T cell subset with high levels of CCR7, CXCR4, and CD127 expression while Cluster B consists of a CD4+ effector memory cell subset positive for CX3CR1 and PD1. CITRUS also identified several populations of T cells that were decreased in IIM patients (**Supplemental Figure S5**).

To confirm this finding, marker enrichment modeling (MEM) computationally identified differentially expressed markers "enriched" in each cluster (45) to guide biaxial gating (**Figures 5C, D**). Biaxial population frequencies approximated

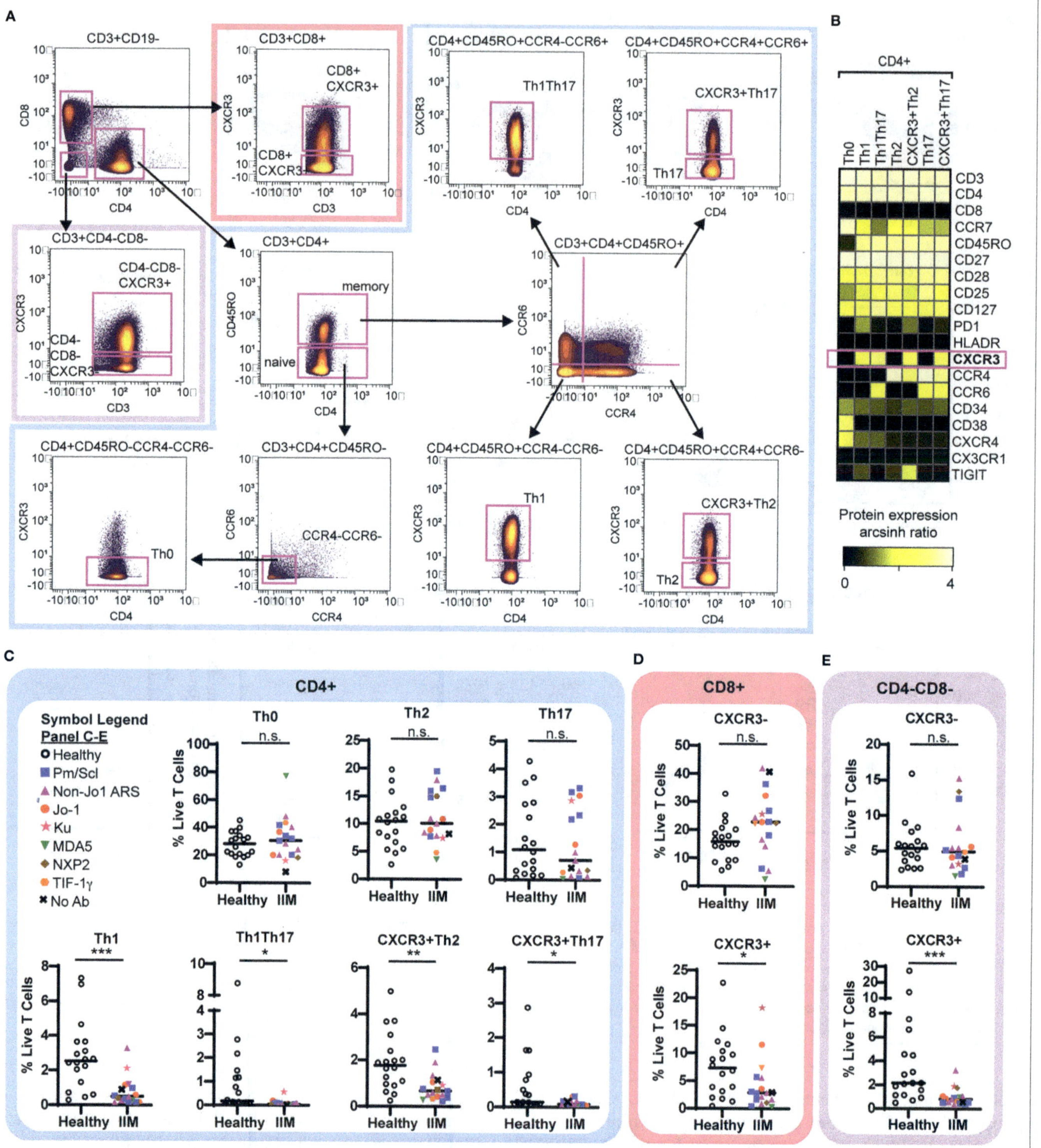

FIGURE 3 | CXCR3+ T cell subsets are decreased in IIM. **(A)** Mass cytometry biaxial gating scheme to identify subsets of CD4-CD8-, CD4+, and CD8+ T cells for healthy controls (n=18) and IIM patients (n=17). **(B)** Expression heatmap of surface markers for CD4+ subsets displaying the arcsinh ratio by table's minimum. **(C–E)** CXCR3- and CXCR3+ T cell populations were examined. Frequencies of biaxially gated T cell subsets are shown for each donor; clinical autoantibody status is indicated as in **Figure 1**; **(C)** CD4+, **(D)** CD8+, and **(E)** CD4-CD8- T cell populations. Statistical comparisons were performed using Mann-Whitney U tests. *p < 0.05, **p < 0.01, ***p < 0.001, not significant (n.s.).

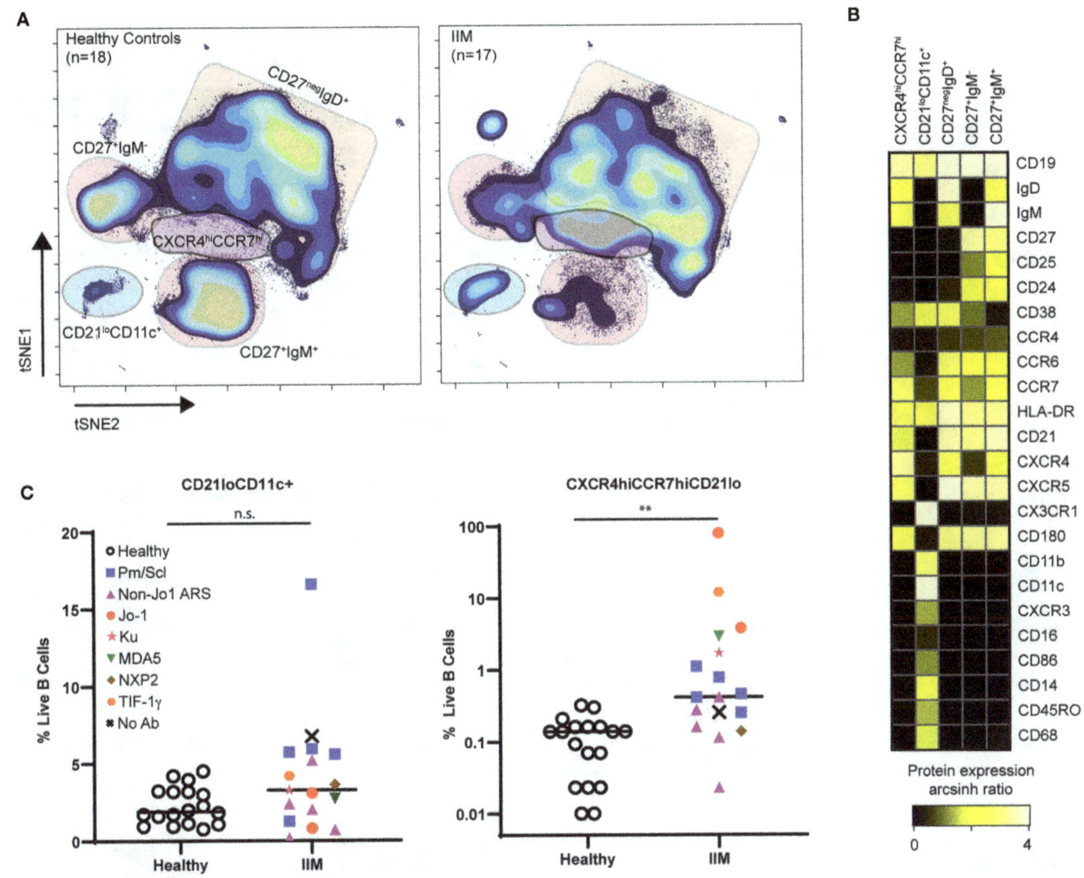

FIGURE 4 | CD21loCD11c+ and CXCR4hiCCR7hi B cell subsets are increased amongst IIM patients. CD3-CD19+ B cells were visualized using t-SNE. **(A)** Concatenated t-SNE maps for all healthy controls (n=18) and IIM patients (n=17) showing traditional B cell subsets and two IIM-associated B cell subsets identified through manual gating of t-SNE plots. **(B)** Expression heatmaps of representative markers for CD21loCD11c+ and CXCR4hiCCR7hi subsets displaying arcsinh ratio by table's minimum of channel median. **(C)** Frequencies of CD21loCD11c+ and CXCR4hiCCR7hi subsets are shown for each donor where various myositis associated and specific autoantibodies are coded as follows: Statistical comparisons were performed using Mann-Whitney U tests, **p < 0.01, not significant (n.s.).

the CITRUS-determined abundances (**Figures 5E, F** and **Table S8**). CD19+CXCR4hiCCR7hi and CD19+CD21loCD11c+ population frequencies were plotted against the biaxially gated frequency of the CD4+CXCR4hiCD38+ and CD4+CD27-PD1+ subsets, respectively (**Supplemental Figure S6**). We calculated Spearman's correlation coefficients (**Table S9**) and confirmed a statistical correlation between CD19+CXCR4hiCCR7hi and CD4+CXCR4hiCD38+populations (r=0.62, p=0.009) and between CD19+CD21loCD11c+ and CD4+CD27-PD1+ populations (r=0.60, p=0.01). Subset frequencies for individual patients are shown in **Tables S10**. These data show that patients defined by specific CD19+ subset perturbations show correlative changes with particular CD4+ T cell subsets.

An Increased Frequency of CD19+CXCR4hiCCR7hi Cells Predicts the Increase of Two Myeloid Populations

Using the previous IIM group assignments (**Table S7**), CITRUS clustered CD3-CD19- cells to correlate myeloid cell abundance with CD19+ cell phenotypes. Two clusters of increased abundance were predicted by having an increased frequency of CD19+CXCR4hiCCR7hi cells (**Figure 6A**). A heatmap of surface marker expression for both populations is shown in **Figure 6B**. While both Cluster C and Cluster D are classical monocytes, differential expression of CXCR4, CD45RO, and CD180 are readily apparent. MEM analysis confirmed Cluster C as a CD180+CXCR4+ classical monocyte and cluster C as a CD180-CXCR4- monocyte (**Figure 6C**). The MEM-derived biaxial gating scheme did not have clear visual cut-offs and final biaxial gating (**Figure 6D**) required the use of a training data set. Thus, myeloid cluster increases were further validated by t-SNE analysis (**Supplemental Figure S7**). Both the biaxial and t-SNE frequencies approximated the CITRUS abundance (**Figures 6E, F** and **Supplemental Figure S7D**). Spearman's correlation coefficients confirmed a statistical correlation of the CD19+CXCR4hiCCR7hi subset with both the biaxially gated classical monocyte (r=0.61, p=0.01) and the CXCR4-CD180- myeloid population (r=0.66, p=0.01). The CD4+CXCR4hiCD38+ population also correlated to both the CD180+CXCR4+ (Spearman r = 0.64, p = 0.007) and CD180-CXCR4- (Spearman r = 0.64, p =

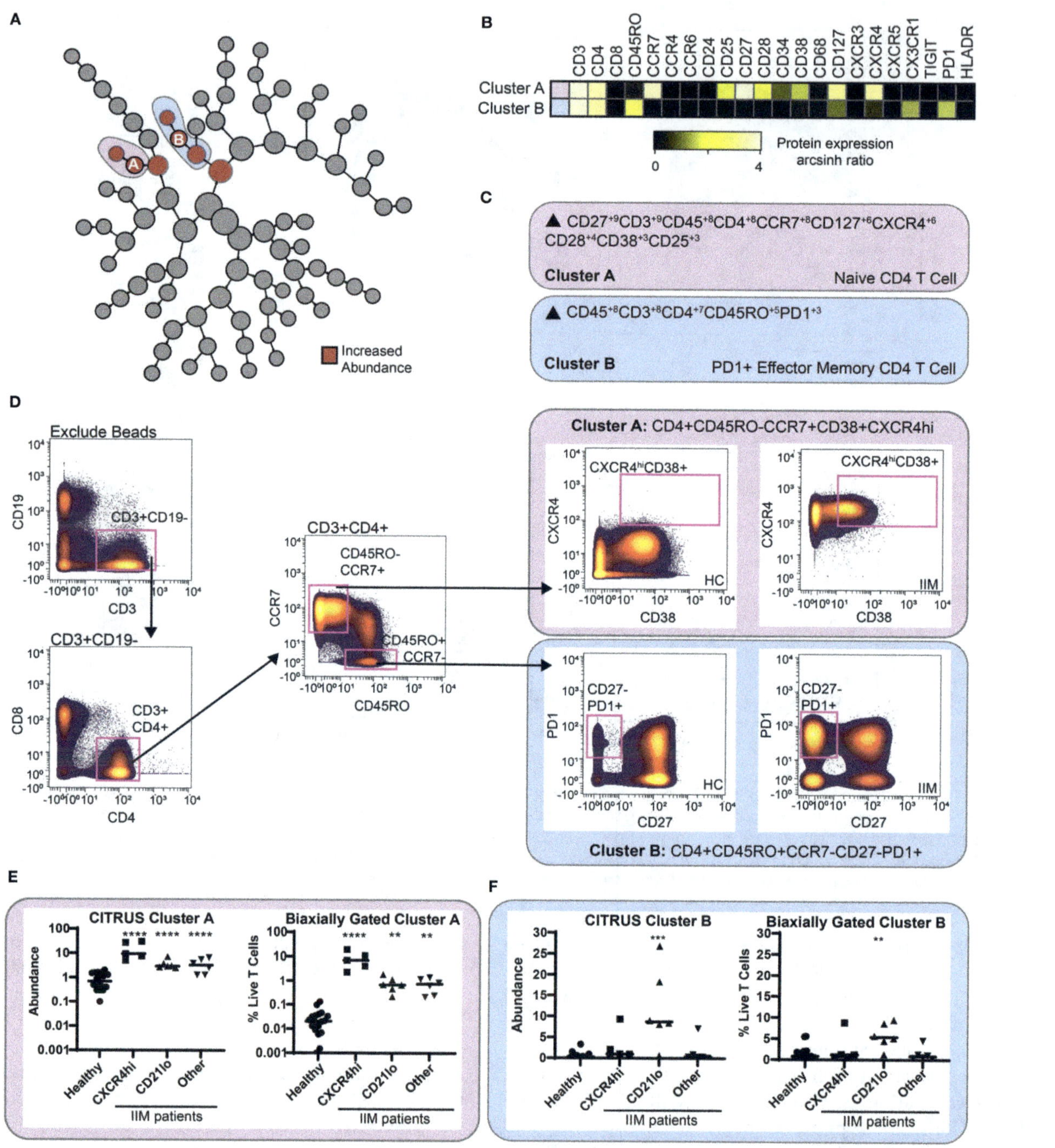

FIGURE 5 | CITRUS identifies T cell clusters associated with abnormal CD19+CXCR4hiCCR7hi and CD19+CD21loCD11c+CD27- populations. CD3+ T cells were clustered *via* CITRUS using four groups (healthy control, n=18, CXCR4hi, n=5, CD21lo, n=6, and other B cell phenotype, n=6) and the nearest shrunken centroid algorithm. **(A)** Increased abundance of clusters A and B are predicted by the presence of the CXCR4hi and CD21lo subsets, respectively. **(B)** Expression heatmap of markers for Clusters A and B displaying arcsinh ratio by table's minimum. **(C)** Algorithmic determination of biaxial gating scheme using marker enrichment modeling (MEM) for Clusters A and B Scale 1-10. **(D)** Biaxial gating scheme derived based on MEM definition; Cluster A: CD4+CD45RO-CCR7+CXCXCR4hiCD38+, and Cluster B: CD4+CR7-CD45RO+CD27-PD1+. Representative healthy control HC and IIM patient plots are shown. **(E, F)** CITRUS determined abundance and corresponding biaxial gating frequency for **(E)** Cluster A and **(F)** Cluster B are plotted for individual donors. If Kruskal-Wallis $p<0.05$, then *post-hoc* Mann-Whitney U tests were used to compare to healthy controls. $^{**}p < 0.01$, $^{***}p < 0.001$, $^{****}p < 0.0001$.

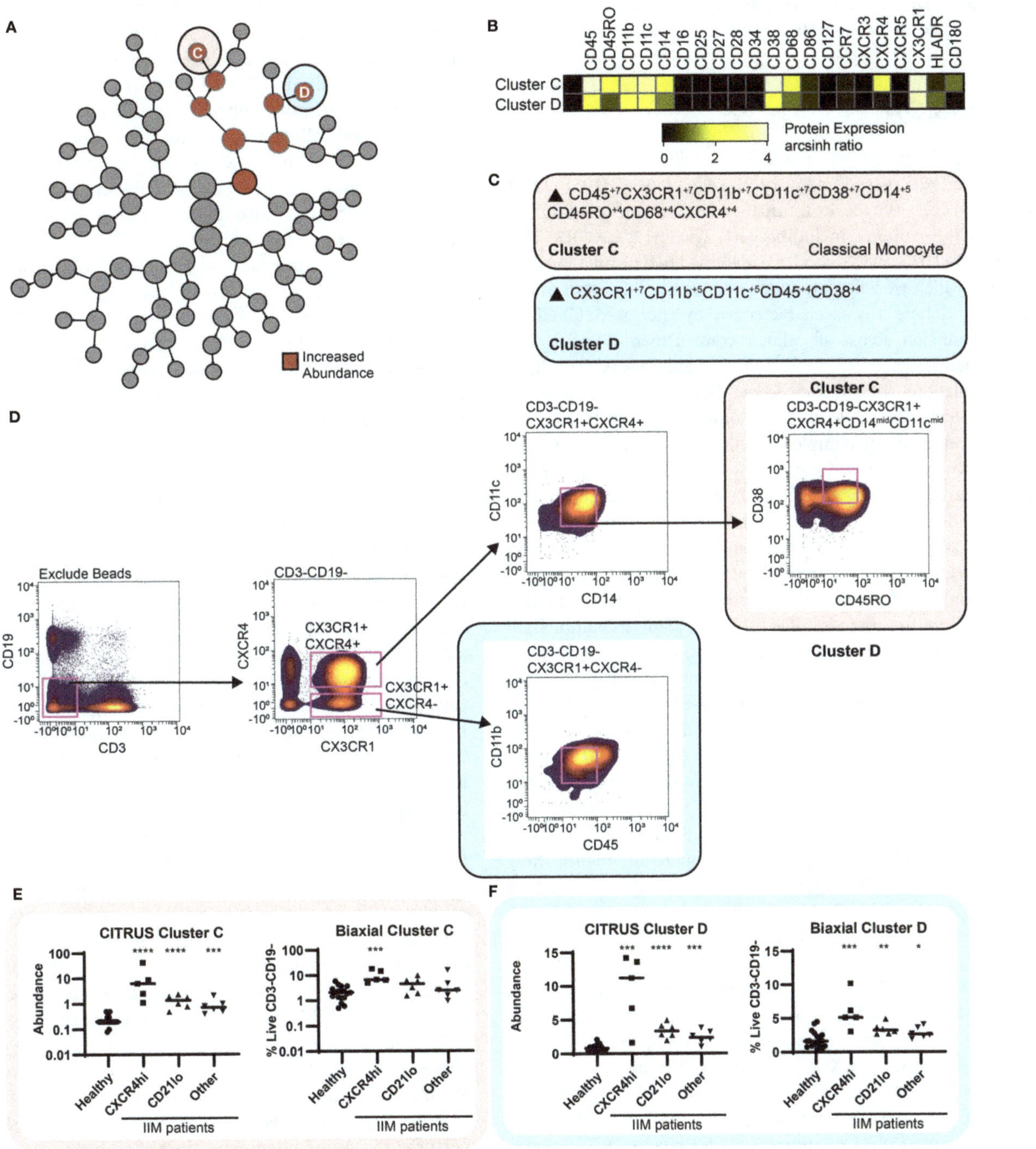

FIGURE 6 | CITRUS identifies myeloid cell clusters that are increased in IIM. CD3-CD19- cells were clustered *via* CITRUS using four groups (healthy control, n=18, CXCR4hi, n=5, CD21lo, n=6, and other B cell phenotype, n=6) and the nearest shrunken centroid algorithm. **(A)** Increased abundance of Clusters C and D are increased across all IIM subsets. No clusters of decreased abundance were identified. **(B)** Expression heatmap of markers for Clusters C and D displaying arcsinh ratio by table's minimum. **(C)** Algorithmic determination of biaxial gating scheme using marker enrichment modeling (MEM) for Clusters C and D. **(D)** Biaxial gating scheme derived based on MEM enrichment shown for a representative IIM patient. Additional t-SNE gating is shown in **Supplemental Figure 4**. **(E)** CITRUS determined abundance and corresponding biaxial gating frequency for Cluster C and **(F)** Cluster D. If Kruskal-Wallis p<0.05, then *post-hoc* Mann-Whitney U tests were used to compare to healthy controls. *p < 0.05, **p < 0.01, ***p < 0.001, ****p < 0.0001.

0.007) classical monocyte populations (**Supplemental Figure S5**). Subset frequencies for individual patients and group assignments are again shown in **Tables S10**.

DISCUSSION

Our key findings are summarized as follows. First, all IIM patients had decreased memory B cells, low RP105/CD180 surface B cell expression, and reduction of circulating CD3+CXCR3+ subsets, including Th1, Th1Th17, CXCR3+Th2, and CXCR3+Th17 cells. Second, we identified two distinct immune signatures, which we will term endotypes, amongst a cohort of IIM patients. Endotype 1 was characterized by increased CXCR4hi surface expression across all cellular compartments. Endotype 2 featured increased CD19+CD21loCD11c+ and CD4+CD27-PD1+ T cell populations. To our knowledge, these are the first immune endotypes to span multiple immune compartments in IIM.

Our B cell findings complement those of prior reports. Jo-1 autoantibody-positive IIM patients were previously reported to have decreased memory B cells (26), which we find across IIM patients independently of which myositis autoantibody was positive or which clinical disease manifestations were observed. Thus, our data suggest decreased peripheral blood memory B cells is a common feature of IIM that extends beyond Jo-1+ IIM patients. While the increase of CD24hiCD38hi (transitional) B cells did not reach statistical significance, some patients did have an increased frequency of this population, as previously observed in juvenile dermatomyositis (27). Decreased surface expression of RP105/CD180 was also found to be a common B cell feature in this clinically heterogeneous IIM patient cohort. CD180 is an alternative B cell signaling cascade capable of activating B cells either independently or synergistically with TLR9 or BCR engagement. CD180 is internalized after binding an unknown ligand, after which signaling occurs through an incompletely elucidated pathway (56). Thus, we postulate decreased surface expression of CD180 may reflect increased CD180 internalization and signaling in IIM patients.

We also identified a general decrease in circulating T cells expressing CXCR3. This may be due to CXCR3+ T cell migration into sites of inflammation. In support of this, interferon gamma and tumor necrosis factor alpha, which are increased in IIM, can induce secretion of the CXCR3 ligand CXCL10 by muscle fibers (57), and CXCR3+ T cells have been identified in the muscle biopsies of polymyositis, dermatomyositis, and inclusion body myositis patients (58). Of interest, CXCR3 ligands, CXCL9 and CXCL10, are increased in the serum of Jo1+ and SRP+ myositis patients (59), and CXCL10 is a validated disease activity biomarker for juvenile dermatomyositis (60).

The two immune endotypes identified here may have clinical correlations. Endotype 1 was hallmarked by increased CXCR4^{hi} surface expression across all immune subsets. Increased surface CXCR4 expression on circulating B and T cells was previously associated with increased disease severity in SLE (61) and 4/5 patients in our IIM cohort with this endotype were enrolled in the inpatient setting. We therefore postulate that the CXCR4^{hi} endotype is also associated with disease severity in IIM. Our sickest patient who was requiring extracorporeal membrane oxygenation also had the highest frequency of CXCR4^{hi} cells. Previously, CD4+CXCR4+ T cells were found to be correlated to high-resolution CT score, % predicted forced vital capacity, and 6-month mortality in IIM-ILD. *In vitro*, CD4+CXCR4+ T cells were found to stimulate fibroblast proliferation *via* IL-21, which was abrogated following co-culture with anti-IL21 blockade or tofacitinib (29). While CXCR4 can be upregulated by several stimuli (62–64), the cause of CXCR4 upregulation in IIM is currently unclear and represents a potential area of future research.

Endotype 2, comprised of the CD19+CD21loCD11c+ and CD4+CD27-PD1+ populations, may represent a pro-fibrotic phenotype. These CD19+ cells may represent DN2 B cells previously reported in SLE amongst patients with RNP antibodies, which are associated with skin and lung fibrosis. In those studies, DN2 B cells were characterized as CD19+CD21loCD27-IgD-CXCR5-CD24-CD11c+Tbet+, appeared to be plasma cell precursors, and were also exquisitely sensitive to TLR7 stimulation (65). The association of DN2 cells with RNP autoantibody positivity is of particular interest as this, like Pm/Scl, is an autoantibody that tends to be associated with features of systemic sclerosis, another fibrotic disease. In our study, most IIM patients with increased CD19+CD21loCD11c+ cells were Pm/Scl+. Alternatively, the numerous myeloid markers observed here raise the possibility that this CD19+ subset may not be of the B cell lineage (66, 67) or that the B cells may have acquired surface markers from follicular dendritic cells (68). CD4+PD1+ T cells have been reported in a number of fibrotic diseases including subglottic stenosis (69), idiopathic pulmonary fibrosis (IPF), and sarcoidosis (70). A trend towards increased frequency of CD4+PD1+ T cells has also been reported in systemic sclerosis (71).

Since these samples were obtained from an observational cohort, potential confounders, including steroid exposure, must be carefully considered. While sample size precluded formal multivariate and confounder analyses, qualitatively, there is no evidence that steroid exposure drove immune endotype. Four of the five patients with endotype 1 and 3/6 patients with endotype 2 were on at least 40 mg/day prednisone. Patients off all medications exhibited both immune endotypes. Additionally, CD180 surface expression and frequency of CXCR3+ T cells was decreased in all IIM patients, regardless of prednisone exposure. Future studies using larger IIM patient cohorts will be required to formally determine whether IIM medications contribute to the perturbed immune phenotypes identified here.

Studies identifying immunophenotypic signatures in rare diseases such as IIM are complicated by limited patient sample numbers, which limits the power to detect changes of modest magnitude or that are heterogeneously represented among the cohort. However, as our study demonstrates, supervised and unsupervised approaches successfully capture larger immune perturbations, which can provide important insight into disease biology. An additional limitation is the lack of concordant muscle or lung sampling precludes us from correlating our peripheral blood findings to end-organ inflammation and damage.

Overall, CyTOF facilitated simultaneous evaluation of multiple PBMC subsets using minimal sample with single cell resolution. Inclusion of hospitalized patients permitted us to investigate the entire spectrum of disease severity. Incorporating unsupervised analysis with traditional biaxial gating confirmed prior findings while also identifying novel subsets in a comprehensive and minimally biased way among IIM patients. The identification of two immune endotypes represents an important step forward in dissecting the immune phenotypes that contribute to clinical manifestations in IIM.

MYSTIC INVESTIGATORS

Ashley Blaske, Division of Rheumatology and Immunology, Vanderbilt University Medical Center, Nashville, TN, United States

Rosemarie B. Dudenhofer, Division of Allergy, Pulmonary, and Critical Care Medicine, Vanderbilt University Medical Center, Nashville TN, United States

Leslie J. Crofford, Division of Rheumatology and Immunology, Vanderbilt University Medical Center, Nashville, TN, United States*

Erin A. Gillaspie, Department of Thoracic Surgery, Vanderbilt University Medical Center, Nashville, TN, United States

Justin C. Hewlett, Division of Allergy, Pulmonary, and Critical Care Medicine, Vanderbilt University Medical Center, Nashville TN, United States

Joseph W. Houston, Division of Rheumatology and Immunology, Vanderbilt University Medical Center, Nashville, TN, United States

Susan Kroop, Division of Rheumatology and Immunology, Vanderbilt University Medical Center, Nashville, TN, United States

Kevin J. Myers, Division of Rheumatology and Immunology, Vanderbilt University Medical Center, Nashville, TN, United States

Stephanie G. Norfolk, Division of Allergy, Pulmonary, and Critical Care Medicine, Vanderbilt University Medical Center, Nashville TN, United States

Kristine Phillips, Division of Rheumatology and Immunology, Vanderbilt University Medical Center, Nashville, TN, United States

Todd W. Rice, Division of Allergy, Pulmonary, and Critical Care Medicine, Vanderbilt University Medical Center, Nashville TN, United States

Carla M. Sevin, Division of Allergy, Pulmonary, and Critical Care Medicine, Vanderbilt University Medical Center, Nashville, TN, United States

Bret Sohn, Division of Rheumatology and Immunology, Vanderbilt University Medical Center, Nashville, TN, United States

Melissa Warren, Division of Allergy, Pulmonary, and Critical Care Medicine, Vanderbilt University Medical Center, Nashville TN, United States

Erin M. Wilfong, Division of Rheumatology and Immunology, Vanderbilt University Medical Center, Nashville, TN, United States*

*Denotes members of the Writing Committee

ETHICS STATEMENT

The studies involving human participants were reviewed and approved by the Vanderbilt University Medical Center IRB#141415. The patients/participants provided their written informed consent to participate in this study.

AUTHOR CONTRIBUTIONS

EW designed the study, performed patient enrolment, clinical chart abstractions, formal analysis of CyTOF data, data interpretation, and wrote the initial draft. TB assisted with CITRUS analysis, performed marker enrichment analysis, and aided in data interpretation. KV designed the CyTOF panel and performed data acquisition. CW performed data analysis and aided in figure creation. JI directed data analysis, interpretation of data, and substantially revised the manuscript. PK designed the study, aided in interpretation of data, and guided data analysis. LC designed the study, performed patient enrolment, directed data analysis and interpretation, and substantially revised the manuscript. RB directed data analysis and interpretation and substantially revised the manuscript. All authors have read and approved the final manuscript.

REFERENCES

1. Bradford Rice J, White A, Lopez A, Galebach P, Schepman P, Popelar B, et al. Healthcare Resource Utilization and Work Loss in Dermatomyositis and Polymyositis Patients in a Privately-Insured US Population. *J Med Econ* (2016) 19(7):649–54. doi: 10.3111/13696998.2016.1151433
2. Johnson C, Pinal-Fernandez I, Parikh R, Paik J, Albayda J, Mammen AL, et al. Assessment of Mortality in Autoimmune Myositis With and Without Associated Interstitial Lung Disease. *Lung* (2016) 194(5):733–7. doi: 10.1007/s00408-016-9896-x
3. Opinc AH, Brzezinska OE, Makowska JS. Disability in Idiopathic Inflammatory Myopathies: Questionnaire-Based Study. *Rheumatol Int* (2019) 39(7):1213–20. doi: 10.1007/s00296-019-04302-y
4. Christopher-Stine L, Casciola-Rosen LA, Hong G, Chung T, Corse AM, Mammen AL. A Novel Autoantibody Recognizing 200-Kd and 100-Kd Proteins Is Associated With an Immune-Mediated Necrotizing Myopathy. *Arthritis Rheum* (2010) 62(9):2757–66. doi: 10.1002/art.27572
5. Mathews MB, Bernstein RM. Myositis Autoantibody Inhibits histidyl-tRNA Synthetase: A Model for Autoimmunity. *Nature* (1983) 304(5922):177–9. doi: 10.1038/304177a0
6. Mathews MB, Reichlin M, Hughes GR, Bernstein RM. Anti-threonyl-tRNA Synthetase, a Second Myositis-Related Autoantibody. *J Exp Med* (1984) 160 (2):420–34. doi: 10.1084/jem.160.2.420

7. Oddis CV, Okano Y, Rudert WA, Trucco M, Duquesnoy RJ, Medsger TA Jr. Serum Autoantibody to the Nucleolar Antigen PM-Scl. Clinical and Immunogenetic Associations. *Arthritis Rheum* (1992) 35(10):1211–7. doi: 10.1002/art.1780351014
8. Sato S, Hoshino K, Satoh T, Fujita T, Kawakami Y, Fujita T, et al. RNA Helicase Encoded by Melanoma Differentiation–Associated Gene 5 Is a Major Autoantigen in Patients With Clinically Amyopathic Dermatomyositis: Association With Rapidly Progressive Interstitial Lung Disease. *Arthritis Rheum* (2009) 60(7):2193–200. doi: 10.1002/art.24621
9. Targoff IN, Mamyrova G, Trieu EP, Perurena O, Koneru B, O'Hanlon TP, et al. A Novel Autoantibody to a 155-Kd Protein Is Associated With Dermatomyositis. *Arthritis Rheum* (2006) 54(11):3682–9. doi: 10.1002/art.22164
10. Cuesta-Mateos C, Colom-Fernández B, Portero-Sainz I, Tejedor R, García-García C, Concha-Garzón MJ, et al. Autoantibodies Against TIF-1-γ and CADM-140 in Spanish Patients With Clinically Amyopathic Dermatomyositis (CADM): Clinical Significance and Diagnostic Utility. *J Eur Acad Dermatol Venereol* (2015) 29(3):482–9. doi: 10.1111/jdv.12591
11. De Lorenzo R, Pinal-Fernandez I, Huang W, Albayda J, Tiniakou E, Johnson C, et al. Muscular and Extramuscular Clinical Features of Patients With Anti-PM/Scl Autoantibodies. *Neurology* (2018) 90(23):e2068-76. doi: 10.1212/WNL.0000000000005638
12. Lega JC, Fabien N, Reynaud Q, Durieu I, Durupt S, Dutertre M, et al. The Clinical Phenotype Associated With Myositis-Specific and Associated Autoantibodies: A Meta-Analysis Revisiting the So-Called Antisynthetase Syndrome. *Autoimmun Rev* (2014) 13(9):883–91. doi: 10.1016/j.autrev.2014.03.004
13. Marie I, Josse S, Decaux O, Dominique S, Diot E, Landron C, et al. Comparison of Long-Term Outcome Between Anti-Jo1- and Anti-PL7/PL12 Positive Patients With Antisynthetase Syndrome. *Autoimmun Rev* (2012) 11(10):739–45. doi: 10.1016/j.autrev.2012.01.006
14. Moghadam-Kia S, Oddis CV, Sato S, Kuwana M, Aggarwal R. Antimelanoma Differentiation-Associated Gene 5 Antibody: Expanding the Clinical Spectrum in North American Patients With Dermatomyositis. *J Rheumatol* (2017) 44(3):319–25. doi: 10.3899/jrheum.160682
15. Petri MH, Satoh M, Martin-Marquez BT, Vargas-Ramírez R, Jara LJ, Saavedra MA, et al. Implications in the Difference of Anti-Mi-2 and -P155/140 Autoantibody Prevalence in Two Dermatomyositis Cohorts From Mexico City and Guadalajara. *Arthritis Res Ther* (2013) 15(2):R48. doi: 10.1186/ar4222
16. Chow KV, Lew AM, Sutherland RM, Zhan Y. Monocyte-Derived Dendritic Cells Promote Th Polarization, Whereas Conventional Dendritic Cells Promote Th Proliferation. *J Immunol* (2016) 196(2):624. doi: 10.4049/jimmunol.1501202
17. Kapsenberg ML. Dendritic-Cell Control of Pathogen-Driven T-Cell Polarization. *Nat Rev Immunol* (2003) 3(12):984–93. doi: 10.1038/nri1246
18. Zhong H, Bao W, Li X, Miller A, Seery C, Haq N, et al. CD16+ Monocytes Control T-Cell Subset Development in Immune Thrombocytopenia. *Blood* (2012) 120(16):3326–35. doi: 10.1182/blood-2012-06-434605
19. DeFuria J, Belkina AC, Jagannathan-Bogdan M, Snyder-Cappione J, Carr JD, Nersesova YR, et al. B Cells Promote Inflammation in Obesity and Type 2 Diabetes Through Regulation of T-Cell Function and an Inflammatory Cytokine Profile. *Proc Natl Acad Sci* (2013) 110(13):5133–8. doi: 10.1073/pnas.1215840110
20. Flores-Borja F, Bosma A, Ng D, Reddy V, Ehrenstein MR, Isenberg DA, et al. CD19+CD24hiCD38hi B Cells Maintain Regulatory T Cells While Limiting TH1 and TH17 Differentiation. *Sci Trans Med* (2013) 5(173):173ra23–ra23. doi: 10.1126/scitranslmed.3005407
21. Li R, Rezk A, Miyazaki Y, Hilgenberg E, Touil H, Shen P, et al. Proinflammatory GM-CSF–producing B Cells in Multiple Sclerosis and B Cell Depletion Therapy. *Sci Trans Med* (2015) 7(310):310ra166–310ra166. doi: 10.1126/scitranslmed.aab4176
22. Wong S-C, Puaux A-L, Chittezhath M, Shalova I, Kajiji TS, Wang X, et al. Macrophage Polarization to a Unique Phenotype Driven by B Cells. *Eur J Immunol* (2010) 40(8):2296–307. doi: 10.1002/eji.200940288
23. Yanaba K, Bouaziz J-D, Haas KM, Poe JC, Fujimoto M, Tedder TF. A Regulatory B Cell Subset With a Unique CD1dhiCD5+ Phenotype Controls T Cell-Dependent Inflammatory Responses. *Immunity* (2008) 28(5):639–50. doi: 10.1016/j.immuni.2008.03.017
24. Torres-Ruiz J, Carrillo-Vazquez DA, Padilla-Ortiz DM, Vazquez-Rodriguez R, Nunez-Alvarez C, Juarez-Vega G, et al. TLR Expression in Peripheral Monocyte Subsets of Patients With Idiopathic Inflammatory Myopathies: Association With Clinical and Immunological Features. *J Transl Med* (2020) 18(1):125. doi: 10.1186/s12967-020-02290-3
25. Dimitri D, Benveniste O, Dubourg O, Maisonobe T, Eymard B, Amoura Z, et al. Shared Blood and Muscle CD8+ T-Cell Expansions in Inclusion Body Myositis. *Brain* (2006) 129(4):986–95. doi: 10.1093/brain/awl020
26. Dzangué-Tchoupou G, Allenbach Y, Preuße C, Stenzel W, Benveniste O. Mass Cytometry Reveals an Impairment of B Cell Homeostasis in Anti-Synthetase Syndrome. *J Neuroimmunol* (2019) 332:212–5. doi: 10.1016/j.jneuroim.2019.04.014
27. Piper CJM, Wilkinson MGL, Deakin CT, Otto GW, Dowle S, Duurland CL, et al. CD19(+)CD24(hi)CD38(hi) B Cells Are Expanded in Juvenile Dermatomyositis and Exhibit a Pro-Inflammatory Phenotype After Activation Through Toll-Like Receptor 7 and Interferon-Alpha. *Front Immunol* (2018) 9:1372. doi: 10.3389/fimmu.2018.01372
28. Lv J, Li L, Li W, Ji K, Hou Y, Yan C, et al. Role of the Chemokine Receptors CXCR3, CXCR4 and CCR7 in the Intramuscular Recruitment of Plasmacytoid Dendritic Cells in Dermatomyositis. *J Neuroimmunol* (2018) 319:142–8. doi: 10.1016/j.jneuroim.2018.01.008
29. Wang K, Zhao J, Chen Z, Li T, Tan X, Zheng Y, et al. CD4+CXCR4+ T Cells as a Novel Prognostic Biomarker in Patients With Idiopathic Inflammatory Myopathy-Associated Interstitial Lung Disease. *Rheumatology* (2019) 58 (3):511–21. doi: 10.1093/rheumatology/key341
30. Fecher P, Caspell R, Naeem V, Karulin AY, Kuerten S, Lehmann PV. B Cells and B Cell Blasts Withstand Cryopreservation While Retaining Their Functionality for Producing Antibody. *Cells* (2018) 7(6):50. doi: 10.3390/cells7060050
31. Jeurink PV, Vissers YM, Rappard B, Savelkoul HFJ. T Cell Responses in Fresh and Cryopreserved Peripheral Blood Mononuclear Cells: Kinetics of Cell Viability, Cellular Subsets, Proliferation, and Cytokine Production. *Cryobiology* (2008) 57(2):91–103. doi: 10.1016/j.cryobiol.2008.06.002
32. Kreher CR, Dittrich MT, Guerkov R, Boehm BO, Tary-Lehmann M. CD4+ and CD8+ Cells in Cryopreserved Human PBMC Maintain Full Functionality in Cytokine ELISPOT Assays. *J Immunol Methods* (2003) 278(1):79–93. doi: 10.1016/S0022-1759(03)00226-6
33. Verschoor CP, Kohli V. Cryopreserved Whole Blood for the Quantification of Monocyte, T-Cell and NK-Cell Subsets, and Monocyte Receptor Expression by Multi-Color Flow Cytometry: A Methodological Study Based on Participants From the Canadian Longitudinal Study on Aging. *Cytom Part A* (2018) 93(5):548–55. doi: 10.1002/cyto.a.23372
34. Maecker HT, McCoy JP, Nussenblatt R. Standardizing Immunophenotyping for the Human Immunology Project. *Nat Rev Immunol* (2012) 12(3):191–200. doi: 10.1038/nri3158
35. Duty JA, Szodoray P, Zheng NY, Koelsch KA, Zhang Q, Swiatkowski M, et al. Functional Anergy in a Subpopulation of Naive B Cells From Healthy Humans That Express Autoreactive Immunoglobulin Receptors. *J Exp Med* (2009) 206(1):139–51. doi: 10.1084/jem.20080611
36. Isnardi I, Ng YS, Menard L, Meyers G, Saadoun D, Srdanovic I, et al. Complement Receptor 2/CD21- Human Naive B Cells Contain Mostly Autoreactive Unresponsive Clones. *Blood* (2010) 115(24):5026–36. doi: 10.1182/blood-2009-09-243071
37. Kikuchi Y, Koarada S, Tada Y, Ushiyama O, Morito F, Suzuki N, et al. Difference in B Cell Activation Between Dermatomyositis and Polymyositis: Analysis of the Expression of RP105 on Peripheral Blood B Cells. *Ann Rheum Dis* (2001) 60(12):1137–40. doi: 10.1136/ard.60.12.1137
38. Kikuchi Y, Koarada S, Tada Y, Ushiyama O, Morito F, Suzuki N, et al. RP105-Lacking B Cells From Lupus Patients are Responsible for the Production of Immunoglobulins and Autoantibodies. *Arthritis Rheum* (2002) 46(12):3259–65. doi: 10.1002/art.10672
39. Nicholas MW, Dooley MA, Hogan SL, Anolik J, Looney J, Sanz I, et al. A Novel Subset of Memory B Cells Is Enriched in Autoreactivity and Correlates With Adverse Outcomes in SLE. *Clin Immunol* (2008) 126(2):189–201. doi: 10.1016/j.clim.2007.10.004
40. Simon Q, Pers JO, Cornec D, Le Pottier L, Mageed RA, Hillion S. In-Depth Characterization of CD24(high)CD38(high) Transitional Human B Cells Reveals Different Regulatory Profiles. *J Allergy Clin Immunol* (2016) 137 (5):1577 84.e10. doi: 10.1016/j.jaci.2015.09.014

41. Amir E-a, Davis KL, Tadmor MD, Simonds EF, Levine JH, Bendall SC, et al. viSNE Enables Visualization of High Dimensional Single-Cell Data and Reveals Phenotypic Heterogeneity of Leukemia. *Nat Biotechnol* (2013) 31 (6):545–52. doi: 10.1038/nbt.2594
42. Bruggner RV, Bodenmiller B, Dill DL, Tibshirani RJ, Nolan GP. Automated Identification of Stratifying Signatures in Cellular Subpopulations. *Proc Natl Acad Sci USA* (2014) 111(26):E2770–7. doi: 10.1073/pnas.1408792111
43. Van Gassen S, Callebaut B, Van Helden MJ, Lambrecht BN, Demeester P, Dhaene T, et al. FlowSOM: Using Self-Organizing Maps for Visualization and Interpretation of Cytometry Data. *Cytom Part A* (2015) 87(7):636–45. doi: 10.1002/cyto.a.22625
44. Weber LM, Robinson MD. Comparison of Clustering Methods for High-Dimensional Single-Cell Flow and Mass Cytometry Data. *Cytom Part A* (2016) 89(12):1084–96. doi: 10.1002/cyto.a.23030
45. Diggins KE, Greenplate AR, Leelatian N, Wogsland CE, Irish JM. Characterizing Cell Subsets Using Marker Enrichment Modeling. *Nat Methods* (2017) 14(3):275–8. doi: 10.1038/nmeth.4149
46. Young-Glazer J, Cisneros A, Wilfong EM, Smith SA, Crofford LJ, Bonami RH. Jo-1 Autoantigen-Specific B Cells Are Skewed Towards Distinct Functional B Cell Subsets in Anti-Synthetase Syndrome Patients. *Arthritis Res Ther* (2021) 23(1):33. doi: 10.1186/s13075-020-02412-8
47. Diggins KE, Ferrell PB Jr, Irish JM. Methods for Discovery and Characterization of Cell Subsets in High Dimensional Mass Cytometry Data. *Methods* (2015) 82:55–63. doi: 10.1016/j.ymeth.2015.05.008
48. McInnes L, Healy J, Melville J. *UMAP: Uniform Manifold Approximation and Projection for Dimension Reduction.* (2020).
49. Lundberg IE, Tjarnlund A, Bottai M, Werth VP, Pilkington C, Visser M, et al. 2017 European League Against Rheumatism/American College of Rheumatology Classification Criteria for Adult and Juvenile Idiopathic Inflammatory Myopathies and Their Major Subgroups. *Ann Rheum Dis* (2017) 76(12):1955–64. doi: 10.1136/annrheumdis-2017-211468
50. Wei C, Anolik J, Cappione A, Zheng B, Pugh-Bernard A, Brooks J, et al. A New Population of Cells Lacking Expression of CD27 Represents a Notable Component of the B Cell Memory Compartment in Systemic Lupus Erythematosus. *J Immunol* (2007) 178(10):6624–33. doi: 10.4049/jimmunol.178.10.6624
51. Wehr C, Eibel H, Masilamani M, Illges H, Schlesier M, Peter HH, et al. A New CD21low B Cell Population in the Peripheral Blood of Patients With SLE. *Clin Immunol* (2004) 113(2):161–71. doi: 10.1016/j.clim.2004.05.010
52. Dirks J, Fischer J, Haase G, Holl-Wieden A, Hofmann C, Girschick H, et al. CD21(lo/-)CD27(-)IgM(-) Double-Negative B Cells Accumulate in the Joints of Patients With Antinuclear Antibody-Positive Juvenile Idiopathic Arthritis. *Front Pediatr* (2021) 9:635815. doi: 10.3389/fped.2021.635815
53. Marrapodi R, Pellicano C, Radicchio G, Leodori G, Colantuono S, Iacolare A, et al. CD21low B Cells in Systemic Sclerosis: A Possible Marker of Vascular Complications. *Clin Immunol* (2020) 213:108364. doi: 10.1016/j.clim.2020.108364
54. Wilfong EM, Vowell KN, Bunn KE, Annapureddy N, Dudenhofer RB, Barnado A, et al. CD19+CD21lo/neg Cells Are Increased in Systemic Sclerosis Associated Interstitial Lung Disease. *Clin Exp Med* (2021). doi: 10.1007/s10238-021-00745-5
55. Pandya JM, Lundell A-C, Hallström M, Andersson K, Nordström I, Rudin A. Circulating T Helper and T Regulatory Subsets in Untreated Early Rheumatoid Arthritis and Healthy Control Subjects. *J Leuk Biol* (2016) 100 (4):823–33. doi: 10.1189/jlb.5A0116-025R
56. Schultz TE, Blumenthal A. The RP105/MD-1 Complex: Molecular Signaling Mechanisms and Pathophysiological Implications. *J Leukoc Biol* (2017) 101 (1):183–92. doi: 10.1189/jlb.2VMR1215-582R
57. Crescioli C, Sottili M, Bonini P, Cosmi L, Chiarugi P, Romagnani P, et al. Inflammatory Response in Human Skeletal Muscle Cells: CXCL10 as a Potential Therapeutic Target. *Eur J Cell Biol* (2012) 91(2):139–49. doi: 10.1016/j.ejcb.2011.09.011
58. De Paepe B, De Keyzer K, Martin JJ, De Bleecker JL. Alpha-Chemokine Receptors CXCR1-3 and Their Ligands in Idiopathic Inflammatory Myopathies. *Acta Neuropathol* (2005) 109(6):576–82. doi: 10.1007/s00401-005-0989-5
59. Richards TJ, Eggebeen A, Gibson K, Yousem S, Fuhrman C, Gochuico BR, et al. Characterization and Peripheral Blood Biomarker Assessment of Anti–Jo-1 Antibody–Positive Interstitial Lung Disease. *Arthritis Rheum* (2009) 60 (7):2183–92. doi: 10.1002/art.24631
60. Wienke J, Bellutti Enders F, Lim J, Mertens JS, van den Hoogen LL, Wijngaarde CA, et al. Galectin-9 and CXCL10 as Biomarkers for Disease Activity in Juvenile Dermatomyositis: A Longitudinal Cohort Study and Multicohort Validation. *Arthritis Rheumatol* (2019) 71(8):1377–90. doi: 10.1002/art.40881
61. Wang A, Guilpain P, Chong BF, Chouzenoux S, Guillevin L, Du Y, et al. Dysregulated Expression of CXCR4/CXCL12 in Subsets of Patients With Systemic Lupus Erythematosus. *Arthritis Rheum* (2010) 62(11):3436–46. doi: 10.1002/art.27685
62. Duchesneau P, Gallagher E, Walcheck B, Waddell TK. Up-Regulation of Leukocyte CXCR4 Expression by Sulfatide: An L-Selectin-Dependent Pathway on CD4+ T Cells. *Eur J Immunol* (2007) 37(10):2949–60. doi: 10.1002/eji.200737118
63. Jourdan P, Abbal C, Noraz N, Hori T, Uchiyama T, Vendrell JP, et al. IL-4 Induces Functional Cell-Surface Expression of CXCR4 on Human T Cells. *J Immunol* (1998) 160(9):4153–7.
64. Jourdan P, Vendrell J-P, Huguet M-F, Segondy M, Bousquet J, Pène J, et al. Cytokines and Cell Surface Molecules Independently Induce CXCR4 Expression on CD4+ CCR7+ Human Memory T Cells. *J Immunol* (2000) 165(2):716–24. doi: 10.4049/jimmunol.165.2.716
65. Jenks SA, Cashman KS, Zumaquero E, Marigorta UM, Patel AV, Wang X, et al. Distinct Effector B Cells Induced by Unregulated Toll-Like Receptor 7 Contribute to Pathogenic Responses in Systemic Lupus Erythematosus. *Immunity* (2018) 49(4):725–39.e6. doi: 10.1016/j.immuni.2018.08.015
66. Baban B, Hansen AM, Chandler PR, Manlapat A, Bingaman A, Kahler DJ, et al. A Minor Population of Splenic Dendritic Cells Expressing CD19 Mediates IDO-Dependent T Cell Suppression *via* Type I IFN Signaling Following B7 Ligation. *Int Immunol* (2005) 17(7):909–19. doi: 10.1093/intimm/dxh271
67. Munn DH, Sharma MD, Hou D, Baban B, Lee JR, Antonia SJ, et al. Expression of Indoleamine 2,3-Dioxygenase by Plasmacytoid Dendritic Cells in Tumor-Draining Lymph Nodes. *J Clin Invest* (2004) 114(2):280–90. doi: 10.1172/JCI21583
68. Suzuki K, Grigorova I, Phan TG, Kelly LM, Cyster JG. Visualizing B Cell Capture of Cognate Antigen From Follicular Dendritic Cells. *J Exp Med* (2009) 206(7):1485–93. doi: 10.1084/jem.20090209
69. Davis RJ, Lina I, Ding D, Engle EL, Taube J, Gelbard A, et al. Increased Expression of PD-1 and PD-L1 in Patients With Laryngotracheal Stenosis. *Laryngoscope* (2020) 131(5):967–74. doi: 10.1002/lary.28790
70. Celada LJ, Kropski JA, Herazo-Maya JD, Luo W, Creecy A, Abad AT, et al. PD-1 Up-Regulation on CD4(+) T Cells Promotes Pulmonary Fibrosis Through STAT3-Mediated IL-17A and TGF-Beta1 Production. *Sci Transl Med* (2018) 10(460):eaar8356. doi: 10.1126/scitranslmed.aar8356
71. Fleury M, Belkina AC, Proctor EA, Zammitti C, Simms RW, Lauffenburger DA, et al. Increased Expression and Modulated Regulatory Activity of Coinhibitory Receptors PD-1, TIGIT, and TIM-3 in Lymphocytes From Patients With Systemic Sclerosis. *Arthritis Rheumatol* (2018) 70(4):566–77. doi: 10.1002/art.40399

20

COVID-19 Disease and Dermatomyositis

Jie Qian and Hui Xu*

Department of Rheumatology, Affiliated Hospital of Nantong University, Nantong, China

***Correspondence:**
Jie Qian
drqianjie@126.com

The pandemic of coronavirus disease 2019 (COVID-19) caused by SARS-CoV-2 has caused a large number of deaths, and there is still no effective treatment. COVID-19 can induce a systemic inflammatory response, and its clinical manifestations are diverse. Recently, it has been reported that COVID-19 patients may develop myositis and interstitial pulmonary disease similar to dermatomyositis (DM). This condition is similar to the rapidly progressive interstitial lung disease associated with $MDA5^+$ DM that has a poor prognosis and high mortality, and this poses a challenge for an early identification. Suppression of the immune system can protect COVID-19 patients by preventing the production of inflammatory cytokines. This article attempts to explore the possibility of a relationship between COVID-19 and DM in terms of the potential pathogenesis and clinical features and to analyze the therapeutic effect of the immunosuppressive drugs that are commonly used for the treatment of both DM and COVID-19.

Keywords: SARS-CoV-2, COVID-19, dermatomyositis, pathogenesis, treatment

INTRODUCTION

In December 2019, a novel infectious disease caused by severe acute respiratory syndrome coronavirus 2 (SARS-CoV-2) was reported (1). Compared with SARS-CoV and MERS-CoV, SARS-CoV-2 is more infectious; therefore, coronavirus disease 2019 (COVID-19) has become a global epidemic. The most common symptoms of COVID-19 are fever, cough, dyspnea, myalgia, and fatigue (2), and pulmonary involvement is significantly associated with a poor prognosis and a high mortality. Viruses can cause a variety of autoimmune diseases, and patients with autoimmune diseases are more susceptible to infection due to the pathogenesis of the autoimmune disease and/or the use of immunosuppressants. Among the potential autoimmune diseases that may be related to COVID-19, the most intriguing is idiopathic inflammatory myopathy (IIM), a heterogeneous disease that primarily affects the skeletal muscles and can be divided into polymyositis, dermatomyositis (DM), immune-mediated necrotizing myopathy, anti-synthase syndrome, and inclusion body myositis (3). During the COVID-19 outbreak, several studies have recognized a striking similarity between COVID-19 and DM due to the lung and muscle involvement and the presence of a rash. DM typically presents with characteristic skin manifestations that accompany or precede muscle weakness, and interstitial lung disease (ILD) is a common complication of DM. The pathogenesis of DM is still unclear, although it is likely associated with inappropriate complement activation and interferon (IFN) response (4, 5), which results in the production of myositis-specific autoantibodies that may be related to unique clinical features. Obviously, COVID-19 is closely related to DM.

COVID-19 AND AUTOIMMUNITY

For many infections, the immune system provides an appropriate response that mediates resistance to the invading microorganism. Appropriate innate and adaptive responses promote the coordinated production of proinflammatory cytokines that can control pathogens. Several environmental factors have been suspected to trigger or even exacerbate existing autoimmune conditions in genetically susceptible patients, and these factors include viral, bacterial, and parasitic infections (6). Viruses can induce autoimmunity in genetically susceptible individuals through multiple mechanisms, including molecular mimicry, epitope spreading, bystander activation, and the immortalization of infected B cells. Chronic relapsing/reactivated infections caused by Epstein-Barr virus (EBV) are associated with the occurrence or onset of various autoimmune diseases, including DM (7). Similar to SARS-CoV, SARS-CoV-2 uses the membranous angiotensin-converting enzyme 2 (ACE2) receptors to enter human cells (8). Then, SARS-CoV-2 can trigger innate and adaptive immune responses, known as cytokine storms. This abnormal elevation of inflammatory cytokines, such as interleukin (IL)-1, IL-6, IL-10, interferon γ (IFN-γ), monocyte chemotactic protein-1 (MCP-1), and granulocyte-macrophage colony-stimulating factor, can interact with the complement and coagulation systems, leading to acute respiratory distress syndrome, disseminated intravascular coagulation, and even multiple organ failure (9). Li et al. demonstrated significant expression of ACE2 receptors on alveolar epithelial cells, which may explain why pulmonary involvement is a hallmark of COVID-19 (10). A retrospective study revealed that SARS-CoV-2 might act primarily on lymphocytes, especially T lymphocytes. Moreover, patients with severe COVID-19 had higher neutrophils and fewer lymphocytes than patients with mild COVID-19, indicating that an increased neutrophil-to-lymphocyte ratio (NLR) in patients with severe COVID-19 and the use of lymphocyte subset monitoring are helpful for early screening, diagnosis, and treatment of severe COVID-19 (11).

PATHOGENESIS AND CLINICAL CHARACTERISTICS OF DM

DM is a rare disease characterized by distinct cutaneous manifestations and a clinically heterogeneous systemic presentation. Pathognomonic skin manifestations such as Gottron's papules and heliotrope rash are conducive to the early diagnosis of DM. Therefore, DM can be difficult to diagnose in the absence of the characteristic dermatologic features. DM has been suggested to occur more frequently in women and African Americans (12), and the age range of the patients at the time of the diagnosis of DM is bimodal, with the peak frequencies occurring in 5- to 14-year-old children and in 40- to 60-year-old adults (13). Epidemiological data has demonstrated that subsets of DM patients that were diagnosed by the presence of different myositis-specific autoantibodies tend to be diagnosed at specific times of the year (14). The pathogeneses of the different types and subtypes of myositis are incompletely understood. Predisposition to IIM are attributable to genetic and environmental factors, and viral or bacterial infections may induce the occurrence of the disease. The seasonal clustering of symptoms suggests that viral or bacterial infections could be common environmental triggers. A case-control study showed that a higher number EBV genomes are present and that anti-Epstein-Barr nuclear antigen 1 antibodies were detected at a higher frequency in DM patients than in healthy control counterparts (15). Autoimmune mechanisms are important in the pathogenesis of IIM, and myositis-specific or associated autoantibodies can be observed in patients with IIM, which is often associated with particular clinical features (16). With the further study of DM, many novel autoantibodies against myositis have been found, including anti-melanoma differentiation-associated gene 5 (MDA5), anti-transcriptional intermediary factor 1 γ, anti-nuclear matrix protein 2, anti-Ku and anti-Mi-2 (17). Anti-MDA5$^+$ DM is typically associated with rapidly progressive interstitial lung disease (RP-ILD), which has a high early mortality (18). It is still controversial whether the immune activation seen in DM is antibody-dependent or is triggered by a classical complement cascade (4). The IFN pathway is activated in the different clinical subtypes of myositis, and type 1 IFN1 is most upregulated in DM patients (5). The expression level of IFN-induced genes was correlated with the indicators of DM disease activity (19). Three different ligand families activate the IFN pathway by binding to cell surface receptors and by stimulating the expression of IFN-inducible genes *via* the Janus kinase (JAK)/signal transducer and the activator of transcription (STAT) signaling pathway (20). A persistent IFN response promotes antigen presentation and lymphocyte responses and induces chemokine expression, and the resulting T and B cell activation may also be responsible for the production of autoantibodies (20).

Approximately 80% of DM patients have myopathy, which usually presents as proximal muscle weakness (4). Extramuscular involvement is common in IIM; the skin, lungs, joints, heart, and gastrointestinal tract can be affected in IIM; and the degree of involvement varies according to the different subtypes of IIM (21). ILD is a common complication of DM, and the severity of the pulmonary symptoms varies among patients with different subtypes (22). Patients with mild ILD are stable and respond well to treatment, while some patients with RP-ILD have more severe disease and have a poor prognosis (23, 24). In addition, the extent of muscle involvement can also be fatal for DM patients because weakness of the intercostal muscles may lead to respiratory disorders and acute respiratory distress syndrome (25).

CORRELATION ON COVID-19 AND DM

The similarity of COVID-19 and DM implies a common underlying mechanism (**Figure 1**). MDA5, a myositis-specific autoantibody, is an intracellular sensor of the intermediates or

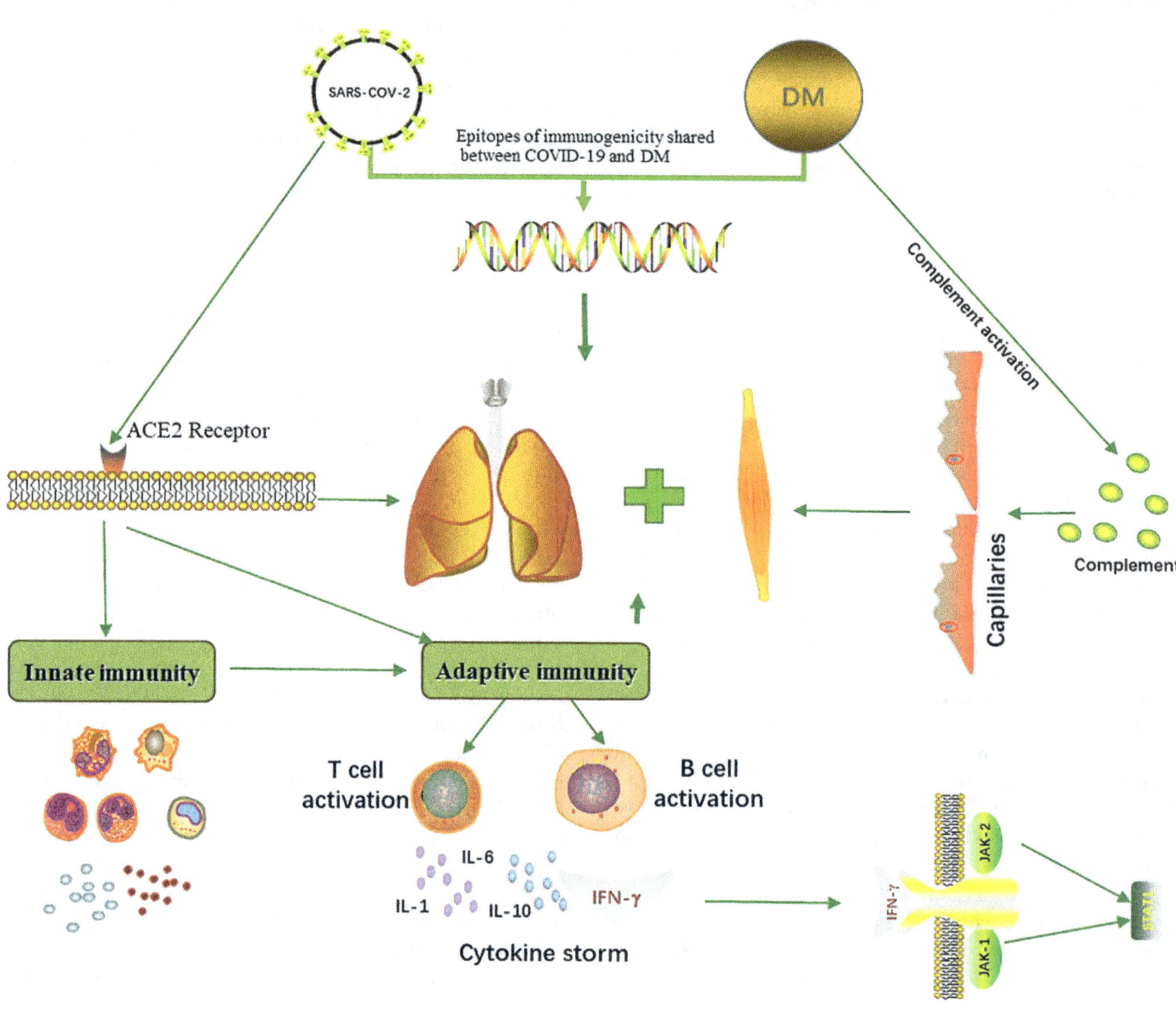

FIGURE 1 | Common pathogenetic mechanisms between COVID-19 and DM. COVID-19 and DM share three immunogenic linear epitopes with high sequence consistency. SARS-CoV-2 enters human cells through the membranous angiotensin-converting enzyme 2 (ACE2) receptors, triggering an innate and adaptive immune response. This initiates the production of cytokines such as IL-1, IL-6, IL-10 and IFN-γ, which can induce lung and muscle damage. The activation of complement in DM patients results in capillary destruction, which further affects multiple organs, and cytokine storms are associated with the occurrence of certain subtypes of DM.

byproducts of double-stranded RNA viral replication that trigger the innate response and subsequent production of cytokines that activate macrophages and helper T cells (26). Increased levels of several cytokines, such as IFN-γ, IL-8, and MCP-1 (which are similar to the cytokine storms seen in severe COVID-19 patients), were found in patients with anti-MDA5^{+} DM (27). IFN1, which plays a major role in the muscle fiber damage in DM patients, is involved in the organ damage seen in COVID-19 (28). Megremis et al. proposed that DM patients have three linear epitopes of immunogenicity that have a high sequence identity with the SARS-CoV-2 protein; thus, a potential exposure to a virus within the coronavirus family may lead to the development of DM (29). An Italian patient study reported a higher prevalence of COVID-19 in patients with autoimmune diseases than in the general population (30). Movahedi et al. noticed a sudden outbreak of new cases of juvenile dermatomyositis during the COVID-19 pandemic, with a higher incidence among women (31). Notably, 76.5% of COVID-19 patients are women (30), and the ratio of males to females in DM is 1:2 (4). Autoimmune diseases are generally more prevalent in women than men, with the strongest sex biases seen in Sjogren's syndrome, systemic lupus erythematosus, autoimmune thyroid disease, and scleroderma (32). Estrogen, especially 17-β estradiol and prolactin, can act as humoral immune enhancers, which causes women to be more susceptible to autoimmune diseases (33). In addition, because of incomplete X chromosome inactivation caused by random silencing in females during the early stages of embryogenesis, several immune-related genes may be upregulated, and their overexpression may influence the immune response (34, 35). Several cases of DM associated with COVID-19 have been summarized (**Table 1**). Of the seven patients that were reported to have both DM and COVID-19, 85.7% were female, and two of these patients were anti-MDA5$^+$. Most patients had distinct cutaneous manifestations, with elevated CK. In addition, the female mortality was 33.3%, even after receiving aggressive treatment. Based on our summary table, we should raise awareness of the fact that women are more susceptible to COVID-19 combined with DM and experience more severe conditions, and effective treatment interventions would help to improve survival. It is increasingly recognized that the features of severe COVID-19 are similar to those of DM, especially anti-MDA5$^+$ DM because these conditions have similar involvement of the lung and are associated with the development of rash, fatigue, and myalgia. In addition, the imaging findings of COVID-19 are comparable to those of the ILD seen in anti-MDA5$^+$ DM because diffuse ground-glass opacifications are often present in both of these diseases, and the presence of the ground-glass opacifications suggest peribronchovascular consolidation (26). Compared with other DM subtypes, the RP-ILD seen in anti-MDA5$^+$ DM usually develops rapidly, rarely relapses, and responds poorly to glucocorticoids and immunosuppressants, which seems to be similar to a viral infection (27). In recent case reports, autoantibodies against myositis, such as anti-MDA5, anti-SAE, anti-Mi2, anti-Ku, and anti-Ro52, have been detected in COVID-19 patients with DM. Viral infections seem to be associated with certain subtypes of DM.

More than 10% of COVID-19 patients were reported to have muscular symptoms and elevated CK levels (43). Muscle biopsies from patients with COVID-19 show abnormal presence of Myxovirus resistance protein A in muscle fibers and capillaries. Myxovirus resistance protein A is one of the IFN1-inducible proteins, is overexpressed in biopsy muscle specimens from DM patients and may be a more sensitive marker of DM (44, 45), suggesting that autoimmune myositis may be caused by COVID-19. The SARS-CoV-2 receptor ACE2 is expressed in a variety of human tissues, including the skeletal muscles, where ACE2 expression is the lowest (10). The expression and distribution of ACE2 remind us that SARS-CoV-2 may cause muscle injury through direct or indirect mechanisms. Beydon et al. reported a case of this type of myositis diagnosed by MRI (46). However, SARS-CoV, which has the same receptor as SARS-CoV-2, was not found in the muscle tissue of the patient at autopsy (47, 48). In addition, the muscle manifestations of COVID-19 patients can be contributed to rhabdomyolysis caused by SARS-CoV-2 (49). Rhabdomyolysis is a life-threatening disease that requires aggressive hydration in order to avoid acute renal failure, which can worsen the oxygenation status in COVID-19 patients (49, 50). Therefore, when patients have focal muscle pain and fatigue, the possibility of rhabdomyolysis should be taken seriously (50). Symptoms of myopathy in severe systemic viral diseases are multifactorial, and further muscle biopsies and antibody screening are required.

TREATMENT OPTIONS

Since hyperinflammation underlies COVID-19 and is associated with the disease severity, anti-inflammatory therapy may be beneficial to patients. Immune impairment may inhibit viral-induced cytokine storm syndrome (11). Immunosuppressive agents have a variety of mechanisms targeting the cellular and humoral immune responses, so the use of immunosuppressive agents may have a protective effect for COVID-19 patients. Along with the increased understanding of COVID-19, several drugs commonly used to treat DM have potential therapeutic effects for COVID-19 patients.

TABLE 1 | Cases of COVID-19-associated DM.

Authors	Year	Sex	Age	Antibody	Clinical characteristics	Treatment	Outcomes
Zhang et al. (36)	2020	F	58	Anti-SSA, Anti-SAE, Anti-Ku	Muscle weakness, dyspnea, myalgia, CK↑	Antiviral drug, MP, HCQ, tocilizumab	Recovered
Kogami et al. (37)	2020	F	46	Anti-MDA5	Erythematous papules	Antiviral drug	Recovered
Cao et al. (38)	2020	F	45	Anti-Ro52	Fever, myalgia, Gottron's sign, RP-ILD, ferritin↑, IL-6↑, CK↑, LDH↑	Antiviral drug, MP, CTX, IVIG	Died
Borges et al. (39)	2021	F	36	Anti-Mi2	Sore throat, fatigue, Gottron's papules, muscle weakness, Raynaud phenomenon, CK↑	MP	Recovered
Quintana-Ortega et al. (40)	2021	F	11	Anti-MDA5, Anti- Ro/SSA	Gottron's papules with calcinosis, heliotrope rash, palmar papules, dysphagia, cervical subcutaneous emphysema, RP-ILD, SF↑, IL-6↑	Antiviral drug, glucocorticoids, HCQ, MMF, TAC, CTX, tocilizumab, tofacitinib, IVIG, PE	Died
Ho et al. (41)	2021	M	58	NA	Fatigue, myalgias, muscle weakness, Gottron's sign, heliotrope rash, CK↑	Glucocorticoids, MTX,	Recovered
Liquidano-Perez et al. (42)	2021	F	4	Anti-RNP/Sm, Anti-Scl-70, Anti-Sm	Muscle weakness, Gottron's papules, heliotrope rash, dysphagia, CK↑	Glucocorticoids, HCQ, MTX, CsA, IVIG	Recovered

CK, creatine kinase; CTX, cyclophosphamide; CsA, cyclosporine; DM, dermatomyositis; F, female; HCQ, hydroxychloroquine; IL-6, interleukin-6; IVIG, Intravenous immunoglobulin; LDH, lactate dehydrogenase; M, male; MMF, mycophenolatemofetil; MP, methylprednisolone; MTX, methotrexate; NA, not available; PE, plasmapheresis; RP-ILD, rapidly progressive interstitial lung disease; TAC, tacrolimus.

Glucocorticoids

Glucocorticoids inhibit inflammatory cytokines and reduce the proliferation and differentiation of lymphocytes and macrophages, and they have immunosuppressive effects on the body and may increase susceptibility to COVID-19 (51). There is no evidence that patients infected with COVID-19 benefit from glucocorticoids, and COVID-19 patients may be more prone to the side effects of glucocorticoid treatment (52). However, retrospective analyses have shown that the use of glucocorticoids reduces hospital mortality in patients with COVID-19 cytokine storms (53). Dexamethasone has been shown to reduce the mortality in patients with COVID-19 who receive invasive mechanical ventilation (54). Strangfeld et al. reported a higher mortality rate in patients receiving higher dosages of glucocorticoids (>10 mg/day prednisolone equivalent dose) than in those who did not receive glucocorticoids (55). The efficacy of glucocorticoids in COVID-19 is controversial, especially in terms of doses and risk of side effects.

Conventional Synthetic Disease-Modifying Antirheumatic Drugs

Some conventional synthetic disease-modifying antirheumatic drugs (csDMARDs), such as methotrexate, hydroxychloroquine (HCQ), and azathioprine, suppress the cytokine storm associated with COVID-19 (11). Methotrexate, a dihydrofolate reductase inhibitor, is widely used in autoimmune diseases because of its pleiotropic therapeutic effects on various immune cells and mediators and its inhibition of the body's overall inflammatory response (56). In patients with DM, the use of HCQ can effectively improve the skin lesions. Chloroquine (CQ) blocks the fusion of the virus to the host cell by interfering with the terminal glycosylation of the cell receptor, ACE2, and by inhibiting sialic acid biosynthesis, which is used as a receptor by the viruses through inhibiting quinine reductase-2 (57). On the other hand, CQ can also play an antiviral role by reducing IFN1 (51). Wang et al. found that CQ played an important role in multiple stages of COVID-19 *in vitro*, and it had immunomodulatory effects that synergically enhanced its antiviral effects (58). However, the mortality of COVID-19 patients treated with HCQ increased, and there was no benefit from CQ (59). In addition, adverse drug reactions associated with CQ and HCQ increased dramatically during the COVID-19 pandemic (60). Mycophenolate mofetil, calcineurin inhibitors, and cyclophosphamide as immunosuppressants have also shown a good therapeutic effect in the treatment of myositis. Mycophenolate mofetil is an inhibitor of purine synthesis that inhibits inosine monophosphate dehydrogenase, reduces lymphocyte proliferation, and has antifibrosis properties (61). Mycophenolate mofetil showed anti-SARS-COV-2 activity and it could be worth considering used for clinical treatment of COVID-19 (62). In addition, tacrolimus and cyclosporine produced dose-dependent inhibitory effects on NK cell degranulation and IFN-γ *in vitro* (63), and tacrolimus also reduced the ability of dendritic cells to stimulate T cells, resulting in decreased production of CXCL-10 and IL-12 (64). Tacrolimus has a positive effect on survival in liver transplant patients with symptoms of COVID-19 compared to other immunosuppressants, including cyclosporine and mycophenolate mofetil (65). Nevertheless, there was no improvement in severe COVID-19 patients who received a combination of methylprednisolone pulses and tacrolimus (66). A prospective study demonstrated that a combination of high-dose glucocorticoids, tacrolimus and intravenous cyclophosphamide improved survival in anti-MDA5$^+$ DM patients complicated with ILD. This regimen also has an increased risk of opportunistic infections, leading to an exacerbation of ILD (67). Some csDMARDs, such as methotrexate, mycophenolate mofetil, and tacrolimus may provide a therapeutic strategy for COVID-19. The efficacy and safety of CQ and HCQ remain controversial and need further research.

Interleukin Receptor Antagonists

Considering the mechanism of COVID-19, cytokine-targeting biologicals and signaling molecule inhibitors are also promising therapeutic approaches (11). Anakinra is a recombinant IL-1 receptor antagonist that can be used to treat autoinflammatory diseases (51). Zong et al. demonstrated that patients with myositis may respond to anakinra, especially DM patients with skin rash (68). Currently, a study is underway that combines anakinra with anti-IFN-γ antibodies for the treatment of patients with COVID-19 (51). IL-6 is a pleiotropic cytokine that plays a key role in the cytokine storm. The IL-6 receptor antagonist tocilizumab is used for the treatment of refractory juvenile DM (69). Tocilizumab may be a salvage therapy for anti-MDA5$^+$ DM associated with RP-ILD patients refractory to an intensive immunosuppressive regimen (70). A retrospective study of patients with severe COVID-19 showed that tocilizumab improved the clinical symptoms and that the early use of tocilizumab effectively controlled the progression of the symptoms (71). Another study also demonstrated that corticosteroids combined with tocilizumab or anakinra reduced mortality in hospitalized patients with COVID-19 and that corticosteroids combined with tocilizumab had better survival outcomes (53). Interleukin receptor antagonists anakinra and tocilizumab may be alternative drugs for COVID-19 patients, but given the intrinsic limitations of retrospective studies, randomized clinical trials are still warranted.

JAK Inhibitors

JAK inhibitors are novel target synthetic immunoregulatory agents that not only inhibit tyrosine kinases, which are involved in intracellular viral transport and epithelial endocytosis, but also inhibit intracellular signal transduction of various inflammatory cytokines (51). A patient with refractory JDM was described as having clinical improvement after treatment with baricitinib. The JAK inhibitor baricitinib binds to cyclin G-associated kinases, a regulator of endocytosis, to block the entry of SARS-CoV-2 into cells and the inflammatory cytokine storm (72). A randomized controlled trial demonstrated that baricitinib combined with remdesivir reduced the recovery time in COVID-19 patients, especially in patients receiving high-flow oxygen or noninvasive ventilation, and it also accelerated the clinical improvement of patients and was associated fewer serious adverse events (73). In the early phase of COVID-19, baricitinib may prevent an excessive inflammatory response and the rapid progression of respiratory failure (74). Kurasawa et al. proposed that tofacitinib combined with conventional treatment might control refractory MDA5$^+$ DM complicated with ILD (75). Furthermore, tofacitinib improved the survival 6 months after the onset of anti-MDA5+ amyopathic DM-associated ILD (76). In a randomized controlled trial, tofacitinib reduced the incidences of mortality and respiratory failure in patients with COVID-19 (77). Baricitinib and tofacitinib can cause thrombosis, and patients with COVID-19 are in hypercoagulable states; therefore, careful monitoring for the development of thrombosis during treatment with JAK inhibitors is necessary (78). JAK inhibitors, such as baricitinib and tofacitinib could be available treatments for COVID-19, thrombosis should be paid extensive attention to.

Intravenous Immunoglobulin and Plasmapheresis

Intravenous immunoglobulin (IVIG) is effective in the treatment of refractory DM (79). IVIG improves patient strength, reduces mortality, and promotes recovery. There is a potential for patients with COVID-19 to respond to early immunotherapy, especially IVIG, which may also provide a variety of potential protective antibodies and anti-cytokine effects (80). Elevated cytokine levels are found in the sera of DM patients with ILD, and plasmapheresis is an option to remove the elevated cytokines as an additional supportive treatment (27, 67). Immunoglobulin and plasmapheresis might be considered in patients affected with SARS-CoV-2. A retrospective study demonstrated that COVID-19 patients who were not treated with DMARDs had a higher mortality rate than those who received methotrexate monotherapy, while leflunomide, antimalarials, TNF inhibitors, abatacept, belimumab, and IL-6 inhibitors were not associated with an increased risk of death (55). The efficacy of high-dose corticosteroids, IVIG, JAK inhibitors, and T-cell modulators for COVID-19 has been reported in a small series of cases, and clinical trials are currently under investigation (81).

CONCLUSION AND PERSPECTIVES

During the recent pandemic, several cases of COVID-19 were reported to be related to DM. In this review article, we discussed the possible relationship between COVID-19 and DM based on the similar potential pathogenic mechanisms and clinical manifestations. More importantly, we provide a direction for the treatment of COVID-19 through an analysis of immunosuppressive agents that are commonly used for DM. We have highlighted that the manifestations of DM, such as ILD and myositis, can also be observed in patients with COVID-19. Therefore, these manifestations of DM are difficult to distinguish in the early clinical stages, and even certain subtypes of DM my involve the same immune response that is caused by COVID-19. It is noteworthy that women have been more susceptible to DM during the COVID-19 pandemic and have more severe clinical symptoms, which means that extensive clinical attention should be given to the possibility of autoimmune diseases in female patients with COVID-19 and that the treatment regimens should be more aggressive in these patients.

In conclusion, infection with SARS-CoV-2 can induce the occurrence of DM. COVID-19 and DM potentially have a common pathogenesis, such as IFN1, which not only participates in organ damage of COVID-19 but also mediates muscle fiber damage in patients with DM. Although there have been some studies supporting the relationship between COVID-19 and DM, the exact mechanism is largely unknown, and more evidence is needed to confirm this association. Routinely available drugs for DM have provided an alternative therapeutic strategy for COVID-19. Further studies should be done to assess the efficacy and safety of the regimen to tackle the inflammatory stages of COVID-19. We recommend that all newly diagnosed DM cases should be tested for COVID-19 during the pandemic, especially for certain subtypes of DM patients, such as anti-MDA5+, and early differential diagnosis is helpful to improve the survival of these patients.

AUTHOR CONTRIBUTIONS

JQ: study design, data analysis, and manuscript revision. HX: literature search, data collection, and article writing. All authors contributed to the article and approved the submitted version.

REFERENCES

1. Zhou P, Yang XL, Wang XG, Hu B, Zhang L, Zhang W, et al. A Pneumonia Outbreak Associated With a New Coronavirus of Probable Bat Origin. *Nat* (2020) 579:270–3. doi: 10.1038/s41586-020-2012-7
2. Meo SA, Alhowikan AM, Al-Khlaiwi T, Meo IM, Halepoto DM, Iqbal M, et al. Novel Coronavirus 2019-Ncov: Prevalence, Biological and Clinical Characteristics Comparison With SARS-CoV and MERS-CoV. *Eur Rev Med Pharmacol Sci* (2020) 24:2012–9. doi: 10.26355/eurrev_202002_20379
3. Vencovský J, Alexanderson H, Lundberg IE. Idiopathic Inflammatory Myopathies. *Rheum Dis Clin North Am* (2019) 45:569–81. doi: 10.1016/j.rdc.2019.07.006
4. DeWane ME, Waldman R, Lu J. Dermatomyositis: Clinical Features and Pathogenesis. *J Am Acad Dermatol* (2020) 82:267–81. doi: 10.1016/j.jaad.2019.06.1309
5. Pinal-Fernandez I, Casal-Dominguez M, Derfoul A, Pak K, Plotz P, Miller FW, et al. Identification of Distinctive Interferon Gene Signatures in Different Types of Myositis. *Neurol* (2019) 93:e1193–204. doi: 10.1212/wnl.0000000000008128
6. Bax CE, Maddukuri S, Ravishankar A, Pappas-Taffer L, Werth VP. Environmental Triggers of Dermatomyositis: A Narrative Review. *Ann Transl Med* (2021) 9:434. doi: 10.21037/atm-20-3719
7. Houen G, Trier NH. Epstein-Barr Virus and Systemic Autoimmune Diseases. *Front Immunol* (2021) 11:587380. doi: 10.3389/fimmu.2020.587380
8. Zhang H, Penninger JM, Li Y, Zhong N, Slutsky AS. Angiotensin-Converting Enzyme 2 (ACE2) as a SARS-CoV-2 Receptor: Molecular Mechanisms and

Potential Therapeutic Target. *Intensive Care Med* (2020) 46:586–90. doi: 10.1007/s00134-020-05985-9

9. Mangalmurti N, Hunter CA. Cytokine Storms: Understanding COVID-19. *Immun* (2020) 53:19–25. doi: 10.1016/j.immuni.2020.06.017
10. Li MY, Li L, Zhang Y, Wang XS. Expression of the SARS-CoV-2 Cell Receptor Gene ACE2 in a Wide Variety of Human Tissues. *Infect Dis Poverty* (2020) 9:45. doi: 10.1186/s40249-020-00662-x
11. Lu C, Li S, Liu Y. Role of Immunosuppressive Therapy in Rheumatic Diseases Concurrent With COVID-19. *Ann Rheum Dis* (2020) 79:737–9. doi: 10.1136/annrheumdis-2020-217460
12. Findlay AR, Goyal NA, Mozaffar T. An Overview of Polymyositis and Dermatomyositis. *Muscle Nerve* (2015) 51:638–56. doi: 10.1002/mus.24566
13. Aussy A, Boyer O, Cordel N. Dermatomyositis and Immune-Mediated Necrotizing Myopathies: A Window on Autoimmunity and Cancer. *Front Immunol* (2017) 8:992. doi: 10.3389/fimmu.2017.00992
14. Nishina N, Sato S, Masui K, Gono T, Kuwana M. Seasonal and Residential Clustering at Disease Onset of Anti-MDA5-Associated Interstitial Lung Disease. *RMD Open* (2020) 6:e001202. doi: 10.1136/rmdopen-2020-001202
15. Chen DY, Chen YM, Lan JL, Chen HH, Hsieh CW, Wey SJ, et al. Polymyositis/dermatomyositis and Nasopharyngeal Carcinoma: The Epstein-Barr Virus Connection? *J Clin Virol* (2010) 49:290–5. doi: 10.1016/j.jcv.2010.08.015
16. Betteridge Z, Tansley S, Shaddick G, Chinoy H, Cooper RG, New RP, et al. Frequency, Mutual Exclusivity and Clinical Associations of Myositis Autoantibodies in a Combined European Cohort of Idiopathic Inflammatory Myopathy Patients. *J Autoimmun* (2019) 101:48–55. doi: 10.1016/j.jaut.2019.04.001
17. Betteridge Z, McHugh N. Myositis-Specific Autoantibodies: An Important Tool to Support Diagnosis of Myositis. *J Intern Med* (2016) 280:8–23. doi: 10.1111/joim.12451
18. Gono T, Sato S, Kawaguchi Y, Kuwana M, Hanaoka M, Katsumata Y, et al. Anti-MDA5 Antibody, Ferritin and IL-18 are Useful for the Evaluation of Response to Treatment in Interstitial Lung Disease With Anti-MDA5 Antibody-Positive Dermatomyositis. *Rheumatol (Oxford)* (2012) 51:1563–70. doi: 10.1093/rheumatology/kes102
19. Walsh RJ, Kong SW, Yao Y, Jallal B, Kiener PA, Pinkus JL, et al. Type I Interferon-Inducible Gene Expression in Blood Is Present and Reflects Disease Activity in Dermatomyositis and Polymyositis. *Arthritis Rheumatol* (2007) 56:3784–92. doi: 10.1002/art.22928
20. Ivashkiv LB, Donlin LT. Regulation of Type I Interferon Responses. *Nat Rev Immunol* (2014) 14:36–49. doi: 10.1038/nri3581
21. Dalakas MC, Hohlfeld R. Polymyositis and Dermatomyositis. *Lancet* (2003) 362:971–82. doi: 10.1016/S0140-6736(03)14368-1
22. Fathi M, Lundberg IE, Tornling G. Pulmonary Complications of Polymyositis and Dermatomyositis. *Semin Respir Crit Care Med* (2007) 28:451–8. doi: 10.1055/s-2007-985666
23. Selva-O'Callaghan A, Pinal-Fernandez I, Trallero-Araguás E, Milisenda JC, Grau-Junyent JM, Mammen AL. Classification and Management of Adult Inflammatory Myopathies. *Lancet Neurol* (2018) 17:816–28. doi: 10.1016/S1474-4422(18)30254-0
24. Sato S, Kuwana M. Clinically Amyopathic Dermatomyositis. *Curr Opin Rheumatol* (2010) 22:639–43. doi: 10.1097/BOR.0b013e32833f1987
25. Selva-O'Callaghan A, Sanchez-Sitjes L, Muñoz-Gall X, Mijares-Boeckh-Behrens T, Solans-Laque R, Angel Bosch-Gil J, et al. Respiratory Failure Due to Muscle Weakness in Inflammatory Myopathies: Maintenance Therapy With Home Mechanical Ventilation. *Rheumatol (Oxford)* (2000) 39:914–6. doi: 10.1093/rheumatology/39.8.914
26. Mehta P, Machado PM, Gupta L. Understanding and Managing Anti-MDA 5 Dermatomyositis, Including Potential COVID-19 Mimicry. *Rheumatol Int* (2021) 41:1021–36. doi: 10.1007/s00296-021-04819-1
27. Xu L, Wang L, Lv C, Tan W. Anti-MDA-5-Positive Dermatomyositis Associated Rapidly Progressive Interstitial Lung Disease, a Virus-Triggered Autoimmune-Like Symptom? *Rheumatol (Oxford)* (2021) 60:4428–9. doi: 10.1093/rheumatology/keab224
28. Tanboon J, Nishino I. COVID-19-Associated Myositis may be Dermatomyositis. *Muscle Nerve* (2021) 63:E9–e10. doi: 10.1002/mus.27105
29. Megremis S, Walker TDJ, He X, Ollier WER, Chinoy H, Hampson L, et al. Antibodies Against Immunogenic Epitopes With High Sequence Identity to SARS-CoV-2 in Patients With Autoimmune Dermatomyositis. *Ann Rheum Dis* (2020) 79:1383–6. doi: 10.1136/annrheumdis-2020-217522
30. Ferri C, Giuggioli D, Raimondo V, L'Andolina M, Tavoni A, Cecchetti R, et al. COVID-19 and Rheumatic Autoimmune Systemic Diseases: Report of a Large Italian Patients Series. *Clin Rheumatol* (2020) 39:3195–204. doi: 10.1007/s10067-020-05334-7
31. Movahedi N, Ziaee V. COVID-19 and Myositis; True Dermatomyositis or Prolonged Post Viral Myositis? *Pediatr Rheumatol Online J* (2021) 19:86. doi: 10.1186/s12969-021-00570-w
32. Ortona E, Pierdominici M, Maselli A, Veroni C, Aloisi F, Shoenfeld Y. Sex-Based Differences in Autoimmune Diseases. *Ann Ist Super Sanita* (2016) 52:205–12. doi: 10.4415/ANN_16_02_12
33. Zandman-Goddard G, Peeva E, Shoenfeld Y. Gender and Autoimmunity. *Autoimmun Rev* (2007) 6:366–72. doi: 10.1016/j.autrev.2006.10.001
34. Selmi C, Brunetta E, Raimondo MG, Meroni PL. The X Chromosome and the Sex Ratio of Autoimmunity. *Autoimmun Rev* (2012) 11:A531–7. doi: 10.1016/j.autrev.2011.11.024
35. Rubtsova K, Marrack P, Rubtsov AV. Sexual Dimorphism in Autoimmunity. *J Clin Invest* (2015) 125:2187–93. doi: 10.1172/JCI78082
36. Zhang H, Charmchi Z, Seidman RJ, Anziska Y, Velayudhan V, Perk J. COVID-19-Associated Myositis With Severe Proximal and Bulbar Weakness. *Muscle Nerve* (2020) 62:E57–60. doi: 10.1002/mus.27003
37. Kogami M, Suzuki S, Nanjo Y, Ikeda K, Tamura N, Sasaki S, et al. Complication of Coronavirus Disease 2019 During Remission Induction Therapy Against Anti-MDA5 Antibody-Positive Dermatomyositis. *Rheumatol Adv Pract* (2020) 4:rkaa068. doi: 10.1093/rap/rkaa068
38. Cao M, Zhang S, Chu D, Xiao M, Liu X, Yu L, et al. COVID-19 or Clinical Amyopathic Dermatomyositis Associated Rapidly Progressive Interstitial Lung Disease? A Case Report. *BMC Pulm Med* (2020) 20:304. doi: 10.1186/s12890-020-01335-z
39. Borges NH, Godoy TM, Kahlow BS. Onset of Dermatomyositis in Close Association With COVID-19 - a First Case Reported. *Rheumatol (Oxford)* (2021) 60:SI96. doi: 10.1093/rheumatology/keab290
40. Quintana-Ortega C, Remesal A, Ruiz de Valbuena M, de la Serna O, Laplaza-González M, Álvarez-Rojas E, et al. Fatal Outcome of Anti-MDA5 Juvenile Dermatomyositis in a Paediatric COVID-19 Patient: A Case Report. *Mod Rheumatol Case Rep* (2021) 5:101–7. doi: 10.1080/24725625.2020.1832755
41. Ho BVK, Seger EW, Kollmann K, Rajpara A. Dermatomyositis in a COVID-19 Positive Patient. *JAAD Case Rep* (2021) 13:97–9. doi: 10.1016/j.jdcr.2021.04.036
42. Liquidano-Perez E, García-Romero MT, Yamazaki-Nakashimada M, Maza-Morales M, Rivas-Calderón MK, Bayardo-Gutierrez B, et al. Juvenile Dermatomyositis Triggered by SARS-CoV-2. *Pediatr Neurol* (2021) 121:26–7. doi: 10.1016/j.pediatrneurol.2021.05.011
43. Mao L, Jin H, Wang M, Hu Y, Chen S, He Q, et al. Neurologic Manifestations of Hospitalized Patients With Coronavirus Disease 2019 in Wuhan, China. *JAMA Neurol* (2020) 77:683–90. doi: 10.1001/jamaneurol.2020.1127
44. Uruha A, Nishikawa A, Tsuburaya RS, Hamanaka K, Kuwana M, Watanabe Y, et al. Sarcoplasmic MxA Expression: A Valuable Marker of Dermatomyositis. *Neurol* (2017) 88:493–500. doi: 10.1212/WNL.0000000000003568
45. Manzano GS, Woods JK, Amato AA. Covid-19-Associated Myopathy Caused by Type I Interferonopathy. *N Engl J Med* (2020) 383:2389–90. doi: 10.1056/NEJMc2031085
46. Beydon M, Chevalier K, Al Tabaa O, Hamroun S, Delettre AS, Thomas M, et al. Myositis as a Manifestation of SARS-CoV-2. *Ann Rheum Dis* (2020). doi: 10.1136/annrheumdis-2020-217573
47. Ding Y, He L, Zhang Q, Huang Z, Che X, Hou J, et al. Organ Distribution of Severe Acute Respiratory Syndrome (SARS) Associated Coronavirus (SARS-CoV) in SARS Patients: Implications for Pathogenesis and Virus Transmission Pathways. *J Pathol* (2004) 203:622–30. doi: 10.1002/path.1560
48. Li W, Moore MJ, Vasilieva N, Sui J, Wong SK, Berne MA, et al. Angiotensin-Converting Enzyme 2 is a Functional Receptor for the SARS Coronavirus. *Nat* (2003) 426:450–4. doi: 10.1038/nature02145
49. Jin M, Tong Q. Rhabdomyolysis as Potential Late Complication Associated With COVID-19. *Emerg Infect Dis* (2020) 26:1618–20. doi: 10.3201/eid2607.200445
50. Parekh R, Care DA, Tainter CR. Rhabdomyolysis: Advances in Diagnosis and Treatment. *Emerg Med Pract* (2012) 14:1–15.

51. Lakota K, Perdan-Pirkmajer K, Hočevar A, Sodin-Semrl S, Rotar Ž, Čučnik S, et al. COVID-19 in Association With Development, Course, and Treatment of Systemic Autoimmune Rheumatic Diseases. *Front Immunol* (2020) 11:611318. doi: 10.3389/fimmu.2020.611318
52. Russell CD, Millar JE, Baillie JK. Clinical Evidence Does Not Support Corticosteroid Treatment for 2019-Ncov Lung Injury. *Lancet* (2020) 395:473–5. doi: 10.1016/S0140-6736(20)30317-2
53. Narain S, Stefanov DG, Chau AS, Weber AG, Marder G, Kaplan B, et al. Comparative Survival Analysis of Immunomodulatory Therapy for Coronavirus Disease 2019 Cytokine Storm. *Chest* (2021) 159:933–48. doi: 10.1016/j.chest.2020.09.275
54. Horby P, Lim WS, Emberson JR, Mafham M, Bell JL, Linsell L, et al. Dexamethasone in Hospitalized Patients With Covid-19. *N Engl J Med* (2021) 384:693–704. doi: 10.1056/NEJMoa2021436
55. Strangfeld A, Schäfer M, Gianfrancesco MA, Lawson-Tovey S, Liew JW, Ljung L, et al. Factors Associated With COVID-19-Related Death in People With Rheumatic Diseases: Results From the COVID-19 Global Rheumatology Alliance Physician-Reported Registry. *Ann Rheum Dis* (2021) 80:930–42. doi: 10.1136/annrheumdis-2020-219498
56. Brown PM, Pratt AG, Isaacs JD. Mechanism of Action of Methotrexate in Rheumatoid Arthritis, and the Search for Biomarkers. *Nat Rev Rheumatol* (2016) 12:731–42. doi: 10.1038/nrrheum.2016.175
57. Tripathy S, Dassarma B, Roy S, Chabalala H. Matsabisa MG. A Review on Possible Modes of Action of Chloroquine/Hydroxychloroquine: Repurposing Against SAR-CoV-2 (COVID-19) Pandemic. *Int J Antimicrob Agents* (2020) 56:106028. doi: 10.1016/j.ijantimicag.2020.106028
58. Wang M, Cao R, Zhang L, Yang X, Liu J, Xu M, et al. Remdesivir and Chloroquine Effectively Inhibit the Recently Emerged Novel Coronavirus (2019-Ncov) *In Vitro*. *Cell Res* (2020) 30:269–71. doi: 10.1038/s41422-020-0282-0
59. Axfors C, Schmitt AM, Janiaud P, Van't Hooft J, Abd-Elsalam S, Abdo EF, et al. Mortality Outcomes With Hydroxychloroquine and Chloroquine in COVID-19 From an International Collaborative Meta-Analysis of Randomized Trials. *Nat Commun* (2021) 12:2349. doi: 10.1038/s41467-021-22446-z
60. Perez J, Roustit M, Lepelley M, Revol B, Cracowski JL, Khouri C. Reported Adverse Drug Reactions Associated With the Use of Hydroxychloroquine and Chloroquine During the COVID-19 Pandemic. *Ann Intern Med* (2021) 174:878–80. doi: 10.7326/m20-7918
61. Broen JCA, van Laar JM. Mycophenolate Mofetil, Azathioprine and Tacrolimus: Mechanisms in Rheumatology. *Nat Rev Rheumatol* (2020) 16:167–78. doi: 10.1038/s41584-020-0374-8
62. Kato F, Matsuyama S, Kawase M, Hishiki T, Katoh H, Takeda M. Antiviral Activities of Mycophenolic Acid and IMD-0354 Against SARS-CoV-2. *Microbiol Immunol* (2020) 64:635–9. doi: 10.1111/1348-0421.12828
63. Morteau O, Blundell S, Chakera A, Bennett S, Christou CM, Mason PD, et al. Renal Transplant Immunosuppression Impairs Natural Killer Cell Function *In Vitro* and *In Vivo*. *PloS One* (2010) 5:e13294. doi: 10.1371/journal.pone.0013294
64. Tiefenthaler M, Hofer S, Ebner S, Ivarsson L, Neyer S, Herold M, et al. *In Vitro* Treatment of Dendritic Cells With Tacrolimus: Impaired T-Cell Activation and IP-10 Expression. *Nephrol Dial Transplant* (2004) 19:553–60. doi: 10.1093/ndt/gfg594
65. Belli LS, Fondevila C, Cortesi PA, Conti S, Karam V, Adam R, et al. Protective Role of Tacrolimus, Deleterious Role of Age and Comorbidities in Liver Transplant Recipients With Covid-19: Results From the ELITA/ELTR Multi-Center European Study. *Gastroenterol* (2021) 160:1151–63.e3. doi: 10.1053/j.gastro.2020.11.045
66. Solanich X, Antolí A, Rocamora-Blanch G, Padullés N, Fanlo-Maresma M, Iriarte A, et al. Methylprednisolone Pulses Plus Tacrolimus in Addition to Standard of Care vs. Standard of Care Alone in Patients With Severe COVID-19. A Randomized Controlled Trial. *Front Med (Lausanne)* (2021) 8:691712. doi: 10.3389/fmed.2021.691712
67. Tsuji H, Nakashima R, Hosono Y, Imura Y, Yagita M, Yoshifuji H, et al. Multicenter Prospective Study of the Efficacy and Safety of Combined Immunosuppressive Therapy With High-Dose Glucocorticoid, Tacrolimus, and Cyclophosphamide in Interstitial Lung Diseases Accompanied by Anti-Melanoma Differentiation-Associated Gene 5-Positive Dermatomyositis. *Arthritis Rheumatol* (2020) 72:488–98. doi: 10.1002/art.41105
68. Zong M, Dorph C, Dastmalchi M, Alexanderson H, Pieper J, Amoudruz P, et al. Anakinra Treatment in Patients With Refractory Inflammatory Myopathies and Possible Predictive Response Biomarkers: A Mechanistic Study With 12 Months Follow-Up. *Ann Rheum Dis* (2014) 73:913–20. doi: 10.1136/annrheumdis-2012-202857
69. Spencer CH, Rouster-Stevens K, Gewanter H, Syverson G, Modica R, Schmidt K, et al. Biologic Therapies for Refractory Juvenile Dermatomyositis: Five Years of Experience of the Childhood Arthritis and Rheumatology Research Alliance in North America. *Pediatr Rheumatol Online J* (2017) 15:50. doi: 10.1186/s12969-017-0174-0
70. Zhang X, Zhou S, Wu C, Li M, Wang Q, Zhao Y, et al. Tocilizumab for Refractory Rapidly Progressive Interstitial Lung Disease Related to Anti-MDA5-Positive Dermatomyositis. *Rheumatol (Oxford)* (2021) 60:e227–8. doi: 10.1093/rheumatology/keaa906
71. Xu X, Han M, Li T, Sun W, Wang D, Fu B, et al. Effective Treatment of Severe COVID-19 Patients With Tocilizumab. *Proc Natl Acad Sci USA* (2020) 117:10970–5. doi: 10.1073/pnas.2005615117
72. Richardson P, Griffin I, Tucker C, Smith D, Oechsle O, Phelan A, et al. Baricitinib as Potential Treatment for 2019-Ncov Acute Respiratory Disease. *Lancet* (2020) 395:e30–1. doi: 10.1016/s0140-6736(20)30304-4
73. Kalil AC, Patterson TF, Mehta AK, Tomashek KM, Wolfe CR, Ghazaryan V, et al. Baricitinib Plus Remdesivir for Hospitalized Adults With Covid-19. *N Engl J Med* (2021) 384:795–807. doi: 10.1056/NEJMoa2031994
74. Puxeddu I, Ferro F, Bartoloni E, Elefante E, Baldini C, Scirè C, et al. COVID-19: The New Challenge for Rheumatologists. One Year Later. *Clin Exp Rheumatol* (2021) 39:203–13.
75. Kurasawa K, Arai S, Namiki Y, Tanaka A, Takamura Y, Owada T, et al. Tofacitinib for Refractory Interstitial Lung Diseases in Anti-Melanoma Differentiation-Associated 5 Gene Antibody-Positive Dermatomyositis. *Rheumatol (Oxford)* (2018) 57:2114–9. doi: 10.1093/rheumatology/key188
76. Chen Z, Wang X, Ye S. Tofacitinib in Amyopathic Dermatomyositis-Associated Interstitial Lung Disease. *N Engl J Med* (2019) 381:291–3. doi: 10.1056/NEJMc1900045
77. Guimarães PO, Quirk D, Furtado RH, Maia LN, Saraiva JF, Antunes MO, et al. Tofacitinib in Patients Hospitalized With Covid-19 Pneumonia. *N Engl J Med* (2021) 385:406–15. doi: 10.1056/NEJMoa2101643
78. Mehta P, Ciurtin C, Scully M, Levi M, Chambers RC. JAK Inhibitors in COVID-19: The Need for Vigilance Regarding Increased Inherent Thrombotic Risk. *Eur Respir J* (2020) 56:2001919. doi: 10.1183/13993003.01919-2020
79. Dalakas MC, Illa I, Dambrosia JM, Soueidan SA, Stein DP, Otero C, et al. A Controlled Trial of High-Dose Intravenous Immune Globulin Infusions as Treatment for Dermatomyositis. *N Engl J Med* (1993) 329:1993–2000. doi: 10.1056/NEJM199312303292704
80. Dalakas MC. Guillain-Barré Syndrome: The First Documented COVID-19-Triggered Autoimmune Neurologic Disease: More to Come With Myositis in the Offing. *Neurol Neuroimmunol Neuroinflamm* (2020) 7:e781. doi: 10.1212/NXI.0000000000000781
81. De Lorenzis E, Natalello G, Gigante L, Verardi L, Bosello SL, Gremese E. What can We Learn From Rapidly Progressive Interstitial Lung Disease Related to Anti-MDA5 Dermatomyositis in the Management of COVID-19? *Autoimmun Rev* (2020) 19:102666. doi: 10.1016/j.autrev.2020.102666

21

Co-Occurrence of Dermatomyositis and Polycythemia Unveiling Rare *de Novo* Neuroendocrine Prostate Tumor

Charalampos Papagoras [1†], Stella Arelaki [2†], Ioannis Botis [1], Ioannis Chrysafis [3], Stavros Giannopoulos [4] and Panagiotis Skendros [1]*

[1] First Department of Internal Medicine, University Hospital of Alexandroupolis, Democritus University of Thrace, Alexandroupolis, Greece, [2] Department of Pathology, University Hospital of Alexandroupolis, Democritus University of Thrace, Alexandroupolis, Greece, [3] Department of Radiology, University Hospital of Alexandroupolis, Democritus University of Thrace, Alexandroupolis, Greece, [4] Department of Urology, University Hospital of Alexandroupolis, Democritus University of Thrace, Alexandroupolis, Greece

***Correspondence:**
Panagiotis Skendros
pskendro@med.duth.gr

† These authors have contributed equally to this work

We present a case of dermatomyositis together with polycythemia as initial manifestations of a particularly rare type of prostate cancer. A 69-year-old man was hospitalized for facial erythema and symptoms of fatigue. Physical evaluation, serum creatinine phosphokinase and electromyography were consistent with dermatomyositis. In parallel, the hemoglobin level was 18.5 g/dL, serum erythropoietin levels were low normal and no *JAK2* mutation was found. Given a strong suspicion of a paraneoplastic syndrome the patient underwent abdominal computed tomography revealing a prostate mass, enlarged iliac lymph nodes and a fracture of L1 due to metastasis. The unusual paraneoplastic manifestations prompted a more thorough immunohistologic examination of the needle biopsy specimen taken from the prostate, which led to the diagnosis of large cell neuroendocrine prostate carcinoma. It is a most rare type of prostate cancer, carrying a poor prognosis. To our knowledge, this is the first case in the literature associating a neuroendocrine cancer of the prostate with dermatomyositis.

Keywords: prostate cancer, neuroendocrine neoplasia, dermatomyositis, polycythemia, erythrocytosis

INTRODUCTION

The association between idiopathic inflammatory myopathies, particularly dermatomyositis, and cancer is a well-established observation. The most common type of cancer underlying dermatomyositis is adenocarcinoma, and the most commonly affected sites are the lung, ovary, breast, colon, uterus cervix, bladder, nasopharynx, esophagus, pancreas, and kidney (1). Although several other less frequent types of malignancy have been reported in patients with myositis, herein we report a case of an extremely rare type of prostate cancer manifesting with dermatomyositis and polycythemia.

BACKGROUND

A 69-year-old man was admitted to the hospital for recurrent facial swelling and redness, accompanied by worsening fatigue during the previous 3 months. The episodes had initially been considered allergic and responded to short courses of glucocorticoids, only to recur a few weeks later. He had a history of arterial hypertension and an endovascular aortic aneurysm repair 6 years ago and his chronic medications included perindopril and low dose aspirin. He reported no significant urinary symptoms. Upon examination he had a reddish periorbital edema and an erythema of the face and the neck V-region (**Figure 1A**). Importantly, there was muscular weakness affecting the trunk and the proximal muscles of the extremities (grade 3 in a 0–5 scale). Apart from raised inflammatory markers (erythrocyte sedimentation rate 56 mm/h, C-reactive protein 6.1 mg/dL), serum creatinine phosphokinase was also elevated (1,819 U/L, normal 32–294). Electromyography of both proximal and distal muscles of the upper and lower limbs revealed scattered myopathic motor unit potentials, spontaneous fibrillations and increased insertional irritability, confirming the diagnosis of dermatomyositis.

In parallel, the patient had polycythemia (hematocrit 54.2%, hemoglobin 18.5 g/dL). Regarding possible causes, the patient's arterial pO_2 was 80 mmHg on room air, serum erythropoietin level was low-normal (5 mU/mL, range 4.3–29) and a test for *JAK2* mutation was negative. The co-occurrence of late-onset dermatomyositis and polycythemia of undefined cause raised strong suspicions of an underlying malignant disease. A subsequent computed tomography scan of the abdomen revealed a large prostate tumor (**Figure 1B**), enlarged left iliac lymph nodes (**Figure 1C**) and a heterogeneous osteosclerosis of the left side of the L1 vertebral body with a collapse of its upper part and paravertebral fat edema, consistent with a metastasis at the L1 vertebra. The serum prostate specific antigen (PSA) was 11.49 ng/mL (normal 0–4). Remarkably, at this time point, symptoms and signs consistent with enlarged prostate were not yet apparent.

Needle core biopsy from the prostate revealed extensive sheets from large sized cells with prominent nucleoli, abundant cytoplasm and no prominent glandular differentiation. The tumor featured plenty of mitoses and apoptotic bodies. Immunohistochemical stains were strongly positive for neuroendocrine markers chromogranin A (**Figure 1D**) and synaptophysin and negative for the CD56 antigen. Interestingly, prostate markers such as PSA and prostatic specific acid phosphatase (PSAP) were positive, but only in a localized and weak pattern. The Ki-67 proliferative index was up to 70% of tumor cells. The histopathological report was of a large cell neuroendocrine prostate carcinoma (LCNPC). Therefore, the patient was diagnosed with metastatic LCNPC with paraneoplastic dermatomyositis and polycythemia and was referred to the Oncology department for treatment. However, the response to treatment was poor and he died 4 months after the diagnosis. Written informed consent was obtained from his wife for the publication of this case report.

Abbreviations: HMGCR, 3- hydroxy-3- methylglutaryl-coenzyme-A reductase; LCNPC, Large cell neuroendocrine prostate carcinoma; PSA, Prostate specific antigen; PSAP, Prostatic specific acid phosphatase ; SRP, signal recognition particle; TIF-1γ , Transcription Intermediary Factor 1 γ.

DISCUSSION

We present a case of a very rare type of prostate cancer that manifested with symptoms of dermatomyositis and concomitant laboratory findings of erythrocytosis. The case is unique, because dermatomyositis or erythrocytosis in the course of large cell neuroendocrine prostate cancer have never been reported in the literature to our knowledge.

Idiopathic inflammatory myopathies are the rheumatologic diseases most strongly associated with cancer. Dermatomyositis seems to carry the highest relative risk compared to the general population, up to 5.5, followed by polymyositis with a relative risk 1.62 (2). Immune-mediated necrotizing myopathy, a recently described type of myositis, has also been linked to cancer, particularly in patients negative for antibodies against signal recognition particle (SRP) or positive against 3- hydroxy-3-methylglutaryl-coenzyme-A reductase (HMGCR) (3), although the latter are associated with statin-associated autoimmune myopathy as well (4). The risk of malignancy is usually highest the year preceding or following the myositis diagnosis and it seems to wane within 1–5 years post myositis diagnosis (1). Therefore, the most important issue is the recognition of prognostic factors to identify patients at risk, in order to screen for cancer and follow up appropriately. In a recent meta-analysis, risk factors for dermatomyositis-associated cancer were male sex, older age, cutaneous necrosis, elevated inflammatory markers and positivity for the anti-p155 antibody, which is thought to be directed against Transcription Intermediary Factor 1 γ (TIF-1γ). On the other hand, the presence of anti-Jo-1 and anti-Nuclear Extractable Antigen antibodies negatively associated with the risk of malignancy (5). Our patient had dermatomyositis with several of those risk factors (male, older age, elevated inflammatory markers), although we did not test for anti-p155/TIF-1γ antibodies. A possible mechanism underlying the paraneoplastic manifestations could be the production of antibodies against tumor antigens cross-reacting with muscle antigens (3, 6).

Erythrocytosis secondary to cancer is a recognized paraneoplastic manifestation of several types of cancer, such as hepatic or renal cancer (7). It may arise due to the ectopic production of erythropoietin or other erythropoiesis-inducing molecules from malignant cells (8). In a case report of a patient with colon adenocarcinoma and erythrocytosis, the colonic malignant cells expressed erythropoietin, although serum erythropoietin levels were also low normal, suggesting that the serum erythropoietin levels might be disproportionately high relative to the level of blood hemoglobin (7). As in our patient serum levels of erythropoietin were low normal as well, ectopic production of erythropoietin from the malignant neuroendocrine cells of the tumor cannot be ruled out, although immunohistochemistry for erythropoietin was not performed in the pathological specimen to confirm it.

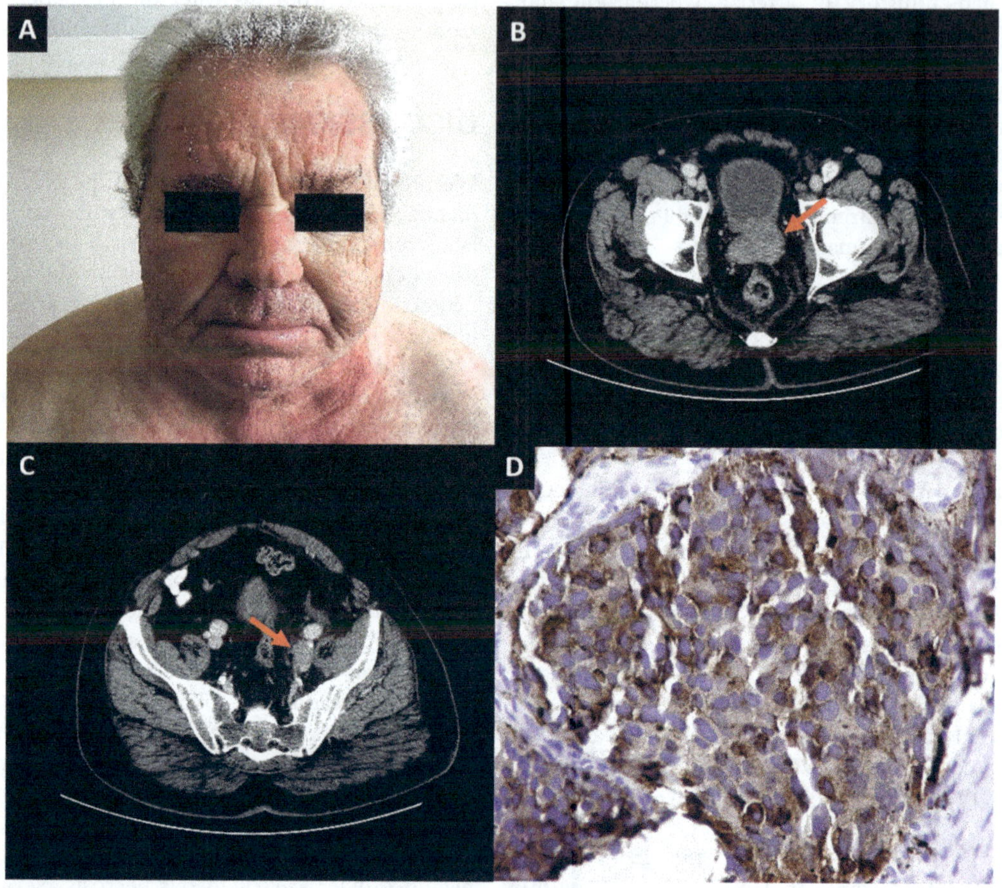

FIGURE 1 | (A) Diffuse erythema of the face and the "V-neck sign," suggestive of dermatomyositis. **(B)** Computed tomography of the abdomen revealing a prostate tumor (arrow) and **(C)** an enlarged left iliac lymph node (arrow) **(D)** Immunohistochemical section of a needle core biopsy from the prostate of the patient showing large cells staining positive for chromogranin A.

Prostate cancer is the second most common malignancy in males and the second urological tumor associated with paraneoplastic manifestations after renal cell carcinoma (9). The vast majority are adenocarcinomas, while only 0.5% of tumors are classified as neuroendocrine (10). Among them, the occurrence of LCNPC is extremely rare, described only in case reports. The etiology of LCNPC is unknown. Most cases occur after androgen deprivation therapy for prostate adenocarcinoma (11). However, there have been reports of very few cases developing either *de novo* (11–14) or with advanced high-grade prostate adenocarcinoma (11, 15). The prognosis is poor with an average survival of <1 year, as they are usually diagnosed in a metastatic stage (10).

The clinical manifestations, as well as the histopathologic features of a prostate neuroendocrine carcinoma may be similar to a high-grade prostatic adenocarcinoma. Moreover, neuroendocrine tumors are often characterized by inappropriate secretion of peptides, amines or other bioactive substances causing related syndromes. For instance, secretion of serotonin is the hallmark of the carcinoid syndrome, which is manifested with flushing of the skin, diarrhea, abdominal pain, right-sided heart-disease including right heart valve fibrosis and rarely myopathy, arthropathy and pigmentation (9). A great variety of other paraneoplastic signs and symptoms, such as hypercalcemia, syndrome of inappropriate antidiuretic hormone production, Cushing syndrome, Lambert-Eaton myasthenic syndrome, peripheral neuropathy or limbic encephalopathy, occur in association with genitourinary cancers, particularly small cell carcinomas, including those of the prostate (9, 16). However, such manifestations have not been reported with large cell neuroendocrine carcinoma of the prostate.

The key to diagnosis of this type of cancers is a neuroendocrine-orientated immunostaining, which, as in this case, should be prompted by the heterogeneous prostate enlargement and, particularly, the unusual symptoms which rarely occur in the common prostate adenocarcinoma (17). Serum PSA, a frequently used marker for prostate cancer screening of at-risk patients (including males over

50 years with myositis), may not be helpful, as there are several cases of neuroendocrine prostate cancer lacking significant PSA elevations despite the existence of a bulky tumor.

CONCLUDING REMARKS

In conclusion, we present an extremely rare case of a *de novo* large cell neuroendocrine prostate carcinoma which manifested with features of dermatomyositis and polycythemia, while urinary symptoms were absent. A high grade of suspicion for an underlying malignancy and the unusual systemic manifestations prompted a deeper scrutiny of the histopathological specimen revealing this rare type of cancer, which is treated through a different approach from classic prostate adenocarcinoma.

ETHICS STATEMENT

This report was in accordance with the rules of Ethics Review Board of the University Hospital of Alexandroupolis.

AUTHOR CONTRIBUTIONS

CP treated the patient and drafted the manuscript. SA performed the histopathological tests and drafted the manuscript. IB and SG treated the patient and reviewed the manuscript. IC performed the imaging tests and reviewed the manuscript. PS treated the patient, reviewed the manuscript and supervised the work.

REFERENCES

1. Tiniakou E, Mammen AL. Idiopathic inflammatory myopathies and malignancy: a comprehensive review. *Clin Rev Allergy Immunol.* (2017) 52:20–33. doi: 10.1007/s12016-015-8511-x
2. Yang Z, Lin F, Qin B, Liang Y, Zhong R. Polymyositis/dermatomyositis and malignancy risk: a metaanalysis study. *J Rheumatol.* (2015) 42:282–91. doi: 10.3899/jrheum.140566
3. Aussy A, Boyer O, Cordel N. Dermatomyositis and immune-mediated necrotizing myopathies: a window on autoimmunity and cancer. *Front Immunol.* (2017) 8:992. doi: 10.3389/fimmu.2017.00992
4. Mohassel P, Mammen AL. The spectrum of statin myopathy. *Curr Opin Rheumatol.* (2013) 25:747–52. doi: 10.1097/01.bor.0000434673.85515.89
5. Lu X, Yang H, Shu X, Chen F, Zhang Y, Zhang S, et al. Factors predicting malignancy in patients with polymyositis and dermatomyostis: a systematic review and meta-analysis. *PLoS ONE* (2014) 9:e94128. doi: 10.1371/journal.pone.0094128
6. Manger B, Schett G. Rheumatic paraneoplastic syndromes-a clinical link between malignancy and autoimmunity. *Clin Immunol.* (2018) 186:67–70. doi: 10.1016/j.clim.2017.07.021
7. Kitayama H, Kondo T, Sugiyama J, Hirayama M, Oyamada Y, Tsuji Y. Paraneoplastic erythrocytosis of colon cancer, with serum erythropoietin within the normal reference range. *Am J Case Rep.* (2016) 17:417–20. doi: 10.12659/AJCR.897904
8. Tandon R, Goel P, Kataria S, Saha PK, Punia RP, Dimri K. Paraneoplastic erythrocytosis in a malignant ovarian steroid cell tumour. *Indian J Hematol Blood Transfus.* (2014) 30:54–5. doi: 10.1007/s12288-012-0193-4
9. Sacco E, Pinto F, Sasso F, Racioppi M, Gulino G, Volpe A, et al. Paraneoplastic syndromes in patients with urological malignancies. *Urol Int.* (2009) 83:1–11. doi: 10.1159/000224860
10. Zaffuto E, Pompe R, Zanaty M, Bondarenko HD, Leyh-Bannurah SR, Moschini M, et al. Contemporary incidence and cancer control outcomes of primary neuroendocrine prostate cancer: a SEER database analysis. *Clin Genitourin Cancer* (2017). 15:e793–e800. doi: 10.1016/j.clgc.2017.04.006
11. Evans AJ, Humphrey PA, Belani J, van der Kwast TH, Srigley JR. Large cell neuroendocrine carcinoma of prostate: a clinicopathologic summary of 7 cases of a rare manifestation of advanced prostate cancer. *Am J Surg Pathol.* (2006) 30:684–93. doi: 10.1097/00000478-200606000-00003
12. Okoye E, Choi EK, Divatia M, Miles BJ, Ayala AG, Ro JY. *De novo* large cell neuroendocrine carcinoma of the prostate gland with pelvic lymph node metastasis: a case report with review of literature. *Int J Clin Exp Pathol.* (2014) 7:9061–6.
13. Acosta-Gonzalez G, Qin J, Wieczorek R, Melamed J, Deng FM, Zhou M, et al. *De novo* large cell neuroendocrine carcinoma of the prostate, case report and literature review. *Am J Clin Exp Urol.* (2014) 2:337–42.
14. Lin D, Tan AJ, De Sousa AF, Singh-Rai R. A rare case of large cell neuroendocrine carcinoma. *BMJ Case Rep.* (2014) 2014:bcr2014206403. doi: 10.1136/bcr-2014-206403
15. Azad AA, Jones EC, Chi KN. Metastatic large-cell neuroendocrine prostate carcinoma: successful treatment with androgen deprivation therapy. *Clin Genitourin Cancer* (2014) 12:e151–153. doi: 10.1016/j.clgc.2014.03.006
16. Kanaji N, Watanabe N, Kita N, Bandoh S, Tadokoro A, Ishii T, et al. Paraneoplastic syndromes associated with lung cancer. *World J Clin Oncol.* (2014) 5:197–223. doi: 10.5306/wjco.v5.i3.197
17. Hong MK, Kong J, Namdarian B, Longano A, Grummet J, Hovens CM, et al. Paraneoplastic syndromes in prostate cancer. *Nat Rev Urol.* (2010) 7:681–92. doi: 10.1038/nrurol.2010.186

22

Dermatomyositis and Immune-Mediated Necrotizing Myopathies: A Window on Autoimmunity and Cancer

Audrey Aussy[1], *Olivier Boyer*[1]* *and Nadège Cordel*[1,2]

[1] *Normandie University, UNIROUEN, INSERM, U1234, Rouen University Hospital, Department of Immunology, Rouen, France,* [2] *Unit of Dermatology and Internal Medicine, Pointe-à-Pitre University Hospital, University of the French West Indies, Fouillole, Pointe-à-Pitre, Guadeloupe*

Correspondence:
Olivier Boyer
olivier.boyer@chu-rouen.fr

Autoimmune myopathies (myositides) are strongly associated with malignancy. The link between myositis and cancer, originally noticed by Bohan and Peter in their classification in 1975 (1), has been evidenced by large population-based cohort studies and a recent meta-analysis. The numerous reports of cases in which the clinical course of myositis reflects that of cancer and the short delay between myositis and cancer onset support the notion that myositis may be an authentic paraneoplastic disorder. Thus, cancer-associated myositis raises the question of cancer as a cause rather than a consequence of autoimmunity. Among myositides, dermatomyositis and more recently, although to a lesser extent, immune-mediated necrotizing myopathies are the most documented forms associated with cancer. Interestingly, the current diagnostic approach for myositis is based on the identification of specific antibodies where each antibody determines specific clinical features and outcomes. Recent findings have shown that the autoantibodies anti-TIF1γ, anti-NXP2 and anti-HMGCR are associated with cancers in the course of myositis. Herein, we highlight the fact that the targets of these three autoantibodies involve cellular pathways that intervene in tumor promotion and we discuss the role of cancer mutations as autoimmunity triggers in adult myositis.

Keywords: cancer, myositis, autoimmunity, TIF1gamma, autoantibody

INTRODUCTION

The link between autoimmunity and cancer has become a topic of unceasing interest over the past decade. Although it is increasingly evident that the risk of cancer is augmented in patients affected by several types of autoimmune diseases (AID), the nature of the interplay between autoimmunity and cancer remains elusive (2–4). One important question here recalls the old egg-and-chicken dilemma: is the autoimmune background in AID a seedbed for cancer development or, alternatively, may cancer cause autoimmunity?

Rheumatic AID such as systemic lupus erythematosus, rheumatoid arthritis, or Sjögren syndrome promote cancer development after several years of chronic inflammation and also exposure to immunosuppressive drugs (2, 5, 6). In the case of lupus for instance, the broadness of cancer type spectrum is striking, including hematological—mostly virus induced—malignancies but also numerous kinds of solid tumors such as vulva, lung, thyroid, and liver cancer (7). Here, the risk of cancer cannot only be ascribed to the sole autoimmune status but also presumably to iatrogenic immunosuppression.

This view is counterbalanced by the examples of paraneoplastic neurological syndromes, systemic sclerosis, and myositis. Paraneoplastic neurological syndromes with anti-neuronal autoantibodies (aAbs) include a most illustrative example, i.e., anti-Hu encephalitis associated with small cell lung carcinoma (SCLC) (8). Anti-Hu aAbs recognize the HuD autoantigen normally restricted to neurons but ectopically expressed on SCLC cells (9). Expression of the immunogenic HuD molecule by SCLC elicits the production of anti-Hu aAb and $CD8^+$ cytotoxic T cells, explaining the parallel clinical course of neurological symptoms and SCLC evolution and demonstrating the direct link between cancer and tissue-specific AID (10). Cancer-induced breakage of tolerance can also be caused by tumoral somatic mutations, as recently highlighted by the case of systemic sclerosis associated with anti-polymerase III (POL3) aAbs. The immunogenic peptides generated by *POLR3* gene mutations induce a POL3-specific $CD4^+$ T cell response with production of specific antibodies that secondarily target wild-type POL3 by epitope spreading (11).

This present review focuses on the forms of myositides, i.e., dermatomyositis (DM) and immune-mediated necrotizing myopathies (IMNMs) which have been identified as associated with cancer and represent a paradigm of cancer-associated AID.

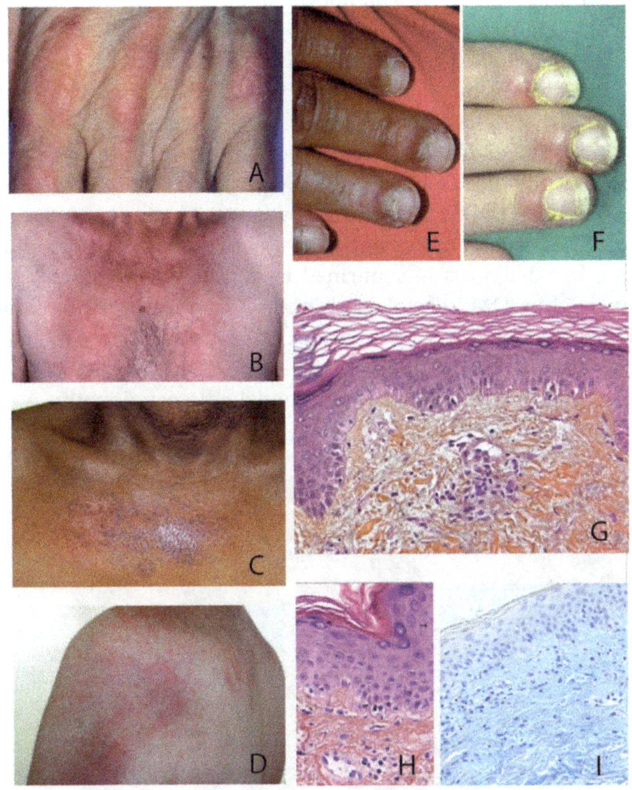

FIGURE 1 | Clinical and histological features of dermatomyositis (DM). **(A)** Gottron's sign: erythematous scaly papules over the metacarpophalangeal joints. **(B)** «V sign» in a white European male patient with DM. **(C)** Poikiloderma (i.e., erythema, atrophy, variable pigmentary changes) on the upper trunk of an African Caribbean female patient with DM. **(D)** Typical centripetal flagellate erythema affecting the upper trunk of a male patient with DM. **(E,F)** Periungual erythema and telangiectatic capillary loops in patients with DM. **(G–I)** Histological feature of a Gottron's papule. **(G)** Slight hyperkeratosis, basal cell vacuolar degeneration, upper dermal edema, and perivascular inflammatory cell infiltrate with enlarged capillaries (HES staining, ×20). **(H)** DM interface dermatitis with vacuolar changes of the basal cell layer, perivascular inflammatory cell infiltrate with capillary dilatation, endothelial cell turgescence, and pigmentary incontinence (HES staining, ×40). **(I)** Positive alcian-blue staining attesting dermal mucin deposits (×20).

DM, RISK OF CANCER, AND DIAGNOSTIC CONTRIBUTION OF AUTOANTIBODIES

Autoimmune myopathies or myositides constitute a heterogeneous group of severe acquired myopathies. They are characterized clinically by symmetrical proximal muscle weakness, associated or not with systemic features, and histologically by various levels of myofiber necrosis/regeneration and interstitial mononuclear infiltrates. Clinical and histopathological patterns define different diseases: polymyositis, DM, overlap myositis, sporadic inclusion-body myositis, and IMNM (12–17).

Dermatomyositis affects both adults and children among all ethnic groups with an unbalanced 1/2-sex-ratio in favor of women. Its annual incidence varies from 1.9 to 7.7 cases per million inhabitants according to data in the literature with a peak of frequency in 40–60-year-old adults and in 5–14-year-old children (13, 18). The appearance of specific cutaneous manifestations is typical of DM and is among its diagnostic criteria. Cutaneous manifestations typically consist of erythematous scaly papules over the metacarpophalangeal knuckles (Gottron's papules) (**Figure 1A**); a symmetrical reddish-violet periorbital edema that predominates on the upper eyelids (heliotrope erythema) but may affect the rest of the face; lupus-like erythema which involves low neck (V sign) (**Figure 1B**), shoulders (shawl sign), extensor surfaces of the limbs, dorsal side of hands and fingers and scalp; poikiloderma of the upper trunk (**Figure 1C**); and centripetal flagellate erythema affecting the trunk and or proximal extremities (**Figure 1D**). Cutaneous manifestations of DM also include non-specific lesions such as (i) vascular lesions, i.e., periungual erythema with telangiectatic capillary loops, nail fold dilated capillaries visible to the naked eye, cuticular hypertrophy (**Figures 1E,F**), vasculitis, cutaneous necrosis, or Raynaud's phenomenon, which are more prevalent in the course of juvenile dermatomyositis and (ii) several other dermatological features such as pruritus (present in 30% of DM), photosensitivity, mucinosis, and calcifications, which are more frequent in children rather than in adults, i.e., 30–70 versus 10%. Dermatological particularities of DM have been reported in several ethnic groups. In Afro-Caribbeans, edema of the face is usually predominant whereas in Eurasians, the Wong-type DM which mimicks a pytiriasis rubra pilaris seems to be more frequent (19).

Specific lesions of DM are histologically characterized by an interface dermatitis with basal layer vacuolar changes that are associated in various degrees with hyperkeratosis, epidermal atrophy, basement membrane thickening, upper dermal edema, pigmentary incontinence, mucine deposits, and light perivascular CD4+ T lymphocyte infiltrate of the superficial dermis (**Figures 1G–I**) (20).

Dermatological features usually precede muscle weakness by 3–6 months but may appear several years before. However, muscular manifestations may be absent, defining the amyopathic form of DM with an associated cancer rate, which is theoretically the same as classic DM (21, 22).

Diagnosis of DM is supported by serum creatine kinase (CK) elevation, which mirrors muscle lysis and by electromyographic data, but diagnosis is confirmed by muscle biopsy except for amyopathic DM. Histological examination of muscle tissue (**Figure 2**) typically shows perifascicular atrophy, necrotic and regenerative muscle fibers, septal and/or perivascular inflammatory cell infiltrate, and endomysial microangiopathy with membranolytic attack complex C5b-9 capillary staining that may also be present in cutaneous lesions. Although these capillary injuries have long been considered as indirect evidence of an initial endothelial target in DM, recent scientific findings demonstrate that capillary lesions might be non-specific in relationship to ischemia-reperfusion injury of perimysial arcade arteries (23). The role for interferons in DM pathogenesis is increasingly evident, since a typical interferon type 1 pathway signature was found in both muscle (24) and skin (25), with a correlation with disease activity (26).

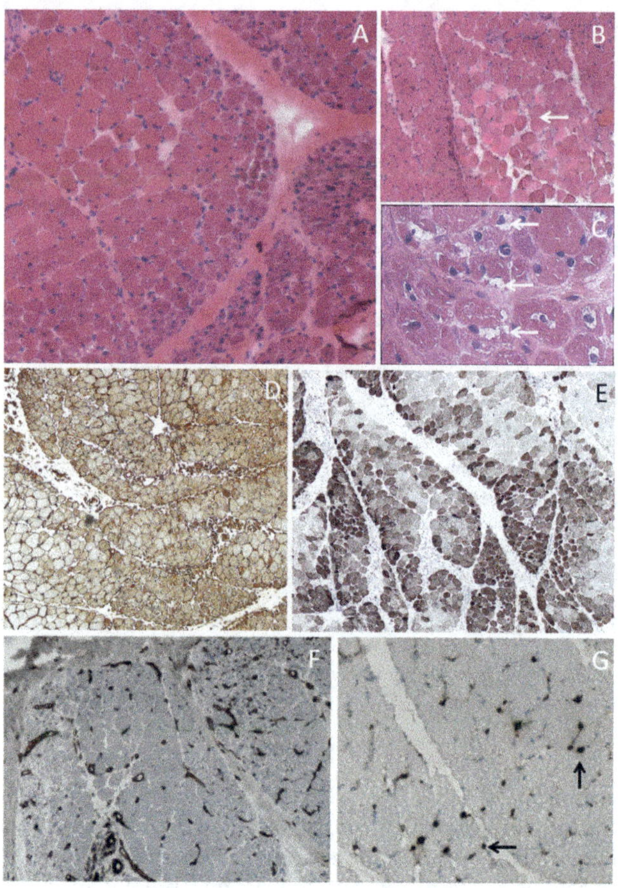

FIGURE 2 | Muscle biopsy of dermatomyositis. **(A)** Perifascicular atrophy. **(B)** Area of contiguous necrotic myofibers (arrow) corresponding to a microinfarct. **(C)** Punch-out vacuoles within myofibers (arrows) assessing focal myosinolysis. **(D)** Ubiquitous myofiber reexpression of MHC-class I with perifascicular reinforcement. **(E)** Neural cell adhesion molecule (NCAM) immunostaining showing large areas of positive myofibers indicating muscle ischemia. **(F)** Platelet endothelial cell adhesion molecule (PECAM) immunostaining for endothelial cells showing marked endomysial capillary drop out. **(G)** Complement activation assessed by the presence of membrane attack complex deposits at the level of endomysial capillaries (arrows). Frozen sections, light microscopy; hematoxylin-eosin **(A–C)**, immunoperoxydase technique **(D–G)**, HLA-ABC **(D)**, CD56/NCAM **(E)**, CD31/PECAM **(F)**, and C5b-9 **(G)**.

The outcome of DM is variable with benign forms highly responsive to treatment and severe forms associated with cardiac or lung involvement and/or malignancies. In juvenile DM, cancer association is uncommon. Nonetheless, a poor prognosis may be due to the intensity of vasculitis and vascular damage that involves the skin and the digestive system. Calcifications on the areas around joints may also lead to severe functional impairment in children.

Interestingly, several dermatological manifestations of DM such as cutaneous necrosis, skin vasculitis or pruritus, or histological patterns such as leucocytoclastic vasculitis are reported to be associated with cancer whatever the ethnic group (27, 28). Conversely, several features seem to protect against cancer such as Afro-Caribbean ethnicity (29).

Globally, myositides are rare diseases and epidemiologic data remain scarce. Studies are limited by their retrospective character and small population size. Yet, since its first descriptions (30, 31), the association between cancer and myositis has been confirmed by several studies published between 1975 and 2012, reporting a global malignancy rate from 6.7 to 32% (32–35). Importantly, several studies also point to cancer as the main cause of death in cancer-associated myositis patients (34, 36, 37). Yet, it may be difficult to distinguish between cancer on the one hand, and myositis exacerbation and its complications on the other hand, as the actual cause of death. Most observations highlighted the short delay between the onset of myositis and the discovery of cancer. In some cases, cancer even preceded myositis, reinforcing the view that myositis might be the consequence rather than the cause of cancer and even leading to individualizing "cancer-associated myositis" in one classification in 2005 (14). Cancer risk is particularly established in DM. A recent meta-analysis confirmed adult (but not juvenile) DM as a risk-factor of cancer, with a standardized incident ratio (SIR) for occurrence of cancer of 5.5 [4.3–6.7], mostly peaking at 1 year around DM diagnosis (38). A limitation to previous studies, including those reviewed in this meta-analysis, is that the classification of myositis was essentially based on the widely used Bohan and Peter classification which tends to classify IMNM, overlap myositis, and polymyositis in a single category (1). Whereas this classification remains popular for its practical value in DM, progress in the definition of clinical, pathological, and serological patterns has led to newer classifications that are useful for the diagnosis of inclusion-body myositis (12), overlap myositis (14), or IMNM (13). In the light of these different existing classifications for myositis, a new unifying classification would provide a much-awaited tool.

The detection of myositis-specific aAbs (MSA) has proved most helpful in classifying the different forms and predicting the outcome of myositis. Indeed, in clinical practice, MSA define particular clinical ± histological patterns (39). In DM, anti-Mi-2 are classically associated with absence of cancer, sensitivity to treatment and, overall, good prognosis (40–42). Anti-melanoma differentiation antigen 5 (MDA-5) identifies a subgroup of DM patients with interstitial lung disease, necrotizing cutaneous lesions, skin ulcerations, and tender palmar papules while muscle signs are minimal (43–45). Anti-SAE (small ubiquitin-like modifier activating enzyme) has a low prevalence (1–4%) and patients have classic cutaneous signs of DM. Interestingly, a significant but low rate of cancer has been reported in this group (46–48). Anti-TIF1γ (transcriptional intermediary factor 1 gamma) is the leader of cancer-associated aAbs, with a rate of associated malignancy ranging from 60 to 80% of patients (49, 50). Anti-NXP2 (nuclear matrix protein 2) is another biomarker of risk of malignancy in adult patients, with a 30% rate of cancer among DM patients (51, 52).

Besides DM, IMNM is another form of myositis recently suggested to be associated with malignancy (53–55). IMNM may be subdivided in three groups: seronegative, anti-HMGCR (3-hydroxy-3-methylglutaryl-coenzyme-A-reductase), and anti-SRP (signal recognition particle). In contrast to anti-SRP positive patients, one study has recently suggested that, among IMNM, seronegative and anti-HMGCR positive patients have a significantly higher risk of cancer (56).

CANCER-ASSOCIATED MYOPATHIES ACCORDING TO AUTOANTIBODIES

DM with Anti-TIF1γ, the Leader in Cancer-Associated Myositis

Anti-TIF1γ was first described in 2006 as an antibody directed against a 155 kDa protein, especially in patients with DM (49, 57). This protein was rapidly identified as TIF1γ. Anti-TIF1γ aAbs scored positive in 20–30% of adult DM and 30–40% of juvenile DM with some differences according to geographical origin (39, 58). HLA DQA1*0301 was associated with anti-TIF1γ DM (49). The high prevalence of cancer was largely confirmed with a rate from 18 up to 80% of adult patients especially in the 2 years surrounding DM (22, 52, 59). A meta-analysis performed by Trallero-Araguás and colleagues estimated a 78% sensitivity and 89% specificity of these antibodies for diagnosing an associated cancer (50). Since 2001, age has been recognized as a risk factor for cancer among DM patients (33). Recently, two publications strengthened the role of advancing age in the increasing risk of cancer among adult anti-TIF1γ positive DM patients (60, 61).

No study found any predominance of one type of cancer; those occurring in adults with DM were generally comparable to those in the general population, stratified by age and sex (breast, lung, colorectal, bladder) as well as to some more rare cancers such as gastric or thymus cancer (59). Anti-TIF1γ DM associates classic but severe cutaneous signs with moderate muscular symptoms, frequent dysphagia but decreased systemic features compared to other DM (60). The specific clinical and histopathological features of anti-TIF1γ DM are summarized in **Table 1**. Regarding juvenile DM, no increased risk of cancer is observed (62). The median age of DM is 6.8 years of age. Anti-TIF1γ juvenile DM more often presents chronic or polycyclic courses associated with more severe prognosis and profuse cutaneous involvement (63).

DM with Anti-NXP2, the Second Actor in Cancer-Associated Myositis

A novel aAb directed against a 140 kDa protein was found in a 1997 cohort of juvenile DM and named anti-MJ (64). The 140 kDa protein was next identified as NXP2, also known as MORC3 (84). Anti-NXP2 aAbs are present in 22–25% of juvenile DM patients and in 1–17% of adults with DM, depending on the method of detection (61, 70). Forms of myositides other than DM may occasionally be associated with anti-NXP2 (67, 84). Cancer was detected in 24–37.5% of adults who scored positive for anti-NXP2 in several retrospective series (60, 61, 67). As for anti-TIF1γ DM, no specific type of tumor was mentioned. Clinical manifestations are partially distinct from anti-TIF1γ DM (**Table 1**). Indeed, classic cutaneous features are less severe but there is a higher prevalence of calcinosis (70). In addition, muscular involvement is constant and more severe. Similarities between anti-TIF1γ and anti-NXP2 include dysphagia and prevalence of peripheral edema (61, 70). Interstitial lung disease has only been reported in one cohort (85) and Raynaud's phenomenon is found in 20% of cases (64, 85).

In children, the median age at onset has been calculated at 5.8 years of age (58). Two series found an increased risk of calcinosis in children and a high prevalence of severe muscular involvement with functional disabilities, muscle cramps, and dysphagia but no cancer (**Table 1**) (39, 51).

IMNMs, NEW PLAYERS IN CANCER-ASSOCIATED MYOSITIS?

Immune-mediated necrotizing myopathies are a recently described entity, based on specific histological pattern with poor inflammatory infiltrate and presence of significant necrotizing and regenerative fibers (13, 72). As mentioned above, three IMNM subsets have been identified according to serologic status: anti-SRP, anti-HMGCR, or negative serology. Anti-HMGCR and seronegative IMNMs seem to be associated with a higher risk of cancer, with a SIR score of 2.79 and 8.35, respectively (56). Between 13 and 36% of anti-HMGCR positive patients have an associated cancer (56, 68, 69). A genetic study found that HLA-DRB1*11:01 is associated with a higher risk of anti-HMGCR IMNM in both white American and African American adult populations, whereas HLA-DRB1*07:01 seem to be associated with a risk of anti-HMGCR myositis in small series of children (86, 87).

Anti-HMGCR aAbs were discovered in 2010 in a group of patients who developed myositis after exposure to statins, without resolution by stopping statins (65, 66). Histological

TABLE 1 | Characteristics of anti-TIF1γ, anti-NXP2, and anti-HMGCR myositis.

	Anti-TIF1γ dermatomyositis (DM)	Anti-NXP2 DM	Anti-HMGCR immune-mediated necrotizing myopathy
Year of discovery of the aAb	2006 (49, 57)	1997 (64)	2010 (65, 66)
Frequency of cancer association in adults	60–80% (22, 52, 59)	24–37.5% (60, 61, 67)	12.9–36% (56, 68, 69)
Clinical features			
Skin involvement	Extensive cutaneous signs Poikiloderma Psoriasis-like lesions Scaly erythema of the scalp No calcinosis	Mild skin involvement Frequency of calcinosis	Generally not
Muscular involvement	Mild weakness Frequent dysphagia	Mild to severe weakness Frequency of distal weakness Myalgia, muscle atrophy Frequent dysphagia mild to severe	Mild to severe weakness Myalgia Inconstant dysphagia
Other characteristics	Peripheral edema Decreased risk of Raynaud phenomenon, arthralgia, and interstitial lung disease (60)	Peripheral edema Low frequency of interstitial lung disease (61, 70)	High frequency of statin exposure (65, 66, 71)
Histological pattern	Dense C5b-9 deposits on capillaries Presence of vacuolated fibers Overexpression of MHC class I Perifascicular atrophy Necrotic/regenerating fibers (59)	Perivascular inflammation Perifascicular atrophy Necrosis in patient with peripheral edema (70)	Necrosis Muscle fiber regeneration Atrophic fibers Little or no inflammatory infiltration C5b-9 deposition (13, 72)
Target of the aAbs			
Name	Transcriptional intermediary factor 1 gamma	Nuclear matrix protein 2 or microrchidia 3 (MORC3)	3-hydroxy-3-methylglutaryl-coenzyme-A-reductase
Protein expression	Ubiquitous	Ubiquitous Immune cells at high level	Ubiquitous Liver
Subcellular locations	Nucleus Cytosol in part	Nucleus	Endoplasmic reticulum Peroxisome
Role	TGFβ pathway Mitosis Embryonic development DNA repair Erythropoiesis Innate immunity (73–76)	Chromatin remodeling DNA repair Epigenetic regulation Cell regulation Activation of p53 Calcium homeostasis Bone remodeling (77–80)	Limiting enzyme for cholesterol synthesis and other mevalonate-dependent pathways (81–83)

features corresponded to IMNM (88–90). While the association with statins was confirmed in recent studies, it involved a wide range between 37 and 94% of patients (56, 91). Thus, statins are not necessarily required to develop anti-HMGR myositis. Clinically, patients present severe and acute muscle weakness, dramatically elevated CK level, but extra-muscular disorders are uncommon (65, 66, 71). Anti-HMGCR aAbs have also been identified in the sera of juvenile myositis, without exposure either to statins or cancer. Clinical features in children may wrongly shift toward muscular dystrophy (92).

TARGETS OF CANCER-ASSOCIATED AUTOIMMUNE RESPONSE IN MYOSITIS

Intriguingly, all three aAb targets in cancer-associated myositis are involved to some extent in cancer pathogenesis.

TIF1γ, Encoded by the *TRIM33* Gene

TIF1γ, also known as ecto, RETfused7, or TRIM33, was discovered in 1999 and identified as the third member of the TIF1 protein (after TIF1α and TIF1β) (73). These three proteins belong to the TRIM (tripartite motif) protein family defined by a particular RING-finger domain (93). TIF1 proteins are a subfamily characterized by several domains from 3′ to 5′, including the RING-finger domain, 1 or 2B-boxes, a coiled-coil domain, a plant homeodomain (PHD), and a bromodomain (94). They are involved in multiple critical biological processes. TIF1γ is particularly known for being involved in embryonic development, hematopoiesis, mitosis and cycle regulation, DNA repair, innate and adaptive immunity, osteoblast differentiation, viral transcription, and oncogenesis in case of dysregulation. TIF1γ can exert its role as an E3-ubiquitin ligase, as a histone-binding protein or by sumoylating proteins.

The main interacting pathways of TIF1γ are the TGF-β canonical (Smad4-dependent) and non-canonical (Smad4-independent) pathways (95–97). In the canonical pathway, TIF1γ acts either as a repressor (*via* ubiquitination), a competitor or a partner of Smad4, depending on the cellular context (96). In the canonical TGF-β pathway, the activation of the TGF-β receptor leads to the recruitment of RSmad (Smad 2 or 3) and phosphorylation allows the formation of a RSmad/Smad4 complex, which next enters the nucleus to activate the transcription of targeted genes. During mammalian embryonic development, TIF1γ plays a major role in patterning and polarizing embryonic cells before gastrulation by inhibiting Nodal/Smad4 signaling, which promotes endodermic proliferation (98). Later in embryonic development, Smad4 and TIF1γ cooperate or act redundantly to promote both proliferation and differentiation of neural stem cells and palate development (99, 100). It has been shown that TIF1γ participates in the differentiation of stem cells in collaboration with Smad4, by direct interaction with histone *via* PHD–bromodomain leading to the assembling of Smad4/Smad2–3 complex on targeted genes (101). In adult tissues, TIF1γ promotes the terminal differentiation of mammary gland and lactation by antagonization of Smad4 (102), supports both osteoblast proliferation and differentiation under stimulation of bone morphogenetic proteins (BMP) *via* the activation of a particular RSmad complex (Smad1/5) (103), regulates granulopoiesis in mice (104), and participates in the development of iNKT cells (105). During erythropoiesis, Smad4 and TIF1γ competitively bind to phosphorylated SMad2/3 (RSmad) in response to TGF-β to promote the proliferation and maturation of erythroblasts (106, 107). Otherwise, TIF1γ is involved in the balance between lymphoid and myeloid lineage and protects hematopoietic stem cells from aging (108), through TAL1 and PU1 DNA-binding protein, whose transcriptional activity depend on TGF-β (109, 110). TIF1γ has many other functions in cells, mediated by different pathways and functions. Regarding the innate immune system, TIF1γ directly represses the transcription of the interferon-b gene (*ifnb*) at late phase of macrophage activation (74). Also, it binds multiple chromatin sites in monocyte to promote production of macrophage, binds other chromatin sites in mature macrophage to regulate the responses after toll-like receptor (TLR) activation by lipo-polysaccharide (LPS) (111), and is directly involved in proteasome activation *via* the ubiquitination of DHX33 (112). TIF1γ also has many roles in cell homeostasis; TIF1γ is strongly involved in antiproliferative cellular effect by (i) mediating ubiquitination and then the degradation of LIM-domain-binding protein which is involved in the transcription of cycle activator genes (113) and (ii) interaction with APC/C (anaphase-promoting complex/cyclosome) to promote the alignment and stability of chromosomes during mitosis and to prevent abnormal metaphase–anaphase transition (75, 76). Moreover, TIF1γ is largely involved in DNA repair by recruiting different proteins promoting chromatin relaxation and repair (114, 115). Next, TIF1γ is a strong tumor suppressor by preventing β-catenin degradation (116), epithelial-to-mesenchymal transition (117, 118), and by regulation of the chromatin (119, 120). The role of TIF1γ as a tumor suppressor has been directly shown in chronic myelomonocytic leukemia (121), pancreatic tumor (122–124), hepatocellular carcinoma (125), renal cell carcinoma (126), and non-small cell lung cancer (127), where TIF1γ decreased expression or inactivation promotes proliferation and probably epithelial-to-mesenchymal transition (97–104). Paradoxically, overexpression of TIF1γ is involved in oncogenesis notably in breast cancer, where TIF1γ interferes with TGF-β to promote poorer prognosis (128). Moreover, hyper-expression of TIF1γ has been shown in a significant proportion of colorectal adenocarcinomas (129).

NXP2, Encoded by the MORC3 Gene

MORC3 (microrchidia3) is a nuclear protein which belongs to a highly conserved nuclear matrix protein family which has recently been identified (77). Four MORC members have been identified and are characterized by three common structural domains (ATPase domain, Zinc finger domain, and coiled-coil domain) involved in chromatin remodeling and epigenetic regulation (77). MORC3 includes two other domains, a nuclear matrix binding site and an RNA binding site, essential for the regulation of transcription (78). Its mRNA expression is relatively ubiquitous but the expression of MORC3 protein is particularly elevated in immune cells (78, 79). MORC3 plays several critical roles in cell regulation, illustrated by an early death at birth or day 1 in MORC3 knockout mice (130). MORC3 promotes the activation of p53, a tumor suppressor inducing cellular senescence in response to oncogenic factors and supports the architecture of the nucleus (78, 130). The ATPase domain of MORC3 interacts with the coiled-coil domain to form homodimers that can bind DNA (131). Zinc finger is implicated in the nucleus localization and binds MORC3 to histone (132). These two mechanisms seem to be involved in DNA repair and epigenetic regulation (77, 80). MORC3 interacts with ROR1, a tyrosine kinase involved in pre-B cell receptor signaling pathway promoting cell proliferation (133). Finally, MORC3 plays a role in the transduction of calcium homeostasis regulator and is involved in bone remodeling (134).

HMGCR, Encoded by the *HMGCR* Gene

HMGCR is a limiting enzyme from the cholesterol biosynthetic chain, catalyzing the reduction reaction of HMGCoA to mevalonate (81). This enzyme has a large transmembrane domain in the endoplasmic reticular membrane and the harbored cytosolic N and C terminal domain. The catalytic domain is in the C-terminal domain (82, 83). This catalytic domain is the target of both statins and specific autoantibodies. Interestingly, it has been recently shown that its functions were indirectly crucial in many pathways. Indeed, HMGCR positively regulates the growth and migration of glioblastoma cells and could play a role in the metastatic capacities of tumoral cells, as well as other enzymes involved in lipidic metabolism (135). The role of HMGCR and the mevalonate pathway in oncogenesis has been suspected for two decades and cases of tumors have been reported to exhibit higher level and activity of HMGCR (136, 137). In 2010, Clendening et al. (138) confirmed this hypothesis by showing that the dysregulation of HMGCR promotes transformation of normal breast epithelial cells and

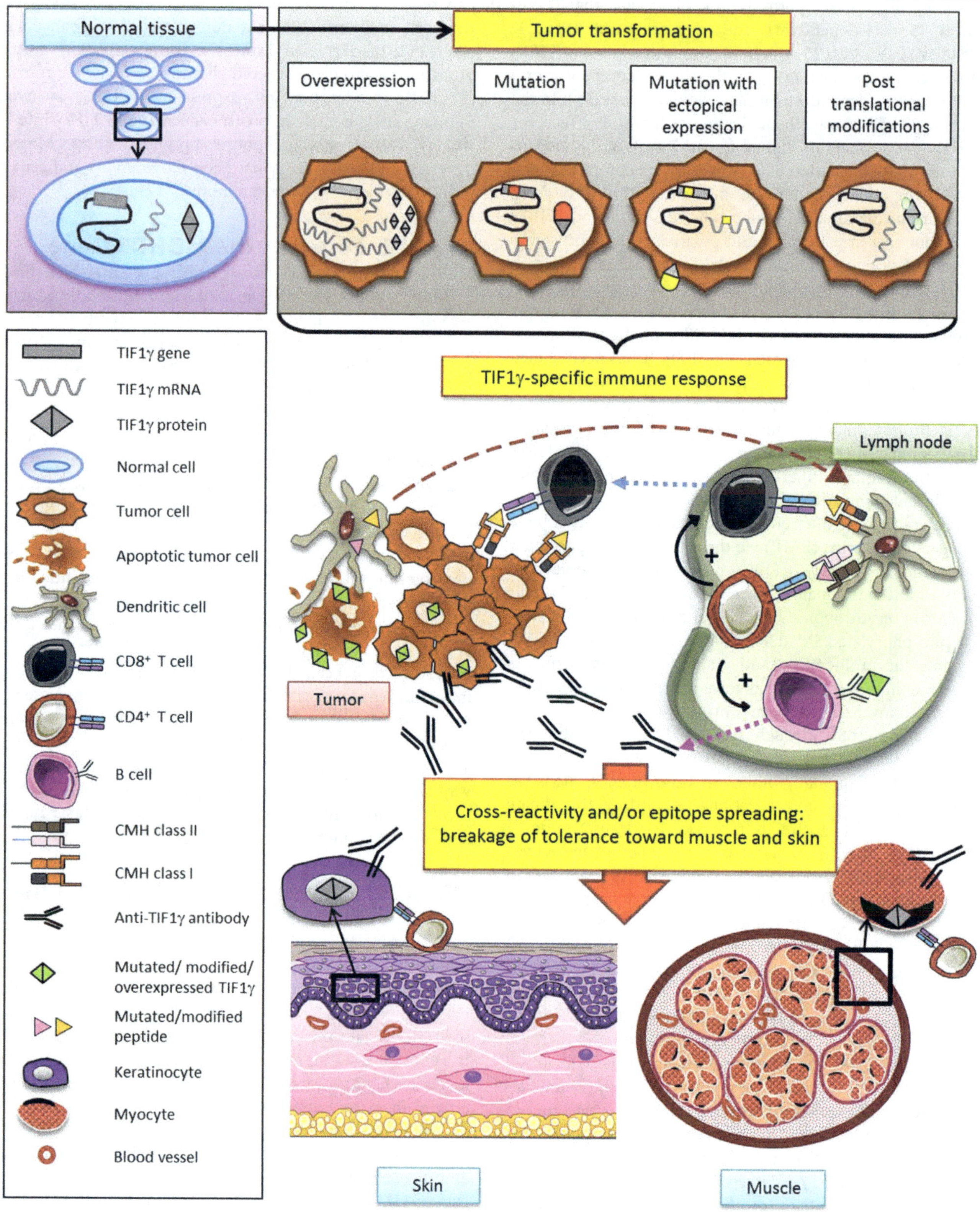

FIGURE 3 | Hypothetical model of specific antitumoral response as a trigger of dermatomyositis through the example of TIF1γ. According to this model, TIF1γ (or NXP2, or HMGCR) is modified in the tumor (gene mutation, overexpression, ectopic expression, posttranslational modification), leading to the development of a TIF1γ- (or NXP2-, or HMGCR-) specific T and B cell antitumor response. Secondarily, breakage of tolerance results from cross-reactivity and/or epitope spreading, promoting a response against muscle and skin.

growth of transformed cells (138). Moreover, different levels of HMGCR are associated with different response to radiotherapy in bladder cancer (139) and upregulation of HMGCR is also known to promote proliferation and migration of malignant cells in both glioblastoma and gastric cancer (135, 140). *In vitro* inhibition of HMGCR performed by specific miRNA limits proliferation, invasion, and metastasis process of breast cancer cells (141).

TIF1γ, NXP2, AND HMGCR: TARGETS OF AN ANTITUMORAL RESPONSE?

In the model proposed by Joseph and colleagues in systemic sclerosis, the immune response directed against POL3 was initially an antitumor immune response. Oncogenesis results from random and additive mutations on several genes some of which are involved in mitotic checkpoint, DNA repair, or differentiation, under the effect of viruses, oncogenes, or radiation. Later, tumoral cells can over-express, ectopically express, or express mutated forms of distinct proteins. The immune system may recognize these newly synthetized forms as neoantigens, which may ultimately lead to T cell and B cell responses (142, 143).

In many human cancers, TIF1γ is considered as a tumor suppressor by inhibiting the TGF-β pathway. HMGCR also seems to be involved to some extent in oncogenesis through its role in metabolic pathways. Today, NXP2 is not directly known to be involved in cancer but it interacts with the well documented p53 tumor suppressor. Therefore, the targets of these three MSA appear to be proteins involved in cellular pathways that intervene in tumor promotion. Thus, it is reasonable to hypothesize that somatic mutations of TIF1γ, NXP2, or HMGCR genes in tumors may provoke a specific antitumoral immune response which may secondarily extend to the target organs of myositis (muscle, skin) by cross-reactivity and/or a process of epitope spreading (**Figure 3**). It is tempting to speculate that absence of cancer in some myositis patients may result from an efficacious antitumoral immune response: in this view, myositis might be the immunological price to pay for tumor eradication.

The hypothesis developed herein implies that the above-mentioned antitumoral response provokes/sustains myositis. How this response could promote myositis is unclear. Indeed, the three TIF1γ, NXP-2, and HMGCR proteins are ubiquitously expressed, raising the question of how they could be muscle/skin-specific. In this regard, it should be remembered that most if not all MSAs, associated with cancer or not, are specific for ubiquitously expressed, intracellular proteins such as t-RNA synthetases, MDA-5, and signal recognition particles.

Some elements support the direct pathogenicity of aAbs in some forms of myositis. For instance, aAb level correlates with clinical evolution in IMNM (72, 144–146). The pathogenic effect of aAbs is particularly real for anti-HMGCR aAb. Indeed, Arouche-Delaperche and colleagues recently demonstrated that anti-HMGCR aAbs promoted muscle atrophy and impaired regeneration and expression of inflammatory cytokines (147). A similar effect could be expected for anti-TIF1γ and NXP2 aAbs. TIF1γ has been shown to be over-expressed in regenerating muscle (148), which could explain the recognition of TIF1γ in muscle by aAb.

THE THERAPEUTIC DILEMMA OF CANCER-ASSOCIATED MYOSITIS

Most myositis clinical trials exclude patients with cancer, limiting the spectrum of our therapeutic knowledge. While beneficial for treating myositis, immunosuppression is of difficult use in the presence of cancer. Reciprocally, myositis alters the patient's condition and complicates the therapeutic strategy, i.e., administering antitumoral drugs or performing surgery. Guidelines will be required to help manage patients in this context. The hypothesis of myositis triggered by cancer, rather than the opposite, supports a therapeutic strategy of performing an active antitumoral treatment compatible with the patient's myositis status. Among new cancer therapies, immune checkpoint inhibitors may expose the patient to an exacerbation of autoimmunity that may yield a myositis flare. Since aAbs may be directly involved in myositis pathogenesis, therapeutic trials evaluating plasma exchanges are welcome.

CONCLUSION

Taken together, available data point to a unicist view of cancer-associated myositis, in which AID may result from an antitumoral response. This response may be triggered by mutations, overexpression, or posttranslational modification of the autoantigen in tumor. Elucidating these mechanisms will provide strong clues to better understand the potential role of cancer as a cause of autoimmunity.

AUTHOR CONTRIBUTIONS

The first version of this review was written by AA and NC. OB revised it critically for important intellectual content. All authors approved the version to be published.

ACKNOWLEDGMENTS

We are grateful to Nikki Sabourin-Gibbs (Rouen University Hospital) for her help in editing the manuscript. We would like to thank Marie Beylot-Barry (Bordeaux University Hospital) for providing clinical images, and Philippe Courville (Rouen University Hospital) and François-Jérôme Authier (Henri Mondor Hospital-APHP) for providing histological images. We also express our gratitude to François-Jérôme Authier, Yves Allenbach (Pitié Salpêtrière Hospital-APHP), and Alain Meyer (Strasbourg University Hospital) for their critical reading of the manuscript and helpful suggestions.

REFERENCES

1. Bohan A, Peter JB. Polymyositis and dermatomyositis (first of two parts). *N Engl J Med* (1975) 292(7):344–7. doi:10.1056/NEJM197502132920706
2. Zintzaras E, Voulgarelis M, Moutsopoulos HM. The risk of lymphoma development in autoimmune diseases: a meta-analysis. *Arch Intern Med* (2005) 165(20):2337–44. doi:10.1001/archinte.165.20.2337
3. Shah AA, Casciola-Rosen L, Rosen A. Review: cancer-induced autoimmunity in the rheumatic diseases. *Arthritis Rheumatol* (2015) 67(2):317–26. doi:10.1002/art.38928
4. Egiziano G, Bernatsky S, Shah AA. Cancer and autoimmunity: harnessing longitudinal cohorts to probe the link. *Best Pract Res Clin Rheumatol* (2016) 30(1):53–62. doi:10.1016/j.berh.2016.03.001
5. Bernatsky S, Ramsey-Goldman R, Joseph L, Boivin JF, Costenbader KH, Urowitz MB, et al. Lymphoma risk in systemic lupus: effects of disease activity versus treatment. *Ann Rheum Dis* (2014) 73(1):138–42. doi:10.1136/annrheumdis-2012-202099
6. Liang Y, Yang Z, Qin B, Zhong R. Primary Sjogren's syndrome and malignancy risk: a systematic review and meta-analysis. *Ann Rheum Dis* (2014) 73(6):1151–6. doi:10.1136/annrheumdis-2013-203305
7. Bernatsky S, Ramsey-Goldman R, Labrecque J, Joseph L, Boivin JF, Petri M, et al. Cancer risk in systemic lupus: an updated international multi-centre cohort study. *J Autoimmun* (2013) 42:130–5. doi:10.1016/j.jaut.2012.12.009
8. Honnorat J, Antoine JC. Paraneoplastic neurological syndromes. *Orphanet J Rare Dis* (2007) 2:22. doi:10.1186/1750-1172-2-22
9. Manley GT, Smitt PS, Dalmau J, Posner JB. Hu antigens: reactivity with Hu antibodies, tumor expression, and major immunogenic sites. *Ann Neurol* (1995) 38(1):102–10. doi:10.1002/ana.410380117
10. Pignolet BS, Gebauer CM, Liblau RS. Immunopathogenesis of paraneoplastic neurological syndromes associated with anti-Hu antibodies: a beneficial antitumor immune response going awry. *Oncoimmunology* (2013) 2(12):e27384. doi:10.4161/onci.27384
11. Joseph CG, Darrah E, Shah AA, Skora AD, Casciola-Rosen LA, Wigley FM, et al. Association of the autoimmune disease scleroderma with an immunologic response to cancer. *Science* (2014) 343(6167):152–7. doi:10.1126/science.1246886
12. Griggs RC, Askanas V, DiMauro S, Engel A, Karpati G, Mendell JR, et al. Inclusion body myositis and myopathies. *Ann Neurol* (1995) 38(5):705–13. doi:10.1002/ana.410380504
13. Hoogendijk JE, Amato AA, Lecky BR, Choy EH, Lundberg IE, Rose MR, et al. 119th ENMC international workshop: trial design in adult idiopathic inflammatory myopathies, with the exception of inclusion body myositis, 10-12 October 2003, Naarden, The Netherlands. *Neuromuscul Disord* (2004) 14(5):337–45. doi:10.1016/j.nmd.2004.02.006
14. Troyanov Y, Targoff IN, Tremblay JL, Goulet JR, Raymond Y, Senecal JL. Novel classification of idiopathic inflammatory myopathies based on overlap syndrome features and autoantibodies: analysis of 100 French Canadian patients. *Medicine (Baltimore)* (2005) 84(4):231–49. doi:10.1097/01.md.0000173991.74008.b0
15. Lundberg IE. New ways to subclassify patients with myositis. *J Intern Med* (2016) 280(1):4–7. doi:10.1111/joim.12515
16. Lundberg IE, Miller FW, Tjärnlund A, Bottai M. Diagnosis and classification of idiopathic inflammatory myopathies. *J Intern Med* (2016) 280(1):39–51. doi:10.1111/joim.12524
17. Simon JP, Marie I, Jouen F, Boyer O, Martinet J. Autoimmune myopathies: where do we stand? *Front Immunol* (2016) 7:234. doi:10.3389/fimmu.2016.00234
18. Oddis CV, Conte CG, Steen VD, Medsger TA. Incidence of polymyositis-dermatomyositis: a 20-year study of hospital diagnosed cases in Allegheny County, PA 1963-1982. *J Rheumatol* (1990) 17(10):1329–34.
19. Francès C, Bessis D. Dermatomyosite. *Manifestations dermatologiques des connectivites, vasculites et affections systémiques apparentées*. 2nd Ed. Paris: Springer (2012). p. 1–15.
20. McKee P, Calonje E, Granter S. *Pathology of the Skin with Clinical Correlations*. 3rd ed. Philadelphia: Elsevier/Mosby (2005).
21. Sontheimer RD. Cutaneous features of classic dermatomyositis and amyopathic dermatomyositis. *Curr Opin Rheumatol* (1999) 11(6):475–82. doi:10.1097/00002281-199911000-00005
22. Iaccarino L, Ghirardello A, Bettio S, Zen M, Gatto M, Punzi L, et al. The clinical features, diagnosis and classification of dermatomyositis. *J Autoimmun* (2014) 4(8–49):122–7. doi:10.1016/j.jaut.2013.11.005
23. Gitiaux C, Kostallari E, Lafuste P, Authier FJ, Christov C, Gherardi RK. Whole microvascular unit deletions in dermatomyositis. *Ann Rheum Dis* (2013) 72(3):445–52. doi:10.1136/annrheumdis-2012-201822
24. Greenberg SA, Pinkus JL, Pinkus GS, Burleson T, Sanoudou D, Tawil R, et al. Interferon-alpha/beta-mediated innate immune mechanisms in dermatomyositis. *Ann Neurol* (2005) 57(5):664–78. doi:10.1002/ana.20464
25. Wong D, Kea B, Pesich R, Higgs BW, Zhu W, Brown P, et al. Interferon and biologic signatures in dermatomyositis skin: specificity and heterogeneity across diseases. *PLoS One* (2012) 7(1):e29161. doi:10.1371/journal.pone.0029161
26. Huard C, Gullà SV, Bennett DV, Coyle AJ, Vleugels RA, Greenberg SA. Correlation of cutaneous disease activity with type 1 interferon gene signature and interferon β in dermatomyositis. *Br J Dermatol* (2017) 176(5):1224–30. doi:10.1111/bjd.15006
27. Hunger RE, Dürr C, Brand CU. Cutaneous leukocytoclastic vasculitis in dermatomyositis suggests malignancy. *Dermatology* (2001) 202(2):123–6. doi:10.1159/000051611
28. Burnouf M, Mahé E, Verpillat P, Descamps V, Lebrun-Vignes B, Picard-Dahan C, et al. [Cutaneous necrosis is predictive of cancer in adult dermatomyositis]. *Ann Dermatol Venereol* (2003) 130(3):313–6.
29. Tersiguel AC, Longueville C, Beltan E, Vincent T, Tressières B, Cordel N. [Prevalence of cancer in the Afro-Caribbean population presenting dermatomyositis and anti-synthetase syndrome: a preliminary study conducted at Pointe-à-Pitre University Hospital, 2000-2012]. *Ann Dermatol Venereol* (2014) 141(10):575–80. doi:10.1016/j.annder.2014.04.112
30. Kankeleit H. Über primaire nichteitrige polymyositis. *Dtsch Arch Klin Med* (1916) 120:335–9.
31. Stertz G. Polymyositis. *Berl Klin Wochenschau* (1916) 53:489.
32. Hill CL, Zhang Y, Sigurgeirsson B, Pukkala E, Mellemkjaer L, Airio A, et al. Frequency of specific cancer types in dermatomyositis and polymyositis: a population-based study. *Lancet* (2001) 357(9250):96–100. doi:10.1016/S0140-6736(00)03540-6
33. Stockton D, Doherty VR, Brewster DH. Risk of cancer in patients with dermatomyositis or polymyositis, and follow-up implications: a Scottish population-based cohort study. *Br J Cancer* (2001) 85(1):41–5. doi:10.1054/bjoc.2001.1699
34. András C, Ponyi A, Constantin T, Csiki Z, Szekanecz E, Szodoray P, et al. Dermatomyositis and polymyositis associated with malignancy: a 21-year retrospective study. *J Rheumatol* (2008) 35(3):438–44.
35. Zahr ZA, Baer AN. Malignancy in myositis. *Curr Rheumatol Rep* (2011) 13(3):208–15. doi:10.1007/s11926-011-0169-7
36. Airio A, Pukkala E, Isomäki H. Elevated cancer incidence in patients with dermatomyositis: a population based study. *J Rheumatol* (1995) 22(7):1300–3.
37. Wakata N, Kurihara T, Saito E, Kinoshita M. Polymyositis and dermatomyositis associated with malignancy: a 30-year retrospective study. *Int J Dermatol* (2002) 41(11):729–34. doi:10.1046/j.1365-4362.2002.01648.x
38. Yang Z, Lin F, Qin B, Liang Y, Zhong R. Polymyositis/dermatomyositis and malignancy risk: a metaanalysis study. *J Rheumatol* (2015) 42(2):282–91. doi:10.3899/jrheum.140566
39. Betteridge Z, McHugh N. Myositis-specific autoantibodies: an important tool to support diagnosis of myositis. *J Intern Med* (2016) 280(1):8–23. doi:10.1111/joim.12451
40. Ghirardello A, Zampieri S, Iaccarino L, Tarricone E, Bendo R, Gambari PF, et al. Anti-Mi-2 antibodies. *Autoimmunity* (2005) 38(1):79–83. doi:10.1080/08916930400022681
41. Selva-O'Callaghan A, Labrador-Horrillo M, Solans-Laque R, Simeon-Aznar CP, Martínez-Gómez X, Vilardell-Tarrés M. Myositis-specific and myositis-associated antibodies in a series of eighty-eight Mediterranean patients with idiopathic inflammatory myopathy. *Arthritis Rheum* (2006) 55(5):791–8. doi:10.1002/art.22237
42. Chinoy H, Fertig N, Oddis CV, Ollier WE, Cooper RG. The diagnostic utility of myositis autoantibody testing for predicting the risk of cancer-associated myositis. *Ann Rheum Dis* (2007) 66(10):1345–9. doi:10.1136/ard.2006.068502

43. Fiorentino D, Chung L, Zwerner J, Rosen A, Casciola-Rosen L. The mucocutaneous and systemic phenotype of dermatomyositis patients with antibodies to MDA5 (CADM-140): a retrospective study. *J Am Acad Dermatol* (2011) 65(1):25–34. doi:10.1016/j.jaad.2010.09.016
44. Hall JC, Casciola-Rosen L, Samedy LA, Werner J, Owoyemi K, Danoff SK, et al. Anti-melanoma differentiation-associated protein 5-associated dermatomyositis: expanding the clinical spectrum. *Arthritis Care Res (Hoboken)* (2013) 65(8):1307–15. doi:10.1002/acr.21992
45. Sato S, Kuwana M, Fujita T, Suzuki Y. Anti-CADM-140/MDA5 autoantibody titer correlates with disease activity and predicts disease outcome in patients with dermatomyositis and rapidly progressive interstitial lung disease. *Mod Rheumatol* (2013) 23(3):496–502. doi:10.1007/s10165-012-0663-4
46. Betteridge ZE, Gunawardena H, Chinoy H, North J, Ollier WE, Cooper RG, et al. Clinical and human leucocyte antigen class II haplotype associations of autoantibodies to small ubiquitin-like modifier enzyme, a dermatomyositis-specific autoantigen target, in UK Caucasian adult-onset myositis. *Ann Rheum Dis* (2009) 68(10):1621–5. doi:10.1136/ard.2008.097162
47. Muro Y, Sugiura K, Akiyama M. Low prevalence of anti-small ubiquitin-like modifier activating enzyme antibodies in dermatomyositis patients. *Autoimmunity* (2013) 46(4):279–84. doi:10.3109/08916934.2012.755958
48. Ge Y, Lu X, Shu X, Peng Q, Wang G. Clinical characteristics of anti-SAE antibodies in Chinese patients with dermatomyositis in comparison with different patient cohorts. *Sci Rep* (2017) 7(1):188. doi:10.1038/s41598-017-00240-6
49. Targoff IN, Mamyrova G, Trieu EP, Perurena O, Koneru B, O'Hanlon TP, et al. A novel autoantibody to a 155-kd protein is associated with dermatomyositis. *Arthritis Rheum* (2006) 54(11):3682–9. doi:10.1002/art.22164
50. Trallero-Araguás E, Rodrigo-Pendás J, Selva-O'Callaghan A, Martínez-Gómez X, Bosch X, Labrador-Horrillo M, et al. Usefulness of anti-p155 autoantibody for diagnosing cancer-associated dermatomyositis: a systematic review and meta-analysis. *Arthritis Rheum* (2012) 64(2):523–32. doi:10.1002/art.33379
51. Gunawardena H, Wedderburn LR, Chinoy H, Betteridge ZE, North J, Ollier WE, et al. Autoantibodies to a 140-kd protein in juvenile dermatomyositis are associated with calcinosis. *Arthritis Rheum* (2009) 60(6):1807–14. doi:10.1002/art.24547
52. Fiorentino DF, Chung LS, Christopher-Stine L, Zaba L, Li S, Mammen AL, et al. Most patients with cancer-associated dermatomyositis have antibodies to nuclear matrix protein NXP-2 or transcription intermediary factor 1γ. *Arthritis Rheum* (2013) 65(11):2954–62. doi:10.1002/art.38093
53. Basharat P, Lahouti HA, Mammen AL, Pinal-Fernandez I, Bichile T, Lloyd TE, et al. Diabetes and atorvastatin are potential risk factors for statin-associated myopathy with autoantibodies against 3-hydroxy-3-methylglutaryl-coenzyme A reductase. *American College of Rheumatology Meeting 2014*. Boston, USA (2014).
54. Limaye V, Bundell C, Hollingsworth P, Rojana-Udomsart A, Mastaglia F, Blumbergs P, et al. Clinical and genetic associations of autoantibodies to 3-hydroxy-3-methyl-glutaryl-coenzyme a reductase in patients with immune-mediated myositis and necrotizing myopathy. *Muscle Nerve* (2015) 52(2):196–203. doi:10.1002/mus.24541
55. Tiniakou E, Mammen AL. Idiopathic inflammatory myopathies and malignancy: a comprehensive review. *Clin Rev Allergy Immunol* (2015) 52(1):20–33. doi:10.1007/s12016-015-8511-x
56. Allenbach Y, Keraen J, Bouvier AM, Jooste V, Champtiaux N, Hervier B, et al. High risk of cancer in autoimmune necrotizing myopathies: usefulness of myositis specific antibody. *Brain* (2016) 139(Pt 8):2131–5. doi:10.1093/brain/aww054
57. Kaji K, Fujimoto M, Hasegawa M, Kondo M, Saito Y, Komura K, et al. Identification of a novel autoantibody reactive with 155 and 140 kDa nuclear proteins in patients with dermatomyositis: an association with malignancy. *Rheumatology (Oxford)* (2007) 46(1):25–8. doi:10.1093/rheumatology/kel161
58. Rider LG, Nistala K. The juvenile idiopathic inflammatory myopathies: pathogenesis, clinical and autoantibody phenotypes, and outcomes. *J Intern Med* (2016) 280(1):24–38. doi:10.1111/joim.12444
59. Hida A, Yamashita T, Hosono Y, Inoue M, Kaida K, Kadoya M, et al. Anti-TIF1-γ antibody and cancer-associated myositis: a clinicohistopathologic study. *Neurology* (2016) 87(3):299–308. doi:10.1212/WNL.0000000000002863
60. Fiorentino DF, Kuo K, Chung L, Zaba L, Li S, Casciola-Rosen L. Distinctive cutaneous and systemic features associated with antitranscriptional intermediary factor-1γ antibodies in adults with dermatomyositis. *J Am Acad Dermatol* (2015) 72(3):449–55. doi:10.1016/j.jaad.2014.12.009
61. Fujimoto M, Watanabe R, Ishitsuka Y, Okiyama N. Recent advances in dermatomyositis-specific autoantibodies. *Curr Opin Rheumatol* (2016) 28(6):636–44. doi:10.1097/BOR.0000000000000329
62. Gunawardena H, Wedderburn LR, North J, Betteridge Z, Dunphy J, Chinoy H, et al. Clinical associations of autoantibodies to a p155/140 kDa doublet protein in juvenile dermatomyositis. *Rheumatology (Oxford)* (2008) 47(3):324–8. doi:10.1093/rheumatology/kem359
63. Habers GE, Huber AM, Mamyrova G, Targoff IN, O'Hanlon TP, Adams S, et al. Brief report: association of myositis autoantibodies, clinical features, and environmental exposures at illness onset with disease course in juvenile myositis. *Arthritis Rheumatol* (2016) 68(3):761–8. doi:10.1002/art.39466
64. Ceribelli A, Fredi M, Taraborelli M, Cavazzana I, Franceschini F, Quinzanini M, et al. Anti-MJ/NXP-2 autoantibody specificity in a cohort of adult Italian patients with polymyositis/dermatomyositis. *Arthritis Res Ther* (2012) 14(2):R97. doi:10.1186/ar3822
65. Christopher-Stine L, Casciola-Rosen LA, Hong G, Chung T, Corse AM, Mammen AL. A novel autoantibody recognizing 200-kd and 100-kd proteins is associated with an immune-mediated necrotizing myopathy. *Arthritis Rheum* (2010) 62(9):2757–66. doi:10.1002/art.27572
66. Mammen AL, Chung T, Christopher-Stine L, Rosen P, Rosen A, Doering KR, et al. Autoantibodies against 3-hydroxy-3-methylglutaryl-coenzyme A reductase in patients with statin-associated autoimmune myopathy. *Arthritis Rheum* (2011) 63(3):713–21. doi:10.1002/art.30156
67. Ichimura Y, Matsushita T, Hamaguchi Y, Kaji K, Hasegawa M, Tanino Y, et al. Anti-NXP2 autoantibodies in adult patients with idiopathic inflammatory myopathies: possible association with malignancy. *Ann Rheum Dis* (2012) 71(5):710–3. doi:10.1136/annrheumdis-2011-200697
68. Basharat P, Christopher-Stine L. Immune-mediated necrotizing myopathy: update on diagnosis and management. *Curr Rheumatol Rep* (2015) 17(12):72. doi:10.1007/s11926-015-0548-6
69. Kadoya M, Hida A, Hashimoto Maeda M, Taira K, Ikenaga C, Uchio N, et al. Cancer association as a risk factor for anti-HMGCR antibody-positive myopathy. *Neurol Neuroimmunol Neuroinflamm* (2016) 3(6):e290. doi:10.1212/NXI.0000000000000290
70. Rogers A, Chung L, Li S, Casciola-Rosen L, Fiorentino DF. The cutaneous and systemic findings associated with nuclear matrix protein-2 antibodies in adult dermatomyositis patients. *Arthritis Care Res (Hoboken)* (2017). doi:10.1002/acr.23210
71. Allenbach Y, Benveniste O. [Autoantibody profile in myositis]. *Rev Med Interne* (2013) 35(7):437–43. doi:10.1016/j.revmed.2013.12.006
72. Allenbach Y, Benveniste O. Acquired necrotizing myopathies. *Curr Opin Neurol* (2013) 26(5):554–60. doi:10.1097/WCO.0b013e328364e9d9
73. Venturini L, You J, Stadler M, Galien R, Lallemand V, Koken MH, et al. TIF1gamma, a novel member of the transcriptional intermediary factor 1 family. *Oncogene* (1999) 18(5):1209–17. doi:10.1038/sj.onc.1202655
74. Ferri F, Parcelier A, Petit V, Gallouet AS, Lewandowski D, Dalloz M, et al. TRIM33 switches off Ifnb1 gene transcription during the late phase of macrophage activation. *Nat Commun* (2015) 6:8900. doi:10.1038/ncomms9900
75. Sedgwick GG, Townsend K, Martin A, Shimwell NJ, Grand RJ, Stewart GS, et al. Transcriptional intermediary factor 1γ binds to the anaphase-promoting complex/cyclosome and promotes mitosis. *Oncogene* (2013) 32(39):4622–33. doi:10.1038/onc.2012.501
76. Pommier RM, Gout J, Vincent DF, Alcaraz LB, Chuvin N, Arfi V, et al. TIF1γ suppresses tumor progression by regulating mitotic checkpoints and chromosomal stability. *Cancer Res* (2015) 75(20):4335–50. doi:10.1158/0008-5472.CAN-14-3426
77. Li DQ, Nair SS, Kumar R. The MORC family: new epigenetic regulators of transcription and DNA damage response. *Epigenetics* (2013) 8(7):685–93. doi:10.4161/epi.24976
78. Kimura Y, Sakai F, Nakano O, Kisaki O, Sugimoto H, Sawamura T, et al. The newly identified human nuclear protein NXP-2 possesses three distinct domains, the nuclear matrix-binding, RNA-binding, and

coiled-coil domains. *J Biol Chem* (2002) 277(23):20611–7. doi:10.1074/jbc.M201440200

79. Su AI, Wiltshire T, Batalov S, Lapp H, Ching KA, Block D, et al. A gene atlas of the mouse and human protein-encoding transcriptomes. *Proc Natl Acad Sci U S A* (2004) 101(16):6062–7. doi:10.1073/pnas.0400782101
80. Hong G, Qiu H, Wang C, Jadhav G, Wang H, Tickner J, et al. The emerging role of MORC family proteins in cancer development and bone homeostasis. *J Cell Physiol* (2017) 232(5):928–34. doi:10.1002/jcp.25665
81. Durr IF, Rudney H. The reduction of beta-hydroxy-beta-methyl-glutaryl coenzyme A to mevalonic acid. *J Biol Chem* (1960) 235:2572–8.
82. Roitelman J, Simoni RD. Distinct sterol and nonsterol signals for the regulated degradation of 3-hydroxy-3-methylglutaryl-CoA reductase. *J Biol Chem* (1992) 267(35):25264–73.
83. Stormo C, Kringen MK, Grimholt RM, Berg JP, Piehler AP. A novel 3-hydroxy-3-methylglutaryl-coenzyme A reductase (HMGCR) splice variant with an alternative exon 1 potentially encoding an extended N-terminus. *BMC Mol Biol* (2012) 13:29. doi:10.1186/1471-2199-13-29
84. Espada G, Maldonado Cocco JA, Fertig N, Oddis CV. Clinical and serologic characterization of an Argentine pediatric myositis cohort: identification of a novel autoantibody (anti-MJ) to a 142-kDa protein. *J Rheumatol* (2009) 36(11):2547–51. doi:10.3899/jrheum.090461
85. Ishikawa A, Muro Y, Sugiura K, Akiyama M. Development of an ELISA for detection of autoantibodies to nuclear matrix protein 2. *Rheumatology (Oxford)* (2012) 51(7):1181–7. doi:10.1093/rheumatology/kes033
86. Mammen AL, Gaudet D, Brisson D, Christopher-Stine L, Lloyd TE, Leffell MS, et al. Increased frequency of DRB1*11:01 in anti-hydroxymethylglutaryl-coenzyme A reductase-associated autoimmune myopathy. *Arthritis Care Res (Hoboken)* (2012) 64(8):1233–7. doi:10.1002/acr.21671
87. Kishi T, Rider LG, Pak K, Barillas-Arias L, Henrickson M, McCarthy PL, et al. Anti-3-hydroxy-3-methylglutaryl-coenzyme a reductase autoantibodies are associated with DRB1*07:01 and severe myositis in pediatric myositis patients. *Arthritis Care Res (Hoboken)* (2017) 69(7):1088–94. doi:10.1002/acr.23113
88. Grable-Esposito P, Katzberg HD, Greenberg SA, Srinivasan J, Katz J, Amato AA. Immune-mediated necrotizing myopathy associated with statins. *Muscle Nerve* (2010) 41(2):185–90. doi:10.1002/mus.21486
89. Allenbach Y, Drouot L, Rigolet A, Charuel JL, Jouen F, Romero NB, et al. Anti-HMGCR autoantibodies in European patients with autoimmune necrotizing myopathies: inconstant exposure to statin. *Medicine (Baltimore)* (2014) 93(3):150–7. doi:10.1097/MD.0000000000000028
90. Watanabe Y, Suzuki S, Nishimura H, Murata KY, Kurashige T, Ikawa M, et al. Statins and myotoxic effects associated with anti-3-hydroxy-3-methylglutaryl-coenzyme A reductase autoantibodies: an observational study in Japan. *Medicine (Baltimore)* (2015) 94(4):e416. doi:10.1097/MD.0000000000000416
91. Bergua C, Chiavelli H, Simon JP, Boyer O, Jouen F, Stenzel W, et al. Immune-mediated necrotizing myopathy. *Z Rheumatol* (2016) 75(2):151–6. doi:10.1007/s00393-015-0029-3
92. Liang WC, Uruha A, Suzuki S, Murakami N, Takeshita E, Chen WZ, et al. Pediatric necrotizing myopathy associated with anti-3-hydroxy-3-methylglutaryl-coenzyme A reductase antibodies. *Rheumatology (Oxford)* (2017) 56(2):287–93. doi:10.1093/rheumatology/kew386
93. Hatakeyama S. TRIM proteins and cancer. *Nat Rev Cancer* (2011) 11(11):792–804. doi:10.1038/nrc3139
94. Reymond A, Meroni G, Fantozzi A, Merla G, Cairo S, Luzi L, et al. The tripartite motif family identifies cell compartments. *EMBO J* (2001) 20(9):2140–51. doi:10.1093/emboj/20.9.2140
95. Agricola E, Randall RA, Gaarenstroom T, Dupont S, Hill CS. Recruitment of TIF1γ to chromatin via its PHD finger-bromodomain activates its ubiquitin ligase and transcriptional repressor activities. *Mol Cell* (2011) 43(1):85–96. doi:10.1016/j.molcel.2011.05.020
96. Andrieux G, Fattet L, Le Borgne M, Rimokh R, Théret N. Dynamic regulation of Tgf-B signaling by Tif1γ: a computational approach. *PLoS One* (2012) 7(3):e33761. doi:10.1371/journal.pone.0033761
97. Dupont S, Inui M, Newfeld SJ. Regulation of TGF-β signal transduction by mono- and deubiquitylation of Smads. *FEBS Lett* (2012) 586(14): 1913–20. doi:10.1016/j.febslet.2012.03.037
98. Morsut L, Yan KP, Enzo E, Aragona M, Soligo SM, Wendling O, et al. Negative control of Smad activity by ectodermin/Tif1gamma patterns the mammalian embryo. *Development* (2010) 137(15):2571–8. doi:10.1242/dev.053801
99. Falk S, Joosten E, Kaartinen V, Sommer L. Smad4 and Trim33/Tif1γ redundantly regulate neural stem cells in the developing cortex. *Cereb Cortex* (2014) 24(11):2951–63. doi:10.1093/cercor/bht149
100. Lane J, Yumoto K, Azhar M, Ninomiya-Tsuji J, Inagaki M, Hu Y, et al. Tak1, Smad4 and Trim33 redundantly mediate TGF-β3 signaling during palate development. *Dev Biol* (2015) 398(2):231–41. doi:10.1016/j.ydbio.2014.12.006
101. Massagué J, Xi Q. TGF-β control of stem cell differentiation genes. *FEBS Lett* (2012) 586(14):1953–8. doi:10.1016/j.febslet.2012.03.023
102. Hesling C, Lopez J, Fattet L, Gonzalo P, Treilleux I, Blanchard D, et al. Tif1γ is essential for the terminal differentiation of mammary alveolar epithelial cells and for lactation through SMAD4 inhibition. *Development* (2013) 140(1):167–75. doi:10.1242/dev.085068
103. Guo J, Qin W, Xing Q, Gao M, Wei F, Song Z, et al. TRIM33 is essential for osteoblast proliferation and differentiation via BMP pathway. *J Cell Physiol* (2017) 232(11):3158–69. doi:10.1002/jcp.25769
104. Chrétien ML, Legouge C, Martin RZ, Hammann A, Trad M, Aucagne R, et al. Trim33/Tif1γ is involved in late stages of granulomonopoiesis in mice. *Exp Hematol* (2016) 44(8):727–39.e6. doi:10.1016/j.exphem.2016.04.009
105. Doisne JM, Bartholin L, Yan KP, Garcia CN, Duarte N, Le Luduec JB, et al. iNKT cell development is orchestrated by different branches of TGF-beta signaling. *J Exp Med* (2009) 206(6):1365–78. doi:10.1084/jem.20090127
106. He W, Dorn DC, Erdjument-Bromage H, Tempst P, Moore MA, Massagué J. Hematopoiesis controlled by distinct TIF1gamma and Smad4 branches of the TGFbeta pathway. *Cell* (2006) 125(5):929–41. doi:10.1016/j.cell.2006.03.045
107. Bai X, Trowbridge JJ, Riley E, Lee JA, DiBiase A, Kaartinen VM, et al. TiF1-gamma plays an essential role in murine hematopoiesis and regulates transcriptional elongation of erythroid genes. *Dev Biol* (2013) 373(2):422–30. doi:10.1016/j.ydbio.2012.10.008
108. Quéré R, Saint-Paul L, Carmignac V, Martin RZ, Chrétien ML, Largeot A, et al. Tif1γ regulates the TGF-β1 receptor and promotes physiological aging of hematopoietic stem cells. *Proc Natl Acad Sci U S A* (2014) 111(29):10592–7. doi:10.1073/pnas.1405546111
109. Kusy S, Gault N, Ferri F, Lewandowski D, Barroca V, Jaracz-Ros A, et al. Adult hematopoiesis is regulated by TIF1γ, a repressor of TAL1 and PU.1 transcriptional activity. *Cell Stem Cell* (2011) 8(4):412–25. doi:10.1016/j.stem.2011.02.005
110. Monteiro R, Pouget C, Patient R. The gata1/pu.1 lineage fate paradigm varies between blood populations and is modulated by tif1γ. *EMBO J* (2011) 30(6):1093–103. doi:10.1038/emboj.2011.34
111. Gallouet AS, Ferri F, Petit V, Parcelier A, Lewandowski D, Gault N, et al. Macrophage production and activation are dependent on TRIM33. *Oncotarget* (2017) 8(3):5111–22. doi:10.18632/oncotarget.13872
112. Weng L, Mitoma H, Trichot C, Tricot C, Bao M, Liu Y, et al. The E3 ubiquitin ligase tripartite motif 33 is essential for cytosolic RNA-induced NLRP3 inflammasome activation. *J Immunol* (2014) 193(7):3676–82. doi:10.4049/jimmunol.1401448
113. Howard PW, Ransom DG, Maurer RA. Transcription intermediary factor 1gamma decreases protein expression of the transcriptional cofactor, LIM-domain-binding 1. *Biochem Biophys Res Commun* (2010) 396(3):674–8. doi:10.1016/j.bbrc.2010.04.160
114. Kulkarni A, Oza J, Yao M, Sohail H, Ginjala V, Tomas-Loba A, et al. Tripartite motif-containing 33 (TRIM33) protein functions in the poly(ADP-ribose) polymerase (PARP)-dependent DNA damage response through interaction with amplified in liver cancer 1 (ALC1) protein. *J Biol Chem* (2013) 288(45):32357–69. doi:10.1074/jbc.M113.459164
115. Oza J, Ganguly B, Kulkarni A, Ginjala V, Yao M, Ganesan S. A novel role of chromodomain protein CBX8 in DNA damage response. *J Biol Chem* (2016) 291(44):22881–93. doi:10.1074/jbc.M116.725879
116. Xue J, Chen Y, Wu Y, Wang Z, Zhou A, Zhang S, et al. Tumour suppressor TRIM33 targets nuclear β-catenin degradation. *Nat Commun* (2015) 6:6156. doi:10.1038/ncomms7156

117. Hesling C, Fattet L, Teyre G, Jury D, Gonzalo P, Lopez J, et al. Antagonistic regulation of EMT by TIF1γ and Smad4 in mammary epithelial cells. *EMBO Rep* (2011) 12(7):665–72. doi:10.1038/embor.2011.78

118. Ikeuchi Y, Dadakhujaev S, Chandhoke AS, Huynh MA, Oldenborg A, Ikeuchi M, et al. TIF1γ protein regulates epithelial-mesenchymal transition by operating as a small ubiquitin-like modifier (SUMO) E3 ligase for the transcriptional regulator SnoN1. *J Biol Chem* (2014) 289(36):25067–78. doi:10.1074/jbc.M114.575878

119. Herquel B, Ouararhni K, Davidson I. The TIF1α-related TRIM cofactors couple chromatin modifications to transcriptional regulation, signaling and tumor suppression. *Transcription* (2011) 2(5):231–6. doi:10.4161/trns.2.5.17725

120. Herquel B, Ouararhni K, Khetchoumian K, Ignat M, Teletin M, Mark M, et al. Transcription cofactors TRIM24, TRIM28, and TRIM33 associate to form regulatory complexes that suppress murine hepatocellular carcinoma. *Proc Natl Acad Sci U S A* (2011) 108(20):8212–7. doi:10.1073/pnas.1101544108

121. Aucagne R, Droin N, Paggetti J, Lagrange B, Largeot A, Hammann A, et al. Transcription intermediary factor 1γ is a tumor suppressor in mouse and human chronic myelomonocytic leukemia. *J Clin Invest* (2011) 121(6):2361–70. doi:10.1172/JCI45213

122. Vincent DF, Yan KP, Treilleux I, Gay F, Arfi V, Kaniewski B, et al. Inactivation of TIF1gamma cooperates with Kras to induce cystic tumors of the pancreas. *PLoS Genet* (2009) 5(7):e1000575. doi:10.1371/journal.pgen.1000575

123. Vincent DF, Gout J, Chuvin N, Arfi V, Pommier RM, Bertolino P, et al. Tif1γ suppresses murine pancreatic tumoral transformation by a Smad4-independent pathway. *Am J Pathol* (2012) 180(6):2214–21. doi:10.1016/j.ajpath.2012.02.006

124. Ligr M, Wu X, Daniels G, Zhang D, Wang H, Hajdu C, et al. Imbalanced expression of Tif1γ inhibits pancreatic ductal epithelial cell growth. *Am J Cancer Res* (2014) 4(3):196–210.

125. Ding ZY, Jin GN, Wang W, Chen WX, Wu YH, Ai X, et al. Reduced expression of transcriptional intermediary factor 1 gamma promotes metastasis and indicates poor prognosis of hepatocellular carcinoma. *Hepatology* (2014) 60(5):1620–36. doi:10.1002/hep.27273

126. Jingushi K, Ueda Y, Kitae K, Hase H, Egawa H, Ohshio I, et al. miR-629 targets TRIM33 to promote TGFβ/Smad signaling and metastatic phenotypes in ccRCC. *Mol Cancer Res* (2015) 13(3):565–74. doi:10.1158/1541-7786.MCR-14-0300

127. Wang L, Yang H, Lei Z, Zhao J, Chen Y, Chen P, et al. Repression of TIF1γ by SOX2 promotes TGF-β-induced epithelial-mesenchymal transition in non-small-cell lung cancer. *Oncogene* (2016) 35(7):867–77. doi:10.1038/onc.2015.141

128. Kassem L, Deygas M, Fattet L, Lopez J, Goulvent T, Lavergne E, et al. TIF1γ interferes with TGFβ1/SMAD4 signaling to promote poor outcome in operable breast cancer patients. *BMC Cancer* (2015) 15:453. doi:10.1186/s12885-015-1471-y

129. Jain S, Singhal S, Francis F, Hajdu C, Wang JH, Suriawinata A, et al. Association of overexpression of TIF1γ with colorectal carcinogenesis and advanced colorectal adenocarcinoma. *World J Gastroenterol* (2011) 17(35):3994–4000. doi:10.3748/wjg.v17.i35.3994

130. Takahashi K, Yoshida N, Murakami N, Kawata K, Ishizaki H, Tanaka-Okamoto M, et al. Dynamic regulation of p53 subnuclear localization and senescence by MORC3. *Mol Biol Cell* (2007) 18(5):1701–9. doi:10.1091/mbc.E06-08-0747

131. Mimura Y, Takahashi K, Kawata K, Akazawa T, Inoue N. Two-step colocalization of MORC3 with PML nuclear bodies. *J Cell Sci* (2010) 123 (Pt 12):2014–24. doi:10.1242/jcs.063586

132. He F, Umehara T, Saito K, Harada T, Watanabe S, Yabuki T, et al. Structural insight into the zinc finger CW domain as a histone modification reader. *Structure* (2010) 18(9):1127–39. doi:10.1016/j.str.2010.06.012

133. Bicocca VT, Chang BH, Masouleh BK, Muschen M, Loriaux MM, Druker BJ, et al. Crosstalk between ROR1 and the Pre-B cell receptor promotes survival of t(1;19) acute lymphoblastic leukemia. *Cancer Cell* (2012) 22(5):656–67. doi:10.1016/j.ccr.2012.08.027

134. Jadhav G, Teguh D, Kenny J, Tickner J, Xu J. Morc3 mutant mice exhibit reduced cortical area and thickness, accompanied by altered haematopoietic stem cells niche and bone cell differentiation. *Sci Rep* (2016) 6:25964. doi:10.1038/srep25964

135. Qiu Z, Yuan W, Chen T, Zhou C, Liu C, Huang Y, et al. HMGCR positively regulated the growth and migration of glioblastoma cells. *Gene* (2016) 576 (1 Pt 1):22–7. doi:10.1016/j.gene.2015.09.067

136. Larsson O. HMG-CoA reductase inhibitors: role in normal and malignant cells. *Crit Rev Oncol Hematol* (1996) 22(3):197–212. doi:10.1016/1040-8428(96)00193-X

137. Mo H, Elson CE. Studies of the isoprenoid-mediated inhibition of mevalonate synthesis applied to cancer chemotherapy and chemoprevention. *Exp Biol Med (Maywood)* (2004) 229(7):567–85. doi:10.1177/153537020422900701

138. Clendening JW, Pandyra A, Boutros PC, El Ghamrasni S, Khosravi F, Trentin GA, et al. Dysregulation of the mevalonate pathway promotes transformation. *Proc Natl Acad Sci U S A* (2010) 107(34):15051–6. doi:10.1073/pnas.0910258107

139. Butt S, Butt T, Jirström K, Hartman L, Amini RM, Zhou W, et al. The target for statins, HMG-CoA reductase, is expressed in ductal carcinoma-in situ and may predict patient response to radiotherapy. *Ann Surg Oncol* (2014) 21(9):2911–9. doi:10.1245/s10434-014-3708-4

140. Chushi L, Wei W, Kangkang X, Yongzeng F, Ning X, Xiaolei C. HMGCR is up-regulated in gastric cancer and promotes the growth and migration of the cancer cells. *Gene* (2016) 587(1):42–7. doi:10.1016/j.gene.2016.04.029

141. Singh R, Yadav V, Kumar S, Saini N. MicroRNA-195 inhibits proliferation, invasion and metastasis in breast cancer cells by targeting FASN, HMGCR, ACACA and CYP27B1. *Sci Rep* (2015) 5:17454. doi:10.1038/srep17454

142. Blank CU, Haanen JB, Ribas A, Schumacher TN. Cancer immunology. The "cancer immunogram". *Science* (2016) 352(6286):658–60. doi:10.1126/science.aaf2834

143. Pandya PH, Murray ME, Pollok KE, Renbarger JL. The immune system in cancer pathogenesis: potential therapeutic approaches. *J Immunol Res* (2016) 2016:4273943. doi:10.1155/2016/4273943

144. Benveniste O, Drouot L, Jouen F, Charuel JL, Bloch-Queyrat C, Behin A, et al. Correlation of anti-signal recognition particle autoantibody levels with creatine kinase activity in patients with necrotizing myopathy. *Arthritis Rheum* (2011) 63(7):1961–71. doi:10.1002/art.30344

145. Drouot L, Allenbach Y, Jouen F, Charuel JL, Martinet J, Meyer A, et al. Exploring necrotizing autoimmune myopathies with a novel immunoassay for anti-3-hydroxy-3-methyl-glutaryl-CoA reductase autoantibodies. *Arthritis Res Ther* (2014) 16(1):R39. doi:10.1186/ar4468

146. Aggarwal R, Oddis CV, Goudeau D, Koontz D, Qi Z, Reed AM, et al. Autoantibody levels in myositis patients correlate with clinical response during B cell depletion with rituximab. *Rheumatology (Oxford)* (2016) 55(6):991–9. doi:10.1093/rheumatology/kev444

147. Arouche-Delaperche L, Allenbach Y, Amelin D, Preusse C, Mouly V, Mauhin W, et al. Pathogenic role of anti-SRP and anti-HMGCR antibodies in necrotizing myopathies: myofiber atrophy and impairment of muscle regeneration in necrotizing autoimmune myopathies. *Ann Neurol* (2017) 81(4):538–48. doi:10.1002/ana.24902

148. Mohassel P, Rosen P, Casciola-Rosen L, Pak K, Mammen AL. Expression of the dermatomyositis autoantigen transcription intermediary factor 1γ in regenerating muscle. *Arthritis Rheumatol* (2015) 67(1):266–72. doi:10.1002/art.38863

Permissions

All chapters in this book were first published by Frontiers; hereby published with permission under the Creative Commons Attribution License or equivalent. Every chapter published in this book has been scrutinized by our experts. Their significance has been extensively debated. The topics covered herein carry significant findings which will fuel the growth of the discipline. They may even be implemented as practical applications or may be referred to as a beginning point for another development.

The contributors of this book come from diverse backgrounds, making this book a truly international effort. This book will bring forth new frontiers with its revolutionizing research information and detailed analysis of the nascent developments around the world.

We would like to thank all the contributing authors for lending their expertise to make the book truly unique. They have played a crucial role in the development of this book. Without their invaluable contributions this book wouldn't have been possible. They have made vital efforts to compile up to date information on the varied aspects of this subject to make this book a valuable addition to the collection of many professionals and students.

This book was conceptualized with the vision of imparting up-to-date information and advanced data in this field. To ensure the same, a matchless editorial board was set up. Every individual on the board went through rigorous rounds of assessment to prove their worth. After which they invested a large part of their time researching and compiling the most relevant data for our readers.

The editorial board has been involved in producing this book since its inception. They have spent rigorous hours researching and exploring the diverse topics which have resulted in the successful publishing of this book. They have passed on their knowledge of decades through this book. To expedite this challenging task, the publisher supported the team at every step. A small team of assistant editors was also appointed to further simplify the editing procedure and attain best results for the readers.

Apart from the editorial board, the designing team has also invested a significant amount of their time in understanding the subject and creating the most relevant covers. They scrutinized every image to scout for the most suitable representation of the subject and create an appropriate cover for the book.

The publishing team has been an ardent support to the editorial, designing and production team. Their endless efforts to recruit the best for this project, has resulted in the accomplishment of this book. They are a veteran in the field of academics and their pool of knowledge is as vast as their experience in printing. Their expertise and guidance has proved useful at every step. Their uncompromising quality standards have made this book an exceptional effort. Their encouragement from time to time has been an inspiration for everyone.

The publisher and the editorial board hope that this book will prove to be a valuable piece of knowledge for researchers, students, practitioners and scholars across the globe.

List of Contributors

Changjian Wang, Lingchao Guo and Fangzhao Li
College of Computer, National University of Defense Technology, Changsha, China

Jinfeng Du and Fen Li
Department of Rheumatology and Immunology, The Second Xiangya Hospital of Central South University, Changsha, China

Xilong Mei
Department of Radiology, The Second Xiangya Hospital of Central South University, Changsha, China

Hong Luo
Department of Respiratory and Critical Care Medicine, The Second Xiangya Hospital of Central South University, Changsha, China

Takashi Matsuo, Tsuneo Sasai, Ran Nakashima, Isao Murakami, Shuji Akizuki, Kosaku Murakami, Akio Morinobu and Hajime Yoshifuji
Department of Rheumatology and Clinical Immunology, Kyoto University, Kyoto, Japan

Yoshihiro Kuwabara
Cancer Control Center, Osaka International Cancer Institute, Osaka, Japan

Eri Toda Kato
Department of Cardiovascular Medicine, Kyoto University, Kyoto, Japan

Hideo Onizawa and Masao Tanaka
Department of Advanced Medicine for Rheumatic Diseases, Kyoto University, Kyoto, Japan

Motomu Hashimoto
Department of Advanced Medicine for Rheumatic Diseases, Kyoto University, Kyoto, Japan
Department of Clinical Immunology, Graduate School of Medicine, Osaka City University, Osaka, Japan

Tsuneyo Mimori
Department of Rheumatology and Clinical Immunology, Kyoto University, Kyoto, Japan
Takeda General Hospital, Kyoto, Japan

Ben Mulhearn and Sarah L. Tansley
Department and Pharmacy and Pharmacology, University of Bath, Bath, United Kingdom
Royal National Hospital for Rheumatic Diseases, Royal United Hospitals, Bath, United Kingdom

Danyang Li, Fionnuala McMorrow, Hui Lu and Neil J. McHugh
Department and Pharmacy and Pharmacology, University of Bath, Bath, United Kingdom

Yu Zuo, Fang Chen, Qinglin Peng, Xin Lu and Xiaoming Shu
Department of Rheumatology, Key Laboratory of Myositis, China-Japan Friendship Hospital, Beijing, China

Lifang Ye and Guochun Wang
Department of Rheumatology, Key Laboratory of Myositis, China-Japan Friendship Hospital, Beijing, China
Peking Union Medical College, Chinese Academy of Medical Sciences, Beijing, China

Hana Štorkánová, Sabína Oreská, Kristýna Bubová, Olga Kryštůfková, Heřman Mann, Karel Pavelka, Ladislav Šenolt, Jiří Vencovský and Michal Tomčík
Institute of Rheumatology, Prague, Czechia
Department of Rheumatology, 1st Faculty of Medicine, Charles University, Prague, Czechia

Maja Špiritović
Institute of Rheumatology, Prague, Czechia, Prague, Czechia
Department of Physiotherapy, Faculty of Physical Education and Sport, Charles University

Barbora Heřmánková
Department of Physiotherapy, Faculty of Physical Education and Sport, Charles University, Prague, Czechia

Martin Komarc
Department of Methodology, Faculty of Physical Education and Sport, Charles University, Prague, Czechia

Kryštof Slabý
Department of Rehabilitation and Sports Medicine, 2nd Faculty of Medicine, Charles University and University Hospital Motol, Prague, Czechia

Josef Zámečník
Department of Pathology and Molecular Medicine, 2nd Faculty of Medicine, Charles University and University Hospital Motol, Prague, Czechia

Anaïs Nombel and Nicole Fabien
Immunology Department, Lyon-Sud Hospital, Hospices Civils de Lyon, Pierre-Bénite, France

Frédéric Coutant
Immunology Department, Lyon-Sud Hospital, Hospices Civils de Lyon, Pierre-Bénite, France
Immunogenomics and Inflammation Research Team, University of Lyon, Edouard Herriot Hospital, Lyon, France

Haixi Wu, Licheng Diao, Ke Xue, Qian Zhao, Xiaoqing Zhao, Qunli Xia, Jie Zheng, Meng Pan and Hua Cao
Department of Dermatology, Ruijin Hospital, School of Medicine, Shanghai Jiao Tong University, Shanghai, China

Chenjia He, Qibing Xie and Geng Yin
Department of Rheumatology and Immunology, West China Hospital, Sichuan University, Chengdu, China

Wenyu Li,
Health Management Center, West China Hospital, Sichuan University, Chengdu, China

Tomislav Ledenko and Iva Sorić Hosman
Department of Pediatrics, Zadar General Hospital, Zadar, Croatia

Marijana Ćorić
Department of Pathology and Cytology, University Hospital Centre Zagreb, Zagreb, Croatia
School of Medicine, University of Zagreb, Zagreb, Croatia

Alenka Gagro
School of Medicine, University of Zagreb, Zagreb, Croatia
Division of Pulmonology, Allergology, Immunology and Rheumatology, Department of Pediatrics, Children's Hospital Zagreb, Zagreb, Croatia

Naoki Hamada, Ayaka Maeda, Kaoru Takase-Minegishi, Yohei Kirino, Yumiko Sugiyama, Ryusuke Yoshimi and Hideaki Nakajima
Department of Stem Cell and Immune Regulation, Yokohama City University Graduate School of Medicine, Yokohama, Japan

Ho Namkoong
Department of Infectious Diseases, Keio University School of Medicine, Tokyo, Japan

Nobuyuki Horita
Chemothrapy Center, Yokohama City University Hospital, Yokohama, Japan

Yu Zuo, Fang Chen, Xin Lu and Xiaoming Shu
Department of Rheumatology, Key Laboratory of Myositis, China-Japan Friendship Hospital, Beijing, China

Lifang Ye and Guochun Wang
Department of Rheumatology, Key Laboratory of Myositis, China-Japan Friendship Hospital, Beijing, China
Peking Union Medical College, Chinese Academy of Medical Sciences, Beijing, China

Yawen Shen
Department of Rheumatology, Beijing Shijitan Hospital, Capital Medical University, Beijing, China

Jia Shi, Mingwei Tang, Shuang Zhou, Dong Xu, Jiuliang Zhao, Chanyuan Wu, Qian Wang, Xinping Tian, Mengtao Li and Xiaofeng Zeng
Department of Rheumatology and Clinical Immunology, Peking Union Medical College Hospital, Peking Union Medical College & Chinese Academy of Medical Sciences, Key Laboratory of Rheumatology & Clinical Immunology, Ministry of Education, Beijing, China
National Clinical Research Center for Dermatologic and Immunologic Diseases (NCRC-DID), Ministry of Science & Technology, Beijing, China

Lijuan Zhao, Junyu Zhou, Honglin Zhu and Hui Luo
Department of Rheumatology, Xiangya Hospital of Central South University, Changsha, China
National Clinical Research Center for Geriatric Disorders, Xiangya Hospital of Central South University, Changsha, China
Provincial Clinical Research Center for Rheumatic and Immunologic Diseases, Xiangya Hospital of Central South University, Changsha, China

Shuoshan Xie
Department of Nephrology, Hunan Provincial People's Hospital and The First Affiliated Hospital of Hunan Normal University, Changsha, China

Bin Zhou
Department of Nephrology, The Affiliated Hospital of Qingdao University, Qingdao, China

Chuyu Shen
Department of Rheumatology, The First Affiliated Hospital, Sun Yat-sen University, Guangzhou, China

Liya Li
Department of Rheumatology, The Third Xiangya Hospital of Central South University, Changsha, China

Weiwei Pi
Department of Oncology, The First People's Hospital of Changde City, Changde, China

Zhen Gong
Department of Rheumatology, Yiyang Central Hospital, Yiyang, China

Jing Zhao
Department of Rheumatology, The First Affiliated Hospital of Jishou University, Jishou, China

Qi Peng
Department of Rheumatology, Yueyang People's Hospital, Yueyang, China

Jiaqi Peng and Liang Song
Huaihua No.1 People's Hospital Affiliated to Nanhua University, Huaihua, China

Yan Zhou
Department of Obstetrics and Gynecology, Zhuzhou Central Hospital, Zhuzhou, China

Lingxiao Zou
Department of Obstetrics and Gynecology, The Third Xiangya Hospital of Central South University, Changsha, China

Kaiwen Wang, Jiangfeng Zhao, Wanlong Wu, Wenwen Xu, Shuhui Sun, Zhiwei Chen, Yakai Fu, Li Guo, Hui Du and Shuang Ye
Department of Rheumatology, Renji Hospital, Shanghai Jiao Tong University School of Medicine, Shanghai, China

Silvia Svegliati
Department of Clinical and Molecular Sciences, Marche Polytechnic University, Ancona, Italy

Maria Giovanna Danieli and Gianluca Moroncini
Department of Clinical and Molecular Sciences, Marche Polytechnic University, Ancona, Italy
Clinica Medica, Department of Internal Medicine, Ospedali Riuniti, Ancona, Italy

Jacopo Umberto Verga
Department of Life and Environmental Sciences, Polytechnic University of Marche, Ancona, Italy
The Science Foundation Ireland (SFI) Centre for Research Training in Genomics Data Science, National University of Ireland, Galway, Ireland

Cristina Mezzanotte
Internal Medicine Residency Program, Marche Polytechnic University, Ancona, Italy

Irene Terrenato
Biostatistics and Bioinformatic Unit, Scientific Direction, IRCCS Regina Elena Cancer Institute, Rome, Italy

Maria Beatrice Bilo
Department of Clinical and Molecular Sciences, Marche Polytechnic University, Ancona, Italy
Allergy Unit, Department of Internal Medicine, Ospedali Riuniti, Ancona, Italy

Lili Zhu, Shiyao Wang, Yanhong Ren, Bingbing Xie, Jing Geng and Huaping Dai Chen Wang
Department of Pulmonary and Critical Care Medicine, China-Japan Friendship Hospital, Capital Medical University, Beijing, China
National Center for Respiratory Medicine, Beijing, China
National Clinical Research Center for Respiratory Diseases, Institute of Respiratory Medicine, Chinese Academy of Medical Sciences, Peking Union Medical College, Beijing, China

Zhong Cao and Changshui Zhang
Institute for Artificial Intelligence, Tsinghua University (THUAI), State Key Lab of Intelligent Technologies and Systems, Beijing National Research Center for Information Science and Technology (BNRist), Beijing, China

Lei Fang
Data Canvas Technology Co., Ltd, Beijing, China

Sheng Xie
Department of Radiology, China-Japan Friendship Hospital, Beijing, China

Ling Zhao
Department of Pathology, China-Japan Friendship Hospital, Beijing, China

Li Ma
Department of Rheumatology, China-Japan Friendship Hospital, Beijing, China

Shuhui Sun, Zhiwei Chen, Danting Zhang, Wenwen Xu, Wanlong Wu, Fangfang Sun, Liyang Gu, Jie Chen, Jiajie Li, Ting Li, Xiaodong Wang and Shuang Ye
Department of Rheumatology, Renji Hospital, Shanghai Jiaotong University School of Medicine, Shanghai, China

Yu-Lan Chen, Cui-Lian Liu, Jing-Yi Xie, Bao-Dong Sun and Dong-Zhou Liu
Department of Rheumatology and Immunology, Shenzhen People's Hospital (The Second Clinical Medical College, Jinan University, The First Affiliated Hospital, Southern University of Science and Technology), Shenzhen, China

Suo Zhang
Department of Rheumatology and Immunology, Shenzhen People's Hospital (The Second Clinical Medical College, Jinan University, The First Affiliated Hospital, Southern University of Science and Technology), Shenzhen, China
Department of Rheumatology and Immunology, Shenzhen Second People's Hospital, Shenzhen, China

Katherine N. Vowell and Camille S. Westlake
Division of Rheumatology and Immunology, Vanderbilt University Medical Center, Nashville, TN, United States

Erin M. Wilfong
Division of Rheumatology and Immunology, Vanderbilt University Medical Center, Nashville, TN, United States
Division of Allergy, Pulmonary, and Critical Care Medicine, Vanderbilt University Medical Center, Nashville, TN, United States
Vanderbilt Institute for Infection, Immunology, and Inflammation, Vanderbilt University Medical Center, Nashville, TN, United States
Human Immunology Discovery Initiative and Vanderbilt Center for Immunobiology, Vanderbilt University Medical Center, Nashville, TN, United States

Todd Bartkowiak
Department of Cell and Developmental Biology, Vanderbilt University, Nashville, TN, United States
Vanderbilt-Ingram Cancer Center, Vanderbilt University Medical Center, Nashville, TN, United States

Jonathan M. Irish
Vanderbilt Institute for Infection, Immunology, and Inflammation, Vanderbilt University Medical Center, Nashville, TN, United States
Human Immunology Discovery Initiative and Vanderbilt Center for Immunobiology, Vanderbilt University Medical Center, Nashville, TN, United States
Department of Cell and Developmental Biology, Vanderbilt University, Nashville, TN, United States
Vanderbilt-Ingram Cancer Center, Vanderbilt University Medical Center, Nashville, TN, United States Deparment of Pathology, Microbiology, and Immunology, Vanderbilt University Medical Center, Nashville, TN, United States

Peggy L. Kendall
Division of Allergy, Pulmonary, and Critical Care Medicine, Vanderbilt University Medical Center, Nashville, TN, United States
Vanderbilt Institute for Infection, Immunology, and Inflammation, Vanderbilt University Medical Center, Nashville, TN, United States
Deparment of Pathology, Microbiology, and Immunology, Vanderbilt University Medical Center, Nashville, TN, United States
Department of Medicine, Division of Allergy and Immunology, Washington University School of Medicine St. Louis, MO, United States

Leslie J. Crofford
Division of Rheumatology and Immunology, Vanderbilt University Medical Center, Nashville, TN, United States
Vanderbilt Institute for Infection, Immunology, and Inflammation, Vanderbilt University Medical Center, Nashville, TN, United States
Human Immunology Discovery Initiative and Vanderbilt Center for Immunobiology, Vanderbilt University Medical Center, Nashville, TN, United States
Deparment of Pathology, Microbiology, and Immunology, Vanderbilt University Medical Center, Nashville, TN, United States

Rachel H. Bonami
Division of Rheumatology and Immunology, Vanderbilt University Medical Center, Nashville, TN, United States
Vanderbilt Institute for Infection, Immunology, and Inflammation, Vanderbilt University Medical Center, Nashville, TN, United States
Human Immunology Discovery Initiative and Vanderbilt Center for Immunobiology, Vanderbilt University Medical Center, Nashville, TN, United States
Vanderbilt-Ingram Cancer Center, Vanderbilt University Medical Center, Nashville, TN, United States
Deparment of Pathology, Microbiology, and Immunology, Vanderbilt University Medical Center, Nashville, TN, United States

Jie Qian and Hui Xu
Department of Rheumatology, Affiliated Hospital of Nantong University, Nantong, China

Charalampos Papagoras, Ioannis Botis and Panagiotis Skendros
First Department of Internal Medicine, University Hospital of Alexandroupolis, Democritus University of Thrace, Alexandroupolis, Greece

Stella Arelaki
Department of Pathology, University Hospital of Alexandroupolis, Democritus University of Thrace, Alexandroupolis, Greece

Ioannis Chrysafis
Department of Radiology, University Hospital of Alexandroupolis, Democritus University of Thrace, Alexandroupolis, Greece

Stavros Giannopoulos
Department of Urology, University Hospital of Alexandroupolis, Democritus University of Thrace, Alexandroupolis, Greece

Audrey Aussy and Olivier Boyer
Normandie University, UNIROUEN, INSERM, U1234, Rouen University Hospital, Department of Immunology, Rouen, France

Nadège Cordel
Unit of Dermatology and Internal Medicine, Pointe-à-Pitre University Hospital, University of the French West Indies, Fouillole, Pointe-à-Pitre, Guadeloupe

Index

www.ingramcontent.com/pod-product-compliance
Lightning Source LLC
LaVergne TN
LVHW060533210926
848485LV00005B/1193